BIOARTIFICIAL ORGANS

SCIENCE, MEDICINE,
AND TECHNOLOGY

ANNALS OF THE NEW YORK ACADEMY OF SCIENCES
Volume 831

BIOARTIFICIAL ORGANS

SCIENCE, MEDICINE, AND TECHNOLOGY

Edited by Ales Prokop, David Hunkeler, and Alan D. Cherrington

The New York Academy of Sciences
New York, New York
1997

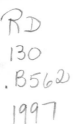

COVER ART Histological section of empty coherent microcapsule containing renal sub-capsular space after 30 days of graft in normal CD-1 mice (courtesy of Ricardo Calafiore). The lower right corner shows a confocal micrograph of an HEMA-MMA microcapsule containing HepG2 cells in the absence of Matrigel at 1 week (Courtesy of Michael Sefton).

Library of Congress Cataloging-in-Publication Data

Bioartificial organs : science, medicine, and technology / editors, Ales Prokop, David Hunkeler, Alan D. Cherrington.
        p.   cm.—(Annals of the New York Academy of Sciences : v. 831)
    This volume is the result of a conference held on July 21–26, 1996 in Nashville, Tenn.
    Includes bibliographical references and index.
    ISBN 1-57331-098-0 (cloth : alk. paper).—ISBN 1-57331-099-9 (pbk. : alk. paper)
    1. Artificial organs—Congresses. 2. Artificial cells——Congresses. 3. Biomedical materials—Congresses. 4. Islands of Langerhans—Transplantation—Congresses. 5. Liver—Transplantation——Congresses. I. Prokop, Aleš. I. Hunkeler, David. III. Cherrington, Alan, 1946-   . IV. Series.
    Q11.N5 vol. 831
    [RD130]
    500 s—dc21
    [617.9′5]
                                                                                  97-46923
                                                                                       CIP

BiC/PCP
Printed in the United States of America
ISBN 1-57331-098-0 (cloth)
ISBN 1-57331-099-9 (paper)
ISSN 0077-8923

ANNALS OF THE NEW YORK ACADEMY OF SCIENCES

Volume 831
December 31, 1997

BIOARTIFICIAL ORGANS [a]

SCIENCE, MEDICINE,

AND TECHNOLOGY

Editors and Conference Organizers
ALES PROKOP, DAVID HUNKELER, AND ALAN D. CHERRINGTON

Sponsor
ENGINEERING FOUNDATION

CONTENTS

[a] This volume is the result of a conference entitled **Bioartificial Organs: Science and Technology,** which was sponsored by the Engineering Foundation and held on July 21–26, 1996 in Nashville, Tennessee.

Financial assistance was received from:

- ENGINEERING FOUNDATION
- JUVENILE DIABETES FOUNDATION
- NATIONAL INSTITUTES OF HEALTH
- NATIONAL SCIENCE FOUNDATION
- NEW YORK ACADEMY OF SCIENCES
- WHITAKER FOUNDATION

Preface

ALES PROKOP

Chemical Engineering Department
Vanderbilt University, 107 Olin Hall
Nashville, Tennessee 37235

DAVID HUNKELER

Laboratory of Polymers and Biomaterials
Department of Chemistry
Swiss Institute of Technology (EPFL)
CH-1015 Lausanne, Switzerland

ALAN D. CHERRINGTON

Department of Molecular Physiology and Biophysics
Vanderbilt University School of Medicine
Nashville, Tennessee 37232

Bioartificial Organs is an interdisciplinary domain comprising biological sciences, chemistry, physical chemistry, material science, polymer chemistry, cell culture, recombinant DNA technology, bioprocess engineering and clinical sciences. To continue and enhance the rate of research progress it is necessary to promote effective communication between these diverse groups. A symposium entitled **Bioartificial Organs: Science and Technology** was held from July 21–26, 1996 in Nashville, Tennessee (USA), under the aegis of the Engineering Foundation Conferences. Approximately 100 scientists, medical professionals, and engineers attended the meeting, with the approximate breakdown of attendees between different categories as follows: medical professionals and biological scientists 54%, polymer scientists 18% and engineers 28%. The conference included representatives from 11 countries, three national regulatory agencies, and 19 private companies. This book is a collection of the majority of papers presented at this meeting grouped under common themes, rather than in the order presented. The book is organized into eight sections. The Overview provides a look at the current state of bioartificial organ research, challenges, as well as emerging regulatory and ethical issues. Part II discusses the synthesis of novel polymeric biomaterials, while Parts III and IV present surface characterization and technological issues, respectively. The second half of the book is medically and clinically oriented, with Part V presenting an overview of artificial cells, immunoisolation and organ regeneration. Specific sections are also dedicated to the bioartificial pancreas (Part VI) and bioartificial liver (Part VII). Finally, the application of tissue engineering to uses involving scaffold matrices for cartilage constructs, bone regeneration, immunoregulation, and gene therapy are discussed in Part VIII.

The editors would like to thank the members of the organizing committee of the symposium consisting of Todd Giorgio (Vanderbilt), Milton Harris (University of Alabama), Kiki Hellman (FDA), Jeffrey Hubbell (Caltech), Robert Langer (MIT), Alan Laskin (Engineering Foundation), Kenneth Luskey (Metabolex), Alvin Powers (Vanderbilt), Paul Kemp (Organogenesis), Anthony M. Sun (University of

Toronto), and Taylor G. Wang (Vanderbilt). The true success of the symposium was due to the efforts of the chairpersons and the co-chairpersons of the different sessions: Jeffrey Hubbell, Milton Harris, T. K. Stevenson (Wichita State University), Buddy Ratner (University of Washington), Shalaby W. Shalaby (Poly-Med), Karel Ulbrich (Czech Academy of Sciences), Clark Colton (MIT), Robert Lanza (BioHybrid Technologies), Alvin Powers, Wei-Shou Hu (University of Minnesota), Paul Kemp, Michael Caldwell (University of Minnesota), Gail Naughton (Advanced Tissue Sciences), and Athanassios Sambanis (GeorgiaTech).

A number of reviewers provided dedicated service to the publication of these proceedings. These reviewers put up with the demands of the editors and provided a rapid turnover of the manuscripts with the critical comments necessary for ensuring the quality of this publication. The editors are thankful to them for their effort. The reviewers are:

James D. Bryers, Montana State University, Bozeman, MT
Riccardo Calafiore, Univ. Degli Studi Di Perugia, Perugia, Italy
Paul Dubin, Indiana-Purdue University, Indianapolis, IN
Kazumori Funatsu, Kyushu University, Fukuda, Japan
Todd D. Giorgio, Vanderbilt University, Nashville, TN
Jorge Heller, APS Research Institute, Redwood City, CA
Ronald S. Hill, Neocrin, Irvine, CA
Wei-Shou Hu, University of Minnesota, Minneapolis, MN
Paul D. Kemp, Organogenesis, Canton, MA
John Lake, UCSF, San Francisco, CA
Robert Lanza, BioHybrid Technologies, Shrewsburry, MA
Charles L. Linden, Jr., Walter Reed Army Institute, Washington, DC
Hans Joerg Mathien, EPFL, Lausanne, Switzerland
Tuoc Tuan Nguyen, EPFL, Lausanne, Switzerland
Alvin C. Powers, Vanderbilt University, Nashville, TN
David T. Rovee, Organogenesis, Canton, MA
Athanassios Sambanis, Georgia Institute of Technology, Atlanta, GA
Michael Sefton, University of Toronto, Toronto, Canada
Ulrike Siebers, Justus-Liebig-Universität, Giessen, Germany
Karel Smetana, Jr., Charles University, Prague, Czech Republic
William T. K. Stevenson, Wichita State University, Wichita, KS
Anthony M. Sun, University of Toronto, Toronto, Canada
Linda A. Tempelman, CytoTheraputics, Lincoln, RI
Marcus Textor, ETH, Zurich, Switzerland
Florence J. Wu, Advanced Tissue Sciences, La Jolla, CA
Ioannis V. Yannas, MIT, Cambridge, MA

Finally, we would like to acknowledge the enormous contributions from the Engineering Foundation, particularly Charles Freiman, Barbara Hickernell, Alan Laskin and Donna McArdle.

The second conference of this series, BIO+AO II, will be held in Banff, Alberta, Canada, in July 1998 with Professor David Hunkeler, EPFL, Lausanne, Switzerland as chairperson. The organizing committee consists of Alan Cherrington, Ales Prokop, Ray Rajotte, and Michael Sefton.

Introduction

ALES PROKOP
Chemical Engineering Department
Vanderbilt University, 107 Olin Hall
Nashville, Tennessee 37235

DAVID HUNKELER
Laboratory of Polymers and Biomaterials
Department of Chemistry
Swiss Institute of Technology (EPFL)
CH-1015 Lausanne, Switzerland

ALAN D. CHERRINGTON
Department of Molecular Physiology and Biophysics
Vanderbilt University School of Medicine
Nashville, Tennessee 37232

For the most part bioartificial organ research has been targeted at several hormone-deficiency and neurodegenerative diseases such as Parkinson's, Alzheimer's, and Huntington's chorea as well as at the control of chronic pain and human growth factors. The encapsulation of hepatocytes for the production of a bioartificial liver and the development of artificial skin are other emerging applications. However, to date, bone marrow transplantation is the only cellular transplantation technique that is currently clinically practiced, although limited clinical trials have been performed with a bioartificial pancreas. A bioartificial organ involves immunoisolation of mammalian cells in order to provide a steric selectivity to the ingress and egress of various molecules. Semipermeable polymeric membranes have been developed with the aim of permitting the transplantation of xenogenic cells, from species with a large phylogenic separation from humans, without recourse to immunosuppression therapy. Several biologically active species have been encapsulated or immobilized and the techniques generally have potential for diseases requiring enzyme or endocrine replacement.

TISSUE- AND HOST-RELATED ISSUES

The most appropriate source for procurement is still being debated, with discordant grafts generally preferred over concordant xenografts. For example, pigs produce an insulin which is structurally similar to human's and they are the only large animals slaughtered in sufficient quantities to supply the estimated demand from Type-I diabetics. However, porcine islets are fragile and have poor long-term stability. Fetal and neonatal sources are under consideration, though these present ethical challenges. To deal with supply-related issues, centers of excellence in cryosuppression have been proposed. However, it remains to be determined if banking will be coordinated on a municipal, regional, national, or continental scale. Recently, viable bioartificial pancreases have been produced from cryopreserved, encapsulated tissue, and this presents another alternative. The long-term suitability of primary tissue is, however, questionable, and many believe that a genetically engineered cell line would be preferred since it would avoid scale-up-related problems in tissue procurement. The issue of co-immobilization has also not been extensively investigated. It remains to be conclusively demonstrated that vascularization can improve the functioning of a bioartificial organ. Furthermore, the issues of the protection of the host from the graft and the recovery of the transplant have not received significant research attention. There is also serious criticism that any bioartificial organ will suffer from long-term bioincompatibility. The tissue immune rejection response is another important issue to resolve. There is also evidence that the site of transplantation influences the release properties of the transplanted device. Studies of sufficient magnitude are therefore required on each chemistry to provide sufficient data to permit biostatistical inferences to be drawn. The resolution of the question of whether an immunoisolation barrier can prevent the destruction of the xenograft is particularly relevant if, as is the case with diabetes mellitus, the disease has an autoimmune etiology.

POLYMER- AND TECHNOLOGY-RELATED ISSUES

Macrophage activation, which participates in foreign-body reactions, is still a problem for many polymers. Therefore, the purity and consistency of batches of polymers used as immunoisolation materials needs to be improved. Furthermore, for any non-conformal transplant, dead volume is unavoidable. The technologies for the scale-up of both tissue procurement and bioartificial organ processing also do not exist. In terms of membrane properties, it is still indeterminate if an immunoisolation barrier can provide a balance between protection and nutrition. Indeed, the optimal MW cutoff remains a source of debate. Some researchers also question if cutoff reduction improves immunological reactions, while the issue of the measurement and control of the breadth of the pore-size distribution is just beginning to be considered. The mechanical and transport properties of several polyelectrolyte-based membranes could be improved if formation occurred at non-neutral pHs. Therefore, it needs to be resolved if tissue can survive a transient deviation in pH, and, if so, for how long and what is the result of the shock on its viability. Design targets in terms of capsule elasticity and internal oxygen levels are also required. Finally, it should be recognized that the membrane stoiciometry and strength are sensitive to the local environment in physiological solution. Overall, while small model testing and preliminary large animal trials are encouraging, the application of semipermeable immunoisolation barriers still presents several challenges to interdisciplinary teams comprised of polymer scientists, engineers, biologists, and medical professionals.

Bioartificial Organs as Outcomes of Tissue Engineering

Scientific and Regulatory Issues

KIKI B. HELLMAN

United States Food and Drug Administration
5600 Fishers Lane
Rockville, Maryland 20852

On behalf of the U.S. Food and Drug Administration (FDA), it is a pleasure to participate in the *International Conference on Bioartificial Organs: Science and Technology*, sponsored by the Engineering Foundation, and to participate in the continuing initiatives for fostering dialogue and cooperation between the public and private sector, academe, governments, and industry, both nationally and internationally, in the development of novel technology(ies) and its promising contributions to clinical medicine.

From the FDA perspective, the conference is representative of endeavors to continually review the research advances in multi-disciplinary technologies and their applications to product development. It is indicative of the many efforts that the FDA has participated in over the last several years in the general area of biotechnology, its application to biomaterials, and novel cell and tissue engineering approaches.

In order to focus on those areas of benefit to the scientific community and to the continued progress in development of bioartificial organs, this communication considers the following topics:

- advances in cell and tissue engineering responsible for major contributions to the field;
- scientific and regulatory issues integral to the translation of technology to products; and
- future challenges for the scientific and regulatory communities which are important for shepherding the field towards realization of its full potential in the armamentarium of clinical medicine.

ADVANCES IN CELL AND TISSUE ENGINEERING

The advances in cell and tissue engineering, and what they encompass, are major contributors that have led to the development of bioartificial organs as potential approaches for ameliorating different medical conditions. Cell and tissue engineering have emerged over the past ten to fifteen years as novel technologies that use the concepts and tools of biotechnology, molecular and cell biology, materials science, and engineering to understand the structure-function relationships in mammalian tissues[1] and to develop biological substitutes for the repair, reconstruction, regeneration, or replacement of tissue or organ function.[2]

1

There are many avenues to reach the desired endpoint, as shown in FIGURE 1, which represents the universe of organ, cell, and tissue engineering applications as medical therapy alternatives. It can be conceived of as a continuum with regard to: 1) the initial source, either cells, tissues, or organs; 2) the level of processing, from minimally processed to modification of structure and/or function; and 3) the end use as a direct implant or incorporation into a device for implantation or use extracorporeally.

As a source of products or systems, cell and tissue engineering technologies have emerged at the interface between the medical devices and biotechnology industries.[3] As bioartificial organs, these biological substitutes generally consist of cells or tissues and biomaterials. The biological component can be either metabolic or non-metabolic and can consist of cells or tissues from either human or animal sources that are isolated, native material or genetically manipulated. Cellular products such as cytokines, and cellular components, such as genes or structural elements, can be used either alone or in conjunction with cells or tissues. The biomaterial component of this biological substitute can consist of natural materials from native body tissues or synthetic materials designed for specific physical or chemical properties. The biomaterial provides the: 1) scaffolding or three-dimensional architecture for tissue regeneration; 2) modulation of a specific cell function; or 3) immunoprotection.

The general development of cell and tissue engineering and of bioartificial organs as outcomes or products of this technology is a result of three critical elements: 1) the progress in cell and tissue culture technology; 2) developments in biomaterials; and 3) the contributions of interdisciplinary research teams in academe and industry.

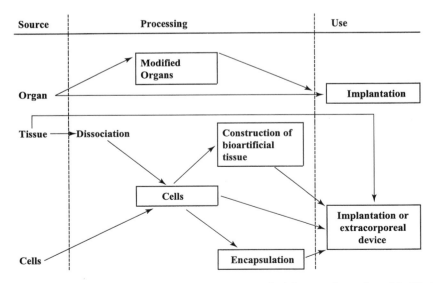

FIGURE 1. Engineering organs, cells, and tissues as medical therapy alternatives. (Modified from Berthiaume *et al.*[4])

TABLE 1. Key Developments in Cell and Tissue Culture Technology: Application to Bioartificial Organs

- Cell growth/regeneration studies
- Cell structure/function modification
  - Surface receptors
  - Genetic manipulation
- Propagation of differentiated cells, tissues, and organs with desired function from:
  - Many organ system sites (skin, bone, cartilage, pancreatic islets, *etc.*)
  - Different host sources (autologous, allogeneic, xenogeneic)
- Cell/tissue growth scale-up in containers for direct clinical application (*e.g.*, biosynthetic skin)
- Progress in stem cell research

PROGRESS IN CELL AND TISSUE CULTURE TECHNOLOGY

The ability to propagate differentiated cells, tissues, and organs with the desired function from many organ system sites, different host sources, and even in closed system containers for direct clinical application, such as biosynthetic skin, is due to the continued progress in cell and tissue culture technology over the last forty years and certain key developments (TABLE 1). These include: propagation of cells *in vitro* indefinitely in continuous culture and under conditions of a steady state as in a bioreactor, to preserve the cells or maintain the lineage, that is, genotype and phenotype; and modification of the cells' structure or function in order to optimize a certain response via effects on cell surface receptors or manipulation of the genotype, and/or via isolated and characterized cytokines, growth factors, and other agents. In addition, the progress being made in stem cell research, such as that in bone marrow cells, will expand to other areas, thereby permitting the culture of pluripotent cells that can be either used for repopulation or manipulated to permit propagation of the desired state of differentiation.

DEVELOPMENTS IN BIOMATERIALS RESEARCH

Owing to the progress made in biomaterials research over the last several years, it is now possible to use either synthetic or naturally derived materials tailored to the specific needs of the system. New materials and/or applications are continually being developed.

Pivotal developments include the modification of materials' surfaces to promote cell adhesion, and the use of resorbable materials that degrade when they are no longer needed, or materials that serve as scaffolding that enables cells to conform to a certain desired shape. The development of biomaterials that serve as membranes of selective permeability for use in cellular implants or extracorporeal systems has been critically important to the development of bioartificial organs. In addition, growth factors and other agents can be used in the system to modify the materials' response, while nano-microfabrication technology enables the design of implants on the same level as that of the cells, permitting cells to communicate with each other and their environment. Further, self-assembly systems based on natural molecular self-assembly show promise for drug/vaccine delivery and, eventually, the delivery of gene or cell therapy (TABLE 2).

TABLE 2. Pivotal Developments in Biomaterials Research

- Modification of material surfaces to promote cell adhesion (*e.g.*, RGD sequence)
- Bioresorbable materials
- Scaffolds to control cell regeneration in a certain shape
- Encapsulation technology applied to cellular implants (*e.g.*, pancreatic islets, adrenal chromaffin cells) and extracorporeal systems (ELADs)
- Response modifiers (*e.g.*, growth factors/other agents)
- Nano/microfabrication technology permits implant design on same level as cells and operation of cell recognition phenomena
- Self-assembly systems via natural molecular self assembly (*e.g.*, for drug/vaccine delivery)

PRODUCT APPLICATIONS

Just as the investment in basic research in molecular biology from the 1950s spawned biotechnology and its products in the 1980s, so has the research investment in cell biology, materials science, engineering and related fields been responsible for the development of cell and tissue engineered products such as bioartificial organs. The interdisciplinary research teams composed of basic scientists, engineers, surgeons, and clinicians have been responsible for the cross-fertilization of ideas and approaches that have contributed to the field's success and future promise.

There are many types of products and systems in different stages of development which promise major advances in clinical medicine. The opportunities/applications in medical therapy range from: wound covering and repair systems, such as biosynthetic skin; bone, cartilage, ligament and tendon repair systems; and encapsulated cells for restoration of tissue and organ function, used either as implants, that is, secretory tissue "organoids" or *ex vivo*, as metabolic support systems; to blood substitutes, such as liposome encapsulated hemoglobin; cardiovascular products, such as replacement heart valves, and endothelialized scaffolds for vascular grafts; human tissue products used either for direct replacement or in sites other than the retrieval site; nerve regeneration approaches; genitourinary products, such as artificial kidney; gene therapy vehicles; and drug delivery systems (TABLE 3). In point of fact, technology is under development to address pathology(ies) of virtually every organ system, owing to the establishment of productive research teams that are foci of imaginative approaches and industries endeavoring to translate the research into medical products and systems.

These initiatives are indicative of the novel therapeutic approaches that are being developed through technological advances that combine the delivery of pharmacologically active substances, elements of medical devices, biological products, and surgical interventions.[3]

SCIENTIFIC AND REGULATORY ISSUES

Cell and tissue engineered products, such as bioartificial organs, are subject to regulatory evaluation by the national agencies responsible for overseeing their approval for commercial distribution and use. Issues of product safety and efficacy as they relate to product manufacture, preclinical evaluation, clinical investigation, and post-market requirements are considered in this evaluation.

FDA InterCenter Tissue Engineering Working Group

The FDA InterCenter Tissue Engineering Working Group (TEWG) was established approximately three years ago to address the scientific and regulatory issues of cell and tissue engineered products. The Working Group has accomplished a great deal in a relatively short time; it has facilitated communication, enhanced cooperation, and promoted regulatory harmonization across the Centers of the Agency, with other national regulatory bodies, and with the research and development community to shepherd the technology and its products.

To accomplish its goals, the Working Group has developed a number of ongoing projects in key areas. These include efforts in: information updates and technology monitoring via the FDA Tissue Engineering Knowledge Base (TEKB) and publications on generic product and review issues; training and education through courses coordinated by the FDA Staff Colleges, and conferences/workshops organized towards specific goals such as the May 1996 Toronto Workshop on global regulatory perspectives for tissue engineered products; and a science-based rationale (SBR) for regulatory decision making (TABLE 4). The SBR effort is interacting with the voluntary guidance initiative of the Tissue Engineering Special Interest Group of the Society for Biomaterials and complements efforts discussed by the representatives at the Toronto Workshop, *i.e.*, Australia, Canada, the European Union, Japan, and the United States.

Taken together, these efforts are pivotal in developing a proper regulatory approach. As these products assume a worldwide marketplace, assurance of consistent regulatory procedures among different countries for their evaluation becomes more important, and a common regulatory approach is critical for reaping the public health benefits worldwide. To this end, an understanding of how the products are

TABLE 3. Cell and Tissue Engineering; Applications in Medical Therapy

- Biological and interactive dressings in wound healing
  Wound covering and repair systems
- Bone, cartilage, ligament/tendon repair systems
- Encapsulated cells for restoration of tissue and organ function
  - *In vitro*: secretory tissue "organoids"
    - Bioartificial pancreas
    - Neurodegenerative disease (Parkinsons)
  - *Ex vivo*: metabolic support systems
    - Bioartificial liver
- Blood substitutes
  - Liposome encapsulated hemoglobin
- Cardiovascular tissue engineered devices
  - Replacement heart valves
  - Endothelialized scaffolds for vascular grafts
- Human tissue products
  - Direct replacement
    - Heart valves, corneas
  - Use in sites other than retrieval site
    - Small bone fragments
- Nerve regeneration approaches
- Genitourinary tissue engineered products
  - Artificial kidney
- Gene therapy vehicles
- Drug delivery systems

TABLE 4. FDA InterCenter Tissue Engineering Working Group (TEWG): Ongoing Projects

- Information Updates/Technology Monitoring
  FDA TE Knowledge Base (TEKB)
  Publications on generic tissue engineering product, review issues
- Training and Education
  FDA Staff Colleges
  Conferences/Workshops
- Science-based Rationale (SBR) for Regulatory Decision Making
  Interaction with Voluntary Guidance Initiatives
- International Regulatory Perspective for Tissue Engineered Products
  Outcome of May 1996 Toronto Workshop between Australia, Canada, European
  Union, Japan, United States
- Cooperative Projects with Public/Private Groups
  Information sharing (databases)
  Research
  Workshops/Courses
  Guidance

regulated, who regulates them, the pre- and post-market requirements, and most importantly, the rationale for decision making are critical for the ultimate development of a global regulatory perspective for establishing the consistent quality of present and future products. Cooperative projects with public and private groups, such as the National Institute for Standards and Technology (NIST), the Pittsburgh and Toronto Tissue Engineering Initiatives, and others in information sharing, research, especially test method development and generic research in enabling technologies, workshops, and guidance for the industry exemplify the importance of a working interchange among all partners of the enterprise devoted to the safe and efficacious application of cell and tissue engineering technology to medical products.

Product Safety and Effectiveness

An important goal of the Working Group is to identify generic safety and effectiveness issues for consideration by the community in its development of products. Examples of these issues are: product consistency and stability in manufacture, including material sourcing, adventitious agents, toxicity testing, and sterility for preclinical safety; material characterization, for example, structural and functional activity, biomaterial compatibility testing, and *in vitro* animal models for preclinical activity/evaluation; and clinical indications, endpoints for clinical efficacy, safety monitoring, and post-market reporting during clinical investigation (TABLE 5).

Combination Products and Regulation

Many tissue engineered products such as bioartificial organs are combination products in the regulatory sense, that is, they may constitute a combination of a drug, device, or biological product. The FDA InterCenter Agreements were established to clarify product jurisdictional issues for such combination products. The Center for Biologics Evaluation and Research (CBER), the Center for Devices and Radiological Health (CDRH), and the Center for Drug Evaluation and Research (CDER) have entered into these agreements, and there are guidance documents between the Centers that describe the allocation of responsibility for certain products and product classes. For example, tissues and tissue engineered products are under the regulatory purview of both the CBER and CDRH. Both Centers are involved in the evaluation of combination products, with the lead Center currently identified by the primary mode of action of the combination product; the other Center acts as a consultant. This approach and others will be evaluated by the FDA Tissue Engineering Working Group as it develops the Science-Based Rationale (SBR) for Regulatory Decision Making.

Certain scientific issues have been identified as important in molecular and cell biology, and biomaterials for continued progress in cell and tissue engineering (TABLE 6). Doubtless, others would add to these lists; they are, by no means, exhaustive and, as is the nature of science, ever-changing.

In the area of molecular and cell biology, by far the most important issues are the control of cellular proliferation and differentiation and modulation for the desired cell function or phenotype, with the development of adequate test methods to monitor cellular activity. As systems are developed with more than one cell type, it will be important to understand how different cells communicate with one another, and how this can be optimized in the desired setting or environment. With the

TABLE 5. Regulatory Issues in Manufacture, Preclinical Evaluation, and Clinical Investigation for Cell and Tissue Engineered Products

- Manufacture
  - Product consistency
  - Product stability
    - Functional
    - Genetic
- Preclinical Safety
  - Material sourcing
  - Adventitious agents
    - Testing
    - Process validation
  - Toxicity testing
    - Short term
    - Chronic/repeated dose
    - Carcinogenicity
    - Immunogenicity
  - Sterility
  - Sterilization by-products
- Preclinical Activity
  - Material characterization structural/functional activity
    - Biological cells/tissues
    - Biomaterial
  - Biomaterial compatibility testing
  - *In vitro*/animal models
    - Efficacy measures
- Clinical
  - Indications
  - Efficacy endpoints
  - Safety monitoring
  - Population exposure
  - Post-market reporting

increased use of allogeneic and xenogeneic cell and tissue sources comes the need to assure graft and host immunocompatibility, or ways to minimize or eliminate the host's untoward immunological reaction or inflammatory response. In addition, it must be remembered that there may be subpopulations of individuals for which the cells or tissues may have altered safety, such as immunosuppressed individuals. If genetically modified cells are utilized, the potential for cell transformation by the vector, vector stability, optimal functioning of the inserted gene, as well as the inflammatory response at the implant site, which is a potential for all implants, must be considered.

For biomaterials, an important issue is whether a naturally derived or a synthetic material is the appropriate choice for a particular application. This will, to some extent, be determined by what the biomaterial is asked to do, that is, its function. Will it last indefinitely or will it degrade or resorb over a period of time? What structural or mechanical characteristics are needed for or dictated by the *in situ* environment?

It is important to minimize or eliminate reactions at the biomaterial-host interface, such as the potential for inflammation and biodegradation, and to identify and characterize the mechanisms of degradation and its byproducts. If a material is designed to biodegrade, it will be important to control and measure the rate of degradation. Will the material induce a fibrotic reaction in the host? How will the fibrotic potential be determined? Are there approaches for preventing fibrosis by testing the host material-product interface? Of course, some inflammation and fibrotic response accompany virtually any soft-tissue implant or surgical procedure. The important question is whether the intensity of the response represents a safety risk to the host or interferes with the product's effectiveness. The host itself, and the individual variations in response, must also be considered. The functional activity of any product must be consistent and predictable from product to product. To that end, variation in a biomaterial must be minimized or eliminated by consistent processing methods and testing parameters.

TABLE 6. Scientific Issues for Bioartificial Organs as Outcomes of Cell Biology and Tissue Engineering

---

Molecular/Cell Biology
- Control of proliferation/differentiation
- Modulation of cell function/phenotype
- Cell-cell communication
- Control of inflammatory response
- Control of immunological responses
- Genetically modified cells
  Optimal gene function
  Vector stability

Biomaterials
- Natural versus synthetic materials
- Minimize/eliminate reactions at biomaterial-host interface
  Potential for inflammation and/or biodegradation
- Control of fibrotic response
- Biomaterial stability
  Understand mechanisms of degradation and its by-products
- If biodegradable, control and measure rate of degradation
- Biomaterial reproducibility
  Minimize and eliminate variation by consistent processing methods/testing parameters

---

TABLE 7. Future Challenges for Bioartificial Organs

Science
• Novel applications for reconstructive surgery
• Union of genetic techniques and tissue engineering
• Novel approaches for delivery of gene/cell therapy
• Development of functional artificial organs
Regulation
• Science-based rationale for decision making
• International regulatory perspective

FUTURE CHALLENGES

What are the future challenges for cell and tissue engineering and bioartificial organs from both the scientific and regulatory perspectives? Although any number of items could be identified, certain approaches, which build on the progress achieved and the successes, hold promise: novel applications for reconstructive surgery that utilize methods developed for biosynthetic skin; the union of genetic techniques with cell and tissue engineering; tissue engineered systems for the delivery of gene and somatic cell therapy; and the development of functional artificial organs, such as the artificial kidney (TABLE 7).

From the regulatory view, certainly a regulatory framework that utilizes a science-based rationale for regulatory decision making and an international regulatory perspective will contribute to establishing the proper niche for tissue engineered products and bioartificial organs in clinical medicine.

ACKNOWLEDGMENTS

The author wishes to thank the members of the Food and Drug Administration (FDA) InterCenter Tissue Engineering Working Group for their many contributions and suggestions, especially Drs. Grace Lee Picciolo, Charles Durfor, and Emma Knight.

REFERENCES

1. HELLMAN, K. B., G. L. PICCIOLO & C. F. FOX. 1994. Prospects for application of biotechnology-derived biomaterials. J. Cell. Biochem. **56:** 210–224.
2. HELLMAN, K. B. 1995. Biomedical applications of tissue engineering technology: Regulatory issues. Tissue Engineering **1**(2): 203–210.
3. GALLETTI, P. M., K. B. HELLMAN & R. M. NEREM. 1995. Tissue engineering: From basic science to products: A preface. Tissue Engineering **1**(2): 147–149.
4. BERTHIAUME, F. et al. 1994. The host response and biomedical devices. In Implantation Biology. R. S. Greco, Ed. CRC Press, Inc. Boca Raton, FL.

Regulatory Considerations in the Development of Encapsulated Cells

MRUNAL S. CHAPEKAR[a]

Division of Application Review and Policy
Office of Therapeutics Research and Review
Center for Biologics Evaluation and Research
FDA, HFM-591
1401 Rockville Pike
Rockville, MD 20852-1448

One of the major tissue engineering strategies for restoration or improvement of the tissue or organ function in humans is to encapsulate the allogenic or xenogeneic cells intended for implantation[1] or *ex vivo* perfusion in a semipermeable membrane[2] to prevent their rejection by the host. The membrane allows the passage of nutrients to the cells and diffusion of the secretory products of the cells out of the capsule for their utilization by the host. The membrane, however, prevents the passage of the host immune cells and immune mediators that induce rejection of the encapsulated cells. The cells may be incorporated into microcapsules or macrocapsules. The macrocapsules may include individual microcapsules containing the cells, or the cells embedded in a matrix such as collagen or agarose. The capsular membrane may be composed of synthetic materials such as polyacrylonitrile/polyvinylchloride (PAN/PVC) and polytetrafluoroethylene, or naturally derived biomaterials such as alginate or agarose. The macrocapsules may be spherical, in the form of hollow fiber tubes, or sheets containing the vascularizing semipermeable membrane.

Encapsulated cells are combination products that include biological and biomaterial components. To provide a mechanism for designating the primary review center for a combination product or any other product where the center jurisdiction is not clear, FDA has promulgated 21 CFR Part 3 Subpart A regulation.[3] As stated in this regulation, the designation of the primary review center for a combination product is based on its primary mode of action. This regulation further announces the availability of the intercenter documents among the Center for Biologics Evaluation and Research (CBER), the Center for Devices and Radiological Health (CDRH), and the Center for Drug Evaluation and Research (CDER), which are working agreements that clarify the center jurisdiction for combination products or other products where there are jurisdictional concerns. For a combination product that is not included in the intercenter agreements, or any other products where the center jurisdiction is unclear, the sponsor may submit a request for designation to the FDA jurisdiction officer or FDA Ombudsman before filing an application for premarket review. The highlights of the CBER/CDRH intercenter agreement and 21 CFR Part 3 Subpart A regulation are included in the publication by Chapekar.[4] Since the primary mode of action of the encapsulated cell products is via the cellular component, CBER is designated as the primary review center, and it reviews the safety and efficacy data for these products in consultation with CDRH and other FDA centers as necessary.

[a] Tel: (301) 827-5102; fax (301) 827-5397; e-mail: Chapekar@A1.CBER.FDA.GOV

Both the cellular and the biomaterial components of the encapsulated cell products raise specific concerns. Somatic cells may be derived from autologous, allogenic, and xenogeneic sources. When the cells are derived from an autologous or a xenogeneic source, the transmission of adventitious agents from the donor of the somatic cells to the recipient is one of the major safety concerns. The somatic cells are highly sensitive to terminal sterilization procedures such as heat, radiation, or filtration. In addition, inactivation or removal of pathogenic organisms is difficult during the cell separation process. Therefore, rigorous controls over donor testing, cell isolation, and propagation procedures are necessary to ensure the safety of the somatic cells. When genetically altered cells are used, there are additional concerns such as viral recombination, cell transformation by the vector, vector stability, and optimal function of the inserted gene. CBER has drafted several guidance documents such as *Points to Consider in Human Somatic Cell and Gene Therapy* and *Points to Consider in the Characterization of Cell Lines Used to Produce Biologicals* that enlist the regulatory concerns and recommendations related to somatic cells intended for human use. The additional considerations related to the clinical use of somatic cells and the list of the FDA guidance documents and guidelines relevant to biologic-biomaterial combinations are described in the publication by Chapekar.[4] These documents can be obtained at no charge from the Congressional and Consumer Affairs Branch (HFM-46), Rockwall 1, 6th floor, 11400 Rockville Pike, Rockville MD 20852-1448.

The mechanical strength of the capsular material is critical, especially when long-term implantation of the capsules is intended. Capsules should be able to withstand the pressures generated by the cells and by the circulating body fluids of the host. The capsular membranes should be permeable to cell-derived mediators, and to O_2 and other nutrients that support cell viability and growth. These membranes should, however, be impermeable to shed antigens from the encapsulated cells, and to host immune cells and other immune mediators that induce rejection of the encapsulated cells. Moreover, the biomaterials used in encapsulated cell products should be sterilized before combining with the cellular component to ensure the sterility of the final product. Importantly, the materials used in the construction of encapsulated cell products should be compatible with the host as well as with the encapsulated cells. Biomaterials such as commercial alginate with high mannuronic acid content[5] and polytetrafluoroethylene[6] have been shown to induce inflammatory mediators in monocyte macrophage cell cultures. These inflammatory mediators may adversely affect the viability and function of the encapsulated cells. For example Pukel, Baquerizo, and Rabinovitch[7] reported synergistic lysis of pancreatic islets by cytokines including TNF and interleukin 1 and Miller, Rose-Caprara, and Anderson[8] have shown induction of inflammatory mediators and the development of a fibrotic reaction after implantation of biomaterials in the animals. A fibrotic capsule around the encapsulated cells may reduce the transport of nutrients and O_2 to the encapsulated cells thus further affecting their growth. The fibrotic capsule may also prevent the passage of the cell-derived mediators to the host thus reducing the efficacy of the encapsulated cells. Therefore, finished biomaterial components should be tested for biocompatibility using appropriate *in vitro* and *in vivo* tests specified in the FDA modified ISO-10993-1.[9]

Encapsulated cell products may be assembled from individual biomaterial and cellular components at the clinical site, or preassembled by the manufacturer and maintained in culture before their shipment to the clinical site. In the latter case, *in vitro* studies should be performed to demonstrate the stability of the encapsulated cells during their storage and transport.

The preclinical safety and efficacy studies of encapsulated cell products may provide useful information on the immunogenicity and inflammatory potential of the final product in humans. If immortalized cells are used, tumorigenicity of the encapsulated cells is a concern, especially when there are questions about the mechanical strength of the capsule and when the cells are implanted in immunocompromised recipients. Moreover, the studies conducted in the animal models of disease may aid in optimizing the cell concentration and the duration and schedule of treatment.

Since encapsulated cells may include multiple components, the development of these products may be complicated and early dialog with FDA is useful in identifying and resolving critical development issues before an Investigational New Drug Application (IND) is submitted. Consultations may be obtained through pre-IND meetings or conference calls involving appropriate FDA reviewers. To schedule a pre-IND meeting for encapsulated cell products, the sponsor needs to submit a pre-meeting request summarizing the manufacturing and preclinical data, the clinical proposal and, most importantly, specific issues for discussion to the Division of Application Review and Policy in the Office of Therapeutics Research and Review in CBER. This request will be reviewed and if adequate, a meeting will be scheduled. To receive optimal input from the FDA reviewers at the pre-IND meeting, the sponsor should submit a pre-meeting package that includes sufficient information on the manufacturing, preclinical data, clinical proposal, and specific issues for discussion at least two weeks before the meeting. The meeting will focus primarily on the issues identified by the sponsor and any additional concerns from the FDA review of the pre-meeting material.

REFERENCES

1. SULLIVAN, S. J., T. MAKI, K. M. BORLAND, M. D. MAHONEY, B. A. SOLOMAN, T. E. MULLER, A. P. MONACO & W. L. CHICK. 1991. Biohybrid artificial pancreas: Long term studies in diabetic dogs. Science 252: 718–721.
2. ROZGA, J., M. D. HOLZMAN & M. RO. 1993. Development of a hybrid bioartificial liver. Ann. Surg. 217(5): 502–511.
3. Code of Federal Regulation, Title 21, Chapter 1, Food and Drug Administration, Department of Health and Human Services, Washington D.C. Office of the Federal Register National Archives and Records Administration, 1996.
4. CHAPEKAR, M. S. 1996. Regulatory concerns in the development of biologic-biomaterial combinations. J. Biomed. Mater. Res. 33: 199–203.
5. OTTERLEI, M., K. OSTGAARD, G. SKJAK-BRAEK, O. SMIDSROD, P. SOON-SHIONG & T. ESPEVIK. 1991. Induction of cytokine production from human monocytes stimulated with alginate J. Immunotherapy 10: 286–291.
6. CHAPEKAR, M. S., T. G. ZAREMBA, R. K. KUESTER & V. M. HITCHINS. 1996. Synergistic induction of tumor necrosis factor α by bacterial lipopolysaccharide and lipoteichoic acid in combination with polytetrafluoroethylene particles in a murine macrophage cell line RAW 264.7. J. Biomed. Mater. Res. 31: 251–256.
7. PUKEL, C., H. BAQUERIZO & A. RABINOVITCH. 1988. Destruction of rat islet cell monolayers by cytokines. Synergistic interactions of interferon γ, tumor necrosis factor, lymphotoxin and interleukin 1. Diabetes 37: 133–136.
8. MILLER, K. M., V. M. ROSE-CAPRARA & J. M. ANDERSON. 1989. Generation of IL-1-like activity in response to biomedical polymer implants: A comparison of in vitro and in vivo models. J. Biomed. Mater. Res. 23: 1007–1026.
9. FDA modified matrix of ISO-10993-1. Biological evaluation of medical devices part I: evaluation and testing. CDRH Blue Memorandum (G95-1), May 1995.

Design and Synthesis of New Biomaterials via Macromolecular Substitution[a]

HARRY R. ALLCOCK

Department of Chemistry
The Pennsylvania State University
University Park, Pennsylvania 16802

Four classes of materials are widely used in artificial organ research and clinical practice—synthetic organic polymers, biopolymers and modified tissues, ceramics, and metals. Of these, metals are strong, impact-resistant, and easily sterilized, but most are heavy, prone to corrosion to toxic metal ions, and lack the physical characteristics of living tissues. Ceramics are rigid and thermally stable, but are usually heavy, brittle, and difficult to fabricate into intricate shapes. Biopolymers and chemically modified tissues can lead to antigenic responses or disease transmission. Synthetic polymers come closest to the ideal biomedical materials because they are lightweight, tough and flexible, can be easily fabricated into a wide variety of intricate shapes that include films, fibers, and microspheres, and they can avoid problems associated with product variability and biological contamination. Moreover, different types of synthesized polymers lend themselves well to uses in membranes, gels, tissue engineering matrices, cardiovascular and renal devices, bioerodible materials, bone composites, artificial skin, and so on.

Hundreds of different polymers exist, but only six or seven are the focus of most biomaterials research—silicone rubber, polyurethanes, poly(hydroxyethyl methacrylate) (HEMA), poly(glycolic-lactic acid), poly(ethylene glycol), poly(tetrafluoroethylene) (Teflon), and polyethylene. Although these polymers *approximate* to some of the properties required for use in artificial organs, they are definitely not ideal. They frequently lack the combinations of properties that are needed—for example, elasticity combined with ease of surface colonization by endothelial cells, or strength, toughness, or elasticity combined with bioerosion to non-toxic products, or hydrogel character combined with control of the activity of immobilized enzymes or cells. Nevertheless, much has been accomplished with polymers that were originally designed or optimized to serve some other, non-biomedical purpose. But it is perhaps too much to expect that, for example, polyurethanes, developed for use in seat cushions or clothing, should behave like human tissue when used in heart pumps, or that poly(tetrafluoroethylene), widely used in mechanical bearings and waterproof clothing, should make an ideal blood vessel.

The main purpose of this article is to emphasize that the field of biomaterials in artificial organs need not be limited to a few "found" polymers that happen to be commercially available off the shelf. Instead, it will be emphasized that the use of modern chemistry and a broad perspective of polymer structure-property relationships now allows polymers to be designed and assembled with a wide

[a] This work was supported mainly by the U.S. Army Research Office, the Office of Naval Research, the National Institutes of Health, and Johnson & Johnson.

13

variety of targeted properties. Fine tuning of the polymer molecular structure allows access to materials that can be optimized for almost any selected biomedical application. Unless advantage is taken of these opportunities, artificial organ research and the subsequent clinical developments may cease to advance, for new materials are not produced by studying long-existing polymers in ever greater detail.

THE BASIS OF NEW POLYMER DESIGN

Polymers are central to the future of artificial organ research because the long macromolecular chains in these species are directly responsible for properties such as flexibility, toughness, ease of fabrication, hydrogel character, and surface behavior. Polymers absorb impact energy and convert it into chain motions rather than bond breakage. The absence of discrete, flexible molecular chains in ceramics is a reason for their brittleness. The molecular flexibility of most polymers allows them to become entangled in the solid state or even to form knots. These entanglements, together with either crystalline segments or covalent cross-links, provide dimensional stability under stress and, for many polymers, enhance elasticity. Cross-links also generate hydrogels from water-soluble polymers. Heavy cross-linking reduces flexibility and can lead to ceramic-like properties. However, some polymers are inherently more flexible than others and this is a key factor in tailoring physical properties for specific biomedical applications.

Most of the properties of polymers can be traced to features of the molecular structure.[1] An understanding of the connection between specific molecular features and the properties of a polymer is the basis of new polymer design. The properties of a polymer can be understood in terms of a) its backbone structure, and b) the types of side groups that are present (FIG. 1).

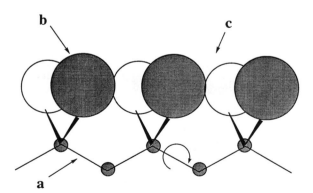

FIGURE 1. a: Bonds and elements in the main chain determine the inherent flexibility of the polymer via their influence on bond torsional freedom. They also control photo- and oxidative stability, and sensitivity to hydrolysis. **b:** The side groups control polymer solubility, reactivity, thermal stability, crystallinity, cross-linking, and (indirectly) chain flexibility. Their hydrophobicity or hydrophilicity has a marked influence on the behavior of the backbone under hydrolytic conditions. **c:** The "free volume" between side groups affects polymer motion, solvent penetration, membrane behavior, and density.

The elements and bond types in the backbone govern the inherent ease of twisting of segments of the polymer chain and hence the overall materials' flexibility. The backbone structure also controls thermal and radiation stability since heat and high energy radiation can damage a polymer primarily through cleavage of backbone bonds. The backbone also controls the inherent stability of the molecule to hydrolysis and hence is a critical factor in bioerodibility. It is possible to look upon the polymer backbone as a platform to which side groups are attached, but a platform that provides the basic properties that the side groups may embellish. CHART 1 lists some representative backbone structures and their characteristics.

The side groups, in general, control solubility, cross-linking processes, crystallinity, and reactivity. Indirectly, they also influence chain stiffness and hydrolytic stability. For example, bulky or polar side groups may increase the stiffness of the polymer by steric interference or dipole-dipole interactions. Bulky hydrophobic side groups can protect a hydrolytically-sensitive backbone against hydrolysis or, conversely, hydrophilic side groups may accelerate the breakdown of such a chain. CHART 1 lists some of the ways in which different chemical units in the side groups influence properties in most polymers.

From the viewpoint of biomaterials' design, it is necessary to consider these factors against a backdrop of three different types of properties that control biomaterials' behavior (CHART 2). These are: 1) the bulk physical properties of the material, 2) the surface properties, and 3) whether the material will be biostable or bioerodible. These factors can be designed into a polymer by three approaches—at the molecular level, via processing methods, and by surface chemistry (CHART 3).

The *bulk properties* of interest revolve around questions such as: a) Is the material to be rigid, flexible, or elastic? b) Will it be a solid or a gel? c) Will it absorb water or will it be impervious to aqueous media? (CHART 4). The *surface characteristics* that can be designed into a material are: a) hydrophobicity, hydrophilicity, or amphiphilicity (CHART 5), b) a bioactive or bioinert surface, c) the surface could be acidic, basic, neutral, charged or uncharged, d) the polymer may yield a physically stable surface, or the surface could undergo turnover, and e) the surface could be rough, smooth, or a hydrogel. The third factor—whether the polymer is biostable or bioerodible—is both a surface phenomenon and a characteristic of the bulk phase. If bioerodibility is required, the hydrolysis products must be nontoxic.

POLYPHOSPHAZENES AND STRUCTURE-PROPERTY TUNING

$$\left[-N = \overset{\displaystyle R}{\underset{\displaystyle R}{P}} - \right]_n$$

STRUCTURE 1

Most synthetic polymer systems make use of backbones based on the element carbon. The main reason for this is the ready availability of inexpensive monomers from the petrochemicals industry. However, a few polymer systems utilize skeletal elements other than carbon. Poly(organosiloxanes) (silicones) possess a skeleton of

CHART 1. Polymer Materials Design Through Molecular Chemistry

Backbones	Side Groups

Chemical Units for Hydrophilicity or Water Solubility

$-CH_2CH_2O-$	$-OH$
$-CH_2O-$	$-NH_2$
$-C(O)NH-$	$-COOH$
$-P(O)O-$	$-COONa$
$-C(O)O-$	$-NR_3^+ Cl^-$
$--P=N-$	$-SO_3H$
	$-SO_3Na$
	$-OCH_3$
	$-CN$

Units for Hydrophobicity and Water Insolubility

$-CH_2CH_2CH_2-$	$-CH_3$
$-CF_2CF_2CF_2-$	$-CH_2CH_2CH_2CH_3$
$-Si(CH_3)_2O-$	$-CF_3$
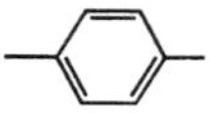	$-CH_2CF_2CF_2CF_3$
	$-Si(CH_3)_3$ 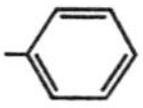

Units for Hydrolytic Instability

$-C(O)OC(O)-$ (anhydride)	Some side groups (hydrophilic) will
$-C(O)NH-$ (amide)	sensitize the backbone to hydrolysis
$-C(O)O-$ (ester)	and others (bulky, hydrophobic) will
$-P=N-$ (phosphazene)	protect it against hydrolysis
$-OC(O)NH-$ (urethane)	

Chemical Units for Polymer Molecular Flexibility

$-CH_2CH_2-$	$-CH_3$
$-CH_2O-$	$-CH_2CH_3$ etc.
$-CH_2CH_2O-$	$-OCH_3$
$-CH_2O-$	$-OCH_2CH_2OCH_3$ etc.
$-P=N-$	
$-Si-O-$	

Units for Polymer Molecular Rigidity

$-C(O)O-$	Polar side groups
$-C(O)NH-$	Ionic side groups
	Side groups that can
	form hydrogen bonds
	Bulky side groups that
	cause intramolecular
	steric interference, eg.

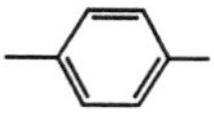

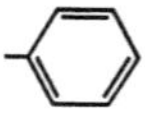

CHART 2. Three Sets of Properties That Need to Be Designed into Any Biomaterial

1. THE BULK PHYSICAL PROPERTIES
   Elasticity, Rigidity, or Flexibility
   Solid or Gel
   Water-absorbing or Water-repelling)

2. THE SURFACE PROPERTIES
   Hydrophobic, Hydrophilic, or Amphiphilic
   Acidic, Basic, Neutral, Charged or Uncharged
   Physically Stable Surface, or Surface Turnover
   Rough, Smooth, or Hydrogel Surface
   Bioactive Surface Groups, or Inactive

3. BIOSTABLE MATERIAL OR BIOERODIBLE
   Hydrolytically Stable or Unstable
   Stable to Enzymic Action or Unstable
   Toxic or Nontoxic Breakdown Products

alternating silicon and oxygen atoms with two organic groups attached to each silicon, and polyphosphazenes have a backbone of alternating phosphorus and nitrogen atoms, with two organic groups attached to each phosphorus (STRUCTURE 1). Of these two "inorganic" backbone polymer systems, the polyphosphazenes comprise by far the broadest class, with more then 700 different variants known. Because of this diversity, they provide an excellent example of how biomedical and other properties can be optimized by control of different aspects of the molecular structure.

The replacement of a traditional carbon-based backbone by a phosphorus-nitrogen skeleton brings about a major shift in bulk-, surface-, and biomedical-related properties and broadens the range of properties that can be achieved. First, contrary to intuition, this backbone is more flexible than those of most organic polymers. The inherent barrier to twisting of the phosphorus-nitrogen bonds is so low that glass transition temperatures as low as $-100°C$ can be achieved. This chain flexibility allows access to elastomers as well as to a wide variety of flexible films and fibers. Second, the backbone is sensitive to hydrolysis to phosphate and ammonia, especially when certain hydrophilic side groups are linked to each phosphorus. Hence, bioerosion can occur to phosphate, ammonia, and the side group, which can be an amino acid, a sugar, or a simple alcohol. However, the vast majority of different organic side groups protect the skeleton against hydrolysis. Hence, the choice of side group allows either total

CHART 3. Methods for the Incorporation of Specific Properties into Biomaterials

1. Through the design and synthesis of a polymer at the molecular level

2. By physical manipulation of the material after it has been synthesized

3. By surface chemistry

CHART 4. Control of Bulk Physical Properties

<u>Materials Flexibility or Elasticity</u>	<u>Materials Rigidity</u>
All the factors that cause molecular flexibility	All the factors that cause molecular rigidity
Presence of small molecules as "plasticizers" including solvents in swollen gels	Extensive crosslinking of chains Presence of crystallinity caused by molecular symmetry A high glass transition temperature (Tg)
<u>Water Absorption</u>	<u>Water Exclusion</u>
Presence of hydrophilic groups such as -OH, -COOH, -COONa NH_2, SO_3H, SO_3Na, etc.	Presence of hydrophobic groups such as benzene rings, fluoroalky groups, or organosilicon groups
<u>Solid</u>	<u>Gel</u>
Absence of water, organic solvents, or plasticizers High molecular weight polymers	Lightly crosslinked polymer swollen by water or organic solvents

resistance to hydrolysis or control over the hydrolysis rate by the use of both sensitizing and protecting side groups in different ratios. But the most important feature of polyphosphazenes is their method of synthesis, which allows an unprecedented number of different side groups to be linked to this one chain structure, and this is the basis of rational design and development of properties.

SYNTHESIS OF POLYPHOSPHAZENES

Polymer structural variations in classical organic polymers are normally accomplished through the polymerization of different monomers. If a new polymer is to be produced, it requires the synthesis of a new monomer and the development

CHART 5. Control of Surface Properties

Hydrophilic	Hydrophobic	Amphiphilic
-OH	$-CH_2CH_2CH_2CH_3$	Mixtures of hydrophilic
-COOH	$-CF_2CF_2CF_3$	and hydrophobic surface
-COONa	$-Si(CH_3)_3$	groups
$-O(CH_2CH_2O)_xCH_3$	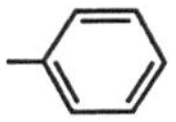	
$-NH_2$		
$-NR_3{}^+ Cl^-$		
$-SO_3H$	etc.	
etc.		

of processes to optimize the polymerization of that monomer. The chain length may vary from polymer to polymer. The method developed in our laboratory is an unusual one. It involves a two-step process as shown in SCHEMES 1 and 2.[2-5] First, the thermal ring-opening polymerization of a cyclic inorganic "monomer" leads to a high molecular weight linear, reactive polymeric intermediate

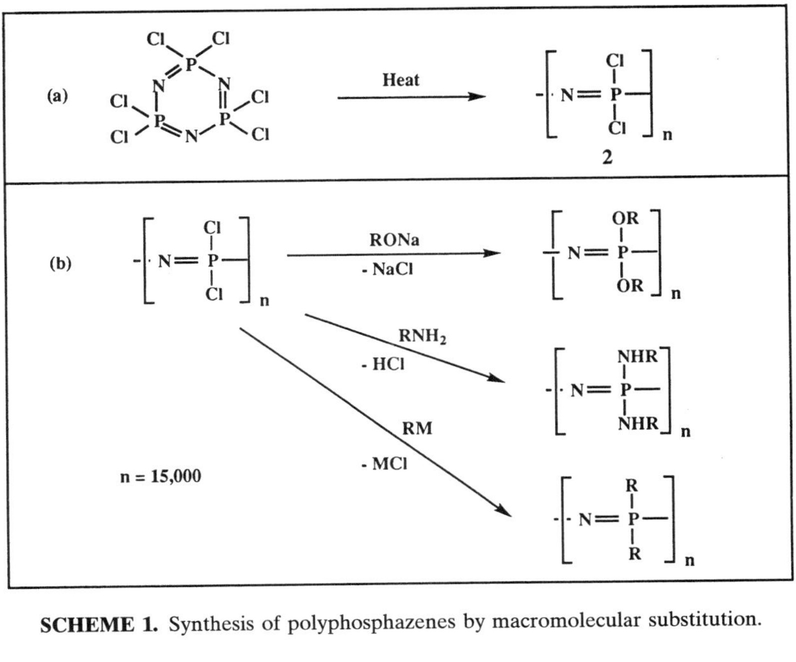

SCHEME 1. Synthesis of polyphosphazenes by macromolecular substitution.

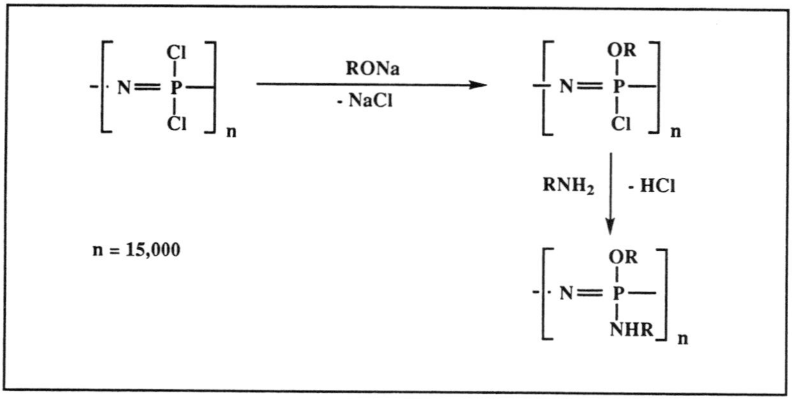

SCHEME 2. Sequential substitution.

known as poly(dichlorophosphazene) **(2)**. This highly reactive macromolecule is then subjected to chlorine replacement reactions in which all the halogen atoms are replaced by organic groups. Because many different organic reagents can participate in this process, and polymers with two or more different types of side groups can be produced readily, an almost infinite variety of structures is accessible. And because different side groups generate widely differing properties, the opportunities for optimization for biomedical research are very broad indeed. For example, different side groups generate elasticity, flexibility or rigidity, hydrophobic or hydrophilic character, bioerosion or hydrolytic stability, bioactivity or inertness, water-solubility or insolubility, low or high glass transition temperatures, amorphous or crystalline characteristics, or the ability to conduct further chemical reactions on the side groups without altering the main chain. A knowledge of the overall property relationships outlined in CHARTS 1–5 allows a measure of rational design of polymer structure and properties. Enough is now known about this system (CHART 6) that considerable reliability is now possible in this predictive process. CHART 7 illustrates some of the design possibilities that have been developed.

Virtually the only restrictions that apply to this synthesis method are: 1) bulky side groups require the use of forcing reaction conditions to bring about total chlorine replacement,[6] and 2) difunctional reagents (for example, p-hydroxybenzoic acid) must be protected initially in the form of p-hydroxyethyl benzoate units to prevent cross-linking, and must then be deprotected (by ester hydrolysis) after linkage to the polyphosphazene chain.[7-9] The success of the synthesis process depends on being able to replace all 30,000 or so chlorine atoms per macromolecule. Failure to do this may yield a polymer that hydrolyzes and cross-links on storage. However, the fact that all the chlorine atoms can be replaced in most instances illustrates the high reactivity of the P—Cl bonds in poly(dichlorophosphazene) **(2)**. A recent new method for the preparation of poly(dichlorophosphazene) allows control over the chain length, and provides access to narrow molecular weight distributions and block copolymers.[10] The following sections illustrate a few of the many examples in which this reaction has been used to prepare biomedical materials with specific properties.

CHART 6. Molecular and Materials Design in Polyphosphazenes by Side Group Variations

For Elastomer Formation	For Fibers and Films
OCH_3, OC_2H_5, OC_3H_7, OC_4H_9 $OCH_2CH_2OCH_3$ $OCH_2CH_2OCH_2CH_2OCH_3$ OCH_2CF_3 / $OCH_2(CF_2)_xCF_2H$ OC_6H_5 / $OC_6H_4CH_3$ OCH_2CF_3 / $CH_2Si(CH_3)_3$	OCH_2CF_3 OC_6H_5 OC_6H_4R
For High T_g's (above 37^0C)	For Solubility in Water
NHC_6H_5 $OC_6H_4C_6H_5$ OC_6H_4COOH OC_6H_4COONa $OC_6H_4N=CHR$ Glucosyl	$NHCH_3$ OCH_3 $OCH_2CH_2OCH_2CH_2OCH_3$ OC_6H_4COONa $OC_6H_4SO_3Na$ Glucosyl, Glyceryl
For Bioerosion	For Biostability
$NHCH_2COOC_2H_5$, etc Imidazolyl Glucosyl Glyceryl Possibly OC_2H_5	OCH_2CF_3 $OCH_2(CF_2)CF_2H$ OC_6H_5R $CH_2Si(CH_3)_3$ $OCH_2CH_2OCH_2CH_2OCH_3$
For Surface Hydrophobicity	For Surface Hydrophilicity
OCH_2CF_3 $OCH_2(CF_2)CF_2H$ OC_6H_6 $CH_2Si(CH_3)_3$	$OCH_2CH_2OCH_2CH_2OCH_3$ OC_6H_4COOH $OC_6H_4SO_3Na$ $OC_6H_4SO_3H$ $OC_6H_4NH_2$
For Radiation Crosslinking	For Linkage of Bioactive Agents
$OCH_2CH_2OCH_2CH_2OCH_3$ $NHCH_3$ Diacetoneglucosyl	$OC_6H_4NH_2$ OC_6H_4COOH $OC_6H_4N^+R_3Br^-$ $OCH_2CH_2OCH_2CH_2NH_2$

BIOSTABLE ELASTOMERS

Three groups of phosphazene elastomers have been synthesized, two of which have been produced on a large scale. The first comprises polymers with two different types of fluoroalkoxy side groups, for example, $-OCH_2CF_3$ and $-OCH_2(CF_2)_{2-10}-CF_2H$ units, arrayed randomly along the chains (11).[11,12] These polymers are highly hydrophobic and are unaffected by water and most organic solvents. The main

CHART 7. Molecular Structure-Property Relationships in Polyphosphazenes

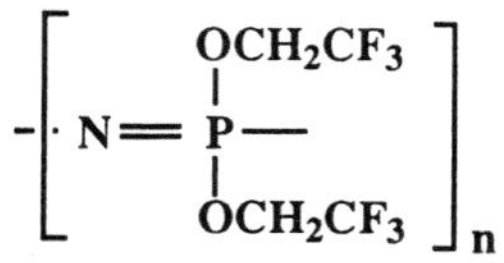

$$\left[-\cdot N=\underset{\underset{OCH_2CF_3}{|}}{\overset{\overset{OCH_2CF_3}{|}}{P}}-\right]_n$$

3
Hydrophobic

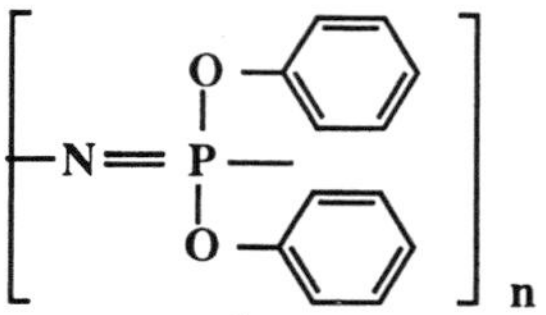

$$\left[-N=\underset{\underset{O-\bigcirc}{|}}{\overset{\overset{O-\bigcirc}{|}}{P}}-\right]_n$$

4
Hydrophobic

$$\left[-N=\underset{\underset{NHCH_3}{|}}{\overset{\overset{NHCH_3}{|}}{P}}-\right]_n$$

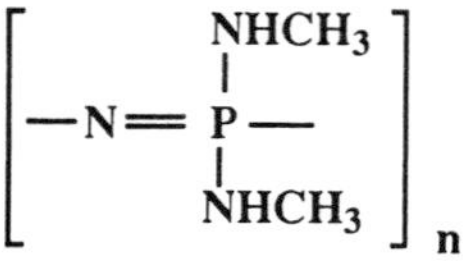

5
Hydrophilic and water-soluble

$$\left[+N=\underset{\underset{OCH_2CH_2OCH_2CH_2OCH_3}{|}}{\overset{\overset{OCH_2CH_2OCH_2CH_2OCH_3}{|}}{P}}-\right]_n$$

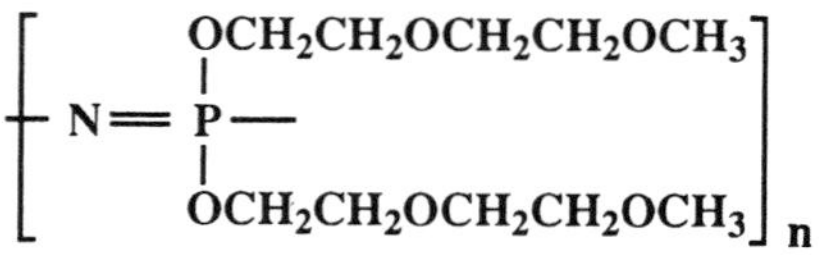

6
Hydrophilic and water-soluble

$$\left[-\cdot N=\underset{\underset{OCH_2CF_3}{|}}{\overset{\overset{NHCH_3}{|}}{P}}-\right]_n$$

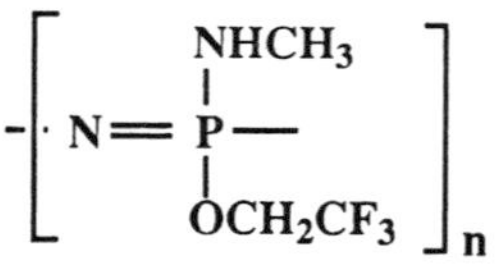

7
Amphiphilic (membranes)

$$\left[-N=\underset{\underset{O-\bigcirc}{|}}{\overset{\overset{NHCH_3}{|}}{P}}-\right]_n$$

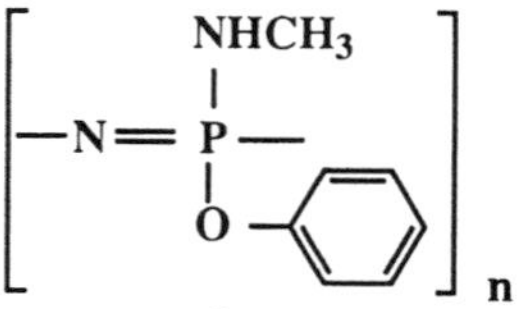

8
Amphiphilic (membranes)

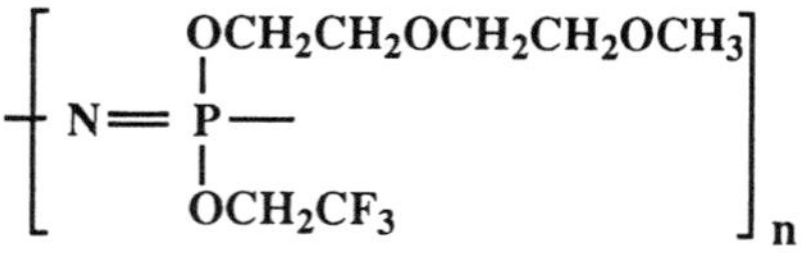

$$\left[+N=\underset{\underset{OCH_2CF_3}{|}}{\overset{\overset{OCH_2CH_2OCH_2CH_2OCH_3}{|}}{P}}-\right]_n$$

9
Amphiphilic

$$\left[+N=\underset{\underset{O-\bigcirc}{|}}{\overset{\overset{OCH_2CH_2OCH_2CH_2OCH_3}{|}}{P}}-\right]_n$$

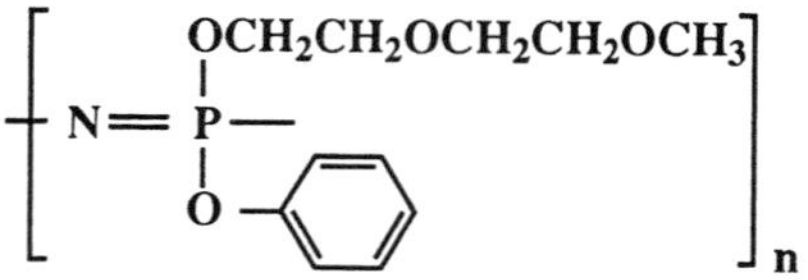

10
Amphiphilic

uses for these polymers so far have been in aircraft and other high performance engineering applications. But at least one biomedical (dental) application has been commercialized.[13] Based on their properties, these elastomers should be excellent candidates for use in cardiovascular applications, especially since surface chemistry has been developed that allows the formation of hydrophilic or hydrogel surfaces on the highly hydrophobic elastomer.

The second biostable elastomer class includes polymers with two different ary-

CHART 7. (*Continued*)

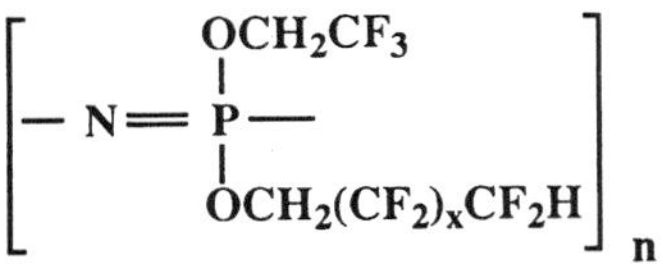

$\left[\begin{array}{c} OCH_2CF_3 \\ \mid \\ -N{=}P- \\ \mid \\ OCH_2(CF_2)_xCF_2H \end{array}\right]_n$ **11** **Hydrophobic elastomer**	$\left[\begin{array}{c} O-\bigcirc \\ \mid \\ -N{=}P- \\ \mid \\ O-\bigcirc-C_2H_5 \end{array}\right]_n$ **12** **Hydrophobic elastomer**
$\left[\begin{array}{c} OCH_2CF_3 \\ \mid \\ -N{=}P- \\ \mid \\ OCH_2Si(CH_3)_3 \end{array}\right]_n$ **13** **Hydrophobic elastomer**	$\left[\begin{array}{c} NHCH_2COOC_2H_5 \\ \mid \\ -N{=}P- \\ \mid \\ NHCH_2COOC_2H_5 \end{array}\right]_n$ **14** **Bioerodible leathery material**
$\left[\begin{array}{c} NHCH_2COOC_2H_5 \\ \mid \\ -N{=}P- \\ \mid \\ O-\bigcirc \end{array}\right]_n$ **15** **Amphiphilic tunable bioerodible material**	$\left[\begin{array}{c} \text{(glucose ring)} \\ -N{=}P- \\ \mid \\ OR \end{array}\right]_n$ **16** **Bioerodible polymer**
$\left[\begin{array}{c} OH \\ \mid \\ OCH_2CHCH_2OH \\ \mid \\ -N{=}P- \\ \mid \\ OCH_2CHCH_2OH \\ \mid \\ OH \end{array}\right]_n$ **17** **Bioerodible**	$\left[\begin{array}{c} O-\bigcirc-COONa \\ \mid \\ -N{=}P- \\ \mid \\ O-\bigcirc-COONa \end{array}\right]_n$ **18** **Water-soluble**

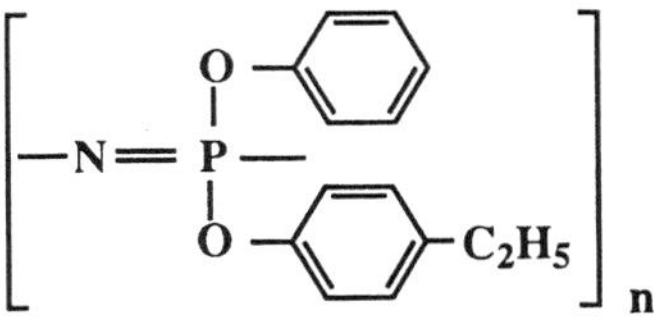

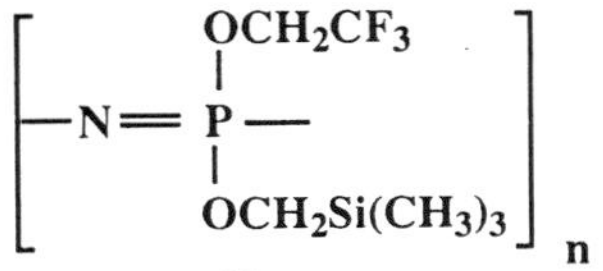

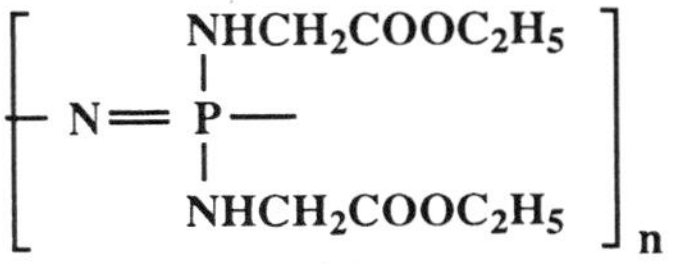

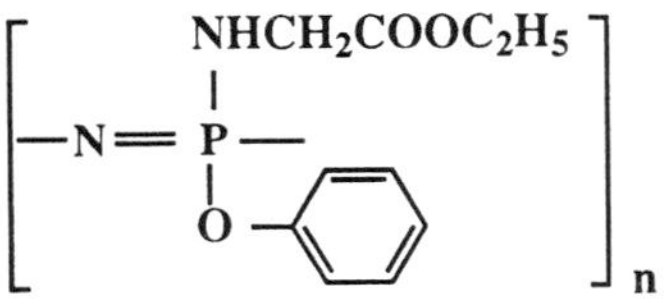

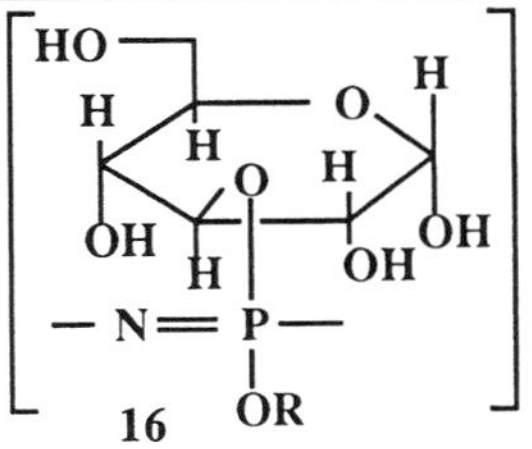

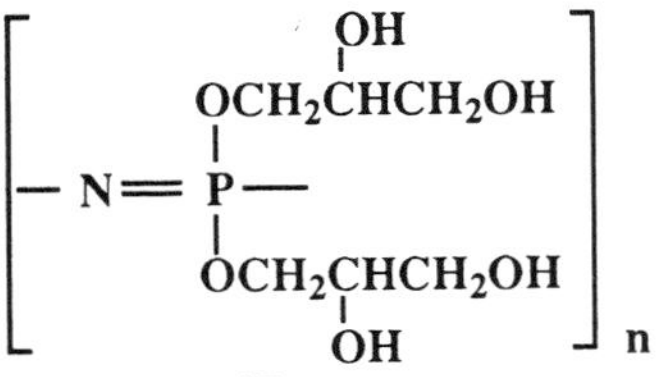

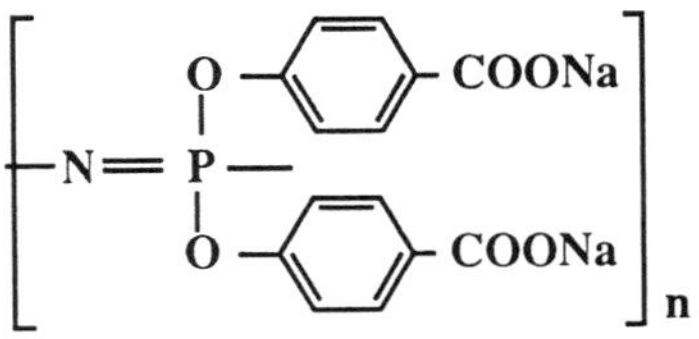

Note that, in the mixed-substituent polymers, the two sets of side groups may be geminal or non-geminal, or be part of random or block arrangements.

loxy side groups **(12)**.[11,12] These too have been commercialized for non-medical engineering uses. They are hydrophobic and chemically inert. Their biomedical potential has not yet been determined, although animal model tests have indicated that they are bioinert.[14] Surface chemistry has been developed for these polymers also for the generation of hydrophilic or bioactive surfaces (see below).

The third class **(13)** comprises a range of polyphosphazenes that bear organosilicon side groups, for example $-CH_2Si(CH_3)_2$, as well as $-OCH_2CF_3$ or $-OC_6H_5$ groups.[15] In a sense, they are hybrid systems that possess the skeletal advantages of phosphazenes and the side group advantages of silicones. These elastomers are hydrophobic materials with potential uses in oxygen transport membranes.

BIOERODIBLE PHOSPHAZENES

Side groups, such as amino acid esters,[16,17] glucosyl,[7] glyceryl,[8] imidazolyl,[18] ethyl lactyl, and ethyl glycolyl units,[19] sensitize the phosphazene backbone to hydrolysis (14–17). It appears that they have this influence first through their hydrophilicity, second, because of the hydrolytic lability of the bond that links the side group to phosphorus, and third, in several cases, because of the presence of carboxylic acid units generated at intermediate stages in the hydrolysis process.

Amino acid ester derivatives have already been shown to be excellent drug release matrices, and animal model studies have shown good biocompatibility in subcutaneous implantation tests.[20] In addition, recent work has shown that polymers that bear both ethyl glycinate and p-alkylphenoxy side groups (15) are supportive matrices for the growth of osteoblasts and thus are promising materials for bone tissue engineering.[21]

HYDROGELS

A number of side groups confer water-solubility on polyphosphazenes. These include glucosyl, glyceryl, methylamino (5), alkyl ether groups such as $-OCH_2OCH_2CH_2OCH_3$ (6), and salts of acid-substituted phenoxy groups such as OC_6H_4COONa (18) or $OC_6H_4SO_3Na$. All but the first two form aqueous solutions that are stable at pH 7 for long periods of time (months to years). The polymers formed with $-OCH_2CH_2OCH_2CH_2OCH_3$ (6) or related groups or with $-OC_6H_4COONa$ side groups (18) are of special interest when cross-linked, since they form hydrogels.[22–26]

Alkyl ether groups linked to a phosphazene chain are sensitive to ~2 megarads of gamma-radiation, while the backbone bonds are radiation-stable. The C–H bonds in the side groups undergo free radical cleavage and the carbon radicals formed in this process cross-combine to form C—C cross-links. Once cross-linked, the polymers absorb water to form hydrogels. They also exhibit lower critical solution temperature (LCST) behavior above which temperature the hydrogel will contract and extrude water.[27,28] The LCST temperature varies with the exact structure of the side group, as illustrated in CHART 8. Enzymes such as urease have been trapped in such hydrogels, and their activity is retained below the LCST, but can be turned off above this temperature. The LCST values shown in CHART 8 show how this phenomenon might be employed for a wider range of biomedical applications.

Polymer 18 is a water-soluble polyelectrolyte that is cross-linked by divalent or trivalent cations,[24,29] as shown in SCHEME 3. This process has been used for the microencapsulation of hybridoma liver cells, proteins, and vaccines, and has the potential for use in a wide range of artificial organ devices. The same polymer has also been used as the polymer matrix in hydroxyapatite composite materials.[30] The

CHART 8. LCSTs for Alkyl Ether Phosphazene Polymers

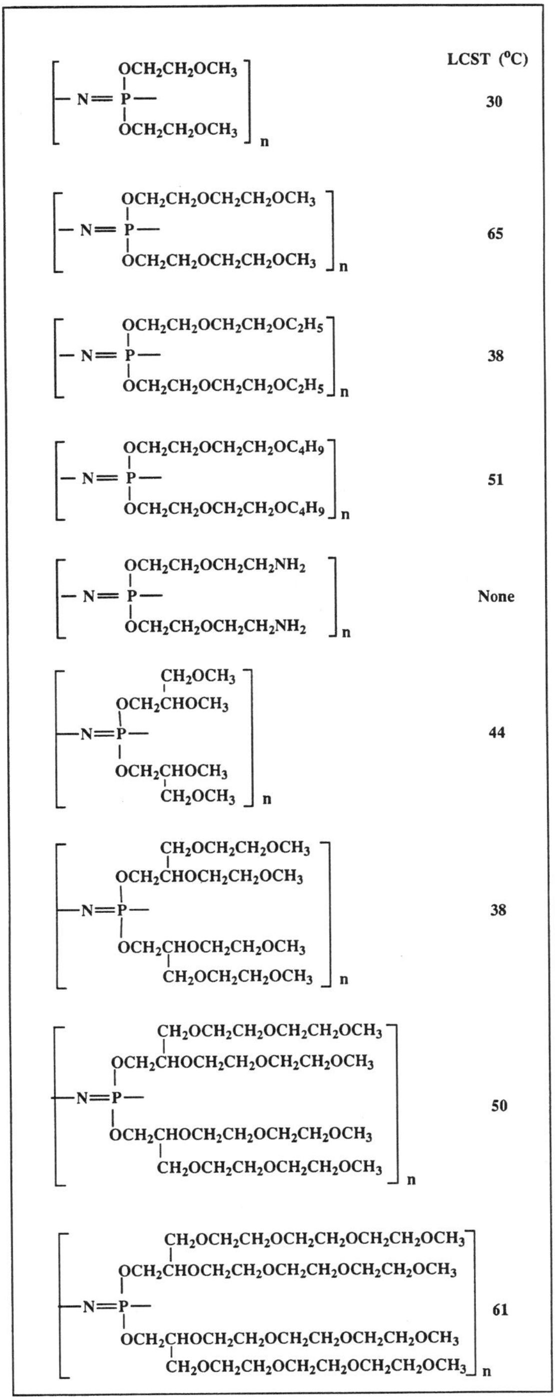

$$\left[-N\!\!=\!\!P\begin{matrix} OCH_2CH_2OCH_3 \\ | \\ | \\ OCH_2CH_2OCH_3 \end{matrix} \right]_n$$

LCST (°C)

30

$$\left[-N\!\!=\!\!P\begin{matrix} OCH_2CH_2OCH_2CH_2OCH_3 \\ | \\ | \\ OCH_2CH_2OCH_2CH_2OCH_3 \end{matrix} \right]_n$$

65

$$\left[-N\!\!=\!\!P\begin{matrix} OCH_2CH_2OCH_2CH_2OC_2H_5 \\ | \\ | \\ OCH_2CH_2OCH_2CH_2OC_2H_5 \end{matrix} \right]_n$$

38

$$\left[-N\!\!=\!\!P\begin{matrix} OCH_2CH_2OCH_2CH_2OC_4H_9 \\ | \\ | \\ OCH_2CH_2OCH_2CH_2OC_4H_9 \end{matrix} \right]_n$$

51

$$\left[-N\!\!=\!\!P\begin{matrix} OCH_2CH_2OCH_2CH_2NH_2 \\ | \\ | \\ OCH_2CH_2OCH_2CH_2NH_2 \end{matrix} \right]_n$$

None

$$\left[-N\!\!=\!\!P\begin{matrix} CH_2OCH_3 \\ OCH_2CHOCH_3 \\ | \\ OCH_2CHOCH_3 \\ CH_2OCH_3 \end{matrix} \right]_n$$

44

$$\left[-N\!\!=\!\!P\begin{matrix} CH_2OCH_2CH_2OCH_3 \\ OCH_2CHOCH_2CH_2OCH_3 \\ | \\ OCH_2CHOCH_2CH_2OCH_3 \\ CH_2OCH_2CH_2OCH_3 \end{matrix} \right]_n$$

38

$$\left[-N\!\!=\!\!P\begin{matrix} CH_2OCH_2CH_2OCH_2CH_2OCH_3 \\ OCH_2CHOCH_2CH_2OCH_2CH_2OCH_3 \\ | \\ OCH_2CHOCH_2CH_2OCH_2CH_2OCH_3 \\ CH_2OCH_2CH_2OCH_2CH_2OCH_3 \end{matrix} \right]_n$$

50

$$\left[-N\!\!=\!\!P\begin{matrix} CH_2OCH_2CH_2OCH_2CH_2OCH_2CH_2OCH_3 \\ OCH_2CHOCH_2CH_2OCH_2CH_2OCH_2CH_2OCH_3 \\ | \\ OCH_2CHOCH_2CH_2OCH_2CH_2OCH_2CH_2OCH_3 \\ CH_2OCH_2CH_2OCH_2CH_2OCH_2CH_2OCH_3 \end{matrix} \right]_n$$

61

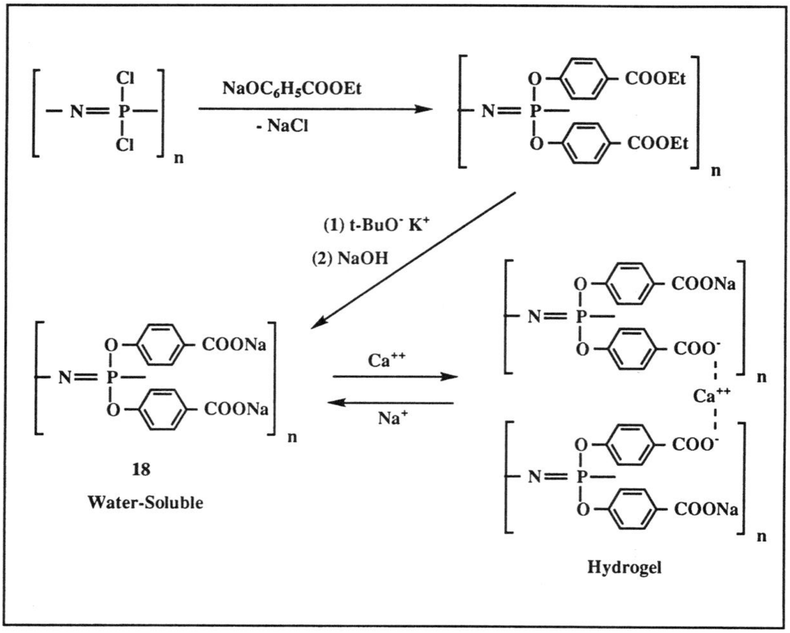

SCHEME 3. Reaction sequence for the formation of calcium-crosslinked hydrogels.

hydroxyapatite is formed at body temperature from an aqueous paste of calcium phosphate precursors in the presence of polymer **18**. The polymer becomes incorporated into the hydroxyapatite matrix through calcium cross-linking and provides strength and impact resistance. Porous structures have been fabricated which should facilitate blood vessel and osteoblast colonization.

SURFACE CHEMISTRY

A final group of examples illustrates the use of the unique possibilities for surface chemistry carried out on polyphosphazenes. Surface reactions that change the interfacial chemistry are known for a variety of organic polymers, such as polyethylene. However, the ability of the chemist to program side groups into the polymer and then carry out targeted surface reactions is one of the strengths of the polyphosphazene systems.[31–38] Four examples are shown in SCHEMES 4–6. All the examples convert a hydrophobic polymer to one in which the bulk hydrophobicity is retained, but the surface becomes hydrophilic or bioactive. This offers wide possibilities for improving the resistance of the surface to protein deposition or for favoring colonization by endothelial cells. The radiation grafting of polymer **6** (MEEP) to the surfaces of a number of organic polymers

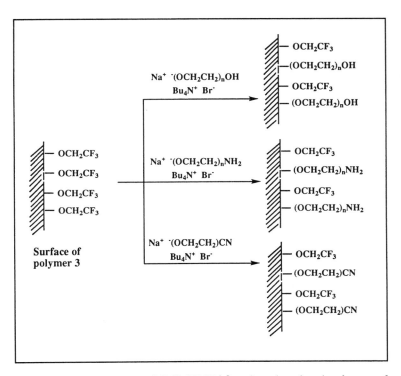

SCHEME 4. Surface reactions on $[NP(OCH_2CF_3)_2]_n$ to introduce functional groups for the linkage of bioactive or biocompatible species.

provides a way to improve the biocompatibility of hitherto non-compatible conventional polymers.

FINAL COMMENTS

Why are the design and synthesis advantages of macromolecular substitution not more widely used? The answer lies in the chemical limitations of most organic polymers. Macromolecular substitution works well for polyphosphazenes because of the high reactivity of the P—Cl bonds in the polymer intermediate. Few bonds to carbon backbones have this level of reactivity. Hence, once an organic polymer such as polyethylene, polyethylene glycol, poly(vinyl chloride), a polyester, or a nylon has been synthesized, only limited changes can be made by subsequent side group chemistry at the molecular level. The macromolecular substitution approach cannot yet be used for silicones because the required polymeric intermediate, $(O-SiCl_2)_n$, is difficult to synthesize. However, some attempts are being made to develop this approach for polymers with alternating silicon and carbon atoms in the backbone.[39]

So, are polyphosphazenes the only macromolecules that can fully exploit the macromolecular substitution approach? Not necessarily. A few classical organic polymers can be modified by macromolecular substitution. The hydrolysis of poly(vinyl acetate) to poly(vinyl alcohol) approaches 99.5% conversion. Cellulose can also be subjected to high yield chemical changes to the hydroxy side groups. Polystyrene, can undergo limited side group reactions without decomposition. But the biomedical polymers that are currently in use are generally not appropriate for modification by this method. Either the side group reactivity is too low, or the backbones are cleaved at the same time as side groups are replaced. However, *surface* reactions are possible with many organic polymers. But, for the present and the foreseeable future, polyphosphazenes offer the widest choice for polymer side group tailoring and rational biomaterials' design for artificial organic research.

One final comment is appropriate. The chemistry of macromolecular substitution for polyphosphazenes has been developed to a high level of sophistication, and the opportunities now exist for these polymers to be used widely in artificial organ research. Yet it is by no means certain that this will happen. The culture of biomaterials research and the regulatory restrictions tend to reinforce the current focus on the characterization or manipulation of the six or seven traditional biopolymers and, virtually all of the available resources are channeled into this specialization in spite of the scientific arguments for a broader approach. Without the concerted

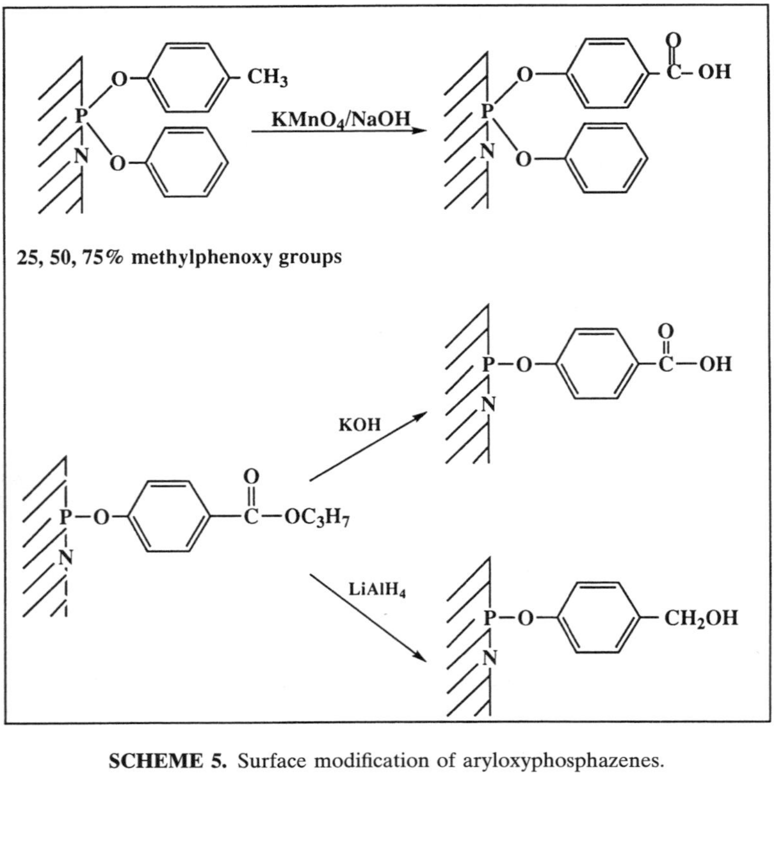

SCHEME 5. Surface modification of aryloxyphosphazenes.

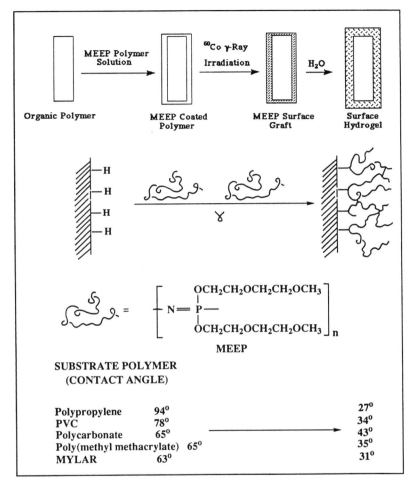

SCHEME 6. Surface-grafted MEEP hydrogels on organic polymers.

utilization of new polymers by bioengineers, physicians, and cell biologists, the full opportunities in artificial organ research will not be realized in the foreseeable future.

ACKNOWLEDGMENTS

It is a pleasure to acknowledge the contributions of the numerous coworkers mentioned in the reference list.

REFERENCES

1. ALLCOCK, H. R. & F. W. LAMPE. 1990. Contemporary Polymer Chemistry, 2nd edit. Englewood Cliffs, NJ. Prentice Hall.
2. MARK, J. E., H. R. ALLCOCK & R. WEST. 1992. Inorganic Polymers. Englewood Cliffs, NJ. Prentice Hall.
3. ALLCOCK, H. R. & R. L. KUGEL. 1965. J. Am. Chem. Soc. **87:** 4216.
4. ALLCOCK, H. R., R. L. KUGEL & K. J. VALAN. 1966. Inorg. Chem. **5:** 1709.
5. ALLCOCK, H. R. & R. L. KUGEL. 1966. Inorg. Chem. **5:** 1716.
6. ALLCOCK, H. R., M. N. MANG, A. A. DEMBEK & K. J. WYNNE. 1989. Macromolecules **22:** 4179.
7. ALLCOCK, H. R. & A. G. SCOPELIANOS. 1983. Macromolecules **16:** 715.
8. ALLCOCK, H. R. & S. KWON. 1988. Macromolecules **21:** 1980.
9. ALLCOCK, H. R. & S. KWON. 1989. Macromolecules **22:** 75–79.
10. HONEYMAN, C. H., I. MANNERS, C. T. MORRISSEY & H. R. ALLCOCK. 1995. J. Am. Chem. Soc. **117:** 7035.
11. TATE, D. P. 1974. J. Polym. Sci., Polym. Symp. **48:** 33.
12. PENTON, H. R. 1988. *In* Inorganic and Organometallic Polymers, Chapter 21. M. Zeldin, K. J. Wynne & H. R. Allcock, Eds. ACS. Symp. Ser. Vol. 360.
13. GETTLEMAN, L., J. M. VARGO, P. H. GELBERT, C. L. FARRIS, R. J. LeBOEUF & H. R. RAWLS. 1987. *In* Advances in Biomedical Polymers, p. 55.
14. WADE, C. W. R., S. GOURLAY, R. RICE & A. HEGYELI. 1978. *In* Organometallic Polymers. C. E. Carraher, Jr., J. E. Sheats & C. U. Pittman, Jr., Eds.: 289. New York. Academic Press.
15. ALLCOCK, H. R., D. J. BRENNAN & B. S. DUNN. 1989. Macromolecules **22:** 1534.
16. ALLCOCK, H. R., T. J. FULLER, D. P. MACK, K. MATSUMURA & K. M. SMELTZ. 1977. Macromolecules **10:** 824.
17. ALLCOCK, H. R., S. R. PUCHER & A. G. SCOPELIANOS. 1994. Biomaterials **15:** 563.
18. LAURENCIN, C. H., J. KOH, T. X. NEENAN, H. R. ALLCOCK & R. LANGER. 1987. J. Biomed. Mater. Res. **21:** 1231.
19. ALLCOCK, H. R., S. R. PUCHER & A. G. SCOPELIANOS. 1994. Macromolecules **1:** 1.
20. deVISSER, A. C., C. W. J. GROLLEMAN, H. van der GOOT, H. TIMMERMAN & J. G. C. WOLKE. 1984. Adv. Biomater. **5:** 373.
21. LAURENCIN, C. T., S. F. EL-AMIN, S. E. IBIM, D. A. WILLOUGHBY, M. ATTAWIA, A. A. AMBROSIO & H. R. ALLCOCK. 1996. J. Biomed. Mater. Res. **30:** 133.
22. ALLCOCK, H. R., P. E. AUSTIN, T. X. NEENAN, J. T. SISKO, P. M. BLONSKY & D. F. SHRIVER. 1986. Macromolecules **19:** 1508.
23. ALLCOCK, H. R., S. KWON, G. H. RIDING, R. J. FITZPATRICK & J. L. BENNETT. 1988. Biomaterials **19:** 509.
24. ALLCOCK, H. R. & S. KWON. 1989. Macromolecules **22:** 75.
25. COHEN, S., M. C. BANO, L. G. CIMA, H. R. ALLCOCK, J. P. VACANTI, C. A. VACANTI & R. LANGER. 1993. Clin. Mater. **13:** 3.
26. ANDRIANOV, A., S. COHEN, R. LANGER, K. B. VISSCHER & H. R. ALLCOCK. 1993. J. Controlled Release **27:** 69.
27. ALLCOCK, H. R., S. R. PUCHER, M. L. TURNER & R. J. FITZPATRICK. 1992. Macromolecules **25:** 5573.
28. ALLCOCK, H. R. & G. K. DUDLEY. 1996. Macromolecules **29:** 1313.
29. COHEN, S., M. C. BANO, K. B. VISSCHER, M. CHOW, H. R. ALLCOCK & R. LANGER. 1990. J. Am. Chem. Soc. **112:** 7832.
30. TenHUISEN, K. S., P. W. BROWN, C. S. REED & H. R. ALLCOCK. 1996. J. Mater. Sci., Mater. Med. **7:** 673.
31. ALLCOCK, H. R., J. S. RUTT & R. J. FITZPATRICK. 1991. Chem. Mater. **3:** 442.
32. ALLCOCK, H. R. & R. J. FITZPATRICK. 1991. Chem. Mater. **3:** 450.
33. ALLCOCK, H. R., S. R. PUCHER & R. J. FITZPATRICK. 1992. Biomaterials **13:** 857.
34. ALLCOCK, H. R. & R. J. FITZPATRICK. 1991. Chem. Mater. **3:** 1120.
35. ALLCOCK, H. R., R. J. FITZPATRICK & L. SALVATI. 1992. Chem. Mater. **4:** 769.

36. ALLCOCK, H. R., R. J. FITZPATRICK & K. B. VISSCHER. 1992. Chem. Mater. **4:** 775.
37. ALLCOCK, H. R. & D. E. SMITH. 1995. Chem. Mater. **7:** 1469.
38. ALLCOCK, H. R., C. T. MORRISSEY, W. K. WAY & N. WINOGRAD. 1996. Chem. Mater. **8:** 2730.
39. RUSHKIN, I. L. & L. V. INTERRANTE. 1996. Macromolecules **29:** 3123.

Elastic Protein-based Materials in Tissue Reconstruction[a]

DAN W. URRY[b,d] AND ASIMA PATTANAIK[c]

[b]*Laboratory of Molecular Biophysics*
The University of Alabama at Birmingham
1670 University Boulevard VH 300
Birmingham, Alabama 35294-0019

[c]*Bioelastics Research, Ltd.*
1075 13th Street South
Birmingham, Alabama 35205-3408

Cells attach to their extracellular matrix by means of receptors (integrins) in the cell membrane which are in turn attached to cytoskeletal fibers running intracellularly between integrins either directly or through intermediate attachment to nuclear material. By means of these attachments and the physicochemical properties of the integrins, cytoskeletal fibers and nuclear components, cells become mechano-chemical transducers that sense the tensional force changes to which their attached extracellular matrix is subjected. These tensional force changes can have three distinguishing features: 1) the magnitude or intensity of the force changes, 2) the range of forces over which the force changes occur, and 3) the temporal characteristics or time course of the force changes.

The urinary bladder fills over a time course of several hours and empties in fractions of a minute as tensional forces change from near zero to pressures of about 30 mm Hg. The artery, on the other hand, cycles approximately every second between a normal low (diastolic) value of about 70 mm Hg to a normal high (systolic) value of about 120 mm Hg. It is believed that these different patterns of tensional force changes result in different chemical signals causing the nucleus to elaborate the appropriate extracellular matrix (ECM) with which to sustain such tensional force changes. This was appreciated early by Glagov and coworkers[1] studying vascular smooth muscle cell attachment to isolated vascular internal elastic lamina and the cellular response to the absence and presence of stretch/relaxation cycles; it was demonstrated in part by van der Lei *et al.*[2,3] using elastic synthetic arteries, and it is more currently given identification with greater molecular biological characterization as the *tensegrity principle.*[4-7]

Thus, the structure and function of a tissue is the integrated result of its constituent cells and the cellular response to the forces to which the tissue is subjected. Functional tissue derives from the efficient mechano-chemical transduction of these external forces by the cells themselves undergoing the tensional

[a] The authors wish to acknowledge the following support: the Office of Naval Research under the grant No. N00014-89-J-1970 and N43-DK-4-2209 from National Institute of Diabetes and Digestive and Kidney Diseases.

[d] Author to whom correspondence should be addressed. Tel: (205) 934-4177; Fax: (205) 934-4256; E-mail: MOBI006@uabdpo.dpo.uab.edu

force changes through their attachments to the extracellular matrix, ECM, components.

The questions regarding the actual cellular responses (from structural elements to biochemical messenger) remain to be answered. Mechanical strain has been shown to increase: 1) the proliferation and differentiation of smooth muscle cells,[8] 2) the synthesis of DNA in different cell types,[9,10] and 3) the synthesis of extracellular proteins.[11,12] In addition to these structural elements, other responses such as increases in the intracellular concentration of Ca^{2+}, $[Ca^{2+}]_i$, have been observed by several researchers.[13,14] The study by Oike et al.[14] demonstrates a relationship between increase in $[Ca^{2+}]_i$ and F-actin turnover or depolymerization by mechanical activation. These observations of the response of cells at the molecular level to tensional force changes have been referred to as *cellular tensegrity* by Ingber and coworkers.[4,5]

Extensive research has been underway towards the improvement of biomaterials for tissue reconstruction and it is important in doing so to be cognizant of this essential dynamic interaction between cell and ECM. Previously, polymers such as polyglycolic acid have been studied as the biomaterial for reconstruction of the ureteral organ.[15-17] Significant limitations of this material are the absence of cell anchoring sites and the absence of elasticity in the polyglycolic acid polymer matrix, that is, the inability of polyglycolic acid to match the compliance of the tissue to be replaced or reconstructed.

Here, we consider preliminary results on the development of elastic protein-based materials for bladder reconstruction. In particular, human ureteral explants are placed on elastic protein-based matrices containing GRGDSP cell attachment sequences; the outgrowth of urothelial cells onto the elastic matrix is compared with and without simulated bladder filling and emptying, and, specifically, the effects of a dynamic as opposed to a static matrix are considered in terms of urothelial cell proliferation and elaboration of extracellular matrix.

Of perhaps more fundamental relevance to the development of an understanding of the molecular processes underlying cellular tensegrity, the present report initially reviews experimental data on elastic protein-based materials that elucidate the mechanism whereby tensional force changes can result in chemical signals and illustrates the effects of different magnitude, range and time course of tensional force changes on the resulting chemical signals.

MECHANO-CHEMICAL TRANSDUCTION IN MODEL ELASTIC PROTEIN-BASED POLYMERS

What is the mechanism whereby extending or stretching a protein or a model elastic protein can result in a chemical signal? In our view, it involves the competition for hydration between hydrophobic and charged species constrained to coexist along a polymer sequence. To demonstrate this mechanism, several experimental results are brought into focus using elastic protein-based polymers that exhibit phase transitional behavior. The starting model protein, (Gly-Val-Gly-Val-Pro)$_n$ or simply (GVGVP)$_n$ with $n \geq 200$, comes from a repeating sequence found in bovine elastin where an n of 11 occurs. This model protein is miscible with water at all proportions below 25°C, but on raising the temperature to physiological values, solutions of this repeating peptide sequence exhibit a phase separation due to hydrophobic folding and assembly to form a more dense phase that is about 50% peptide and 50% water by weight.

Temperature Dependence of the Phase Separation of Hydrophobic Assembly

The most fundamental experimental finding concerning these phase transitions is the dependence of the transition temperature on hydrophobicity. Poly(GVGVP) is miscible with water in all proportions below 25°C, and it begins to aggregate hydrophobically on raising the temperature above 25°C, that is, its phase separation begins at 25°C. When the polymer is made more oil-like, as when one of the Val (V) residues with the side chain, $-CH(CH_3)_2$, is replaced by an Ile (I) residue, with the added CH_2 moiety, *i.e.*, $-CH(CH_3)CH_2CH_3$, the temperature for the phase transition of poly(GIGVP) begins at a lower temperature, that is, at 10°C.[18,19]

When the polymer, poly[f_V(GVGVP),f_F(GFGVP)] where f_V and f_F are mole fractions with $f_V + f_F = 1$, is studied containing the even more hydrophobic Phe (F) residue with the aromatic hydrocarbon side chain, $-CH_2C_6H_5$, only one Phe per 25 residues (an f_F of 0.2) is sufficient to lower the temperature for the onset of phase separation to 10°C.[19] Accordingly, when replacing the Val residue, the Phe residue is five times more hydrophobic than the Ile residue.

When a glutamic acid (E) residue is introduced into the repeating sequence as in the polymer, poly[f_V(GVGVP),f_E(GEGVP)], even with an f_E of 0.2 giving four Glu (E) residues per 100 residues, the transition temperature is above 100°C in distilled water but reduces to 70°C in the presence of phosphate buffered saline (0.15 N NaCl and 0.01 M phosphate at pH 7.4). On the other hand, when the pH is lowered to 3 where all of the carboxylates of Glu residues become protonated, the phase transition returns to near 25°C.

It should be apparent from the preceding paragraphs that the temperature of the phase separation becomes a practical measure of the relative hydrophobicity of the amino acid residues. In fact, a T_t-based hydrophobicity scale, where T_t is the temperature for the onset of the phase separation as the temperature is raised, has been developed as listed in TABLE 1.[18,19] To the best of our knowledge, this is the only hydrophobicity scale to be based directly on the hydrophobic folding process of interest. In the development of the scale the model protein of the composition, poly[f_V(GVGVP),f_X(GXGVP)], was used in which low values of f_X ranging from about 0.1 to 0.5 provided the data points, and then these were extrapolated in a plot of f_X versus T_t to $f_X = 1$ as a convenient reference state. The complete data, on which the T_t-based hydrophobicity scale of TABLE 1 is based, are contained in references 18 and 19 and in references cited therein.

Our interpretation of this observed temperature dependence of the phase separation contains three components. Firstly, there occur more-ordered waters surrounding hydrophobic groups, waters of hydrophobic hydration, that become destructured to form less-ordered bulk water as an integral part of undergoing the phase transition of hydrophobic folding and assembly. Secondly, when there is more water of hydrophobic hydration, the transition temperature is lower and when there is less water of hydrophobic hydration, the transition temperature is higher. And thirdly, in order for the carboxyl of a glutamic acid or aspartic acid residue to ionize and for the resulting carboxylate to obtain an adequate hydration shell, the carboxylate must destructure the waters of hydrophobic hydration (waters more ordered than bulk water) that are the basis for the phase separation, and the decreased quantity of waters of hydrophobic hydration results in a higher transition temperature.

If this is the case, then there should be an associated shift in the pKa of the carboxyl group as a certain amount of work or free energy is required in order to destructure the waters of hydrophobic hydration. The associated pKa shifts are considered in some detail after the diverse energy conversions are demonstrated, and, in particular, after chemo-mechanical transduction is demonstrated which on

TABLE 1. T_t-Based Hydrophobicity Scale for Proteins T_t = Temperature of Inverse Temperature Transition for poly[f_V(VPGVG),f_X(VPGXG)]

Residue X		T_t, Linearly Extrapolated to $f_X = 1$	Correlation Coefficient
Lys (dihydro NMeN)[a]		−130°C	1.000
Trp	(W)	−90°C	0.993
Tyr	(Y)	−55°C	0.999
Phe	(F)	−30°C	0.999
His (imidazole)	(H°)	−10°C	1.000
Pro	(P)[b]	(−8°C)	calculated
Leu	(L)	5°C	0.999
Ile	(I)	10°C	0.999
Lys (6-OH tetrahydro NMeN)[a]		15°C	1.000
Met	(M)	20°C	0.996
Val	(V)	24°C	reference
Glu(COOCH$_3$)	(E^m)	25°C	1.000
Glu(COOH)	(E°)	30°C	1.000
Cys	(C)	30°C	1.000
His (imidazolium)	(H$^+$)	30°C	1.000
Lys (NH$_2$)	(K°)	35°C	0.936
Pro	(P)[c]	40°C	0.950
Asp (COOH)	(D°)	45°C	0.994
Ala	(A)	45°C	0.997
HyP		50°C	0.998
Asn	(N)	50°C	0.997
Ser	(S)	50°C	0.997
Thr	(T)	50°C	0.999
Gly	(G)	55°C	0.999
Arg	(R)	60°C	1.000
Gln	(Q)	60°C	0.999
Lys (NH$_3^+$)	(K$^+$)	120°C	0.999
Tyr (ϕ-O$^-$)	(Y$^-$)	120°C	0.996
Lys (NMeN, oxidized)[a]		120°C	1.000
Asp (COO$^-$)	(D$^-$)	170°C	0.999
Glu (COO$^-$)	(E$^-$)	250°C	1.000
Ser (PO$_4^=$)		1000°C	1.000

[a] NMeN is for N-methyl nicotinamide pendant on a lysyl side chain, *i.e.*, N-methyl-nicotinate attached by amide linkage to the ε-NH$_2$ of Lys and the most hydrophobic reduced state is N-methyl-1,6-dihydronicotinamide (dihydro NMeN), and the second reduced state is N-methyl-6-OH, 1,4,5,6-tetrahydronicotinamide (6-OH tetrahydro NMeN).

[b] The calculated T_t value for Pro comes from poly(VPGVG) when the experimental values of Val and Gly are used. This hydrophobicity value of −8°C is unique to the β-spiral structure where there is hydrophobic contact between the Val$_i^1$ γCH$_3$ and the adjacent Pro$_i^2$ δCH$_2$ and the interturn Pro$_{i+3}^2$$\beta$CH$_2$ moieties.

[c] The experimental value determined from poly[f_V(VPGVG),f_P(PPGVG)].

reversal becomes the mechano-chemical transduction of interest in cellular tensegrity.

Diverse Energy Conversions by Changing the Temperature Interval of the Phase Transition

Depending on the composition of the model protein and the operating temperature, five different energy inputs can drive hydrophobic folding and assembly, that is, can result in the mechanical work of contraction. The first of these is the thermal energy input of raising the temperature from below to above the onset temperature, T_t, of the transition. The additional four energy inputs lower T_t from above to below the operating temperature to drive hydrophobic folding and the performance of mechanical work; this is called the ΔT_t-mechanism. The four energy inputs that change the value of T_t to perform mechanical work, that is, that change the temperature interval over which the transition occurs, are 1) changes in pressure, 2) changes in the concentration of a chemical (chemical energy), 3) changes in electrical energy, for example, the reduction of a prosthetic group attached to the model protein, and 4) changes in electromagnetic energy, *e.g.*, the absorption of a photon of light by a chromophore attached to the model protein.

These energy conversions are depicted in the hexagon of FIGURE 1, as are all of the additional pairwise free energy transductions involving these energies that

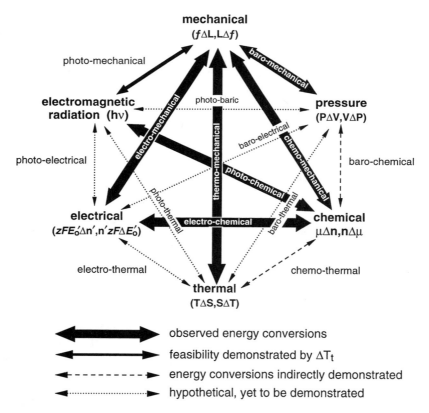

FIGURE 1. Schematic representation of the set of energy conversions possible when using the hydrophobic folding and assembly transition of elastic protein-based polymers. (Adapted with permission from Urry.[19])

are considered possible by model proteins capable of inverse temperature transitions of hydrophobic folding and assembly. The arrow interconnecting a pair of apices indicates a single pairwise free energy transduction, and the bold-faced arrows indicate those pairwise energy conversions that have been demonstrated by model proteins designed using inverse temperature transitions and the understanding of the ΔT_t-mechanism.

Hydrophobic-induced pKa Shifts

In order to address the anticipated hydrophobic-induced pKa shifts arising from the proposed competition between apolar (hydrophobic) and polar (e.g., charged) groups, some forty polymers were synthesized with the general composition, poly[f_V(GVGIP),f_X(GXGIP)] where X was Glu (E), Asp (D) or Lys (K). In all cases as f_X approached zero from a value of 0.75, that is, as the ionizable X residue was systematically replaced by a more hydrophobic Val (V) residue, the pKa values of the remaining E and D residues became higher, up to values of 6.7 and 6.0, respectively,[20,21] and the pKa of K lowered to 8.4.[22] This is the case at the dilution level of $f_X = 0.06$, i.e., for 1.2 residues per 100.

Next, it is instructive to consider a series of poly-30-mers of the formula, poly(GVGVP GVGβP GXGβP GVGVP GVGβP GβGβP) with the ionizable group kept constant, i.e., one X (Glu or Asp) per 30-mer, but with an increasing number (from 2 to 3 to 4 and to 5 wherein the latter case all β = F) of the more hydrophobic Phe (F) residue replacing the less hydrophobic Val (V) residues. There occurs a progression of the pKa shifts for the steps in which 2, 3, 4 and 5 Val residues are replaced by Phe of 0.4, 0.7, 1.4, and 6.1 for Asp and 0.3, 0.6, 1.1, and 3.8 for Glu.[23] *Clearly stepwise increases in hydrophobicity result in increasingly larger shifts in pKa.*

Stretch-induced pKa Shifts (Mechano-chemical Transduction)

Effects of Magnitude of Tensional Force Changes

The contracted state of the elastic protein-based materials is the hydrophobically folded and assembled state. When stretching this state, hydrophobic groups buried away from the water become exposed and surrounded by waters of hydrophobic hydration. As might be expected from the above hydrophobic-induced pKa shifts, this exposure of hydrophobic groups on stretching and the formation of waters of hydrophobic hydration result in the pKa shifts shown in FIGURE 2 for γ-irradiation cross-linked poly[0.82(GVGIP),0.18(GEGIP)].[24] For the unstretched matrix under conditions of physiological pH and 23°C, as seen in FIGURE 2, the Glu (E) side chains are ionized because the pKa is 6.2. On stretching, however, the pKa increases up to 9.5, and the side chains must become protonated. *The mechanical energy input of stretching has resulted in a chemical energy output of picking up protons.*

Effects of Range of Tensional Force Changes

Significantly with respect to the diversity of the resulting mechano-chemical transduction, the magnitude of the pKa shifts are non-linear with increasing mechanical force, as seen in FIGURE 3. As the stress/strain curve is essentially linear (see

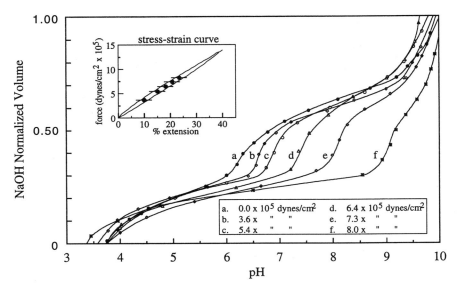

FIGURE 2. Acid-base titration curves of X^{20}-poly[0.82(GVGIP),0.18(GEGIP)] at the % extensions and associated forces given by the insert. Increasing the tensional force causes dramatic increases in the pKa which are non-linear, as shown in the plot of FIGURE 3. The step from curve a to b represents a five fold greater increase in force than the step from curve e to f, and yet gives only one-third the pKa shift. (Reproduced with permission from Urry & Peng.[24])

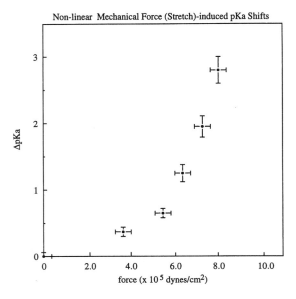

FIGURE 3. Plot of ΔpKa versus force in units of 10^5 dynes/cm^2 for the data of FIGURE 2. Note the marked non-linearity which indicates a more efficient chemical energy output at greater forces for a given change in tensional force.

insert of FIG. 2), the pKa shifts are non-linear with the amount of mechanical energy input. It is possible, therefore, to cycle the tensional force between 0 and 10% extension and obtain a small, 0.5 pH unit, shift in the pKa (*i.e.*, a small chemical energy output) whereas the same tensional force change but cycling between 10 and 20% extensions results in a large, greater than 2 pH units, shift in the pKa. This is where a difference in range of tensional force change can, with the same sensor, bring about a significantly different chemical signal as a result. This would have obvious relevance to the effects of high blood pressure on the proteins elaborated to renew cardiovascular tissue.

Temporal Aspects of Tensional Force Changes

The data of FIGURE 3 were obtained using a time period of 3 hours per data point. This means that each titration required more than two days to complete. The titrations themselves were repeated at least three times at each force level. Also, a repeat run at a given force level was interspersed with runs at different force levels. The approximately twenty titrations were taken in random order and the pKa values at a given force value were reproducible. This demonstrates the reversibility of the mechano-chemical transduction exhibited by this model protein for the same time period for each data point.

If, however, curve d of FIGURE 2 were run at a shorter period per data point, say 30 minutes, the apparent pKa would be higher, that is, in this matrix it takes time for the chemical response of proton release to occur. The finding, that the time to reach equilibrium is so long with this elastic matrix, is not considered a necessary feature for the mechanism but only a feature of these thick isotropic matrices through which protons diffuse only very slowly. The responsiveness of those functional groups at the surface of the matrix would be faster, as would be the energizing of a phosphate near the surface but the time dependence would still occur.

Thus, this mechanism of mechano-chemical transduction, demonstrable in elastic model proteins (a mechanism which we refer to as an apolar-polar repulsive free energy of hydration) inherently contains the three distinguishing features so very useful for understanding the differential responsiveness of cells to 1) the magnitude, 2) the range, and 3) the time course of the tensional force change.

Equivalence between Stretch-induced pKa Shifts and Energizing Phosphates

Our description of the hydrophobic-induced pKa shifts is that it arises from the competition between apolar (hydrophobic) and polar (*e.g.*, charged) groups for the limited hydration arising, even in relatively dilute solutions, from being constrained as part of the primary structure of the protein or model protein. This apolar-polar repulsive free energy of hydration, symbolized as ΔG_{ap}, occurs whether the charged group is positive or negative, although the effect appears to be more pronounced for negatively charged species.

Another expression of the competition for hydration between hydrophobic and charged species is seen in the shifting of T_t, the temperature at which the inverse temperature transition of hydrophobic folding and assembly occur. As is apparent in TABLE 1, the T_t-based hydrophobicity scale, the increase in the value of T_t on formation of a carboxylate of Glu, *i.e.*, the ΔT_t, is 250°C, whereas it is 85°C for the conversion of the Lys side chain from $-NH_2$ to $-NH_3^+$. The effect of forming an anionic species appears to be substantially greater than the effect of forming a cationic species. It would seem, therefore, that the effect of a multivalent anion might be most profound.

In fact, the most dramatic way to increase the value of T_t is to phosphorylate a functional hydroxyl side chain of the model protein. For the model protein poly[30(IPGVG),(RGYSLG)] the change due to 50% phosphorylation of the Ser (S) residue results in a calculated ΔT_t of greater than $1000°C$,[25] some four times greater than that for the formation of the Glu carboxylate. From the pKa shift of Glu due to stretching becoming 9.5 in FIGURE 1 when the normal pKa is about 4, it is possible to calculate ΔG_{ap} ($= 2.3RT\Delta pKa$) to be about 8 kcal/mole. This means that the free energy of an attached phosphate can also increase by a similar amount as the result of similar increases in the hydrophobicity due to stretching. Thus, we take the data of FIGURE 1, combined with the T_t-based hydrophobicity scale of TABLE 1, to indicate that a phosphate attached to a stretched protein structure such as cytoskeletal fibers could readily become energized by 8 to 10 kcal/mole or more and, therefore, be capable of phosphorylating an appropriate species in order to effect a particular gene expression.

PROPERTIES OF ELASTIC, PLASTIC AND HYDROGEL PROTEIN-BASED POLYMERS FOR TISSUE RECONSTRUCTION

There are four properties of elastic protein-based polymers and their related plastic and hydrogel analogues, collectively called bioelastic materials, that auger well for their application to tissue reconstruction: 1) the bioelastic materials tested to date exhibit remarkable biocompatibility, 2) the physical properties of bioelastic materials span continuously from plastic to elastic to hydrogel and as such can be designed with a range of elastic moduli and tensile strengths with which to match the tissue to be reconstructed, 3) these bioelastic materials can be designed to contain cell attachment sequences as an integral part of their primary structure such that the attached cells can sense the correct tensional force changes of the natural tissue in order that the cell can function normally in a physically natural site, and 4) these protein-based polymers are biodegradable and have the potential to be designed with the desired lifetimes *in vivo*.

Thus, the approach is to design temporary functional scaffoldings into which the tissue cells can migrate, to which the cells can attach, within which the cells can sense the correct tensional forces that the natural tissues are subjected in order that the cells function normally in remodeling into a natural tissue.

Biocompatibility of Elastic, Plastic and Hydrogel Protein-based Polymers

Complete biocompatibility studies have been carried out on three representative compositions and their γ-irradiation cross-linked matrices, and in addition, favorable anecdotal information is available on the biocompatibility of numerous elastic, plastic and hydrogel protein-based polymers of quite varied composition. The three representative compositions for which complete biocompatibility studies have been published also provide three representative physical states: elastic, plastic and hydrogel. Representative of the elastic state are poly(GVGVP) and X^{20}-poly(GVGVP), the 20 Mrad, γ-irradiation cross-linked matrix. The set of eleven tests recommended for materials in contact with tissue, tissue fluids and blood demonstrated a remarkable biocompatibility.[26] Representative of the plastic state are poly(AVGVP) and X^{20}-poly(AVGVP) and for the same set of tests the material showed good biocompatibility.[27] Representative of the hydrogel state is poly(GGAP), and the biocompatibility of this protein-based polymer, again using the same set of tests, is really quite extraordinary.[28]

Elastic Moduli and Tensile Strengths of Elastic, Plastic and Hydrogel Protein-based Polymers

The elastic moduli of 20 Mrad γ-irradiation cross-linked (X^{20}) protein-based polymers varies over a wide range depending on the composition. For hydrogels like X^{20}-poly(GVGVP) and X^{20}-poly(AVGVP) below 25°C, X^{20}-poly(GGVP) below 45°C, and X^{20}-poly(GGAP) at all temperatures, the elastic moduli are in the range of 10^4 N/m². For elastomers like X^{20}-poly(GVGVP) above 35°C and X^{20}-poly(GVGIP) above 15°C, the elastic moduli are in the range of 10^5 to 10^6 N/m² with a tensile strength for the latter of 1.1×10^5 N/m². By way of comparison, the elastic modulus of femoral artery is about 5×10^5 N/m². For plastics like X^{20}-poly(AVGVP), the elastic modulus is greater than 10^7 N/m², and the tensile strength of poly(FVGVP) is 5×10^7 N/m². Accordingly, the elastic moduli and tensile strengths of elastic, plastic and hydrogel protein-based polymeric materials suggest a broad range of potential applications in the general area of tissue reconstruction.

Cell Attachment to Elastic Protein-based Matrices

Bovine aortic endothelial cells (BAECs) and bovine ligamentum nuchae fibroblasts (LNFs) are not adherent to X^{20}-poly(GVGVP) in cell culture media[29] nor do they appear to attach in vivo while in the peritoneal cavity of the rat in a bloodied-contaminated model for the prevention of post-operative adhesions,[30,31] nor under the conjunctiva of the rabbit eye in a model for strabismus surgery.[28] Neither LNFs nor human umbilical vein endothelial cells (HUVECs) adhere to X^{20}-poly(GGAP) even when in cell culture media containing serum.[32] This is interpreted to mean that serum proteins such as fibronectin do not adhere to this matrix, to X^{20}-poly(GGAP), as such adsorbed protein would be expected to impart some cell attachment even though suboptimal. Submaximal cell attachment by BAECs and LNFs to X^{20}-poly(GVGVP) does occur in the presence of fetal bovine serum but significant growth does not occur.[29,32]

When the RGD cell attachment sequence from fibronectin is incorporated into the sequence of the protein-based polymer, as in X^{20}-poly[40(GVGVP), (GRGDSP)], all cells so far tested, BAECs, LNFs, HUVECs, and the A375 human melanoma cell line[33] attach, spread where relevant and grow to confluence.[29–33]

It is of further interest that in the matrix, X^{20}-poly[40(GVGVP),(GRGDSP)], the cell attachment is by means of a vitronectin-like receptor rather than to the expected fibronectin receptor.[33] This is of significance for use of the material as vascular prosthesis as platelets contain the fibronectin receptor and would normally be expected to bind and be activated by a GRGDSP sequence. Since platelets did not react in this way to the X^{20}-poly[40(GVGVP),(GRGDSP)] matrix, the above noted studies were carried out to determine which integrin attached to the X^{20}-poly[40(GVGVP),(GRGDSP)] matrix.

Programming Biodegradability of Elastic and Plastic
Protein-based Polymers and Matrices

Ideally what we are attempting to achieve is tissue reconstruction by starting with a temporary functional scaffolding that can provide for the correct implementation of cellular tensegrity and that, once an adequate natural tissue has been reconstructed by the natural cells, the temporary functional scaffolding will gracefully degrade and be gone. In order to achieve this it is necessary to be able to program the rate of degradation of the scaffolding.

Fortunately the 20 naturally occurring amino acid residues contain among them the capacity to introduce chemical clocks for the controlled degradation of the temporary functional scaffoldings made of protein-based polymers. The amino acid residues asparagine (Asn, N) and glutamine (Gln, Q) contain carboxamides in their side chains. As shown by Robinson,[34] depending on the residues preceding and following the N or Q residue, the carboxamides hydrolyze to form carboxylates, and the half-lives for the breakdown can vary from a few days to a decade.

As discussed above carboxylates raise the temperature, T_t, of the inverse temperature transition of hydrophobic folding and assembly. When the value of T_t is raised above body temperature, 37°C, a matrix basically of X^{20}-poly[40(GVGVP), (GRGDSP)] but also containing Asn or Gln, for example, would swell, and non-cross-linked coacervate phases would disperse.[35] Now, it has been our experience that the hydrophobic folded and assembled state is resistant to proteolytic degradation, whereas the swollen state is subject to slow proteolytic degradation in the peritoneal cavity, for example.[36] Thus, with available half-lives in the range of a few days to decades, it becomes possible to program the biodegradability of elastic and plastic protein-based polymers and matrices for virtually the full range of biological tissue reconstruction.

APPROACH TO RECONSTRUCTION OF A UROLOGICAL PROSTHESIS

Urothelial Cell Attachment to Bioelastic Matrices

The sequence of the protein based polymer has been designed for urothelial cell growth such that the elastic modulus of the cross-linked matrix would be comparable to that of natural tissue. The elastic modulus of the human bladder strips have been reported to be about 1.9×10^5 N/m^2.[37] The elastic modulus of the 20 Mrad γ-irradiation cross-linked protein-based polymer, poly(GVGVP), i.e., X^{20}-poly(GVGVP), is 1.6×10^5 N/m^2 and that of X^{20}-poly(GVGIP) is 4.8×10^5 N/m^2. The cell attachment site, GRGDSP, has been incorporated into both sequences by means of gene construction. The genes for [(GVGVP)$_{10}$–GVGVP**GRGDSP**–(GVGVP)$_{10}$]$_{18}$(GVGVP) and for [(GVGIP)$_{10}$–GVGVP**GRGDSP**–(GVGIP)$_{10}$]$_{18}$(GVGVP) have been constructed and expressed at high levels. These polymers, each of 2003 residues in length with a molecular weight of ~170 kilodalton, have been expressed, purified and cross-linked to obtain elastic matrices. The cross-linked matrix of the former gave an elastic modulus of 1.5×10^5 N/m^2 and has been prepared with a remarkable 900% extensibility. This matrix, incorporated with GRGDSP and exhibiting an elastic modulus comparable to that of natural bladder tissue, therefore, holds significant promise for consideration as a biomaterial for urological prostheses. Previously, chemically synthesized and cross-linked X^{20}-poly[40(GVGVP),(GRGDSP)] has been used for the urothelial cell growth study.

In the urothelial cell attachment studies, pieces of normal human ureter explants were placed on the bioelastic matrices. The urothelial cells outgrew from the explant on to the bioelastic matrix. The morphology of the sheet of urothelial cells on the bioelastic matrix was similar to the outgrowth onto collagen coated substrates, a more commonly used substrate for urothelial cells (See FIG. 4, A and B). The expression of cytokeratin-8, a marker of the urothelial cell, by these cells on the bioelastic matrix identifies the cells of the outgrowth as epithelial cells. This indicates that urothelial cells grow on the bioelastic matrices in a normal fashion.

Preliminary Studies on Urinary Bladder Simulation

To mimic normal micturition, the natural filling and emptying process of the bladder, an apparatus with a chamber has been designed and constructed. This apparatus is controlled by computer in such a way that the pressure in the chamber increases by a slow filling of the cell culture media over a 3-hour period followed by a rapid release of volume and pressure in 23 seconds. The bioelastic matrix, with an outgrowth of cells placed in this computer-controlled chamber, can undergo this cyclic pressure change for several days. Because of the elasticity and remarkable extensibility, the bioelastic matrix experiences the pressure change giving stretched and relaxed states. The cells grown on and attached to this matrix are expected to experience the similar tensional force changes as the matrix. The design of this experiment is, of course, made possible by these properties of the bioelastic matrix.

In a preliminary study, urothelial cells grown on X^{20}-$(GVGVP)_{251}$ adsorbed with fibronectin were subjected to the stretch/relaxation cycle for several days. The cell outgrowth, after undergoing the stretch/relaxation cycle (FIG. 4, D and F), has been increased to a larger area and became more dense compared to the cell outgrowth before the stretch/relaxation (FIG. 4, C and E). This result indicates that cells have been growing, dividing and responding to the tensional force change. Qualitatively, increased cell density and cell-cell contact have been observed as the effects of the stretch/relaxation cycle. Similar results, such as increase in cell-cell contact and the number of desmosomes, have been observed by others.[10]

SUMMARY

In natural tissues, cells form multiple attachment sites to their extracellular matrix. By means of those attachments, cells deform as the tissue deforms in response to the natural mechanical stresses and strains that the tissue must sustain during function. These mechanical forces are the energy input that instruct the cells to produce the extracellular matrix sufficient to sustain those forces. Thus, an ideal artificial material should have both the attachment sites for the natural cells and a compliance that matches the natural tissue.

Elastic protein-based polymers have been designed to provide both cell attachment sites and to exhibit the required elastic modulus of the tissue to be replaced. Thus, this introduces the potential to design a temporary functional scaffolding that will be remodeled, while functioning, into a natural tissue. A feasibility study applies this concept to the problem of urinary bladder reconstruction in terms of the filling and emptying of a simulated bladder comprised of an elastic protein-based matrix containing cell attachment sites with human urothelial cells growing out onto the dynamic matrix.

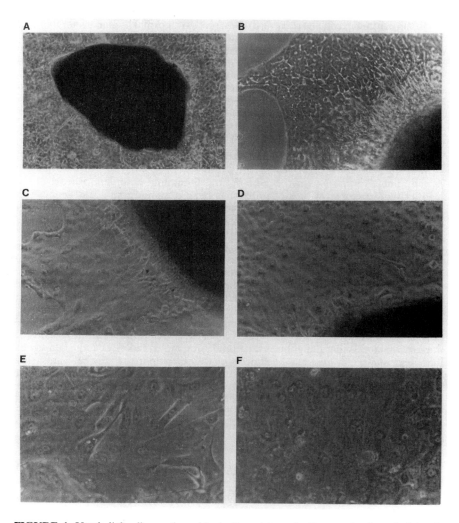

FIGURE 4. Urothelial cell growth on bioelastic matrices. **A:** Outgrowth of urothelial cells from a human ureteral explant (dark area) onto a bioelastic matrix containing the RGD cell attachment sequence. Note the dense outgrowth of cells and extracellular matrix. **B:** Outgrowth of urothelial cells from a human ureteral explant (dark area) onto a collagen-coated surface. It appears the urothelial cells grow fully as well onto the bioelastic matrix as onto the traditional collagen-coated surface. **C** and **D:** Comparison of the urothelial cell outgrowth onto the bioelastic matrix under static conditions, **C,** and under conditions of simulated bladder filling and emptying, **D,** as described in the text. **E** and **F:** The outgrowths of C and D, respectively, at higher magnification.

Furthermore, the elastic protein-based materials themselves have been designed to perform the set of energy conversions that occur in living organisms and, in particular, to convert mechanical energy into chemical energy with the result of chemical signals of the sort that could provide the stimuli to turn on the genes for producing the required extracellular proteins.

REFERENCES

1. LEUNG, D. Y. M., S. GLAGOV & M. B. MATHEWS. 1976. Cyclic stretching stimulates synthesis of matrix components by arterial smooth muscle cells *in vitro*. Science **191:** 475–477.
2. VAN DER LEI, B. *et al.* 1985. Regeneration of the arterial wall in microporous, compliant, biodegradable vascular grafts after implantation into the rat abdominal aorta. Cell & Tissue Res. **242:** 569–578.
3. VAN DER LEI, B. *et al.* 1986. Compliance and biodegradation of vascular grafts stimulate the regeneration of elastic laminae in neoarterial tissue: An experimental study in rats. Surgery: 45–52.
4. INGBER, D. E. 1994. Cellular tensegrity: Exploring how mechanical changes in the cytoskeleton regulate cell growth, migration, and tissue pattern during morphogenesis. Int. Rev. Cytol. **150:** 173–224.
5. INGBER, D. E. 1993. Cellular tensegrity: Defining new rules of biological design that govern the cytoskeleton. J. Cell Sci. **104:** 613–627.
6. WANG, N., J. P. BUTLER & D. E. Ingber. 1993. Mechanotransduction across the cell surface and through the cytoskeleton. Science **260:** 1124–1127.
7. GIRARD, P. R. & R. M. NEREM. 1995. Shear stress modulates endothelial cell morphology and F-actin organization through the regulation of focal adhesion-associated proteins. J. Cell. Physiol. **163:** 179–193.
8. BIRUKOV, K. G. *et al.* 1995. Stretch affects phenotype and proliferation of vascular smooth muscle cells. Mol. Cell. Biochem. **144:** 131–139.
9. KARIM, O. M. A. *et al.* 1992. Stretch-mediated visceral smooth muscle growth *in vitro*. Am. J. Physiol. **262:** 895–900.
10. BRUNETTE, D. M. 1984. Mechanical stretching increases the number of epithelial cells synthesizing DNA in culture. J. Cell Sci. **69:** 35–45.
11. THOUMINE, O. *et al.* Changes in organization and composition of the extracellular matrix underlying cultured endothelial cells exposed to laminar steady shear stress. Laboratory Invest. **75:** 565–576.
12. BASKIN, L. *et al.* 1993. Effect of physical forces on bladder smooth muscle and urothelium. J. Urol. **150:** 601–607.
13. HELMLINGER, G. *et al.* 1995. Calcium responses of endothelial cell monolayers subjected to pulsatile and steady laminar flow differ. Am. J. Physiol. **269:** 367–375.
14. OIKE, M. *et al.* 1994. Cytoskeletal modulation of the response to mechanical stimulation in human vascular endothelial cells. Pflügers Arch. (Eur. J. Physiol.) **428:** 569–576.
15. LANGER, R. & J. P. VACANTI. 1993. Tissue engineering. Science **260:** 920–926.
16. ATALA, A. *et al.* 1993. Implantation *in vivo* and retrieval of artifical structures consisting of rabbit and human urothelium and human bladder muscle. J. Urol. **150:** 608–612.
17. ATALA, A. *et al.* 1992. Formation of urothelial structures *in vivo* from dissociated cells attached to biodegradable polymer scaffolds *in vitro*. J. Urol. **148:** 658.
18. URRY, D. W. *et al.* 1992. Hydrophobicity scale for proteins based on inverse temperature transitions. Biopolymers **32:** 1243–1250.
19. URRY, D. W. 1993. Molecular machines: How motion and other functions of living organisms can result from reversible chemical changes. Angew. Chem. (German) **105:** 859–883; Angew. Chem. Int. Ed. (English) **32:** 819–841.
20. URRY, D. W. *et al.* 1993. Delineation of electrostatic- and hydrophobic-induced pKa shifts in polypentapeptides: The glutamic acid residue. J. Am. Chem. Soc. **115:** 7509–7510.
21. URRY, D. W. *et al.* 1993. Relative significance of electrostatic- and hydrophobic-induced

pK$_a$ shifts in a model protein: The aspartic acid residue. Angew. Chem. (German) **105:** 1523–1525; Angew. Chem. Int. Ed. (English) **32:** 1440–1442.

22. URRY, D. W. *et al.* 1994. Comparison of electrostatic- and hydrophobic-induced pKa shifts in polypentapeptides: The lysine residue. Chem. Phys. Lett. **225:** 97–103.

23. URRY, D. W. *et al.* 1995. Non-linear hydrophobic-induced pKa shifts: Implications for efficiency of conversion to chemical energy. Chem. Phys. Lett. **239:** 67–74.

24. URRY, D. W. & S. Q. PENG. 1995. Non-linear mechanical force-induced pKa shifts: Implications for efficiency of conversion to chemical energy. J. Am. Chem. Soc. **117:** 8478–8479.

25. PATTANAIK, A. *et al.* 1991. Phosphorylation and dephosphorylation modulation of an inverse temperature transition. Biochem. Biophys. Res. Commun. **178:** 539–545.

26. URRY, D. W. *et al.* 1991. Biocompatibility of the bioelastic materials, poly(GVGVP) and its γ-irradiation cross-linked matrix: Summary of generic biological test results. J. Bioactive Compatible Polym. **6:** 263–282.

27. URRY, D. W. *et al.* 1995. Elastic and plastic protein-based polymers: Potential for industrial uses. *In* Industrial Biotechnological Polymers. C. Gebelein and C. E. Carraher, Jr., Eds.: 259–281. Technomic. Lancaster, PA.

28. URRY, D. W. *et al.* 1995. Properties, preparations and applications of bioelastic materials. *In* Enclyclopedic Handbook of Biomaterials and Bioengineering—Part A Materials, Volume 2: 1619–1673. Marcel Dekker, Inc. New York.

29. NICOL, A. *et al.* 1992. Cell adhesion and growth on synthetic elastomeric matrices containing Arg-Gly-Asp-Ser-[3]. J. Biomed. Mater. Res. **26:** 393–413.

30. URRY, D. W. *et al.* 1993. Properties and prevention of adhesions applications of bioelastic materials. Mat. Res. Soc. Symp. Proc. **292:** 253–264.

31. HOBAN, L. D. *et al.* 1994. The use of polypenta-peptides of elastin in the prevention of postoperative adhesions. J. Surgical Res. **56:** 179–183.

32. NICOL, A. *et al.* 1993. Elastomeric polytetrapeptide matrices: hydrophobicity dependence of cell attachment from adhesive, (GGIP)$_n$, to non-adhesive, (GGAP)$_n$, even in serum. J. Biomed. Mater. Res. **27:** 801–810.

33. NICOL, A. *et al.* 1994. Cell adhesive properties of bioelastic materials containing cell attachment sequences. *In* Biotechnology and Bioactive Polymers. C. G. Gebelein & C. E. Carraher, Jr., Eds.: 95–113. Plenum. New York.

34. ROBINSON, A. B. 1974. Evolution and the distribution of glutaminyl and asparaginyl residues in proteins. Proc. Natl. Acad. Sci. USA **71:** 885–888.

35. URRY, D. W. *et al.* 1997. Transductional protein-based polymers as new controlled release vehicles, Part VI: New biomaterials for drug delivery. *In* Controlled Drug Delivery: The Next Generation. Kinam Park, Ed. Am. Chem. Soc. Professional Reference Book, Washington, DC in press.

36. URRY, D. W. *et al.* 1997. Transductional elastic and plastic protein-based polymers as potential medical devices. *In* Handbook of Biodegradable Polymers. A. J. Domb, J. Kost & D. Wiseman, Eds. Harwood. Chur, Switzerland. In press.

37. VAN MASTRIGT, R. *et al.* 1981. First results of stepwise straining of the human urinary bladder and human bladder strip. Invest. Urol. **19:** 58–61.

Synthesis of Biodegradable Polymers for Controlled Drug Release[a]

KAREL ULBRICH,[b] MICHAL PECHAR,[b] JIŘÍ STROHALM,[b]
VLADIMÍR ŠUBR,[b] AND BLANKA ŘÍHOVÁ[c]

[b]Institute of Macromolecular Chemistry
Academy of Sciences of the Czech Republic
Heyrovský Square 2,
162 06 Prague 6, Czech Republic

[c]Institute of Microbiology
Academy of Sciences of the Czech Republic
Vídeňská 1083
142 20 Prague 4, Czech Republic

The study and development of controlled drug release and drug delivery systems means a qualitative change in the approach to the development of new drugs.[1] These systems, depending on their chemical basis and physical design, can be classified as simple drug-releasing systems (oil droplets, encapsulation, dissolution-limited and matrix-diffusion-limited devices, membrane diffusion-controlled systems, microreservoir systems, activation-controlled systems) or more sophisticated targetable systems, facilitating controlled drug release preferably at the target site in the body (modified liposomes, particles or soluble polymeric drug carriers).[2] Biodegradable polymers have been frequently used as a basic material in the development of a number of advanced drug delivery systems. The main advantage of the use of biodegradable polymers is the degradability of the dosage form and elimination of the material from the body once the device is no longer needed. Biodegradability of the system or its part can be also employed as a rate-controlling factor in the controlled drug-release systems. Most of the research on biodegradable drug delivery systems has used hydrophobic polymers such as poly(cyanoacrylates), poly(orthoesters) or polyanhydrides.[3] In this paper we discuss the potential of some hydrophilic polymers to be used in the water-soluble form as targetable carriers of drugs or in the crosslinked form as hydrogel matrixes for controlled drug release.

Three degradable polymer systems will be discussed (FIG. 1). First is the system consisting of a nondegradable polymer backbone with pendant biodegradable oligopeptide side chains (spacers) terminated in the drug molecules. In this case, the rate of biodegradation of the oligopeptide sequence used as a spacer controls the rate of release of a drug from the carrier and thus the biological efficiency of the system. As a practical example of this system, copolymers of N-(2-hydroxypropyl)methacrylamide (HPMA), developed as targetable water-soluble carriers of anti-cancer drugs and immunosuppressants, will be mentioned.[4,5]

Secondly, we will discuss the system consisting of a polymer backbone containing

[a] The authors thank the Grant Agency of the Czech Republic (grant No 307/96/K226) and the Grant Agency of the Academy of Sciences of the Czech Republic (grant No. 72 04 07) for financial support.
[b] Tel: (+4220) 360 341.
[c] Tel: (+4220) 475 2267.

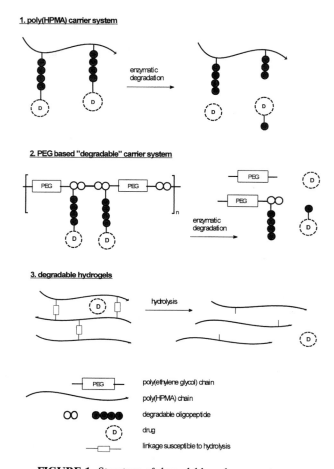

FIGURE 1. Structure of degradable polymer systems.

biodegradable linkages and bearing drug molecules connected with the polymer molecule by means of spacers susceptible to enzymic degradation. Biodegradation of this system results in free drug molecules and low-molecular-weight polymer fragments. Recently, using this principle, new systems based on poly(ethylene glycol) (PEG) block copolymers have been developed.[6] In these systems, the blocks of PEG are linked by biodegradable oligopeptide linkages. The drug is attached to the polymer via an oligopeptide spacer susceptible to lysosomal cleavage. The rate of degradation of the polymer backbone, the rate of drug release from the carrier and the exact site of degradation are controlled by changing the detailed structure of the oligopeptides used.

Finally, we will describe the hydrogel system in which nondegradable polymer chains are connected by linkages susceptible to hydrolytic or enzymic degradation. Hydrolysis of such a hydrogel results in a water-soluble polymer. The feasibility of this approach will be demonstrated using the example of poly(HPMA) hydrogels.[7]

SOLUBLE POLYMER CARRIER SYSTEMS

Poly(HPMA)-drug Conjugates

Synthesis and Structure of Conjugates

HPMA copolymers were developed as water-soluble targetable carriers of drugs, in particular of cancerostatics.[4,5] *In vivo* anti-tumor activity of poly(HPMA) conjugates containing doxorubicin or daunomycin against a number of model tumors (L 1210 leukemia,[5] P 388 leukemia,[8] Walker sarcoma[8] or B16F10 melanoma[9,10]) has been demonstrated previously. In all cases, a prerequisite to *in vivo* anti-cancer activity of conjugates was the susceptibility of the spacer between a drug molecule and polymer carrier to enzymic hydrolysis (cathepsin B, tritosomes).[5] The structure of doxorubicin (DOX)-poly(HPMA) conjugate, targeted by D-galactose and containing tetrapeptide GlyPheLeuGly spacer susceptible to enzymic degradation by lysosomal enzymes, is shown in FIGURE 2. The synthesis of poly(HPMA) conjugates is, in principle, a two-step process. In the first step, a polymeric precursor is prepared by the radical precipitation copolymerization of HPMA with methacryloylated oligopeptide terminated in 4-nitrophenyl ester (ONp), carboxylic, or amino group.[11] In certain cases, also methacryloylated oligopeptide terminated in the drug molecule can be used as a comonomer in polymerization.[11] The second step of the synthesis involves the binding reaction of a drug, combination of drugs, or both drug and targeting moieties to the precursor. A broad variety of polymerization and binding reactions enables the preparation of a number of polymer-drug conjugates differing in their detailed structure. The simplest structure is represented by conjugates in which a single drug is attached to the carrier via an oligopeptide spacer. Susceptibility of the spacer to enzymic degradation is a rate-controlling factor in drug release. More complicated systems consist of two different drugs or combination of a drug

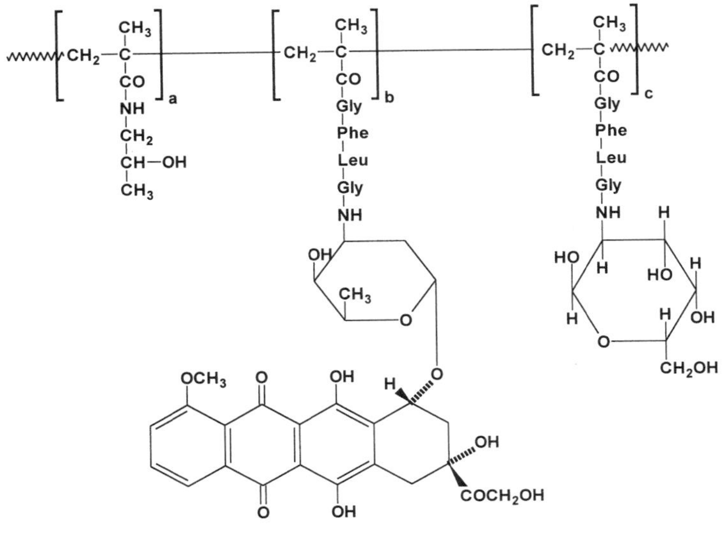

FIGURE 2. Structure of poly(HPMA)-DOX conjugate.

and targeting moieties, both attached to the carrier via the spacer of the same composition, *i.e.*, of the same substrate specificity. In the most complex system, each component (drug or combination of drugs and targeting moieties) is attached to the carrier via special spacers of different substrate specificity. In this case, the release profile of each component (drug) from the carrier will differ depending on the structure of the respective oligopeptide spacer.

The effect of the composition and detailed structure of the spacer as well as of the presence of antibody in the conjugate molecule on the rate of *in vitro* degradation of an oligopeptide spacer and DOX release after incubation with thiolproteinase cathepsin B or the mixture of lysosomal enzymes (tritosomes), isolated from rat liver, has been studied in detail.[12]

Polymeric conjugates of DOX, differing in the structure of the spacer, were prepared by a two-step synthesis.[13] In the first step, polymeric precursors were prepared by radical precipitation copolymerization of HPMA with methacryloylated ONp ester of respective oligopeptide. In the second step, DOX-containing conjugates were prepared by simple aminolytic reaction of the polymeric precursor with the primary amino group of DOX (conjugates without antibody) or by consecutive aminolytic reaction of the polymeric precursor with DOX and anti-CD$_3$ antibody. Conjugates containing the following spacers were synthesized: -GlyGly-, -Gly-DL-PheGly-, -GlyLeuGly-, -Gly-DL-LeuPheGly-, and -Gly-DL-PheLeuGly-, all of them with or without targeting antibody incorporated into conjugate structure. The conjugates contained bound anti-CD$_3$ antibody (25 wt-%) and/or DOX (6–7.1 wt-%), the weight-average molecular weight of polymer carriers was 18 000–27 000 and their polydispersity 1.4–1.5.

Biodegradation of Conjugates and Drug Release

Biodegradation of the oligopeptide spacer is a prerequisite to the DOX release from a polymer-drug conjugate. Oligopeptide spacers were tailor-made as substrates for lysosomal enzyme cathepsin B and susceptibility of the conjugates to lysosomal hydrolysis was verified *in vitro* by incubation with a solution of a model enzyme cathepsin B or with tritosomes[12] (a mixture of enzymes isolated from animal cells) and by measuring the rate of DOX release from the respective conjugate.

The results of DOX-release experiments are given in TABLE 1. They demonstrate that all conjugates were degradable and released DOX, except for the conjugate containing -GlyGly- spacer. The rate of DOX release can be modified in a very broad range by changing the length and detailed structure of the spacer used. The highest rates of degradation and DOX release were obtained for both conjugates containing tetrapeptide spacers. The relation between the structure of the oligopeptide spacer and the rate of DOX release from conjugates incubated with cathepsin B was very similar to that obtained for tritosomes. The effect of glycoprotein (anti-CD$_3$ antibody) incorporated into the polymer-DOX conjugate on the rate of DOX release is not very significant, but the presence of the bulky antibody in a conjugate molecule leads to a decrease in DOX release, probably due to steric hindrance to the enzymic reaction. In the case of conjugates containing tetrapeptide spacers, some amounts (up to 15%) of amino acid derivatives of DOX (-Gly-DOX , -LeuGly-DOX or -PheGly-DOX) were detected by HPLC as a product of cathepsin B degradation in addition to DOX. In contrast to the cathepsin B experiments, no significant amounts of these derivatives were detected after incubation with tritosomes. This indicates that a broad spectrum of peptidase activities of enzymes

TABLE 1. Release of DOX from Poly(HPMA)-DOX Conjugates

Structure	DOX Released (%)				Enzyme
	Time of Incubation				
	5 h	12 h	33 h	46 h	
P-GLFG-DOX	7.5	16.3	38.6	50.2	Cathepsin B
	18.5	33.5	63.3	78.1	Tritosomes
P-GFLG-DOX	2.6	9.6	27.8	41.6	Cathepsin B
	10.5	22.2	46.4	57.6	Tritosomes
P-GLG-DOX	2.9	7.1	15.4	23.3	Cathepsin B
P-GFG-DOX	1.3	2.8	7.6	9.3	Cathepsin B
P-GG-DOX	—	—	0.6	0.7	Cathepsin B
P⟨ GLFG-DOX / GLFG-Ab	5.6	17.6	42.6	57.5	Tritosomes
P⟨ GLG-DOX / GLG-Ab	1.7	5.9	17.6	24.5	Tritosomes
P⟨ GG-DOX / GG-Ab	1.4	1.4	1.5	1.2	Tritosomes

The conjugates with final substrate (DOX) concentration 1×10^{-3} mol l^{-1} were incubated at 37°C in either a solution of cathepsin B (4×10^{-7} mol l^{-1}) in 0.1 mol l^{-1} phosphate buffer containing 1×10^{-3} mol l^{-1} ethylenediaminetetraacetic acid (EDTA) and 5×10^{-3} mol l^{-1} reduced glutathion (GSH), pH 6.0 or in a mixture of 0.3 ml tritosomes and 0.7 ml 0.1 mol l^{-1} phosphate/citric acid buffer containing 1×10^{-3} mol l^{-1} EDTA and 5×10^{-3} GSH, pH 5.5.

present in tritosomes allows to release only free drug from its conjugates after internalization in the living cell.

The results of evaluation of biological activity of poly(HPMA)-DOX conjugates will be a subject of special paper (B. Říhová *et al.*, in preparation).

Biodegradable PEG Block Copolymers

Nondegradability of the polymer chain in poly(HPMA)-drug conjugates limits the use of poly(HPMA) carriers to molecular weights below the threshold estimated for elimination of synthetic polymers from the body via glomerular filtration, *i.e.*, below 40 000–50 000. This partial disadvantage is avoided in the PEG block copolymer carrier system[6] (for a scheme, see FIG. 1). In this system, the same oligopeptide spacers as designed for poly(HPMA) conjugates were used for attachment of drug molecules and thus, the susceptibility of the spacer to enzymic degradation should be the rate-controlling factor in the intracellular release of the drug also in this case. Degradability of the main polymer chain was achieved by connecting relatively short blocks of PEG (M_w 800–5 000) via diamine linkers, consisting of a central diamine molecule modified at both amino ends by amino acids to give the structure susceptible to enzymic degradation. First, feasibility of the synthesis and biodegradability of the system based on PEG block copolymers were verified in model studies, in which the enzymes chymotrypsin[6] and cathepsin B[14] were used. The PEG carrier system was susceptible to enzymic degradation and released the model of drug (4-nitroaniline) from the carrier at a wide range of rates controlled by the length and detailed structure of the oligopeptide spacer. At the same time, the carrier was degraded to PEG chains of the original molecular weight used in the synthesis. The prerequisite to the drug release and the main chain degradation was the optimal structure of oligopeptides, tailor-made as a substrate for the respective enzyme.

On the basis of the results of model biodegradation experiments with cathepsin B, we designed the structure of a PEG conjugate bearing in its side chains the anticancer drug DOX. The conjugate was synthesized using the strategy and methods described for the 4-nitroaniline models.[6,14] In this conjugate, two α-methyl-ω-hydroxypoly(oxyethylene) (mPEG) chains (M_w 5 000) were connected via the biodegradable oligopeptide -PheGluNH(CH_2)$_2$NHGluPhe-, in which some of the carboxylic groups were modified by -GlyPheLeuGly- spacer terminating in DOX molecule (for the structure see FIG. 3). The rate of DOX release and the rate of main chain degradation were determined using HPLC (column TSK 3 000, 50% methanol, 0.1% trifluoroacetic acid, flow rate 0.7 ml min^{-1}) after incubation of the conjugate in the cathepsin B solution. As demonstrated in FIGURE 4, -GlyPheLeuGly- spacer was degraded and approximately 50% of total DOX was released from the carrier within 48 hours of incubation. Amino acid analysis of the degradation products showed that DOX is released in two forms, free DOX (40%) and its glycyl derivative (60%). This finding differs from that obtained for the degradation of analogous poly(HPMA)-DOX conjugate incubated with cathepsin B (10% glycyl derivative) under similar conditions. Degradation of the main chain also took place but at a lower rate (20% in 48 h).

Feasibility of the synthesis of PEG-DOX conjugate having higher molecular weight of the backbone was verified using diamine reagents H-Glu(OBzl)Lys(OBzl)Glu(OBzl)-H and PEG (M_w 2 000) activated by the reaction with di(N-succinimidyl) carbonate.[15] The condensation of activated PEG with trifluoroacetate of the tripeptide was carried out in water-methylene chloride emulsion[15] and benzyl-ester protecting groups were removed from the polymer by catalytic hydrogenation on Pd/C (10%) in methanol.[6] Acetate of the -GlyPheLeuGly- derivative of DOX was prepared using the methods described for its 4-nitroaniline analogue[14] and the final conjugation of the DOX derivative with the polymer carrier was accomplished in dimethylformamide using the dicyclohexylcarbodiimide coupling method.[6] The polymer-DOX conjugate (FIG. 3) was purified chromatographically (Sephadex LH-20, methanol). Molecular weight of the conjugate, a prodrug with potential anticancer activity, was 24 000 (estimated by size-exclusion chromatography, FPLC Pharmacia, Superose 6) and the content of DOX was 9 wt-% (determined spectrophotometrically[8]). Promising results of testing of the anti-cancer activity of this conjugate (mice, colon sarcoma) lead us to further development of this PEG-drug carrier system.

DEGRADABLE HYDROGEL

Copolymers of HPMA with N,O-dimethacryloylhydroxylamine (DMHA) were developed as hydrolytically degradable hydrogels[7] and, consequently, their use as a matrix for controlled drug release was studied.[7] These hydrogels are stable under acid conditions (pH 5 and lower) and undergo hydrolytic degradation both in buffers at physiological pH (7.4) and in vivo, resulting in a water-soluble polymeric product.[7] For the structure of the hydrogel and its polymeric degradation product, see FIGURE 5. The rate of hydrolytic degradation of gels depends on their shape and size and pH of the microenvironment and can be controlled by changing the crosslinking density of the gel and hydrogel structure.[7]

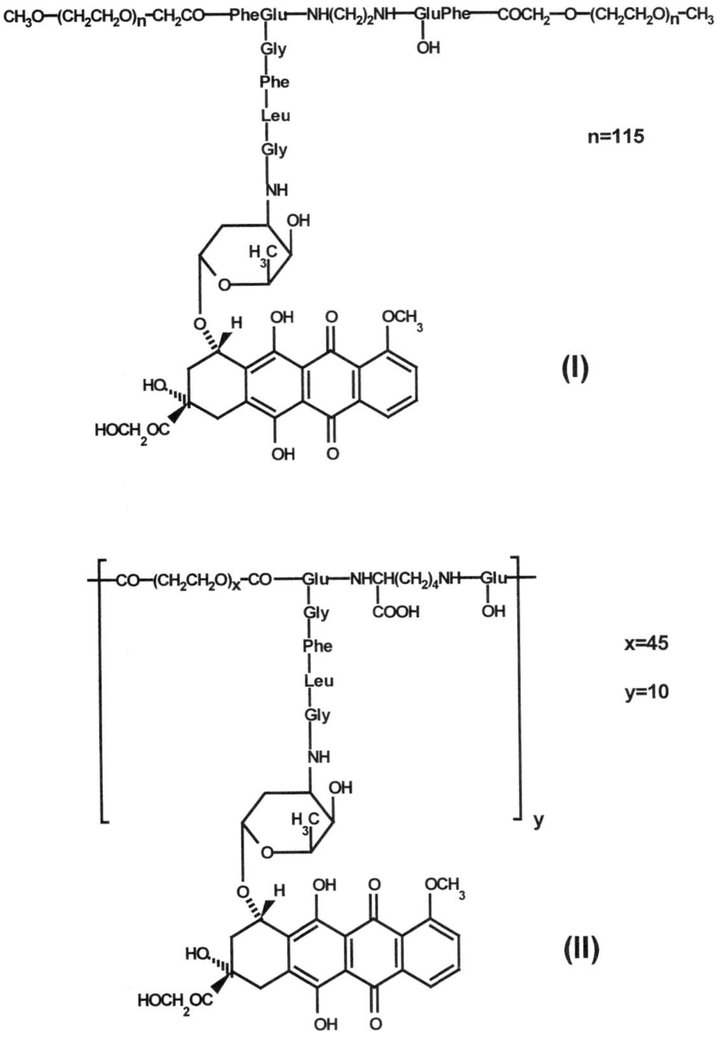

FIGURE 3. Structure of PEG block copolymers.

The hydrogels, prepared in the form of rods and discs as described,[15] were used in degradation and drug-release experiments. Discs (10×1.5 mm) prepared from the hydrogels of different crosslinking density (equilibrium degree of swelling) were dried and the dry polymer samples were soaked in aqueous ethanol solutions of the anti-cancer drug doxorubicin hydrochloride (DOX.HCl) of various concentrations. The hydrogels containing poly(HPMA)-DOX conjugate (M_w 29 200, spacer GlyPheLeuGly, DOX content 5.5 wt-%) were prepared by the radical copolymeriza-

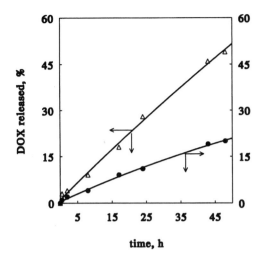

FIGURE 4. Release of doxorubicin and polymer chain degradation of PEG-DOX conjugate incubated in a cathepsin B buffer solution at 37°C (0.1 mol l^{-1} phosphate buffer containing 1 10^{-3} mol l^{-1} ethylenediaminetetraacetic acid (EDTA) and 5 10^{-3} mol l^{-1} reduced glutathion (GSH), pH 6.0).

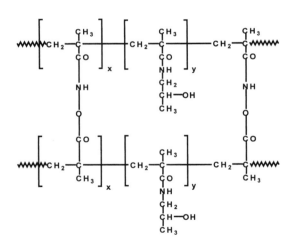

FIGURE 5. Structure of poly (HPMA) hydrogel.

Assumed structure of the product of the in vitro hydrolysis of the hydrogel

TABLE 2. Characteristics of Hydrogels Containing Doxorubicin and Doxirubicin-Polymer Conjugates

Sample	H_2O Content (wt %)	DOX Content (wt %)	Degradation Time (h)
1	95	0.00	16
2	95	0.50	16–17
3	95	1.10	17
4	95	1.80	18
5	94	1.05	17
6	91	0.80	26–28
7	87	0.90	48–52

tion of HPMA and DMHA in an ethanol solution of the conjugate.[7] The hydrolytic degradation of gel samples and drug release were studied in 0.1 mol l^{-1} phosphate buffer saline (0.15 mol l^{-1}), pH 7.4 at 37°C as described.[7] The characteristics of hydrogels are given in TABLE 2 and the results of drug-release experiments in TABLE 3. All hydrogels swell in water to a high degree (more than 85 wt-% of water) and the time required for degradation of a hydrogel to soluble products increases with the decreasing degree of swelling (increasing crosslinking density). The rate of DOX release from a hydrogel depended on the degree of swelling of that gel; the higher the amount of water in the gel swollen to equilibrium and the higher loading of the gel with DOX, the faster the drug release. The drug release is faster than hydrogel degradation and the process is predominantly diffusion-controlled. The high-molecular-weight poly(HPMA)-DOX conjugate (sample 5) was released with an approximately constant but lower rate, similar to the rate of hydrogel degradation. All hydrogels under study released most DOX within ten hours, *i.e.*, within the time used in medicine for long-term drug infusion.

The results of study of the effect of HPMA-based hydrogel samples containing DOX.HCl or poly(HPMA)-DOX on tumor growth, animal life span, leukocyte populations in peripheral blood, and bone marrow function after inoculation of the model tumor EL4 mouse T-cell lymphoma in mice are given elsewhere in this issue.

CONCLUSION

The structure and properties of three different drug release systems have been described. In the first system, the rate of release of a drug from nondegradable

TABLE 3. Release of DOX and Poly(HPMA)DOX from Hydrogels

Sample	DOX Released (%)			
	1 h	2.5 h	6 h	8 h
2	32	64	78	84
3	51	76	88	91
4	62	83	94	97
5	14	25	40	50
6	48	70	85	91
7	35	55	76	78

In 0.1 mol l^{-1} phosphate-buffered saline solution (0.15 mol l^{-1} NaCl) at pH 7.4, 37°C.

synthetic polymer carrier is controlled by a detailed structure of the oligopeptide spacer. In the second system, the degradability of the carrier chain and controlled drug release is achieved analogously by introducing oligopeptide spacers and links into the conjugate structure, tailor-made as substrates for lysosomal enzymes. Both systems have been designed for the use as lysosomotropic pro-drugs. The third hydrogel system is based on hydrophilic polymer chains linked in three-dimensional structures via linkages susceptible to hydrolytic degradation. A drug can be released from this system by the rate-controlled degradation, by diffusion, or by the combination of diffusion and hydrogel degradation. Biological evaluation of all the three systems containing anti-cancer drug doxorubicin is under way.

REFERENCES

1. CHIEN, Y. W., Ed. 1992. Novel Drug Delivery Systems. Marcel Dekker, Inc. New York, Basel, Hong Kong.
2. DUNCAN, R. & L.W. SEYMOUR. 1989. Controlled Release Technologies. A Survey of Research and Commercial Applications. Elsevier Advanced Technology. Mayfield House, 256 Branbury Road, Oxford, UK.
3. ALLÉMANN, E., R. GURNEY & E. DOELKER. 1993. Drug-loaded nanoparticles— preparation methods and drug targeting issues. Eur. J. Pharm. Biopharm. **39:** 173–191.
4. ULBRICH, K. 1991. Water soluble polymeric carriers of drugs. J. Bioact. Compat. Polym. **6:** 348–357.
5. DUNCAN, R. 1992. Drug polymer conjugates—potential for improved chemotherapy. Anti-Cancer Drugs **3:** 175–210.
6. PECHAR, M., J. STROHALM & K. ULBRICH. 1995. Synthesis of poly(ethylene glycol) block copolymers as potential water-soluble drug carriers. Collect. Czech. Chem. Commun. **60:** 1765–1780.
7. ULBRICH, K., V. ŠUBR, P. PODPĚROVÁ & M. BUREŠOVÁ. 1995. Synthesis of novel hydrolytically degradable hydrogels for controlled drug release. J. Controlled Release **34:** 55–165.
8. DUNCAN, R., L. W. SEYMOUR, K. B. O'HARE, P. FLANAGAN, S. WEDGE, I. C. HUME, K. ULBRICH, J. STROHALM, V. ŠUBR, F. SPREAFICO, M. GRANDI, M. RIPAMONTI, M. FARAO & A. SUARATO. 1992. Preclinical evaluation of polymer bound doxorubicin. J. Controlled Release **19:** 331–346.
9. SEYMOUR, L. W. 1994. Soluble polymers for lectin-mediated drug targeting. Adv. Drug Delivery Rev. **14:** 89–111.
10. O'HARE, K. B., R. DUNCAN, J. STROHALM, K. ULBRICH & P. KOPEČKOVÁ. 1993. Polymeric drug-carriers containing doxorubicin and melanocyte-stimulating hormone: *in vitro* and *in vivo* evaluation against murine melanoma. J. Drug Targeting **1:** 217–229.
11. ULBRICH, K., M. PECHAR, J. STROHALM, V. ŠUBR & B. ŘÍHOVÁ. 1997. Polymeric carriers of drugs for site-specific therapy. Macromol. Symp. **118:** 577–585.
12. ULBRICH, K., J. STROHALM, V. ŠUBR, D. PLOCOVÁ, R. DUNCAN & B. ŘÍHOVÁ. 1996. Polymeric conjugates of drugs and antibodies for site-specific drug delivery. Macromol. Symp. **103:** 177–192.
13. ŘÍHOVÁ, B., J. STROHALM, D. PLOCOVÁ & K. ULBRICH. 1990. Selectivity of antibody targeted anthracycline antibiotics on T-lymphocytes. J. Bioact. Compat. Polym. **5:** 249–266.
14. PECHAR, M., J. STROHALM, E. SCHACHT & K. ULBRICH. 1997. Biodegradable drug carriers based on poly(ethyleneglycol) block copolymers. Macromol. Chem. Phys. **198:** 1009–1020.
15. ZALIPSKY, S. 1993. Synthesis of an end-group functionalized polyethylene glycol-lipid conjugate for preparation of polymer-grafted liposomes. Bioconjugate Chem. **4:** 296–299.
16. ŘÍHOVÁ, B., J. SROGL, M. JELINKOVA, M. BURESOVA, V. SUBR & K. ULBRICH. 1997. HPMA-based biodegradable hydrogels containing different forms of doxorubicin: Antitumor effects and biocompatibility. Ann. N. Y. Acad. Sci. **8:** xx–xx. This volume.

HPMA-based Biodegradable Hydrogels Containing Different Forms of Doxorubicin

Antitumor Effects and Biocompatibility[a]

BLANKA ŘÍHOVÁ,[b,d] JAN ŠROGL,[b]
MARKÉTA JELÍNKOVÁ,[b] O. HOVORKA,[b]
MAGDA BUREŠOVÁ,[c] VLADIMÍR ŠUBR,[b]
AND KAREL ULBRICH[c]

[b]Institute of Microbiology
Academy of Sciences of the Czech Republic
Videnska 1083
142 20 Prague 4, Czech Republic

[c]Institute of Macromolecular Chemistry
Academy of Sciences of the Czech Republic
Heyrovskeho sq.2
162 06 Prague 6, Czech Republic

Synthetic polymers are used in various areas of medicine, such as the cardiovascular system, orthopedics, dentistry, ophthalmology, artifical organs and drug delivery. The use of biomaterials to deliver biologically active agents is an attractive concept because local administration of certain therapeutic agents is often the most effective method of treatment.

The development of different strategies for the controlled release of active compounds from polymeric systems is of increasing importance in the treatment of many diseases, cancer being one of them. The application of drug-loaded hydrogels can improve the therapeutic efficacy and reduce the side-effects of biologically active compounds.[1,2] The utility of matrix devices has been proposed for the oral delivery of drugs, hormones and peptides,[3-6] orally administered vaccine[7] or for the controlled release of drugs and proteins.[1,2,8,9]

Nanoparticles, which are defined as solid particles that exist in the nanometer size, have been also reported as potential delivery systems for targeting drugs to specific sites in the organism.[10] Nanoparticles may be composed of either natural polymers, e.g., gelatin, albumin or collagen[11] or synthetic compounds such as polyalkylcyanoacrylates or polyalkylmethacrylates.[10,12]

Considerable literature exists regarding novel hydrogels designed to hydrolyze or break in the presence of physiological fluids. Biodegradation of such hydrogels enables the selective release of the entrapped active drugs from the matrix. The availability of drug imbedded in such a matrix is affected by the rate at which the polymer dissolves.[2,13]

[a] This research was supported by the Grant Agency of the Academy of Sciences of the Czech Republic (grant No. 720 407) and by the Grant Agency of the Czech Republic (grant No. 307/96/K226).

[d] Author to whom correspondence should be addressed: (+4220) 475 2267; Fax (+4220) 472 11 43; E-mail: Rihova@biomed.cas.cz

Water-soluble synthetic polymers based on N-(2-hydroxypropyl)methacrylam-ide (HPMA), which are nontoxic and highly biocompatible have been proven as carrier systems with optimal characteristics for drug delivery.[14–21] HPMA-based polymeric anti-cancer or immunosuppressive prodrugs are pharmacologically active *in vitro* and *in vivo* and show considerably decreased non-specific side toxicity.[19,20] Two forms of prodrugs consisting of HPMA-bound doxorubicin have already reached phase I-II clinical trials.[21]

Based on a copolymer of N-(2-hydroxypropyl)methacrylamide (HPMA) and using N,O-dimethacryloyl hydroxylamine (DMHA) as a crosslinking agent a biode-gradable hydrogel has been developed.[22] The hydrophilic polymeric chains are crosslinked via-COONHCO-linkages, which are sensitive to hydrolytic cleavage *in vitro* at physiological pH 7.4 and also susceptible to hydrolysis *in vivo*.[23] By varying the density of crosslinkages, various rates of gel degradation and thus drug release is achieved. The hydrogel structure is a biodegradable three-dimensional mesh.[23,24] Biodegradation is complete and results in water-soluble HPMA polymers bearing 0.3–1.2 mol% of carboxyl and amino groups depending on the content of DMHA in the polymerization mixture,[24] which are similar to those used in our previous studies as soluble polymeric carriers of drugs.[14,19–21,25–27] The rate of hydrogel degrada-tion in the physiological environment depends on the crosslinking density of the gel and on the chemical structure of the main polymer chain. The degradation both *in vitro* and *in vivo* has been demonstrated previously.[23,24] The release rate of drugs from biodegradable HPMA hydrogels also depends on the kind and molecular weight of the drug, and is controlled by diffusion, gel biodegradation or a combina-tion of both processes.[23]

HPMA hydrogel matrices were loaded with different amounts of the anti-cancer drug doxorubicin or doxorubicin bound to the water-soluble HPMA copolymer carrier (HPMA-DOX). Owing to its high toxicity, DOX is a good candidate for controlled release technology in order to obtain a therapeutic effect *in situ* and to minimize its serious toxic side-effects.

We investigated the *in vivo* antitumor activity of these hydrogels differing in crosslinking density and in the DOX or HPMA-DOX content. Their antitumor activities were compared with those detected after application of soluble targeted or nontargeted drug. As an experimental tumor model, EL4 mouse T-cell lymphoma was used which is known to be rather nonsensitive to treatment with free DOX.[28] In addition to the effect on tumor growth, basic hematological parameters were monitored to draw a parallel to the data obtained in human patients undergoing chemotherapy. The results obtained *in vivo* confirmed the therapeutic efficacy of this novel system of drug release and revealed a direct correlation between the antitumor activity and parameters of the gels used, *i.e.*, degradation rate and drug content. Moreover, the biocompatibility and immunocompatibility of the tested water-soluble and cross-linked HPMA copolymers was confirmed using standard immunological techniques (CFU-s assay, [³H]-TdR incorporation, antibody produc-tion and IL-1 and IL-6 cytokine release).

MATERIAL AND METHODS

Chemicals

1-Amino-2-propanol, methacryloyl chloride (freshly distilled), azo-bis-isobuty-ronitrile (AIBN), hydroxylamine hydrochloride, 4-nitrophenol, glycyl-L-phenyl-alanine, L-leucyl-glycine and dicyclohexylcarbodiimide were from Fluka A.G.

Switzerland, solvents (all used after distillation) and other chemicals were of analytical grade quality, Lachema Brno, Czech Republic. Doxorubicin hydrochloride (DOX) was a kind gift from Farmitalia Carlo Erba, Italy.

Monomers

Synthesis of monomers was described earlier. Briefly, N-(2-hydroxypropyl)methacrylamide (HPMA) was prepared by the reaction of methacryloyl chloride with 1-amino-2-propanol in acetonitrile,[29] N,O-dimethacryloylhydroxylamine (DMHA) by the reaction of hydroxylamine hydrochloride with methacryloyl chloride in pyridine,[23] and N-methacryloylglycyl-phenylalanyl-leucyl-glycyl-4-nitrophenyl ester (MaGlyPheLeuGlyONp) was prepared by the reaction of methacryloylglycyl-phenylalanyl-leucyl-glycine with 4-nitrophenol in dimethylformamide in the presence of dicyclohexylcarbodiimide.[30]

Synthesis of Polymeric Conjugate of Doxorubicin

Polymeric conjugate of DOX (P-GlyPheLeuGly-DOX; HPMA-DOX) was prepared by aminolytic reaction of polymeric precursor-copolymer of HPMA and MaGlyPheLeuGlyONp with DOX.[30,31] In this conjugate DOX was bound to the water-soluble poly(HPMA) carrier via the tetrapeptidic spacer Gly-Phe-Leu-Gly susceptible to enzymatic cleavage. HPMA-DOX used in experiments in its free soluble form or in hydrogel loaded form contained 5.52 wt% DOX, Mw 29200 and Mw/Mn 1.33.

Hydrogels

The biodegradable hydrogels were prepared by radical copolymerization of HPMA with crosslinking agent (DMHA) in ethanol using AIBN as initiator.[23,24] The residual monomers and initiator were removed from hydrogels by extraction in ethanol. Hydrogels were prepared in the shape of discs or rods. Dry gels were loaded with the free drug by soaking in a solution of DOX in ethanol-water (3 : 1) followed by drying in the air. Hydrogels containing HPMA-DOX conjugate were prepared by copolymerization of HPMA and DMHA in ethanol carried out in the presence of P-GlyPheLeuGly-DOX conjugate. The drug content in the gel was determined spectrophotometrically (at 485 nm) after hydrogel degradation was completed. For details of the synthesis and characterization see ref.[24]

Hydrogel Degradation

Hydrolytic degradation of gel samples (discs, size 1.0×1.5 or 5×2 mm) was studied at 37°C in 0.1M phosphate buffered saline (0.15 M NaCl), pH 7.4. The hydrolysis of gels swollen to equilibrium was examined after incubation of the drug-free gel in 20 ml of a buffer and the time needed for their total degradation into soluble polymers was estimated.[24] In principle, three types of hydrogels differing in crosslinking density were used for experiments. The gel with degradation time 16–17 h contained 95 wt% water in its equilibrium swollen state, the gel with degradation time 26–27 h contained 91 wt% and the gel with degradation time 48–52 h, 87 wt% water.

Antitumor Activity

Animals

Male C57BL/10 ScSn (B10, H-2^b) 11- to 13-week old mice were obtained from the Institute of Physiology of the Academy of Sciences of the Czech Republic, Prague and kept under standard conditions with food and water *ad libitum*.

EL4 Mouse T-Cell Lymphoma

The C57BL/10 mice were inoculated subcutaneously with 10^6 cells of EL4 mouse T-cell lymphoma on day 0 on the left side of the back. The tumor growth was apparent macroscopically on day 9–10. It was then quantified by measuring its largest diameter and the one orthogonal to it.

In the studies of therapeutic efficacy, the hydrogels in forms of rods or discs were implanted subcutaneously on day 1 (the day after tumor inoculation) or 9 (just before or at the time when the tumor is macroscopically detectable) on the right side of the back of the mice (opposite to the site of tumor inoculation). The wound was then closed using a tissue adhesive (Histocryl, B. Braun, Melsungen, Germany).

In the studies comparing the therapeutic efficacy of different forms of doxorubicin the soluble forms of the drug or its polymeric derivative (P-GlyPheLeuGly-DOX) in 300 μl saline were administered intraperitoneally on days 1, 4, 7 (parallel to gel administration on day 1) or 9, 12, 15 (parallel to gel administration on day 9).

Flow Cytometry

Flow cytometry analysis was performed on a FACSorter (Becton Dickinson, Mountain View, CA) as previously described.[32] Dead cells were excluded from analysis by a combination of gates set on forward/side scatter and by cell staining with propidium iodide. Fluorescence intensity was determined on 5,000–10,000 cells from each sample using logarithmic amplification, which was converted to the linear equivalent by Becton Dickinson Lysis II software.

In Vivo *Effect on the Bone Marrow*

Reticulocyte Count

Fifty μl of blood was taken from the lateral tail vein of each mouse twice a week, between 8 and 10 a.m. to minimize the influence of circadian rhythms, using heparin as an anticoagulant. The blood of all mice from the same treatment group was then pooled and used for flow cytometry analysis.

The bone marrow function was evaluated by monitoring the percentage of reticulocytes in the whole blood, which is a standard method used in human patients undergoing chemotherapy. The samples of pooled blood were stained by thiazole orange (Retic-count, Becton-Dickinson, San Jose, CA, USA) using the standard protocol recommended by the manufacturer. Briefly, 5 μl of each sample of whole blood was pipetted into 1ml of Retic-Count solution or into 1ml of PBS with 0.1% sodium azide as a negative control. The samples were then incubated in the dark for a minimum of 30 min and 30,000 cells per sample were scanned on the flow cytometer (FACSort, Becton-Dickinson). The data analysis was performed by using the same software by comparing the unstained sample with the stained one. Thus, the relative amount of reticulocytes in peripheral blood was obtained.

Colony-Forming Unit-Spleen Technique, CFU-s Assay

The method of Till and McCulloch[33] was used modified according to Říhová *et al.*[15] Briefly, after exsanguination, the bone marrow was isolated from both femurs of treated mice and after repeated washing with tissue culture medium (RPMI 1640, Sigma), the concentration of cells was adjusted to 5×10^5 cells/ml. The donor bone marrow cell suspension was injected i.v. (0.2 ml containing 1×10^5 cells) into syngeneic recipient mice which were irradiated by ^{60}Co (8 Gy). Transplanted mice were sacrificed 8 days after transplantation, the spleens were removed and fixed in Bouin, and the number of CFU-s was enumerated. The suspension of cells for transfer was a pool from bone marrow of 3–4 immunized mice, injected in one experiment into 5–10 recipients.

Biocompatibility and Immunogenicity Evaluation

Determination of IL-1 and IL-6

Levels of IL-1 and IL-6 interleukins in the serum of mice treated with hydrogel matrix without drug were measured using commercially available ELISA kits (purchased from PharMingen, San Diego, CA, USA)

Antibody Formation

Determination of antibody formation was done according to Říhová *et al.*[34,35] and detected by ELISA.

[³H]-Thymidine Incorporation

Determination of [³H]-thymidine incorporation was done according to Říhová *et al.*[30,36]

RESULTS AND DISCUSSION

In Vivo *Antitumor Effect of Different Forms of Doxorubicin*

The effect of hydrogels containing doxorubicin or doxorubicin bound to HPMA copolymer carrier (P-GlyPheLeuGly-DOX) on the tumor growth and life span of experimental animals inoculated with EL4 mouse T-cell lymphoma was compared with the effect of the identical drugs administered in a soluble form, dissolved in

TABLE 1. Scheme of Therapeutic Regimens in Comparing the *in Vivo* Effect of Different Forms of Doxorubicin; Hydrogel Degradation Rate 16–17 Hours

Form of the Drug	Administration on Days(s)	Total Equivalent Dose of DOX (mg/kg)
Free DOX in hydrogel	1	29.2
P-GlyPheLeuGly-DOX in hydrogel	1	35.2
Free DOX (soluble)	1-4-7	13.9
P-GlyPheLeuGly-DOX (soluble)	1-4-7	13.9
Free DOX in hydrogel	9	28.0
P-GlyPheLeuGly-DOX in hydrogel	9	33.8
Free DOX (soluble)	9-12-15	14.4
P-GlyPheLeuGly-DOX (soluble)	9-12-15	13.9

saline. The hydrogels with degradation rate of 16–17 hours were tested according to the scheme given in TABLE 1. The soluble forms of the drugs were administered in three consecutive doses in order to decrease their toxicity. Therapy administered on day 9 after the tumor implantation tested the therapeutic effect of different forms of the drug in the stage when the tumor has already begun expansive growth and is about to be apparent macroscopically. The effect of the hydrogels and soluble forms of doxorubicin on the tumor growth is shown in FIGURES 1 and 2. Both hydrogels (hydrogel with free doxorubicin or with doxorubicin bound to HPMA) showed better antitumor activity than soluble drug administered on day 1 (FIG. 1). The dose of soluble doxorubicin, which was according to the previous experiments (results not shown), approximately the maximal therapeutic dose, showed moderate

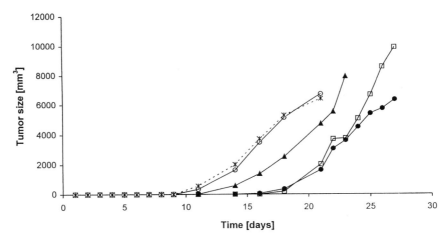

FIGURE 1. *In vivo* effect of different forms of doxorubicin administered on day 1 after inoculation of experimental mice with EL4 mouse T-cell lymphoma. Degradation rate of hydrogels = 16–17 hours. □———□ free DOX in hydrogel; ●———● P-GlyPheLeuGly-DOX in hydrogel; ▲———▲ soluble DOX; ○———○ soluble P-GlyPheLeuGly-DOX; ✻———✻ control (animals with implanted hydrogel matrix without drug).

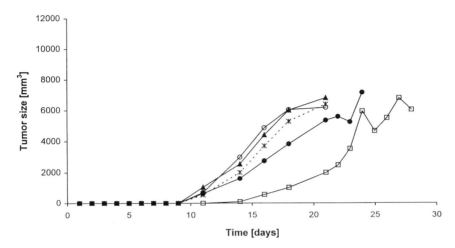

FIGURE 2. *In vivo* effect of different forms of doxorubicin administered on day 9 after inoculation of experimental mice with EL4 mouse T-cell lymphoma. Degradation rate of hydrogels = 16–17 hours. □———□ free DOX in hydrogel; ●———● P-GlyPheLeuGly-DOX in hydrogel; ✱———✱ soluble DOX; ○———○ soluble P-GlyPheLeuGly-DOX; ▲———▲ control (animals with implanted hydrogel matrix without drug)

activity on the tumor growth. However, it was also toxic and led to earlier death of the experimental animals. In mice given the drugs on day 9 (FIG. 2), neither soluble forms (free doxorubicin or doxorubicin bound to HPMA carrier) had any effect on the growth of the experimental tumor. This is probably due to the need of a higher bolus dose of the cytotoxic agent when the solid tumor has been already established. However, the gel containing free doxorubicin showed significant antitumor activity even when implanted on day 9 (FIG. 2). This might suggest a better *in vivo* effect of doxorubicin being released continuously from the hydrogel matrix. Increased antitumor activity of liposomal daunorubicin compared with free drug was reported also by Forssen *et al.*[37] However, they reported that at earlier treatment times free daunorubicin is more toxic than liposome encapsulated drug. At 24 h, free daunorubicin has more than three times the activity of liposomal daunorubicin. Liposomal drug becomes increasingly more cytotoxic than the free drug over time. Thus, by 48 h liposomal daunorubicin is nearly seven times more potent than the free drug. The authors suggest that the increased efficacy is due to increased tumor concentration of daunorubicin and depends also on the rate of drug release from liposomes.

Doses of doxorubicin administered in a form of HPMA hydrogel were almost threefold higher than the maximal tolerated therapeutic doses of the soluble forms without any signs of unwanted toxic side-effects. This is most probably due to a gradual continuous release of the drugs and thus their lower myelosuppressive effect.

Influence of the Degradation Rate of Hydrogels on their Antitumor Efficacy

Hydrogels with identical total content 14 mg/kg of free doxorubicin but different degradation rates (16–17 h; 26–28 h; 48–52 h) were implanted in C57BL/10 mice

TABLE 2. Characteristics of Hydrogels with Different Degradation Rates

Hydrogel No.	Content of DOX.HCl (wt%)	Degradation Rate (hr)	Total Dose of DOX Administered (mg/kg)
1.	1.1	16–17	14
2.	0.8	26–28	14
3.	0.9	48–52	14

with experimental EL4 T-cell lymphoma (TABLE 2). Two control groups were used. Animals of the first one were implanted with EL4 T-cell lymphoma and simultaneously implanted with the hydrogel matrix without active drug. In animals of the second control group no surgery involved in hydrogel implantation was performed and the mice were only inoculated with the EL4 T-cell lymphoma cells. There was a noticeable negative effect of the trauma caused by surgery involved in the hydrogel implantation on the tumor growth and animal life span. Despite this fact the therapeutic effect of the hydrogels is significant. It was shown that the *in vivo* antitumor effect of the hydrogel is directly related to the degradation rate. The shorter the gel degradation rate the better is the antitumor effect. Thus, the best antitumor efficacy was the hydrogel with degradation rate 16–17 h (FIG. 3). It was reported that anthracycline drugs are released from their HPMA hydrogel matrix with a rate comparable to that of matrix degradation.[23] The slow rate of DOX release compared with 5-FU or MTX can probably be attributed to interactions between hydrophobic DOX and the polymer network[8,38] and poor solubility of the drug at pH 7.4.[23]

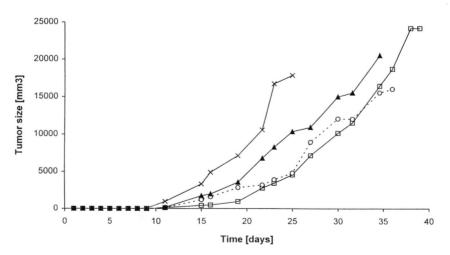

FIGURE 3. Influence of degradation rate of the hydrogels on their *in vivo* antitumor activity. □——□ degradation rate 16–17 h; o——o degradation rate 26–28 h; ▲——▲ degradation rate 48–52 h; ✕——✕ control (animals with implanted hydrogel matrix without drug).

TABLE 3. Characteristics of Hydrogels with Different Doxorubicin Loads

Hydrogel No.	Content of DOX.HCl (wt%)	Degradation Rate (hr)	Total Dose of DOX Administered (mg/kg)
1.	1.1	16–17	14
4.	0.5	16–17	10
5.	1.8	16–17	35
6.	0.0	16–17	0

Influence of Doxorubicin Load on the Antitumor Efficacy of HPMA-based Hydrogels

Hydrogels with identical degradation rates (16–17 h) differing in the total load of free doxorubicin (10 mg/kg; 14 mg/kg; 35 mg/kg) were tested (TABLE 3). The antitumor effect of the gels was directly related to the doxorubicin content in the hydrogels. The gel with the highest doxorubicin content (1.8 wt%) proved to have the best therapeutic effect (FIG. 4). These results show that higher loading of the hydrogels with the drug does not affect their ability to effectively release the drug *in vivo*.

In Vivo *Effect of HPMA-based Hydrogels on Bone-Marrow Function*

Bone Marrow Stem Cells Detected in Vivo *as Colony-Forming Unit-Spleen (CFU-s)*

The toxicity of free doxorubicin, polymer-bound doxorubicin and the hydrogel form of both drugs was compared using a CFU-s assay. Bone marrow cells were

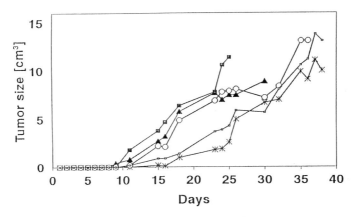

FIGURE 4. Influence of doxorubicin load on antitumor activity of hydrogels. Hydrogels with identical degradation rate (16–17 hours) differing in doxorubicin content. o———o 10 mg/kg; ᴑ———ᴑ 14 mg/kg; ✕———✕ 35 mg/kg; □———□ control (animals without gel); ▲———▲ control (animals with implanted gel matrix without drug).

TABLE 4. Spleen Colony-Forming Units (CFU-s) Detected in Irradiated Recipients after Injection of Bone Marrow Harvested from Mice Implanted with Drug Containing HPMA Hydrogels or with Injected Soluble Drugs

Sample (structure)	Total Dose of DOX (mg)	Number of CFU-s per spleen (mean ± SE)
DOX (soluble)	0.30	6 ± 2
P-GlyPheLeuGly-DOX (soluble)	0.29	29 ± 4
DOX (in hydrogel)	0.34	21 ± 5
P-GlyPheLeuGly-DOX (in hydrogel)	0.38	31 ± 3
Control (hydrogel matrix)	0.0	27 ± 3

isolated from both femurs of treated mice 24 h after the last application of the free drugs and 41 h after the application of drugs in the form of hydrogel with the degradation rate of 16–17 h (17 h + 24 h). The results (TABLE 4) show that free doxorubicin eliminates a part of the subpopulation of bone marrow stem cells, leading to a considerable decrease in the number of CFU-s. Free drug incorporated in hydrogel is substantially less myelosuppressive causing only a limited decrease of the CFU-s number. Both forms of polymer-bound drug, *i.e.*, soluble or incorporated into hydrogel is nontoxic to bone marrow stem cells.

Reticulocyte Count

The normal values of reticulocyte count in the mouse strain used for the experiment (C57BL/10) are higher than those in humans and they vary between 5–7%. This method allows continuous monitoring of the toxic effects because it does not require sacrifice of experimental animals as is the case with the CFU-s assay. The results obtained strongly correlate with the values obtained by using the technique of colony-forming units.

The effect of the hydrogels containing doxorubicin was compared to three different controls. Mice with tumor without gel implantation, mice with tumor implanted with hydrogel without drug, and normal mice without tumor and with no gel implantation. Since 50 μl of blood was taken twice a week, which was the minimum amount of blood necessary for all the flow cytofluorometric measurements, we used the last control group to estimate the influence of the chronic blood loss on the reticulocyte count.

Results of the reticulocyte count measurement are shown on FIGURE. 5. Chronic blood loss led to a maximum increase of 5% whereas the toxic effect of the doxorubicin released from the hydrogels and a subsequent "overshoot" was much higher. The development of reticulocyte count values monitored over a period of 30 days correlated with the doxorubicin content in the implanted hydrogels. The bone marrow recovery in a group administered 55 mg/kg is much slower (27 days to return to normal values) and the bone marrow suppression stronger than in animals given half of the dose (20 days to return to normal values).

The hydrogel matrix alone does not show any bone marrow toxicity. On the contrary it may have caused moderate bone marrow stimulation between days 12 and 20 similarly as was observed in the CFU-s assay.[15]

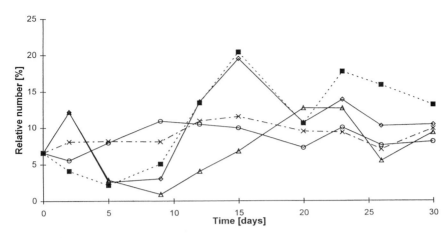

FIGURE 5. Effect of hydrogels on bone marrow function evaluated by the reticulocyte count. Hydrogels with identical degradation rate (40–44 h) differing in doxorubicin content. ◇——◇ 27 mg/kg; ■----■ 35 mg/kg; △——△ 55 mg/kg; ×·---·× control (animals with implanted hydrogel matrix without drug); ○——○ control (animals with no tumor).

Biocompatibility and Immunogenicity of HPMA-based Copolymers

Biocompatibility of HPMA Hydrogels

No release of IL-1 or IL-6 cytokines into peripheral blood and no antibody formation was observed after implantation of the hydrogel matrix without drug. Antibody formation was detected in the peripheral blood by ELISA using a soluble HPMA carrier[23,24] as an antigen. Using [³H]-thymidine incorporation no mitogenic activity was observed *in vitro* after a 3-day incubation of mouse splenocytes or human peripheral blood leukocytes with the HPMA gel matrix in cell culture. From the results obtained so far it can be concluded that HPMA hydrogels showed satisfactory biocompatibility and nonimmunogenicity. However, the real concentration of degradation products *in vivo* is not fully known. Biocompatibility could be influenced by the amount of implanted polymer and the local ability of tissues to clear degradation products.[39]

Immunogenicity of Soluble HPMA Copolymers

The biocompatibility and immunocompatibility of HPMA copolymers developed as carriers and/or matrices for anti-cancer drugs is of fundamental importance to their possible therapeutic uses. It has been demonstrated that after a massive and chronic treatment soluble HPMA copolymers do not disturb the phagocytic activity of peripheral blood leukocytes, do not damage the bone marrow stem cells tested as CFU-s, do not activate alternative or classical pathways of complement, and do not influence the antibody-forming capacity of the recipient of HPMA copolymers to thymus-dependent and thymus-independent antigens.[40]

There is no measurable antibody response to an HPMA homopolymer, *i.e.*, polymer without the oligopeptide side chains. The modification of the homopolymer with oligopeptidic side chains (or side chains terminating in haptens as a model of drugs) results in a very weak thymus-independent, IgM-restricted antibody response which is influenced by many factors including the copolymer molar mass, dose and composition of oligopeptidic side chains, nature of modifying haptens and of the genetic background of the immunized animals. HPMA copolymer carriers are not mitogens and do not activate the classical or alternative complement activation pathway.[34,35,41,42]

HPMA copolymers not only fail to induce a significant immune response against themselves, they have also the capacity to reduce the antibody response against proteins bound to them as a targeting moiety. We have compared the immunogenicity of rabbit IgG, rabbit polyclonal anti-thymocyte serum, bovine gamma globulin and human transferrin bound to HPMA carrier with the immunogenicity of original free antigens. It was found that HPMA carrier decreases immunogenicity of bound proteins more than 200 times.[26,30,41,43]

The mechanisms of reduction of protein immunogenicity after binding to HPMA carrier is not fully understood. HPMA copolymer might simply mask the antigenic determinants of the targeting protein by sterically hindering the accesibility, a mechanism ascribed to PEG reduction of protein immunogenicity following conjugation.[44] Alternatively, the immune system may be specifically suppressed by specific activation of T_S as was described by Sehon et al.[45] for protein-PEG conjugates.

STATISTICAL ANALYSIS

Data were evaluated statistically using the non-parametric Wilcoxon-Mann-Whitney test for unpaired samples. The confidence limit was predetermined at an α value of 0.05. The mean and the standard deviations of at least eight replicates were calculated for each data point.

CONCLUSION

From the above results the following conclusions can be drawn: a) novel HPMA-based biodegradable hydrogels for controlled delivery of anti-cancer drugs proved their *in vivo* antitumor efficacy; b) they showed better *in vivo* antitumor activity than the soluble forms of the drug; c) their *in vivo* antitumor activity is dependent on their degradation rate (hydrogels with shorter degradation rates show better antitumor activity); d) antitumor activity of the hydrogels also directly correlates with the doxorubicin content: the higher the doxorubicin content, the better the activity; e) use of doxorubicin in the form of HPMA-based hydrogels allows a several-fold increase of the administered dose; and f) the hydrogel matrix itself has no toxic effects on the bone marrow.

We conclude that the use of HPMA-based hydrogels containing anti-cancer drugs represents a promising strategy of local chemotherapy in improving cancer treatment and should be a subject of further research.

ACKNOWLEDGMENTS

Authors would like to thank Ms. Hana Semoradova and Dr. David Putnam, for their excellent technical assistance and also for helpful discussions.

SUMMARY

Novel hydrogels based on N-(2-hydroxypropyl)methacrylamide (HPMA) and N,O-dimethacryloylhydroxylamine containing either doxorubicin (DOX) or water-soluble HPMA carrier-bound doxorubicin (P-GlyPheLeuGly-DOX; HPMA-DOX) were synthesized. The cross-linkages are susceptible to hydrolytic cleavage at physiological pH 7.4. Hydrogels in the form of rods or discs loaded with DOX or P-GlyLeuGly-DOX were implanted subcutaneously on the back of C57BL/10 mice on day 1 or on day 9 after inoculation with EL4 mouse T-cell lymphoma. The implanted hydrogels varied in the total load of DOX and rate of hydrolysis, which is dependent on the crosslinking density of the gels. The effect of HPMA based hydrogels containing DOX or HPMA carrier-bound DOX on tumor growth, animal life span, leukocyte populations in peripheral blood and bone marrow function evaluated by reticulocyte count was investigated.

It was shown that: a) DOX and HPMA carrier-bound DOX administered in the form of HPMA-based hydrogels has better antitumor activity against experimental EL4 mouse T-cell lymphoma than soluble forms of the drug, b) hydrogels with shorter degradation rate (16–17 h) show better antitumor activity than hydrogels with longer duration time (48–52 h), c) the therapeutic effect of hydrogels with rate 16–17 h is directly related to the doxorubicin content; the higher the doxorubicin content, the better antitumor activity, d) the gel containing free doxorubicin showed significant antitumor activity even when implanted on day 9, *i.e.*, in the time when tumor growth is already established, e) the hydrogel matrix without drug does not induce release of IL-1 or IL-6 into peripheral blood, does not induce formation of antibodies, and it is not mitogenic.

Use of doxorubicin in the form of HPMA-based hydrogels allows a several-fold increase in the administered dose compared to soluble forms without detectable serious toxic side-effects.

REFERENCES

1. PEPPAS, N. A., Ed. 1987. Hydrogels in Medicine and Pharmacy, vols. 1–3. CRC Press. Boca Raton, FL.
2. LEE, P. I. 1988. Synthetic hydrogels for drug delivery: Preparation, characterization, and release kinetics. *In* Controlled Release Systems: Fabrication Technology, vol. 2. D. Hsieh, Ed. CRC Press. Boca Raton, FL.
3. BRØNDSTED, H. & J. KOPEČEK. 1991. Hydrogels for site-specific drug delivery to colon: In vitro and in vivo degradation. Pharm. Res. **9:** 584–592.
4. PARK, K. 1988. Enzyme-digestible swelling hydrogels as platforms for long term oral drug delivery: Synthesis and characterization. Biomaterials **9:** 435–441.
5. SHALABY, W. S. W., W. E. BLEVINS & K. PARK. 1991. Gastric retention of enzyme-digestible hydrogels in the canine stomach under fasted and fed conditions. ACS Symp. Ser. Polym. Drugs and Drug Deliv. Syst. **469:** 237–248.
6. SAFFRAN, M., G. S. JUMAR & C. SAVARIAR. 1986. A new approach to the oral administration of insulin and other peptide drugs. Science **233:** 1081–1084.
7. BOWERSOCK, T. L., W. S. W. SHALABY, M. Levy, M. L. SAMUELS, R. LALLONE, M. R. WHITE, D. L. BORIE, J. LEHMEYER & K. PARK. 1994. Evaluation of an orally administered vaccine, using hydrogels containing bacterial exotoxins of *Pasteurella haemolytica*, in cattle. Am. J. Vet. Res. **55:** 502–509.
8. ANTONSEN, K. P., J. L. BOHNERT, Y. NABESHIMA, M-S. SHEU, X-S. WU & A. S. HOFFMAN. 1993. Controlled release of proteins from 2-hydroxyethyl methacrylate copolymer gels. Biomat. Art. Cells & Immob. Biotech. **21:** 1–22.

9. KIM, S. W., Y. H. BAE & T. OKANO. 1992. Hydrogels: Swelling, drug loading, and release.
    Pharm. Res. **9:** 283–290.
10. FRESTA, M., G. CAVALLARO, G. GIAMMONA, E. WEHRLI & G. PUGLISI. 1996. Preparation
    and characterization of polyethyl-2-cyanoacrylate nanocapsules containing antiepilep-
    tic drugs. Biomaterials **17:** 751–758.
11. MARTHY, J. J., R. C. OPPENHEIM & P. SPEISER. 1978. Nanoparticles-a new colloidal drug
    delivery system. Pharm. Acta Helv. **53:** 17–23.
12. BONDI, H. V. & D. G. POPE. 1987. Drug delivery systems. *In* Drug Discovery and
    Development. M. Williams & J. B. Malick, Eds.: 291–315. The Humana Press, Inc.
    Clifton, NJ, 1987.
13. HELLER, J. 1984. Bioerodible systems. *In* Medical Applications of Controlled Release,
    vol. 1. R. S. Langer & D. L. Wise, Eds. CRC Press. Boca Raton, FL.
14. KOPEČEK, J. 1984. Synthesis of tailor-made soluble polymeric drug carriers. In Recent
    Advances in Drug Delivery Systems. J. M. Anderson & S. W. Kim, Eds.: 41–62.
    Plenum Press. New York.
15. ŘÍHOVÁ, B., P. KOPEČKOVA, J. STROHALM, P. ROSSMANN, V. VĚTVIČKA & J. KOPEČEK.
    1988. Antibody directed affinity therapy applied to the immune system: In vivo effec-
    tiveness and limited toxicity of daunomycin conjugates to HPMA copolymers and
    targeting antibody. Clin. Immunol. Immunopathol. **46:** 100–114.
16. KOPEČEK, J. 1990. The potential of water-soluble polymeric carriers in targeted and site-
    specific drug delivery. J. Cont. Rel. **11:** 279–290.
17. ULBRICH, K. 1991. Water soluble polymeric carriers of drugs. J. Bioact. Compat. Polym.
    6: 348–357.
18. SEYMOUR, L. W., K. ULBRICH, S. R. WEDGE, I. C. HUME, L. A. MCCORMICK, J. STRO-
    HALM & R. DUNCAN. 1991. N-(2-hydroxypropyl)methacrylamide copolymers targeted
    to the hepatocyte galactose-receptor: Pharmacokinetics in DBA$_2$ mice. Br. J. Cancer
    63: 859–866.
19. DUNCAN, R. 1992. Drug-polymer conjugates: potential for improved chemotherapy. Anti-
    cancer Drugs **3:** 175–210.
20. ŘÍHOVÁ, B. 1995. Antibody-targeted polymer-bound drugs. Folia Microbiol. **40:** 367–384.
21. DUNCAN, R., L. W. SEYMOUR, K. B. O'HARE, P. A. FLANAGAN, S. WEDGE, I. C. HUME,
    K. ULBRICH, J. STROHALM, V. ŠUBR, F. SPREAFICO, M. GRANDI, M. RIPAMONTI, M.
    FARAO & A. SURATO. 1992. Preclinical evaluation of polymer-bound doxorubicin. J.
    Cont. Rel. **12:** 331–346.
22. ŠUBR, V. & K. ULBRICH. Hydrolytically degradable hydrophilic gels and the method for
    preparation thereof, Eur. Pat. O 434 438 A2. U.S. Pat. 5, 124, 421.
23. ULBRICH, K., V. ŠUBR, L. W. SEYMOUR & R. DUNCAN. 1993. Novel biodegradable
    hydrogels prepared using the divinylic crosslinking agent N,O-dimethacryloylhydrox-
    ylamine. 1. Synthesis and characterisation of rates of gel degradation, and rate of
    release of model drugs, in vitro and in vivo. J. Cont. Rel. **24:** 181–190.
24. ULBRICH, K., V. ŠUBR, P. PODPĚROVÁ & M. BUREŠOVA. 1995. Synthesis of novel hydrolyti-
    cally degradable hydrogels for controlled drug release. J. Cont. Rel. **34:** 155–165.
25. KOPEČEK, J. 1984. Controlled biodegradability of polymers-a key to drug delivery systems.
    Biomaterials **5:** 19–25.
26. ŘÍHOVÁ, B. & J. KOPEČEK. 1985. Biological properties of targetable poly-[N-(2-
    hydroxypropyl)methacrylamide]-antibody conjugates. J. Cont. Rel. **2:** 289–310.
27. KOPEČEK, J. & R. DUNCAN. 1987. Poly-[N-(2-hydroxypropyl)methacrylamide] macromol-
    ecules as drug carrier systems. *In* Polymers in Controlled Drug Delivery, L. Illum &
    S. S. Davis, Eds. John Wright. Bristol, UK.
28. TARNOWSKI, G. S., P. RALPH & C. CH. STOCK. 1979. Sensitivity to chemotherapeutic and
    immunomodulating agents of two mouse lymphomas and of a macrophage tumor.
    Cancer Res. **39:** 3964–3967.
29. J. STROHALM & J. KOPEČEK. 1978. Poly-N-(2-hydroxypropyl)methacrylamide. I. Radical
    polymerization. Agnew. Makromol. Chem. **70:** 109–118.
30. ŘÍHOVÁ, B., M. BILEJ, V. VĚTVIČKA, K. ULBRICH, J. STROHALM, J. KOPEČEK & R.
    DUNCAN. 1989. Biocompatibility of N-(2-hydroxypropyl)methacrylamide copolymers
    containing adriamycin. Biomaterials **10:** 335–342.

31. ŘÍHOVÁ, B., J. STROHALM, D. PLOCOVÁ & K. ULBRICH. 1990. Selectivity of antibody-targeted anthracycline antibiotics on T lymphocytes. J. Bioact. Compat. Polym. **5:** 249–266.
32. ŘÍHOVÁ, B., J. STROHALM, D. PLOCOVÁ, V. ŠUBR, J. ŠROGL, M. JELÍNKOVÁ, M. ŠÍROVÁ & K. ULBRICH. 1996. Cytotoxic and cytostatic effects of anti-Thy 1.2 targeted doxorubicin and cyclosporin A. J. Cont. Rel. **40:** 303–319.
33. TILL, J. E. & E. A. MCCULLOCH. 1961. A direct measurement of the radiation sensitivity of normal mouse bone marrow cells. Radiat. Res. **14:** 213–222.
34. ŘÍHOVÁ, B., K. ULBRICH, J. KOPEČEK & P. MANČAL. 1983. Immunogenicity of N-(2-hydroxypropyl) methacrylamide copolymers-potential hapten or drug carriers. Folia Microbiol. **28:** 217–227.
35. ŘÍHOVÁ, B., J. KOPEČEK, K. ULBRICH, M. POSPÍŠIL & P. MANČAL. 1984. Effect of the chemical structure of N-(2-hydroxypropyl)methacrylamide copolymers on their ability to induce antibody formation in inbred strains of mice. Biomaterials **5:** 143–148.
36. ŘÍHOVÁ, B., A. JEGOROV, J. STROHALM, V. MATHA, P. ROSSMAN, L. FORNŮSEK & K. ULBRICH. 1992. Antibody-targeted cyclosporin A. J. Cont. Rel. **19:** 25–39.
37. FORSSEN, E. A., R. MALE-BRUNE, J. P. ADLER-MOORE, M. J. A. LEE, P. G. SCHMDT, T. B. KRASIEVA, S. SHIMIZU & B. J. TROMBERG. 1996. Fluorescence imaging studies for the disposition of daunorubicin liposomes (DaunoXome) within tumor tissue. Cancer Res. **56:** 2066–2075.
38. GAYET, J. CH. & G. FORTIER. 1995. Drug release from new bioartificial hydrogel. Art. Cells. Blood Subs. and Immob. Biotech. **23:** 605–611.
39. IGNATIUS, A. A. & L. E. CLAES. 1996. In vitro biocompatibility of bioerobatle polymers: poly(L,D,L-lactide) and poly(L-lactide-co-glycolide). Biomaterials **17:** 831–839.
40. VOLFOVÁ, I., B. ŘÍHOVÁ, V. VĚTVIČKA, P. ROSSMAN, & K. ULBRICH. 1992. Biocompatibility of biopolymers. J. Bioact. Compat. Polymers **7:** 175–190.
41. ŘÍHOVÁ, B. & I. ŘÍHA. 1984. Immunological problems of polymer-bound drugs. CRC Crit. Rev. Therap. Drug Carrier System **1:** 311–374.
42. ŠIMEČKOVÁ, J., B. ŘÍHOVÁ, D. PLOCOVÁ & J. KOPEČEK. 1986. Activity of complement in the presence of N-(2-hydroxypropyl)methacrylamide copolymers. J. Bioact. Compat. Polymers **1:** 20–31.
43. FLANAGAN, P. A., R. DUNCAN, B. ŘÍHOVÁ, V. ŠUBR & J. KOPEČEK. 1990. Immunogenicity of protein-N-(2-hydroxypropyl)methacrylamide copolymer conjugates in A/J and B10 mice. J. Bioact. Compat. Polymers **5:** 151–166.
44. ABUCHOWSKI, A. & F. F. DAVIS. 1979. Preparation and properties of polyethylene glycol-trypsin adducts, Biochim. Biophys. Acta **578:** 41–46.
45. SEHON, A. H. 1978. Conversion of Xenogeneic Monoclonal Antibodies to Specific Tolerogens, from Advances in the Applications of Monoclonal Antibodies to Clinical Oncology. Royal Post Graduate Medical School. University of London.

Synthetic Strategies for the Preparation of Precursor Polymers and of Microcapsules Suitable for Cellular Entrapment by Polyelectrolyte Complexation of Those Polymers[a]

TANIA A. DYAKONOV,[b] LEI ZHOU,[b] ZENG WAN,[b.]
BIN HUANG,[b] ZHIZHONG MENG,[b] XIAOYAN GUO,[b]
HOLLY ALEXANDER,[c] WAYNE V. MOORE,[d] AND
WILLIAM T. K. STEVENSON[b,e]

[b]Department of Chemistry
Wichita State University
Wichita, Kansas, 67260-0051

[c]Department of Pathology
HCA Wesley Medical Center
Wichita, Kansas, 67214

[d]Department of Pediatrics
University of Kansas Medical Center
Kansas City, Kansas, 66160-7148

Recent advances in medical science has allowed for a better appreciation and, therefore, management of metabolic disorders associated with the endocrine system. Until the genetic and infectious underpinnings of these ailments can be unraveled and proper "cures" or interventions be designed, the best potential stopgaps continue to reside in the realm of transplantation therapy. The strategy behind immunoisolation as a prelude to transplantation will be discussed elsewhere, as will alternative means to that end.

The phenomenon of polyelectrolyte (PE) complexation may be traced to the pioneering work of Fuoss,[1] since "rediscovered" by Michaels.[2] Polyelectrolyte complexes have been the subject of a number of investigations aimed at the discovery and characterization of new bio-materials.[3,4] Essentially, it was found that oppositely charged PE polymers with appropriate structure, after dissolution in aqueous solution, will form a complex (polyelectrolyte complex/complex coacervate, *etc.*) on mixing of the two solutions. The process is very nearly athermal and is driven by the entropy gain associated with the release of small, previously bound, counterions

[a] The authors wish to acknowledge the financial assistance of NIH (Award # R15 DK 46551), of NSF (Awards # OSR-9255223 and OSR-9550487), and of the Great Plains Diabetes Research Foundation, without which this work would not have been possible.

[e] Author to whom correspondence should be addressed at the Department of Chemistry and NIAR, Wichita State University, Wichita, KS, 67260–0051, USA. Tel: (316) 978 3120; Fax: (316) 978 3431; E-mail stevenso@wsuhub.uc.twsu.edu

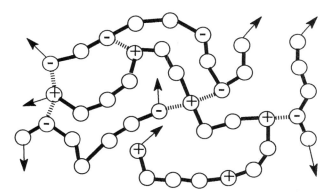

FIGURE 1. A stylized representation of a polyelectrolyte complex between random copolymers of opposite charge. Note that the polymers do not dimerize but form a three dimensional network. Coulombic attractions ("salt bridges") are visualized via hatched lines between the chains.

into the bulk of the solution.[5] The complexation event is illustrated in FIGURE 1. The microencapsulation event consists of adding droplets of dissolved PE polymer to a receiving bath containing another dissolved PE polymer with opposite charge, as illustrated in FIGURE 2.

We have chosen to prepare microcapsules through the polyelectrolyte complexation of methacrylate based polymers as a consequence of their proven bio-compatibility, compositional flexibility, and ease of synthesis. Polymers were prepared under nitrogen in organic solution with azobisisobutyronitrile (AIBN) free radical initiator, or in mixed organic/aqueous solution with azobis 4-cyanopentanoic acid (ACPA) free radical initiator. Almost without exception, co- and ter-polymers were random in composition with only small compositional drifts. Polymer molecular weights were varied by changing monomer and initiator levels in the reactor. Polymers were characterized by application of proton [^{1}H] and by carbon-13 [^{13}C] N.M.R spectroscopy, by conductometric titration, by dilute solution viscometry, and by Infrared (IR) spectroscopy. Polymers were purified by repeated precipitation from solution, by dialysis, and (for the cell culture studies) by sterile filtration. A listing of relevant monomer residues, acronyms, and structures is made in FIGURES 3a and 3b.

DISCUSSION

Microcapsules by Polyelectrolyte Complexation of Weak Polyelectrolyte Polymers Containing a High Charge Density

Our earliest attempts at designing microcapsulation systems around the concept of polyelectrolyte complexation led to the preparation of weakly acidic polymers containing MAA[6] and weakly basic polymers containing DMAEMA,[7] both containing a high mole% of charged functionality. The acidic polymers were prepared at higher molecular weights to ease capsule penetration into the receiving bath. (This preliminary concept was later shown to be misguided, in that best capsules

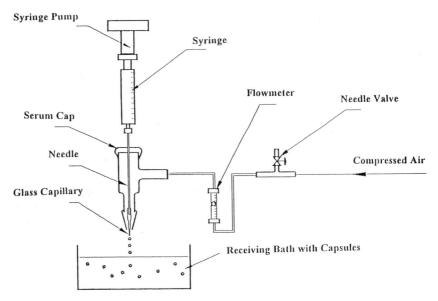

FIGURE 2. A drawing of the capsule forming assembly. Droplets containing dissolved anionic polyelectrolyte polymer are blown from the needle tip by a stream of compressed air and enter the receiving bath which contains dissolved cationic polymer. Capsules are formed by polyelectrolyte complexation at the solution interface.

are almost always created using the highest molecular weight analogues of both polymers which remain soluble in aqueous solution). We prepared polymers with similar composition but with differing molecular weight, others with differing charge content but with a similar molecular weight; and yet others with a similar charge content and molecular weight but with a differing hydrophobic/hydrophilic balance in the remainder of the chain (TABLE 1). These polymers were tested exhaustively as capsule formers in distilled water, PBS, and in cell culture medium, with/without added serum. Best capsules were formed through complexation of polymers 1-3 and 1-12.[8,9] An anchorage independent cell line was successfully encapsulated in capsules made through reaction of these polymers. The cells divided to completely fill the intra capsular space and could be subcultured to confluence after removal from the capsules,[10-12] *thus validating the concept of capsule formation through polyelectrolyte complexation of synthetic methacrylate based weak polyelectrolyte polymers.* Although suitable for cell culture, the capsules so formed were soft and sticky and would be (in our estimation) unable to withstand the rigors of implantation in a mammalian host.

Microcapsules by Polyelectrolyte Complexation of a Weakly Acidic Polyelectrolyte and a Strongly Basic Polyelectrolyte, Both Containing a Low Charge Density

The previous system needed to be improved on a number of fronts. We were concerned about the high osmotic activity of residual dissolved polymer within the

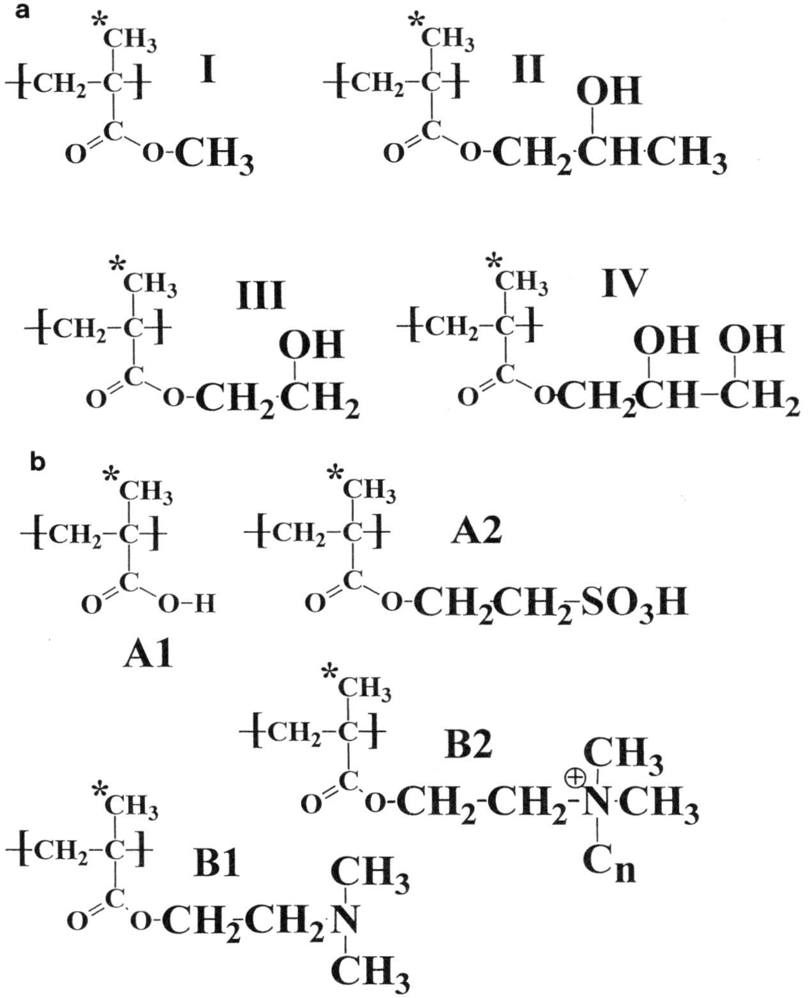

FIGURE 3. a: Uncharged methacrylate residues listed in ascending order of polarity. (The corresponding acrylate residue may be had by replacing *CH$_3$ in the figure by a hydrogen atom.) (I). Methyl methacrylate (MMA), (II) Hydroxypropyl methacrylate (HPMA, one isomer shown), (III) 2-Hydroxyethyl methacrylate (HEMA), (IV) Glyceryl methacrylate (GMA). **b:** Charged methacrylate residues, (A): acidic, (B): basic. (The corresponding acrylate residue may be had by replacing *CH$_3$ in the figure by a hydrogen atom.) (A1): Weakly acidic methacrylic acid (MAA,) shown in protonated form. (A2): The strong acid 2-sulfonyl ethyl methacrylate (SEMA), shown in protonated form. (B1): The weak base, dimethylamino ethyl methacrylate (DMAEMA), shown in deprotonated form. (B2): Quaternized DMAEMA (DMAEMA-Qn). The "n" refers to the length of the linear alkyl iodide residue coupled to the monomer residue. For example, reaction with ethyl iodide would yield a quaternary ammonium ion with n = 2.

TABLE 1. Candidate Polymers for Capsule Formation through Polyelectrolyte Complexation of Weakly Acidic and Basic Functionality, Both Possessing a High Charge Density[a]

Polymer Number	Mole % HEMA[b,c]	Mole % MMA[b,c]	Mole % MAA[b,d]	Mole % DMAEMA[b,c]	Intrinsic Viscosity[e]	% S[f]	Comments
1-3	25	53	22		56.6	57	g, h
1-2	53	26	21		60.3	60	g, h
1-5	20	44	36		56.0	61	g, h
1-4	46	23	31		65.1	60	g, h
1-8	10	36	54		59.4	60	g, h
1-9	34	12	54		70.2	58	g, h
1-6	none	29	71		64.7	67	g, h
1-7	36	none	64		60.8	63	g, h
1-11	27	50		23	14.9	57	g, i
1-19	54	25		21	23.0	58	g, i
1-12	22	40		38	18.8	59	g, i
1-17	46	20		34	22.2	59	g, i
1-13	12	28		60	19.4	60	g, i
1-14	31	10		59	19.2	59	g, i
1-16	none	24		76	12.5	61	g, i
1-15	28	none		72	17.3	59	g, i

[a] This material is condensed from Wen et al.[8]
[b] Monomer acronyms are as defined in FIGURES 3a and 3b.
[c] Determined by proton N.M.R. spectroscopy.
[d] Determined by conductometric titration.
[e] Measured by dilute solution viscometry at 35°C in DMF containing 0.2% LiBr (in units of ml/g).
[f] Mole % syndiotactic content measured by proton N.M.R. spectroscopy.
[g] Synthesized at 70°C by solution polymerization in ethanol for 4 hours using azobisisobutyronitrile as initiator.
[h] Weakly acidic polymer, mole % MAA increases from 1-3 through 1-7. Polymers with similar MAA content are further ordered with respect to increasing HEMA content.
[i] Weakly basic polymer, mole % DMAEMA increases from 1-11 through 1-15. Polymers with similar DMAEMA content are further ordered with respect to increasing HEMA content.

capsule. We were also concerned about the high concentration of salt bridges in the capsule membrane which could lead to rejection of charged solutes. We also wished to strengthen the capsules mechanically. We chose to alleviate these problems by lowering the charge density in both the acidic and basic polymer and to compensate for this by increasing the hydrophilicity of the remainder of the polymer to retain solubility and permeability. Polymers prepared to this end are described in TABLE 2. Other than ease of monomer purification prior to polymerization,[13] we could establish by these tests no compelling reason to incorporate HPMA into capsule forming systems. The best capsules were prepared through complexation of polymers 2-10b and 2-20b.[9,14] *The mechanical stability of these capsules was superior to that of capsules from weak polyelectrolytes containing a high mole % of charged functionality.*

Carboxylic acid functionality in MAA containing polymers is about 100% ionized at physiological pH.[6,8,14] In contrast, DMAEMA containing functionality is only partly ionized at physiological pH,[7,8,14] leading to a limited solubility at low concentrations of DMAEMA in the polymer, *and giving a transient aspect to salt bridge formation at high pH* (as sketched in FIG. 4a). This concept was subjected to preliminary testing by following changes in the dilute solution viscosity of polyampholytes containing MAA and DMAEMA or quaternized DMAEMA.[10,15] These polyampholytes engage in intramolecular salt bridging at neutral pH leading to a compact configuration and a low solution viscosity. In both instances, intramolecular salt bridges were attenuated at low pH due to protonation of the carboxylate anion, and the polymer coil expanded significantly over dimensions at neutral pH. At high pH, attenuation of the salt bridge occurred also with DMAEMA containing polymers due to deprotonation of the DMAEMA residue, leading again to coil expansion. In contrast, polyampholytes containing quaternized DMAEMA residues retained a compact configuration at high pH.

Encouraged by the behavior of this model system, weakly basic polymers containing DMAEMA were transformed into strongly basic polymers by quaternization of the DMAEMA residues with linear alkyl halides (FIG. 4b). Our earliest attempts involved post quaternization with methyl iodide. Polymers containing quaternized DMAEMA could be made soluble at lower DMAEMA contents and could be

TABLE 2. Candidate Polymers for Capsule Formation through Polyelectrolyte Complexation of a Weakly Acidic and either a Weakly Basic or a Strongly Basic Polyelectrolyte Polymer, Both Possessing a Low Charge Density[a]

Polymer Number	Mole % HEMA[b,c]	Mole % HPMA[b,c]	Mole % MMA[b,c]	Mole % MAA[d]	Mole % DMAEMA[b,c]	Intrinsic Viscosity[e]	Comments
2-23	95.3			4.7		91.2	*f, g, k*
2-28	93.5			6.5		73.2	*f, g, k*
2-1	42		48	9		60.4	*f, g, k*
2-10a	91.2			8.8		72.0	*f, g, k*
2-10b	91.5			8.5		114	*f, g, k*
1-24		90.1		9.9		41.0	*f, h, k*
1-27		89.9		10.1		104	*f, h, k*
1-30		86.9		13.1		159	*f, h, k*
2-25	95.9				4.1	54.6	*f, i, k*
2-29	94.3				5.7	71.4	*f, i, k*
2-18	47		44		9	20.6	*f, i, k*
2-20a	91.8				8.2	26.2	*f, i, k, l*
2-20b	91.6				8.4	66.8	*f, i, k, l*
2-26		89.4			10.6	66.7	*f, j, k*
2-31		84.8			15.2	193	*f, j, k*

[a] This material is reproduced from Wen *et al.*[14]
[b] Monomer acronyms are as defined in FIGURES 3a and 3b.
[c] Determined by proton N.M.R. spectroscopy.
[d] Determined by conductometric titration.
[e] Measured by dilute solution viscometry at 35°C in DMF containing 0.2% LiBr (in units of ml/g).
[f] Synthesized at 70°C by solution polymerization for 4 h in ethanol using azobisisobutyronitrile as initiator.
[g] Weakly acidic polymer containing MAA and HEMA.
[h] Weakly acidic polymer containing MAA and HPMA.
[i] Weakly basic polymer containing DMAEMA and HEMA.
[j] Weakly basic polymer containing DMAEMA and HPMA.
[k] Syndiotactic content ~ 60 mole %.
[l] Post-quaternized with methyl iodide.

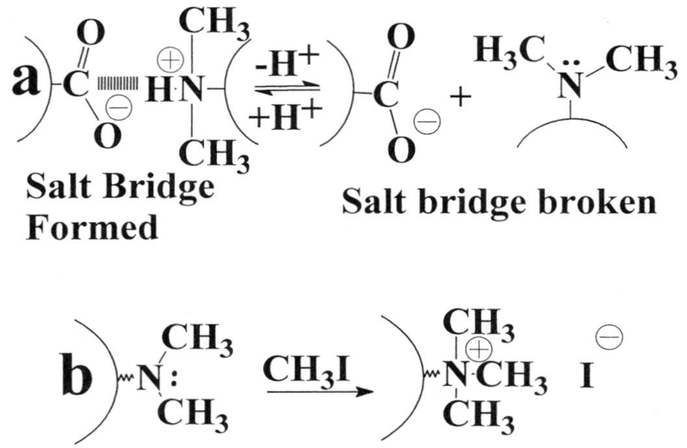

FIGURE 4. The arcs represent a polymer chain. (a) The formation and decomposition of a salt bridge between a carboxylate anion and dimethylamino functionality which is reversibly protonated at pH = 7. (b). The Menschutkin reaction between a dimethylamino functional group and (in this instance) methyl iodide, to form a quaternary ammonium ion.

solubilized at higher molecular weights than unquaternized polymers. Quaternization also appeared to remove the tendency of DMAEMA containing polymers to cross link during storage. Best capsules were made using high molecular weight versions of polymers containing about 10 mole% charged functionality with the balance as HEMA, and designated as 2-10b (the acid polymer) and [C1 quaternized] 2-20b or 2-20b-Q (the basic polymer). These capsules were stable at neutral and high pH but unstable at low pH, as would be expected from examination of the solution behavior of the model polyampholyte polymers.[10,15] Anchorage-independent cells were encapsulated and continued to divide to fill the capsule in much the same manner as cells entrapped in capsules from polyelectrolyte polymers containing a high charge density.[10–12]

To summarize, quaternized DMAEMA containing polymers produced stronger (and less "sticky") capsules on complexation with MAA containing polymers, than did non-quaternized polymers, presumably owing to a lowering of the pH sensitivity of the salt bridges, *thus validating our conjecture that capsule stability could be further improved by transforming the weakly basic center into a strong base.*

Enhancing Capsule Strength by Modifying the Quaternary Ammonium Ion Structure through Quaternization with Differing Alkyl Iodides

We have shown previously that salt bridges, and, therefore, membrane stability, are enhanced through quaternization of dimethylamino functionality prior to capsule formation. A further enhancement of capsule integrity was sought by enhancing the hydrophobicity of the salt bridge through quaternization of the basic residue with higher alkyl iodides. Solvating water would then be more efficiently excluded and $K_{formation}$ for the ion pair would be increased. A number of weakly acidic and weakly basic polymers were synthesized to test this supposition. Dihydroxypropyl methacrylate (DHPMA), an uncharged monomer, more hydrophilic than HEMA, was prepared through simple hydrolysis of glycidyl methacrylate (FIG. 5a). In some instances, polymer solubility was enhanced through the incorporation of DHPMA into terpolymers, to allow for quaternization with (up to) C7 linear Alkyl iodides. Polymers were also quaternized with mixtures of alkyl iodides (not discussed here). Polymer compositions are summarized in TABLE 3. The solubilities of 5% quaternized basic polymer solutions in αMEM medium are also listed in the table. Solubilities can be summarized as (solubility in pH adjusted distilled water) > (in pH adjusted isotonic saline) > (in PBS) ~ (in αMEM medium) due to charge shielding effects. In all instances, derivatization with higher alkyl iodides led to a less soluble polymer.

If the acid polymer is held constant, increasing the hydrophobicity of the quaternary ammonium ion on the basic polymer through quaternization with a longer alkyl iodide and increasing the molecular weight of the basic polymer both lead to an increase in capsule stability. If the modified basic polymer is held constant, capsule stability increases through reaction with a weak polyacid with a higher molecular weight.

In all instances, strongest capsules are formed when the basic polymer is close to precipitation. This can be achieved through many combinations of basic polymer charge density, quaternary ammonium ion structure, and basic polymer molecular weight.

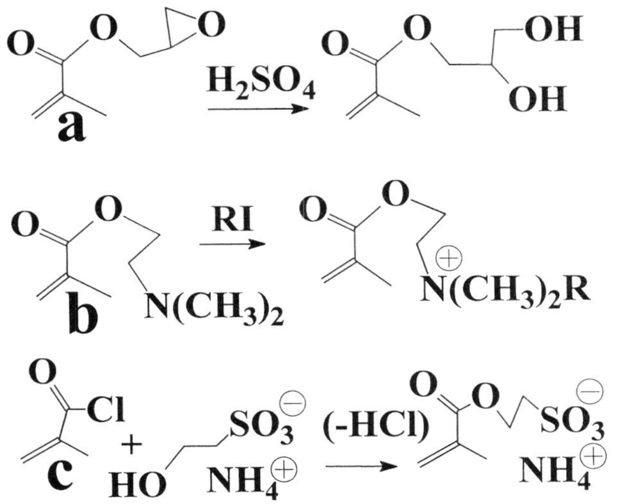

FIGURE 5. The derivatization of commercially available methacrylate monomers. **a:** The hydrolysis of glycidyl methacrylate with concentrated sulfuric acid to form dihydroxypropyl methacrylate (DHPMA). **b:** The alkylation of dimethylaminoethyl methacrylate (DMAEMA) monomer with a generic alkyl iodide to form the quaternary ammonium salt. **c:** Reaction of methacryloylchloride with the ammonium salt of isethionic acid to form the ammonium salt of 2-sulfonyl ethyl methacrylate (SEMA).

TABLE 3. Acidic and Basic Polyelectrolyte Polymers for Capsule Formation through Polyelectrolyte Complexation as a Function of Quaternary Ammonium Ion Structure

Polymer Number	Mole % HEMA[a]	Mole % DMAEMA[b,c]	Mole % DHPMA[a]	Mole % MAA[a]	Intrinsic Viscosity[b]	Comments	Solubility of Quaternized Basic Polymer in αMEM			
							C1	C2	C4	C7
3-1	92.2[d]			7.8[d]	59.8	e, f, i				
3-2	92.5[d]			7.5[d]	113.6	e, f, i				
3-3	95.1[d]			4.9[d]	99.3	e, f, i				
3-4	89[c]			11[c]	21.7	e, f, i				
3-5	89.3[d]			10.7[d]	24.4	e, f, i				
3-6	85.5[d]			14.5[d]	151.5	e, f, i				
3-7	90[c]	10[c]			33.7	e, g, i	s		i	i
3-8	93.4[d]	6.6[d]			83.1	e, g, i	s		i	i
3-9	91.0[d]	9.0[d]			71.6	e, g, i	s	s	i	i
3-10	91.3[d]	8.7[d]			55.8	e, g, i		s		
3-11	91.2[d]	8.8[d]			146.3	e, g, i		i		
3-12	84.0[d]	16.0[d]			27.6	e, g, i	s		s	
3-13	84.1[d]	15.9[d]			67.5	e, g, i	s		s	i
3-14	70[c]	10[c]	20[c]		76.8	e, h, i	s		s	
3-15	80[c]	10[c]	10[c]		44.4	e, h, i	s		i	i
3-16	70[c]	10[c]	20[c]		40.6	e, h, i	s		i	i

[a] Monomer acronyms are as defined in Figures 3a and 3b.
[b] Measured by dilute solution viscometry at 35°C in DMF containing 0.2% LiBr (in units of ml/g).
[c] Monomer charge into reactor.
[d] Determined by proton N.M.R. spectroscopy.
[e] Synthesized at 70°C by solution polymerization in ethanol using azobisisobutyronitrile as initiator.
[f] Weakly acidic copolymer containing MAA and HEMA.
[g] Basic copolymer containing DMAEMA and HEMA, post quaternized with alkyliodides.
[h] Basic terpolymer containing DMAEMA and HPMA, post quaternized with alkyliodides.
[i] Syndiotactic content ~ 60 mole %.
[s,i] soluble and insoluble, respectively, in αMEM cell culture medium.

Creating a More Hydrophilic Capsule Wall through Polyelectrolyte Complexation of Acrylate-based Polyelectrolytes

We have demonstrated that capsule stability may be improved by reacting a weakly acidic polyelectrolyte with a basic polyelectrolyte containing more hydrophobic quaternary ammonium centers. In theory, a stronger salt bridge would further stabilize the capsule membrane and allow, us to create capsules using more hydrophilic comonomers, thus enhancing the diffusion characteristics of the capsule wall. Unfortunately, we are limited, by the solubility in aqueous media of quaternized basic methacrylate co- and ter- polymers containing around 10 mole% charged functionality (our self-imposed upper limit), to a quaternized center created through reaction of DMAEMA residues with (around) heptyl iodide. We circumvented this limitation through the complexation of more hydrophilic *acrylate* based polyelectrolytes. (As with methacrylate based systems, we found that all acrylate polymer compositions closely mirrored monomer charges into the polymerization reactor.)

To this point, all "post" quaternization reactions had been performed on preformed polymers (FIG. 4b). The reactive site (the DMAEMA or DMAEA residue) in "post" quaternized polymers is incorporated randomly into the polymer. However, we can never assume 100% quaternization in the polymer. At this point, we began preparing polymers with pre-quaternized DMAEMA and DMAEA (FIG. 5b). Quaternization of the monomer proved easy and the quaternized monomer appeared to be incorporated into the polymer in random fashion at the low (circa 10 mole%) levels of monomer used in this work. The "pre-quaternized" polymers were 100% quaternized and possessed a long shelf life. "Pre" and "post" quaternized DMAEA containing acrylate-based polymers and corresponding weakly acidic acrylic acid (AA) containing polymers, prepared to test this conjecture, are detailed

TABLE 4. Acrylate Based Polyelectrolytes with a Low Charge Density for Encapsulation

Polymer Number	Mole % HEA[a]	Mole % DMAEMA[b]	Mole % AA[c]	Intrinsic Viscosity[d]	Comments
4-1	83.7		16.3	17.1	e, h
4-2	93.9		6.1	20.5	e, h
4-3	90.0		10.0	29.3	e, h
4-4	92.6		7.4	58.1	e, h
4-5	92.5		7.5	68.7	e, h
4-6	94.6	5.4		15.1	e, f{C1, C4, and C10}
4-7	95.8	4.2		24.7	e, g{C1}
4-8	89.0	11.0		34.9	e, g{C1}

[a] 2-hydroxyethyl acrylate, determined by proton N.M.R. spectroscopy.

[b] dimethylaminoethyl acrylate, determined by proton N.M.R. spectroscopy.

[c] acrylic acid, determined by difference.

[d] Measured by dilute solution viscometry at 35°C in DMF containing 0.2% LiBr (in units of ml/g).

[e] Synthesized at 70°C by solution polymerization in ethanol for 4 hours using azobisisobutyronitrile as initiator.

[f] {Cn}: Polymer was post quaternized with methyl (C1), n-butyl (C4), and n-heptyl (C7) iodide. All derivatives were water soluble or dispersable.

[g] {C1}: Polymer was prepared using DMAEA which had been pre-quaternized with methyl (C1) iodide.

[h] Weakly acidic polyelectrolyte copolymer.

TABLE 5. Candidate Polymers for Capsule Formation through Polyelectrolyte Complexation of a Strongly Acidic and a Strongly Basic Polyelectrolyte Polymer, Both at a Low Charge Density

Polymer Number	Mole % HEMA[a]	Mole % MMA[a]	Mole % Pre-quaternized DMAEMA[b] X-Cn[c]	Mole % SEMA[a]	Intrinsic Viscosity[b]	Comments
5-1	89[d]			11[d]	"low"	f, g
5-2	89[d]			11[d]	"medium"	f, g
5-3	89[d]			11[d]	"high"	f, g
5-4	80[d]	10[d]		10[d]	182.4	f, h
5-5	80[d]	10[d]	10-C1[c,d]		93.7	f, i
5-6	91.6[e]		8.4-C2[c,e]		123.5	f, j
5-7	90.9[e]		9.1-C2[c,e]		65.9	f, j
5-8	89.9[e]		10.1-C3[c,e]		120.7	f, j
5-9	90.1[e]		9.9-C3[c,e]		58.5	f, j
5-10	85.3[e]		14.7-C4[c,e]		92.5	f, j

[a] Monomer acronyms are as defined in FIGURES 3a and 3b.
[b] Measured by dilute solution viscometry at 35°C in DMF containing 0.2% LiBr (in units of ml/g).
[c] Polymer prepared from quaternized DMAEMA, X: Mole % quaternized DMAEMA residue in polymer, -Cn: alkyl iodide used to quaternize DMAEMA residue, ex. 14.7-C4 → 14.7 mole% of butyl iodide quaternized DMAEMA in polymer.
[d] Monomer charge into reactor.
[e] Determined by proton N.M.R. spectroscopy.
[f] Synthesized at 70°C by solution polymerization for 4 hours in a mixed (50/50 by volume) ethanol/water solvent using azobis-4-cyanopentanoic acid as initiator.
[g] Strong acid polyelectrolyte copolymer containing HEMA and SEMA.
[h] Strong acid polyelectrolyte terpolymer containing HEMA, SEMA, and MMA.
[i] Strong base polyelectrolyte terpolymer containing quaternized DMAEMA, HEMA, and MMA.
[j] Strong base polyelectrolyte copolymer containing quaternized DMAEMA and HEMA.

in TABLE 4. We were able to quaternize DMAEA-based polymers with up to decyl iodide. These polymers remained dispersable but developed "detergent-like" characteristics. Unfortunately, we were unable to form capsules using these very soluble acrylate based polyelectrolytes. *We, therefore, determined by these means that there exists an upper limit to the averaged hydrophilic character of the uncharged comonomers in the acidic and basic polymers, above which capsules will not form. That upper limit appears to correspond to a minimum hydrophilic character in the uncharged portions of the chain which would produce a water soluble polymer in the absence of added charged comonomers.*

Microcapsules by Polyelectrolyte Complexation of a Strongly Acidic Polyelectrolyte and a Strongly Basic Polyelectrolyte, Both Containing a Low Charge Density

It has been determined previously see above, that a reduction in the pH sensitivity of the salt bridge at high pH leads to a mechanically stronger capsule at neutral pH. We next surmised that capsule strength could be further enhanced

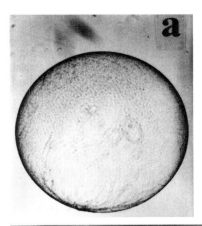

FIGURE 6. All capsules were examined by phase contrast microscopy. **a:** A capsule prepared through complexation of polymer 5-4 and polymer 5-9 (both 5% wt/vol in PBS) after 30 days storage in PBS. **b** and **c:** Capsules prepared from acidic polymer 5-4 (5% wt/vol) and basic polymer 5-7 (4% wt/vol), both in αMEM cell culture medium containing 10% FBS. The acid polymer solution contained initially about 10^6 cells/ml. **b:** Three days after encapsulation. The cells (*see arrow*) have clustered and begun to divide. **c:** Seventeen days after encapsulation. The cells continue to divide within the capsule. The vertical axis of photograph **(a)** = 2.6 mm. The horizontal axis of photographs **(b)** and **(c)** = 1.0 mm.

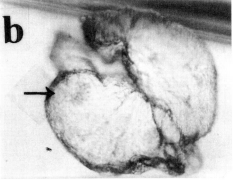

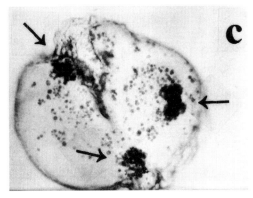

by removing the pH sensitivity of the salt bridge at low pH also. As a preliminary test of this idea, we replaced carboxylic acid functionality by sulfonic acid functionality in a model polyampholyte containing C1 quaternized DMAEMA and measured dilute solution viscosities as a function of pH. As hoped for, the intramolecular salt bridges in this polyampholyte were retained *at high and at low pH*. Encouraged by the behavior of this model system, we prepared a range of sulfonic acid containing polyelectrolytes as candidate polymers for capsule formation. The preparation of the ammonium salt of 2-sulfonyl ethyl methacrylate (SEMA) monomer, subsequently used to prepare the polyampholyte and the strongly acidic co- and ter- polyelectrolytes used to test this "theorem," is sketched in FIGURE 5c. Characteristics of the pre-quaternized basic polyelectrolytes and SEMA containing acidic polyelectrolytes, we prepared to test this "theory," are summarized in TABLE 5. *Capsules from these polymers were stable throughout the normal pH range, could be prepared with 100% efficiency, were considerably tougher and less sticky than capsules from previous systems, and stable over time periods ranging from months to years.* Anchorage independent cells were successfully cultured in the presence of dissolved SEMA containing polyelectrolyte and so the toxicity of the sulfonyl anion in these polymers could be assumed to be low. A phase contrast photograph of a capsule from these polymers is reproduced in FIGURE 6a. Human Burkitt Lymphoma cells are shown in FIGURE 6, b and c to continue to divide within these capsules.

CONCLUSIONS

We have demonstrated that the physical properties of microcapsules prepared through polyelectrolyte complexation/coacervation of synthetic methacrylate based random polyelectrolyte co- and ter- polymers may be improved through suitable adjustments, as driven by a cause and effect analysis based on simple chemical principals, of structural elements within both polymers to enhance the complexation event. We have demonstrated also that nucleated cells may be cultured within those capsules without apparent significant loss of viability.

ACKNOWLEDGMENTS

The authors are grateful for the support of the Clinical Pathology Laboratory, HCA Wesley Medical Center (Wichita, KS) in which facility the cell culture studies were performed. Finally, the authors gratefully acknowledge the help of Mr. Les. Colyott, Dept. Of Physics, Oklahoma State University, for the use of the γ source at that facility.

SUMMARY

The production of microcapsules suitable for the entrapment of mammalian cell by means of polyelectrolyte complexation has, of a necessity, led to the development of novel strategies for the preparation of relatively bioinert polymers which complex efficiently under unique conditions to produce a mechanically resilient membrane with efficient transport properties. In this communication we relate a brief overview of capsule-membrane forming systems for the immunoisolation (or potential immunoisolation) of mammalian cells, which are based upon the complexation of polyelectrolyte (PE) polymers; with emphasis on precursor synthesis and relationships between precursor polymer structure and capsule membrane stability.

REFERENCES

1. FUOSS, R. M. & H. SADEK. 1949. Mutual interactions of polyelectrolytes. Science **110:** 552–554.
2. MICHAELS, A. S. & R. G. MIEKKA. 1961. Polycation-polyanion complexes. **65:** 1765–1773.
3. TSUCUIDA, E. 1994. Formation of polyelectrolyte complexes and their structures. J.M.S.-Pure Appl. Chem. **A31(1):** 1–15.
4. PETRAK, K. 1986. Polyelectrolyte complexes in biomedical applications. J. Bioact. Compat. Polymers **1:** 202–219.
5. BIXLER, H. J. & A. S. MICHAELS. 1969. Polyelectrolyte complexes. *In* Encyclopedia of Polymer Science and Technology, vol. 10: 765–780. H. F. Mark, N. Gaylord & N. M. Bikales, Eds. Wiley Interscience. New York.
6. WEN, S., Y. XIAONAN & W. T. K. STEVENSON. 1991. Preparation and characterization of polyelectrolyte copolymers containing methyl methacrylate and 2-hydroxyethyl methacrylate, Part 1: Polymers based on methacrylic acid. J. Appl. Polym. Sci. **42:** 1399–1406.
7. WEN, S., Y. XIAONAN & W. T. K. STEVENSON. 1991. Preparation and characterization of polyelectrolyte copolymers containing methyl methacrylate and 2-hydroxyethyl methacrylate, Part 2: Polymers based on dimethylaminoethyl methacrylate. J. Appl. Polym. Sci. **43:** 205–112.
8. WEN, S., Y. XIAONAN & W. T. K. STEVENSON. 1991. Microcapsules through polymer complexation, Part 1: By complex coacervation of polymers containing a high charge density. Biomaterials **12:** 374–384.
9. STEVENSON, W. T. K. & M. V. SEFTON. 1992. Development of polyacrylate microcapsules. *In* Fundamentals of Animal Cell Encapsulation and Immobilization, Chapter 7: 143–181. M. F. A. Goosen, Ed. CRC Press. Boca Raton, FL.
10. WEN, S., H. ALEXANDER, A. INCHIKEL & W. T. K. STEVENSON. 1995. Microcapsules through polymer complexation, Part 3: Encapsulation and culture of human Burkitt lymphoma cells in vitro. Biomaterials **16:** 325–335.
11. SEFTON, M. V. & W. T. K. STEVENSON. 1993. Encapsulation of live animal cells using polyacrylates. *In* Advances in Polymer Science #107, Biopolymers. N. A. Peppas & R. S. Langer, Eds.: 143–197. Springer-Verlag. Heidelberg.
12. STEVENSON, W. T. K. & M. V. SEFTON. 1994. Recent developments in polymer based controlled release technology for therapeutic purposes. Trends in Polymer Sci. **2(3):** 98–104.
13. STEVENSON, W. T. K., R. A. EVANGELISTA, R. L. BROUGHTON & M. V. SEFTON. 1987. Preparation and characterization of thermoplastic copolymers from hydroxyalkyl methacrylates. J. Appl. Polym. Sci. **34:** 65–83.
14. WEN, S., Y. XIAONAN, W. T. K. STEVENSON & H. ALEXANDER. 1991. Microcapsules through polymer complexation, Part 2: By complex coacervation of polymers containing a low charge density. Biomaterials, **12:** 479–488.
15. WEN, S. & W. T. K. STEVENSON. 1993. Synthetic pH sensitive polyampholyte hydrogels: A preliminary study. Colloid & Polym. Sci. **271:** 38–49.

Regular Polyelectrolytes with Pyrrolidinium Units

Novel Precursors for Complexes of Charged Polymers

W. JAEGER[a]

[a]Fraunhofer-Institut für Angewandte Polymerforschung
Kantstraße 55
D-14513 Teltow, Germany

A typical feature of water soluble polyelectrolytes is their tendency to form aggregates by interaction with suitable counterpart species. These processes often result in highly organized colloid structures, mainly due to Coulombic interactions. Additionally, other intermolecular forces can play an important role. The aggregation phenomena by interaction with inorganic counter ions, ionic surfactants, macroions, colloidal particles or solid surfaces are the basis of a large number of polyelectrolyte applications in daily life as well as in industrial processes.

Typical examples are[1]

- the formation of gels via crosslinking of polyions with inorganic counter ions used as gelling agents in the food industry,
- the interaction of polyelectrolytes with surfactants leading to products with membrane properties,
- the flocculation of colloids in water purification processes and the retention of fibers and fillers during paper manufacturing as well as
- the conductive coating of surfaces thus avoiding electrostatic charging like with antistatic hair care preparations.

The interaction of soluble polyelectrolytes with oppositely charged macromolecules results in polyanion-polycation-complexes (symplexes). This phenomenological well-known process with many application features is studied extensively by many research groups.[1,2] Rate-determining steps are diffusion processes by forming a symplex gel and rearrangements of the already formed aggregates via conformational changes as well as disentanglements. Depending on the molecular and electrochemical parameters of the macroions involved the complex formation can proceed with increasing polymer concentration by the following steps[1,2]:

- homogeneous one-phase system ($C_{polymer}$ about 10^{-4} g/ml),
- turbid dispersion (surface-charged stabilized primary aggregates),
- complex precipitation ($C_{polymer}$ about 1 wt-%), and
- one-phase system (higher polymer concentration, high ionic strength).

[a] Tel: +49-3328-46401; Fax: +49-3328-46344; E-mail: jaeger@iap.fhg.de

With suitable polymers the aggregation usually leads to insoluble, stable, swellable, and porous polyanion-polycation-complexes. The stoichiometry depends on the type of polyions and the procedure of interaction. The aggregation process can be used to obtain different membranes. Self-supporting or composite flat membranes result from a simultaneous interfacial reaction of a polyanion and a polycation in a suitable mixed solvent or on a microporous support. Mainly cellulose sulfate and polycations containing quaternary N-atoms are used. They are applicable for the dehydration of organic solvents as well as a model in biochemistry and biophysics for investigations of the permeability of ions and other compounds.[1,3] Furthermore, globular shell polymer membranes with sufficient mechanical stability are available by a similar technique using a simple and convenient one-step procedure.[1,4,5] This process can be used for the encapsulation of dissolved or suspended matter. As an example, with cellulose sulfate (CS) and poly(diallyldimethylammonium chloride) (Poly-DADMAC) the encapsulation of sensitive biological matter (enzymes, hepatic microsomes, pancreatic islands, cattle embryos, drugs and many others) takes place at "quasiphysiological" conditions (neutral pH, aqueous systems, moderate ionic strength).

Several other polyelectrolyte component pairings like alginate/poly-L-lysine, polyphosphate/chitosan, polystyrene sulfonate/cationic esters of acrylic acid and polyacrylic acid/polyethylene imine were employed for this process,[1] but the combination of CS and Poly-DADMAC has the advantage of forming capsules with extraordinary mechanical strength.[4,5] Kinetics of formation of the capsule wall and capsule properties (morphological features, cut-off, size, mechanical stability) depend not only on special reaction conditions like concentration of low molecular mass compounds controlling osmotic effects but also to a high extent on the chemical structure of the polyelectrolytes, their charge density, charge strength, molecular mass and molecular mass distribution.[1,4,5]

In the past the optimization of the membrane properties often was carried out with simple and not well-characterized polyelectrolytes. Therefore, the important influences of the different structural elements of the polymers mentioned above could not be investigated precisely and separately. To overcome these difficulties well-characterized polyelectrolytes in terms of molecular and electrochemical parameters as well as polyelectrolytes with regular structure are required. In this paper we summarize results on the synthesis and the characterization of cationic polyelectrolytes mainly based on diallylamine derivatives as monomers or co-monomers concerning this topic. The polymers were selected due to the good application properties of capsules and other types of membranes from complexes containing poly-DADMAC.[1,3-5]

RESULTS AND DISCUSSION

Homopolymers

Poly(diallyldimethylammonium chloride) (poly-DADMAC) is an often used polycation for model investigations as well as for the preparation of symplex membranes. Free radical polymerization of the monomer in aqueous solution proceeds as cyclopolymerization resulting in soluble linear polymers with configurational isomers of pyrrolidinium rings (*cis-trans* ratio 6 : 1) as structural units of the polymer chain. Additionally, the polymers contain a small amount of uncyclized structures

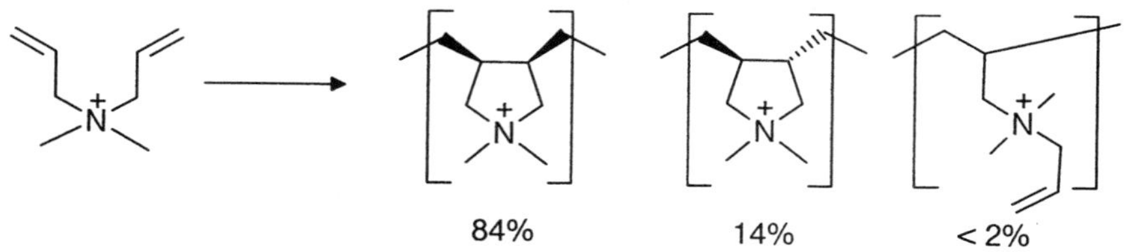

84%   14%   < 2%
cis   trans

FIGURE 1. Cyclopolymerization of DADMAC.

with pendant double bonds (ref. 1, pp. 11–30 and cited literature) (FIG. 1). The kinetics of this process has been studied extensively (refs. 1, pp. 11–30, 6 and 7). The synthesis of strongly linear polymers must avoid side reactions of the pendant double bonds resulting in branches as well as side reactions including the initiator. This can be carried out simply by initiating the polymerization with water soluble cationic azo initiators [2,2'-Azobis(2-amidinopropane)dihydrochloride], termination at low conversion and purification by ultrafiltration and freeze drying. By this procedure really linear polymers with narrow molecular mass distribution covering a broad range of average molecular masses are available (TABLE 1). The absence of microgels and branched structures was indicated by light scattering measurements.

Random Copolymers

Random copolymers with variable charge density but equal molecular mass are avaible by solution copolymerization of charged and uncharged vinyl monomers.

Depending on the monomer reactivity ratios (r-value; ratio of rates of chain propagation between equal and different monomers) of the monomers involved the synthesis of copolymers with constant composition over the whole process can proceed by a batch (equal r-values) or fed polymerization (different r-values). The formation of homogeneous copolymers with variable composition but equal

TABLE 1. Molecular Parameters of Poly-DADMAC

No.	$[\eta]$ cm^3/g^a	$M_n \cdot 10^{-3}$ g/mol^b	$M_n \cdot 10^{-3}$ g/mol^c	$M_w \cdot 10^{-3}$ g/mol^c	$M_w \cdot 10^{-3}$ g/mol^d
1	265	435	423	580	574
2	175	249	272	357	351
3	106	100	116	174	164
4	44	42	54	89	69
5	34	31	30	44	45

[a] 1N NaCl, 30 °C.
[b] Membrane osmometry.
[c] GPC.
[d] Light scattering.

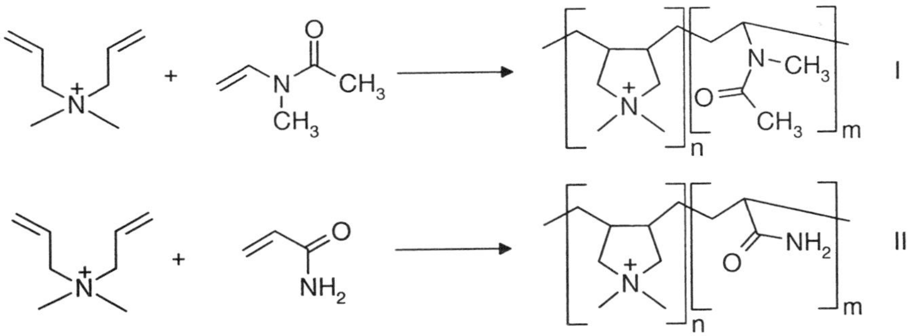

FIGURE 2. Copolymerization of DADMAC with N-methyl-N-vinylacetamide (I) and acrylamide (II).

molecular mass additionally requires knowledge of the kinetics of the polymerization.

The copolymerization of DADMAC (M_1) and N-methyl-N-vinylacetamide (NMVA; M_2) (FIG. 2) in aqueous solution proceeds with nearly equal monomer reactivity ratios. With a total monomer concentration of 1 mol/L values of $r_1 = 0.48$ and $r_2 = 0.66$ are valid. This results in copolymers with variable charge density but equal molecular mass and narrow molecular mass distribution. The copolymers synthesized by a simple batch process are homogenous in compositon up to high conversion (TABLE 2).

Random copolymers with variable charge density are also readily available by copolymerization of DADMAC (M_1) and acrylamide (AAM; M_2) (FIG. 2). Here, the batch polymerization usually leads to a pronounced conversion dependence of the copolymer composition, owing to the large difference of the reactivity ratios. At 50°C increasing values of r_1 (0.02–0.04) but decreasing values of r_2 (6.6–4.6) were found with increasing total monomer concentration (0.5–3.0 mol/L).[7,8] The reason of the concentration dependence of the r-values are electrostatic interactions in the polymerizing system. A fed polymerization with dosage of the more reactive AAM was developed to synthesize copolymers with equal molecular mass as well as variable charge densities but uniform charge distribution along the chains.[8] The polymerization proceeds in n steps, starting with an initial monomer ratio F_0 and an initial concentration C_0. Every step stands for a constant conversion X within a constant reaction time t. X is small to avoid significant changes of the comonomer composition during the reaction. At the end of any step the necessery amount of AAM is added to restore the initial monomer ratio F_0. Termination of the reaction at comparatively low conversion results in copolymers with nearly the calculated composition. Also the M_n-values are nearly constant as expected. The second virial coefficients increase with increasing content of the quaternary compound due to the increase of the charge density (TABLE 3).

Block Copolymers

Block copolymers are available using macroazoinitiators.[9] Azo initiators containing polyethyleneglycol (PEG) moieties can easily be synthesized by a Pinner

TABLE 2. Synthesis of Poly(DADMAC-co-NMVA)

No.	Monomer		Polymer		$[\eta]$ cm³/g	k_H	$M_n \times 10^{-3}$ g/mol[a]	$M_n \times 10^{-3}$ g/mol[b]	$M_w \times 10^{-3}$ g/mol[b]
	DADMAC mol/L	NMVA mol/L	DADMAC mol%	NMVA mol%					
1	1.125	0.375	75	25	73	0.34	71	74	107
2	0.750	0.750	53	47	63	0.32	58	66	98
3	0.281	0.844	24	76	64	0.37		65	92

$[I] = 10^{-2}$ mol/L; T = 50 °C; purification: ultrafiltration and freeze-drying.
[a] Membrane osmometry.
[b] GPC.

TABLE 3. Fed Copolymerization of DADMAC and AAM

c_0 mol/L	$[I] \cdot 10^{-3}$ mol/L	F_1	x mol%	t min	n	DADMAC Content of the Copolymer, mol%		$M_n \cdot 10^{-6}$ g/mol[a]	$M_w \cdot 10^{-6}$ g/mol[b]	$A_2 \cdot 10^7$ mol·L/g[b]
						Experiment	Calculation			
3	1	0.35	2.5	10	2	8	10	0.59	4.22	5.5
3	1	0.77	1.0	6	12	35	30	0.49	2.31	6.3
3	1	0.86	1.0	7	14	47	40	0.54	1.44	6.8
3	1	0.98	1.0	19	14	73	70	0.21	0.58	9.5

[a] Membrane osmometry.
[b] Light scattering.

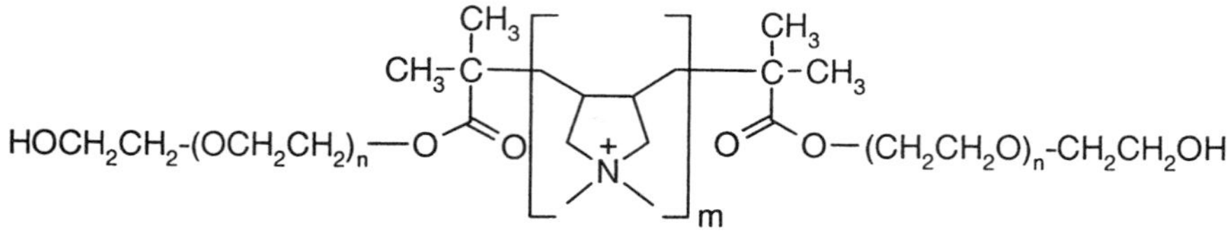

FIGURE 3. Triblock copolymers by polymerization of DADMAC with PEGA-initiators.

reaction of azobis(isobutyronitril) with PEG and subsequent hydrolysis of the iminoether. Pure monomeric products (PEGA) with different PEG-chain lengths were obtained.[7] Polymerization of different cationic vinyl monomers with these PEGA-initiators results in block copolymers AB or ABA type. A is a polyethyleneglycol block, B stands for the cationic block. The structure of the block copolymers depends on the termination reaction. Disproportionation leads to AB type, combination results in ABA type. With DADMAC as a cationic vinyl monomer the polymerization termination occurs exclusively by termination (ref. 1, pp. 11–30). Therefore, the macroinitiated polymerization results in triblock-copolymers (Fig. 3). Copolymers with nearly equal block length, determined by both elemental analysis and ^{1}H-NMR-spectroscopy, were obtained and the values of the molecular weight are nearly as expected (TABLE 4). The reaction conditions for the synthesis of these block-copolymers were established using published kinetic data (refs. 1, pp. 11–30 and 6) of the DADMAC polymerization.

Polyampholytes

Regular polyampholytes with alternating positively and negatively charged units were obtained by radical cyclocopolymerization of ampholytic ionic monomer pairs of maleic acid[10] as well as of maleamic acids[7] with diallylamine derivatives (Fig. 4). In both cases the initial monomer solution only contains the monomers, the vinylic cation is the counter ion of the vinylic anion.

TABLE 4. Synthesis of Triblock-Copolymers PEG-DADMAC-PEG (PDP)

Polymer[a]	Ratio of Block Length PEG:pDADMAC		$M_n \cdot 10^{-3}$ g/mol			$M_w \cdot 10^{-3}$ g/mol
	CHN	^{1}H-NMR	Calculation[b]	MO[c]	GPC	GPC
PDP 2000	0.8:1	0.8:1	22	24	30	47
PDP 1000	0.6:1	0.55:1	14	21	25	40
PDP 600	0.65:1	0.55:1	8.1		14	21
PDP 400	0.65:1	0.45:1	5.5		7.5	15
PDP 200	0.55:1	0.25:1	3.2		4.3	7

[a] Number = molecular weight of the polyethyleneglycol chain.
[b] Calculated from element analysis.
[c] Membrane osmometry.

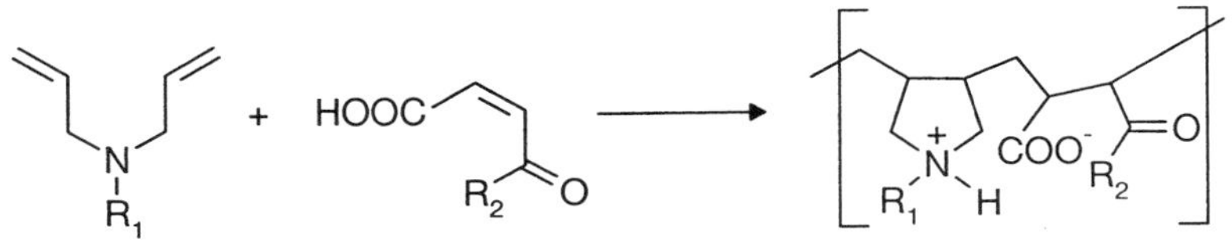

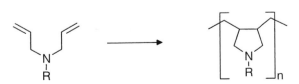

FIGURE 4. Alternating copolymerization of diallylamine derivatives and maleamic or maleic acid

R_1 = H, CH_3 R_2 = OH, NH_2, NHC_3H_7, NHC_4H_9, NHC_6H_{13}, $NHC_{10}H_{21}$, NHC_6H_5

The chemical structure was proofed by ^{13}C-NMR-spectroscopy. The alternating structure results from kinetic measurements, too. The rate of the copolymerization increases strongly with increasing chain length of the alkyl substituent of the maleamic acid. The reason may be the formation of ordered structures in the monomer solution.

Novel polymeric aminophosphonic acids are readily available by cyclopolymerization of the corresponding monomeric betaines (FIG. 5). Like the alternating polyampholytes these polyphosphobetaines are only partly soluble in water depending on the pH.

SUMMARY

Polyelectrolytes with well defined structure are required for investigations of the interaction of charged polymers with low molecular or polymer counter ions and with the surfaces of colloids and macroscopic solids, often resulting in structures of interest in life science. This paper summarizes investigations on the synthesis of water soluble polyelectrolytes with regular structure by free radical cyclopolymerization of diallylamine derivatives in aqueous solution, thereby varying molecular parameters, molecular architecture and electrochemical parameters. The following polymers will be described: well defined copolymers of charged and uncharged monomers, block copolymers consisting of monomer units with different hydrophilicity, alternating polyampholytes, polymeric phosphobetaines.

FIGURE 5. Polymeric aminophosphonic acids

R = $CH_2-PO_3H_2$, $CH(PO_3H_2)_2$

REFERENCES

1. DAUTZENBERG, H., W. JAEGER, J. KÖTZ, B. PHILIPP, CH. SEIDEL & D. STSCHERBINA. 1994. Polyelectrolytes—Formation, Characterization, Application, pp. 248–269, 277–306, and cited literature. Carl Hanser Publications. Munich.
2. KÖTZ, J. 1997. Polyelectrolyte complexes. *In* Polymeric Materials Encyclopedia. J. C. Salomone, Ed. CRC Press, Boca Raton, FL. In press.
3. SCHARNAGEL, N., K.-V. PEINEMANN, A. WENZLAFF, H.-H. SCHWARZ & R.-D. BEHLING. 1996. Dehydration of organic compounds with SYMPLEX composite membranes. J. Membrane Sci. **113:** 1–5
4. DAUTZENBERG, H., G. ARNOLD, B. TIERSCH, B. LUKANOFF & U. ECKERT. 1996. Polyelectrolyte complex formation at the interface of solutions. Progr. Colloid Polym. Sci. **101:** 149–156.
5. DAUTZENBERG, H., B. LUKANOFF, U. ECKERT, B. TIERSCH & U. SCHULDT. 1996. Immobilisation of biological matter by polyelectrolyte complex formation. Ber. Bunsenges. Physical Chem., Chem. Physics **100:** 1045–1053.
6. HAHN, M. & W. JAEGER. 1992. Kinetics of the free radical polymerization of dimethyl diallyl ammonium chloride. Applied Macromol. Chem. **198:** 165–178
7. JAEGER, W., M. HAHN, A. LIESKE, A. ZIMMERMANN & F. BRAND. 1996. Polymerization of water soluble cationic vinyl monomers. Macromol. Symp. **111:** 95–106
8. BRAND, F., H. DAUTZENBERG, W. JAEGER & M. HAHN. 1997. Polyelectrolytes with various charge density. Applied Macromol Chem. **248:** 41–71.
9. NUYKEN, O. & B. VOIT. 1994. Polymeric azo initiators. *In* Macromolecular Design, Concept and Practice. M. K. Mishra, Ed.: 313–343. Polymer Frontiers Int. New York.
10. HAHN, M., W. JAEGER, R. SCHMOLKE & J. BEHNISCH. 1990. Synthesis of regular polyampholytes by copolymerization of maleic acid with allyl and diallyl amine derivatices. Acta Polymerica **41:** 107–112.

Anionic Polymers for Implantation

KAREL SMETANA, JR.[b,c] AND JIŘÍ VACÍK[c]

[b]Institute of Anatomy
1st Faculty of Medicine
Charles University
U nemocnice 3
12800 Prague 2, Czech Republic

[c]Institute of Macromolecular Chemistry
Academy of Sciences of the Czech Republic
Heyrovského náměstí 2
160 00 Prague 6, Czech Republic

Synthetic polymers are more and more frequently used in clinical medicine for the reconstruction of seriously damaged tissues and organs. Unfortunately, they are recognized by immune cells. This process includes the adsorption of bioactive proteins such as fibronectin, vitronectin, complement, fibrinogen or immunoglobulins on foreign surfaces and their recognition by receptors on immune cells.[1] This usually influences the activity and phenotypic characteristics of immune cells colonizing the implant.

Numerous data from the area of anti-infectious immunity demonstrated the distinct effect of chemistry of the surface of bacterial cells on their recognition by non-specific immunity. Bacteria containing the anionic sialic acids in both, monomeric and polymeric form are known as poor activators of the alternative complement pathway, which is also of a great importance in the non-self recognition of synthetic materials.[2] Sialic acids are a quite wide family of derivatives of *N*-acetylneuraminic acid, which are characterized by the presence of carboxylate anions and are normally expressed on the surface of cells in vertebrates. This monosaccharide is recognized by specific populations of macrophages in lymphatic nodes and in the spleen by endogenous lectin sialoadhesin which is participating in immune cell maturation in lymphoid organs.[3] However, the knowledge about the sialoadhesin expression in inflammatory macrophages is only minimal.

In this study we demonstrate the *N*-acetylneuraminic acid (Neu)-binding sites in inflammatory macrophages colonizing the surface of implants in the rat, to estimate the binding capacity of macrophages for this anionic monosaccharide with described biomimetic properties.

The effect of carboxylate anions on hydrogel supports or implants on monocyte adhesion *in vitro* and macrophage adhesion and fusion on surfaces of strips subcutaneously implanted into the rat was tested for a better understanding of the effect of this anion on the non-self recognition of synthetic hydrogels. An intraperitoneal injection of beads prepared from the same polymers was used for the phenotypic characterization of red pulp spleen macrophages and so for an estimation for any

[a] This research was supported by grant No 304/93/0666 of the Grant Agency of the Czech Republic.
[b] Tel: +420 2 24 91 50 03; Fax: +420 2 29 76 92.
[c] Tel: +420 2 36 03 41; Fax: +420 2 36 79 81.

systemic effect of implanted polymers, because these macrophages are not in direct contact with injected polymers.

The results obtained in these experiments were used in the development of a hydrogel posterior-chamber intraocular lens for patients after cataract surgery.

DETECTION OF BINDING SITES FOR *N*-ACETYLNEURAMINIC ACID IN INFLAMMATORY MACROPHAGES

Strips of cellophane or polystyrene (of bacteriological grade) were subcutaneously implanted into Wistar rats of both sexes. The strips were removed 9 days after the surgery, when the foreign body reaction in the subcutaneous region is maximal.[4] Neu-recognizing endogenous lectin was detected by the reverse glycohistochemical reaction employing a neoglycoprotein of structure Neu-bovine serum albumin-biotin as a probe.[5] Biotinylated asialofetuin with β-D-galactoside (Gal) specificity was used for the control reaction. The macrophages as well as MGCs colonizing both used types of implant were negative for Neu-binding site expression. Both the cell types on the surface of cellophane and/or polystyrene were clearly positive for binding sites recognizing Gal.[6]

ADHESION OF MONOCYTES TO POLYMER SURFACES
AN *IN VITRO* STUDY

The influence of molecular structure of hydrogel on human monocyte adhesion was tested by use of glass coverslips coated with non-crosslinked hydrogels. The cells were visualized by the use of immunohistochemical detection of CD14 antigen, or by histochemical visualization of acid phosphatase. The monocytes adhered very intensively to copolymers of 2-hydroxyethylmethacrylate (HEMA) with 10 mol% of 2-dimethylaminoethyl methacrylate (DMAEMA). The pure poly(HEMA) induced only a very low adhesion of monocytes while the adhesivity of these cells to copolymer of HEMA with 3 mol% of sodium methacrylate (NaMA) was only negligible. The adhesivity was somewhat higher in the presence of human plasma than in serum or heat-inactivated serum (TABLE 1).[7]

FOREIGN BODY REACTION TO HYDROGEL IMPLANTS
THE EFFECT OF POLYMER STRUCTURE

The panel of hydrogel implants (4 × 8 mm) was subcutaneously implanted into the rat. The strips were removed 9 days after the surgery. The strips were evaluated

TABLE 1. Numbers of Human Monocytes Adherent to Polymer-Coated Coverslips after 90 Minutes

	Number of CD14[+] Monocytes (%)	
Polymer	Plasma	Heat-inact.-serum
poly(HEMA)	100	75
poly(HEMA-*co*-NaMA)	35	12
poly(HEMA-*co*-DMAEMA)	408	243

The number of monocytes on the surface of polyHEMA is set at 100%.

cytologically with respect to the typing of inflammatory cells on the implant surface and macrophage fusion into foreign-body giant multinucleate cells (MGC). These elements are very important markers for poor biocompatibility of the implant. All implanted hydrogels induced a foreign body reaction and the implants were colonized predominantly by macrophages. MGCs were observed in all types of implants except those with 3 mol% of (NaMA) in copolymers with HEMA. The fusion of macrophages into MGC was clearly inhibited by the increasing concentration of NaMA in these copolymers. On the other hand, the copolymers of HEMA with DMAEMA stimulated formation of MGCs and the macrophage fusion was facilitated by the increasing concentration of this monomer in copolymers with HEMA. The copolymers of HEMA with diethylene glycol dimethacrylate (DEGMA) or with N-(2-pyrrolidonylethylacrylamide) (PEAA) induced approximately the same degree of foreign body reaction including MGC formation as pure poly(HEMA). After alkaline hydrolysis, poly(HEMA) strips have on the surface a very thin layer of methacrylic acid (COO⁻ anions). If these strips are subcutaneously implanted, the extent of the foreign body reaction including MGC formation is very similar to that of copolymer of HEMA with 3 mol% of NaMA (polyHEMA-co-NaMA) (TABLE 2).[8]

INTRAPERITONEAL APPLICATION OF POLYMER BEADS INFLUENCES CARBOHYDRATE-BINDING SITE EXPRESSION IN RED PULP MACROPHAGES IN THE SPLEEN

Microbeads prepared from poly(HEMA), copolymer poly(HEMA-co-NaMA) (3wt%) and copolymer poly(HEMA-co-DMAEMA) (10wt%) were intraperitoneally injected into the rat. A physiological saline injection was applied as a control. The rats were sacrificed 2 days later and the splenic macrophages were phenotypically characterized. The macrophages were immunohistochemically stained by ED-1 antibody (SEROTEC, Oxford). The carbohydrate-binding sites for Neu, Gal, and α-D-mannoside (Man) were detected by reverse glycohistochemical reaction employing biotinylated ASF (Gal) and neoglycoproteins (Sial, Man). The total number of spleen macrophages (ED-1⁺) was not affected by the intraperitoneal injection

TABLE 2. Incidence of Foreign Body Multinucleate Cells Expressed as a Fusion Index[a]

Implanted Polymer	Fusion Index (%)
poly(HEMA)	100
poly(HEMA-co-DEGMA) (30 mol%)	79
poly(HEMA-co-PEAA) (5 mol%)	66
poly(HEMA-co-PEAA) (30 mol%)	113
poly(HEMA-co-NaMA) (1 mol%)	82
poly(HEMA-co-NaMA) (3 mol%)	0
poly(HEMA) hydrolyzed	0
poly(HEMA-co-DMAEMA) (10 mol%)	123
poly(HEMA-co-DMAEMA) (30 mol%)	190

[a] Fusion index = number of nuclei in MGCs: number of nuclei in MGCs + number of nuclei in mononuclear macrophages. Fusion index of macrophages on the surface of polyHEMA is set at 100%.

of polymer beads. The number of macrophages expressing binding sites for all three tested carbohydrate moieties was almost the same after the physiological saline and poly(HEMA-co-NaMA) bead application. Beads from polyHEMA somewhat increased the number of macrophages positive for tested carbohydrate-binding sites and beads from poly(HEMA-co-DMAEMA) significantly elevated the number of positive cells (TABLE 3).[9]

INTRAOCULAR BIOCOMPATIBILITY OF polyHEMA-co-NaMA
AN EXPERIMENTAL STUDY AND CLINICAL TRIALS

Strips prepared from these copolymers were implanted into the anterior eye chamber of rabbits. A long term-testing of the biocompatibility exhibited favorable results. Colonization of strips by inflammatory elements was only minimal. No signs of calcification and damage of intraocular tissues were observed.[10]

A posterior chamber full size lens from poly(HEMA-co-NaMA) (1wt%) was developed. These lenses were implanted into the lens capsule of more than 300 patients after cataract surgery. The results of clinical trials 6 years later are very encouraging.[11]

CONCLUDING REMARKS

The present data demonstrate that inflammatory macrophages are not able to recognize Neu by endogenous lectins. This result agrees very well with numerous observations showing the failure of the activation of the alternative pathway for complement activation by bacteria containing Neu on their surface. Carboxylate is the most prominent functional chemical group of all derivatives of Neu, and the masking effect of the Neu derived saccharides is generally accepted. Our results clearly demonstrated that carboxylate anions as a characteristic functional chemical group of tested hydrogels have an inhibitory effect on the non-self recognition of implanted polymers by the non-specific immunity of the host. The experiments with intraperitoneal injection of polymer beads suggest the possible systemic effect of polymer implantation on the immune system because the polymer beads influenced

TABLE 3. Influence of Chemical Structure of Polymer Beads Intraperitoneally Injected into the Rat on the Phenotypic Characteristics of Red-pulp Spleen Macrophages

| | Number of Positive Macrophages (%) | | | |
Injected Substance	ED1	ASF (Gal)	Man	Neu
Physiol. Saline	100	100	100	100
poly(HEMA) beads	98	142	129	220
poly(HEMA-co-NaMA) (3wt%) beads	95	92	105	153
poly(HEMA-co-DMAEMA) (30wt%) beads	102	171	168	322

The values of macrophages after the injection of physiological saline is set at 100%.

the macrophages in the red pulp of spleen which were not in direct contact with injected particles. The effect of beads containing NaMA with COO⁻ anions on spleen macrophages was very low. The encouraging results of clinical trials of intraocular lenses support hypotheses about the favorable biocompatibility of hydrogels with carboxylate anions in clinical practice.

SUMMARY

The biocompatibility of hydrogels containing carboxylate anions was studied by a panel of tests *in vitro* and *in vivo*. In comparison with other types of similar hydrogels, those with COO⁻ anions induced a lower extent of foreign body reaction, and their systemic effect on the immune system also seems lower. The biomimetic effect of carboxylate anions on biocompatibility of synthetic materials could be explained by a similar biomimetic effect of *N*-acetylneuraminic acid inhibiting the non-self recognition of bacterial cells by non-specific immunity. The encouraging long-term results of clinical trials of intraocular lenses prepared from copolymer of 2-hydroxyethyl methacrylate and sodium methacrylate support this hypothesis.

ACKNOWLEDEGMENTS

The authors are grateful to Dr. Vladimír Hořejší (Institute of Molecular Genetics of the Czech Academy of Sciences, Prague) for anti-CD14 antibody, to Professor Hans-Joachim Gabius (Institute for Physiological Chemistry, Faculty of Veterinary Medicine, Ludwig-Maximilians-University, Munich) for asialofetuin and neoglycoproteins, and to Mrs. Eva Vancová for excellent technical assistance.

REFERENCES

1. SMETANA, K., JR. 1993. Cell biology of hydrogels. Biomaterials **14:** 1046–1050.
2. WETZLER, L. M., K. BARRY, M. S. BLAKE & E. G. GOTSCHLICH. 1992. Gonococcal lipooligosaccharide sialylation prevents the complement-dependent killing by immune sera. Infect. Immun. **60:** 39–43.
3. POWELL L. D. & A. VARKI. 1995. I-type lectins. J. Biol. Chem. **270:** 1243–1246.
4. SMETANA, K., JR. 1987. Multinucleate foreign-body giant cell formation. Exp. Mol. Pathol. **46:** 271–278.
5. GABIUS, H.-J., S. GABIUS, T. V. ZEMLYANUKHINA, N. V. BOVIN, U. BRINCK, A. DANGUY, S. S. JOSHI, K. KAYSER, K. SCHOTTELIUS, F. SINOWATZ, L. F. TIETZE, F. VIDAL-VANACLOCHA & J.-P. ZANETTA. 1993. Reverse lectin histochemistry: Design and application of glycoligands for detection of cell and tissue lectins. Histol. Histopathol. **8:** 369–383.
6. SMETANA, K., JR., H.-J. GABIUS, J. VACÍK, M. JELÍNKOVA & J. LUKÁŠ. 1995. Mapping of endogenous lectins in macrophages colonizing an implanted polymer surface—Effect of polymer structure. Biomaterials **16:** 1149–1152.
7. JIROUŠKOVÁ, M., J. BARTÚŇKOVÁ, K. SMETANA, JR., J. LUKÁŠ, J. VACÍK & J. E. DYR. 1997. Comparative study of human monocyte and platelet adhesion to hydrogels in vitro—Effect of polymer structure. J. Mater. Sci. Mater. Med. **8:** 19–23.
8. SMETANA, K., JR., J. VACÍK, D. SOUČKOVÁ, Z. KRČOVÁ & J. ŠULC. 1990. The influence of hydrogel functional groups on cell behavior. J. Biomed. Mater. Res. **24:** 463–470.

9. SMETANA, K., JR., M. JELÍNKOVA, J. VACÍK, J. FISCHER & H.-J. GABIUS. 1996. Will intraperitoneal injection of synthetic polymer beads of different net charge influence the expression of carbohydrate-binding sites like endogenous lectins in spleen macrophages? Biomaterials. **17:** 2335–2341.
10. SMETANA, K., JR. , J., ŠULC, Z. KRČOVÁ & Š. PITROVÁ. 1987. Intraocular biocompatibility of hydroxyethyl methacrylate and methacrylic acid copolymer/partially hydrolyzed poly(2-hydroxyethyl methacrylate). J. Biomed. Mater. Res. **21:** 1247–1253.
11. PITROVÁ, Š., K. SMETANA, JR., O. WICHTERLE, J. VACÍK, J. KORYNTA & J. CENDELÍN. 1992. First stage of clinical trials of hydrogel lenses manufactured in Czechoslovakia. Cs. Oftal. **48:** 241–246 (in Czech with English abstract).

Scanning Probe Microscopy for the Characterization of Biomaterials and Biological Interactions[a]

MICHAEL D. GARRISON AND BUDDY D. RATNER

Departments of Bioengineering and Chemical Engineering
University of Washington
Seattle, Washington 98195

The 1982 invention of the scanning tunneling microscope (STM) by Binnig and Rohrer precipitated the development of a whole family of proximal probe or scanning probe microscopies (SPMs) to study interfaces at the molecular and atomic scale. Binnig and Rohrer won a Nobel Prize just a few years later in 1986, a measure of the impact these relatively simple and elegant methods have had on science and technology. By 1990, these methods were in widespread use with many commercial vendors. The scanning probe microscopies have unquestionably revolutionized the ability to characterize materials at the nanoscale.

Rapid and widespread acceptance of these new techniques can be attributed to a number of factors. The relative simplicity of the SPMs translates to an apparatus that is easily understood and readily assembled from commercially available components. Typically, little or no special sample preparation is needed before SPM observation. The ability to operate in air, under vacuum, or in fluids leads to wide application and creativity in experimental design. The feature sizes that can be probed, ranging from almost visible to the naked eye to atomic, leads to a unique appreciation of the scaling of surface topography (FIG. 1, A, B, C). The sub-angstrom resolution in the z (height) direction offers a perspective that is difficult to achieve by any other means. Since the data are always processed by a computer, the ability to present those data in a way best suited to communicate the message of importance is an attractive feature. A three-dimensional image of the surface is almost universally appreciated, in contrast to a spectroscopic output that most often requires specific training to interpret. Finally, the basic principles behind these methods (*e.g.*, quantum tunneling, Hooke's Law) are well established and can be exploited to give quantitative information.

With so many positive attributes to these SPM methods, the concerns are also worthy of discussion. Since the SPM data are digital and can be readily manipulated for scaling and esthetics, the information communicated to the viewer can be perhaps too readily manipulated. Six views of one surface, each with differing data presentation and scaling, are offered in FIGURE 1 to illustrate the role of the computer in presenting data. As we have little experience with observing individual molecules based upon their electron clouds, shapes, and mechanics, we often do not know

[a] Generous funding has been received from the Whitaker Foundation, NIH NCRR grant RR01296, and the NSF-funded Engineering Research Center, University of Washington Engineered Biomaterials (UWEB). M. D. Garrison is supported through a US Department of Education GAANN fellowship and NESAC/BIO.

101

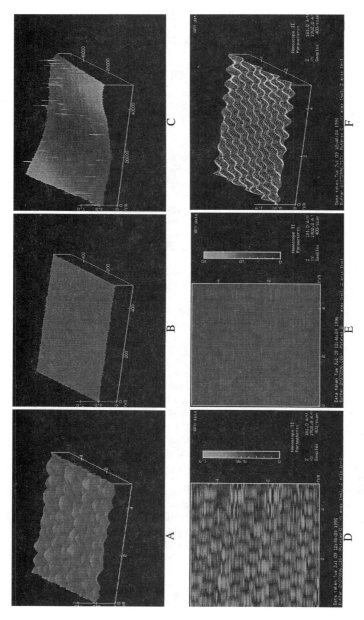

FIGURE 1. Some possibilities for digital AFM image representations. **A-F** are image presentations of cleaved mica analyzed in contact mode in air. **(A)** 5 nm² scan size; atoms are clearly visible. At this scale, the surface appears hilly. **(B)** 500 nm² scan size; atoms are no longer visible. Each pixel has a width of 1.25 nm, larger than the lattice spacing. At this scale, the surface appears extremely smooth. **(C)** 50 μm² scan size; surface particulates are present. Also, image pitch and bow artifacts are prominent. Which representation is the best description of the surface? **(D-E)** Topview representations of the mica atoms in **(A)**. Vertical scales in **(D)** and **(E)** are 2 nm and 20 nm respectively. In **(E)** the atom periodicity is barely visible. **(F)** Lineplot after FFT filtering of the atoms imaged in **(A)**. The lineplot representation reflects the analog signal trace of each pass of the AFM stylus over the surface, as the lines are stacked together into an image. Passband filtering of the spectral period containing the atomic spacing results in clearer distinction of the surface lattice.

precisely what we are observing. This lack of intuition, combined with the ability of the tip to mechanically or electrically induce sample damage or image artifacts, requires rigorous controls for proper interpretation. AFM control experiments should include changing the scan direction by 90° to confirm oriented structures and varying the tip/sample force to understand mechanical damage.

This overview will concentrate on just two of the SPMs, scanning tunneling microscopy and atomic force microscopy (AFM), focusing on their application in biology, medicine and biomaterials. These methods provide unique insights into surface topography (roughness, texture, pattern), and readily image adsorbates ranging in size from atoms to proteins to micro-particles. These SPMs, however, can do more than generate images. Mechanical and electrical properties of surfaces are easily measured at the sub-micron scale. Furthermore, measurements of inter-molecular forces at the nanoscale can be quantified. Specific examples to be presented in this article include the imaging of surface textures, the imaging of protein molecules, studies of self-assembly, the measurement of forces between DNA nucleotide bases and the measurement of forces between biotin and streptavidin. The use of the AFM for nanolithography and creating recognition images of surfaces will also be presented.

STM AND AFM—INSTRUMENTATION BASICS

The STM permits atomic, nano or micro-scale imaging of electrically conductive surfaces and adsorbates on those surfaces. A schematic diagram of an STM system is presented in FIGURE 2. A metal tip terminating in one or a few atoms is brought within angstroms of a metallic or semiconducting surface. At such distances, the probability for an electron to tunnel from an atom in the tip to an atom on the surface is reasonably high. An electrical potential is set up between the tip and surface further increasing the probability of electron tunneling. Under these conditions, the electron tunneling current between tip and surface is described by:

$$J_T \propto V_T exp(-A\phi^{1/2}s) \tag{1}$$

where J_T is the tunneling current, V_T is the voltage between tip and surface, ϕ is the work function (eV), $A \approx 1$ and s is the distance between the tip and surface in angstroms. Note that a change in the distance from the tip to the surface of 1Å can lead to an order of magnitude change in tunneling current, hence the superb (sub-angstrom) resolution in the z direction. The resolution in the x and y directions is approximately 1 ångstrom. As the tip is scanned over the surface, the tunneling current is plotted as function of position on the surface. Changes in tunneling current are a function of both surface topography (tip-sample distance) and the electron density at a given point on a surface.

Whereas the STM measures an electron current between a conducting tip and a conducting surface, the AFM measures forces of interaction between a tip and a surface. The tip and the surface can be electrically conducting or insulating. The attractive or repulsive interactive force between atoms comprising the tip and atoms or molecules on the surface is observed via the deflection of a cantilever onto which the tip is fastened. These ideas are clarified in FIGURE 3. Many outstanding references detail the operation and design theory of STM and AFM.[1,2]

In practice, a lithographically fabricated silicon nitride tip on a thin silicon or silicon nitride cantilever is used to probe the surface. Tip diameters range from 50 to 1000Å. The surface under study is moved in the x, y and z directions via a

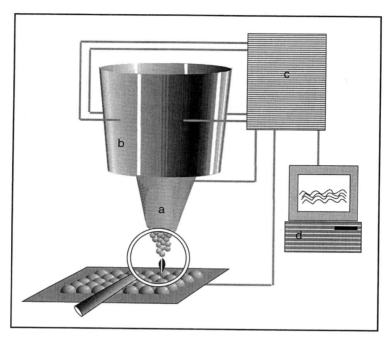

FIGURE 2. Schematic diagram of an STM. **a:** Electron tunneling from the tip to the surface occurs primarily through a single proximal atom. **b:** In STM, the tip is coupled to a piezo positioner, which scans the tip in x, y and z directions. **c:** Hardware and software control algorithms act in feedback mode to read in and react to the position of the piezotube and the tunneling current sensed by the tip. **d:** The digital computer builds the image from successive line scans into a three-dimensional representation of the surface electron density.

platform connected to a piezoelectric crystal. When the tip and the surface are within molecular distances, the tip and surface can undergo attractive, repulsive, or adhesive interactions (FIG. 3). These interactions provide information on surface topography and composition. As the AFM image is generated by the interaction of a tip with the surface as the tip travels at some speed relative to the sample, the size of the image, tip shape and size, scan speed, and tip-sample interaction force are all important parameters for generating an accurate image of the surface. Capillary forces caused by adsorbed water on the tip and sample surface are important when imaging in air, but can be removed by imaging in liquids.

Other modes of SPM operate in a related fashion. A lateral force measurement that codes compositional information can be made by monitoring the torsional (twisting) forces induced in the cantilever. By vibrating the tip in the vicinity of the surface and studying the phase relationships of the tip, information on the nanomechanics and interactive forces can be acquired. Modification of the tip material can lead to images that are reflective of the electrochemistry or magnetic properties of the surface. Chemically modified tips can probe specific aspects of surface chemical structure at the molecular scale.

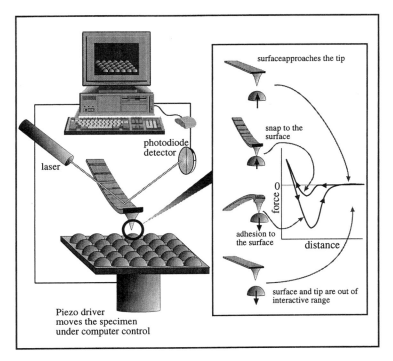

Piezo driver
moves the specimen
under computer control

FIGURE 3. Schematic diagram of an AFM. In contrast to STM, the AFM stylus is non-conducting, interacts with the surface over a discrete area, and remains stationary while the sample is rastered beneath. The deflection of the cantilever is often sensed by the reflection of a laser beam from the back of the cantilever onto a position sensitive photodiode. The piezo position and photodiode response are fed into feedback loops similar to the STM case in order to respond to the surface topography.

STM OF BIOMOLECULES AT INTERFACES

Because of the need for an oxide-free conducting substrate, there are limited, but still important, applications for STM in biology and biomaterials. Adsorption of biomolecules on gold, platinum and graphite constitute the majority of this literature. For example, there are many publications looking at DNA on graphite and gold.[3] However, owing to a lattice defect on the surface of graphite with a periodic spacing similar to the subunits making up DNA, images on graphite are suspect. In contrast, atomically smooth gold has proven to be an excellent substrate for biomolecular imaging. Individual protein molecules have been imaged by a few groups.[4] Molecules such as phthalocyanines and nucleotide bases that form ordered arrays at the gold surface have also been studied.[5] DNA images of astonishing resolution have been obtained.[6] Even though AFM has replaced STM as the method of choice for biomolecule investigation, these original experiments are the foundation of SPM use in the study of biomolecule/biomaterials interactions.

ASSESSING SURFACE TOPOGRAPHY

Perhaps the most straightforward use of the AFM for biomaterials characterization is the assessment of surface topography. Surface roughness of a biomaterial may influence adsorbed protein layers, inflammatory response, cellular ingrowth, and, ultimately, biocompatibility.

A material may be interrogated as to its surface roughness on the basis of measured topographic information. Surface roughness (R_a) of a given region is defined as the variance of the topographic data array, $f(x,y)$, relative to a surface plane parallel to the plane of minimum height variance about the mean region height, and calculated to have equal volume above and below the plane surface.[7] Therefore the calculated surface roughness of an image is dependent upon the image size relative to the height of the features of interest, and the relative size of one pixel within the image as compared to the size of the AFM tip.

An image pixel has a finite width, and an intensity determined by the highest point in that pixel area. Therefore the surface roughness over different scan length scales will vary. This would be analogous to a hiker walking the rugged Bright Angel Trail from the rim to the bottom of the Grand Canyon. The mule trail is rough on the size scale of the hiker's feet, but is smooth relative to the depth variation in the canyon. Similarly, surfaces that appear smooth and defect-free to our naked eye can actually be quite rough at the size scale of a cell or protein.

In addition, for smaller scan sizes where the pixel width is less than the tip radius, sharper tips (smaller radius and apex angle) may reveal more features than a blunted tip simply due to the ability to probe between features.[8] Conventional tips have a 35° apex angle, but specialized tips can be produced with needlelike shapes that have a tip radius of ≈5nm and allow for imaging of sharper features. For measuring vertical or greater than vertical sidewalls, rectangular or flared "boot" shaped tips can be used.[9] The geometry of the AFM tip is always convoluted in the measurement of sample topology. An area of active research involves removal of the influence of the probe from an image by applying a deconvolution algorithm to mathematically eliminate the tip shape contribution.[10,11]

When imaging biomaterials, one must also account for the surface modulus. Imaging of compressible, pliable samples can be difficult and the resolution available is reduced due to the movement of the sample under the pressure of the tip. Often, imaging of such pliant or fragile materials precludes the use of the conventional contact mode AFM, and must be performed at reduced forces. There are many ways to reduce the tip-sample interaction force, such as working in liquids or imaging with intermittent contact ("tapping") of the surface. Recent investigation of gelatin films shows that as the Young's modulus "softens," the effective pixel resolution decreases greatly.[12] Another application of the AFM and surface roughness measurement was demonstrated in the field of dental biomaterials where researchers have followed the progress of various cleaning agents and corrosives on dentin using the AFM.[13] Similarly, Cassinelli and Morra were able to infer a mechanism of action of a dental adhesive by examining the change in the dentin topology as a function of time following treatment.[14]

MEASURING INTERMOLECULAR FORCES

In addition to revealing topography, the AFM can also be used to measure discrete intermolecular forces.[15] Rather than creating an image by rastering the sample in a plane, the surface is held at a fixed x,y position and advanced and retracted vertically into contact with the AFM tip. This vertical oscillation (typically 0.1–25 Hz) causes the tip to engage and disengage from the sample creating a force versus separation loop. Since the cantilever acts as the force transducer in this application, it is essential to accurately measure the spring constant to obtain quantitative values. A standard force curve (FIG. 4) illustrates the approach, an attractive jump-in point, a repulsive region, an adhesive force that holds the tip on the sample, and a snap-off point where the force pulling the tip off the surface becomes greater than the interactions holding it to the surface. General colloidal forces and specific intermolecular forces account for this behavior.[16]

AFM tips can be modified by a number of methods to probe specific intermolecular forces. Gold coated tips provide a useful substrate for self-assembled monolayers (SAMs) of alkane thiols and nucleotide bases. Other methods such as plasma deposition,[17] silane chemistry,[18] and lipid coating,[19] have also been exploited for chemically derivatizing the bare silicon or silicon nitride AFM tips. With an AFM tip functionalized with a molecule of specific polarity, electronegativity, or hydrogen bonding ability, these properties of a surface can be quantitatively probed. Through tip derivatization with $COOH$, CH_3, CH_2OH, NH_2, CH_2Br, and CF_3 groups, the forces of interaction with similarly derivatized surfaces have been studied.

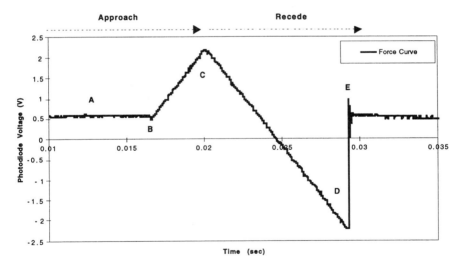

FIGURE 4. Typical force curve (mica in air). The x axis represents the time course of the approach and receding cycle, the y axis represents the resulting photodiode voltage. Increase in the photodiode voltage reflects an increase in the tip/sample interaction repulsive force, while a decrease in voltage would represent the presence of an attractive force. The small DC offset can be controlled by adjustment of the operating setpoint voltage. **A:** The piezo positioner is disabled and the sample is advanced toward the tip. **B:** When the surface reaches the tip, the capillary forces pull the tip down into contact with the surface with a slight attraction. **C:** The tip contacts the surface, and the atoms of the surface and tip repel each other in a near linear fashion. The linearity is evident during the receding part of the curve. **D:** During retraction, the capillary forces hold the tip onto the surface until the force of the cantilever spring breaks the surface bonds, **(E)** and the cantilever snaps off the surface. In fluids, the capillary forces are greatly reduced.

One of the biological interactions most studied with force curve analysis has been that of streptavidin-biotin binding.[20-22] Streptavidin-biotin binding affinity is on the order of $K_a = 10^{15}$, one of the highest known. TABLE 1 summarizes the intermolecular forces measured for this biological pair. It is interesting to note the agreement in the forces measured, and the influence of side-chain modification of the streptavidin or biotin. It is also interesting to note the variation between different cantilevers, tips, and arrangement of the interacting molecules.

In both chemical and biological force interactions, numerous force curves must be obtained to quantitate a single bond dissociation. This is due to the area of interaction between the tip and the sample being much larger than a single molecule. One method of quantitation involves the measurement of the snap off force for each force curve and plotting a histogram.[20] The force histogram will display peaks in integer multiples of a single discrete bond force. Another method assumes that the number of bonds broken for each snap off follows a Poisson statistical distribution, and, as such, the single quantized force is equal to the ratio of the mean to the variance of the forces measured.[23,24] Both models suggest similar bond strengths.

NANOLITHOGRAPHY

Nanolithography refers to the directed manipulation and fabrication of features on the nanometer scale. Both the STM and AFM have been widely applied to nanolithography on semiconductor materials, but recently nanolithography of biological materials has also been demonstrated. During "normal" operation, a sample scans beneath an AFM tip at the lowest force possible ($\approx$10nN for contact mode in air) in order to reduce surface damage and/or deformation. Since images are usually scanned at the lowest possible force, increasing that force is easily done in a controllable manner. As the tip-sample force is increased, the sample may fail in compression or shear and be ruptured, etched, or eroded by the tip pressure. By

TABLE 1. Streptavidin (Avidin)–Biotin Interaction Forces

Interaction		Force (pN)	Reference
WT SA-biotin	(tip 1), (tip 2)	(253 ± 20), (393 ± 10)	20[a]
W79A	(tip 1), (tip 2)	(158 ± 17), (332 ± 31)	
W79F	(tip 1), (tip 2)	(294 ± 10), (439 ± 11)	
W108F		443 ± 33	
W120A		257 ± 28	
W120F		92 ± 19	
Avidin-Biotin		160 ± 20	18[b]
Avidin-Iminobiotin		85 ± 15	
SA-Biotinylated BSA		340 ± 120	19[c]
Blocked w/excess biotin in solution		60 ± 40	

[a] SA mutants on surface, biotinylated tips, 100 force curves averaged.
[b] Avidin tip, biotinylated agarose beads as the surface, 300 force curves averaged,
[c] Biotinylated BSA glass microsphere tips, SA surface, 42 force curves averaged.
Abbreviations: SA: streptavidin, WT: wild type SA, BSA: bovine serum albumin.

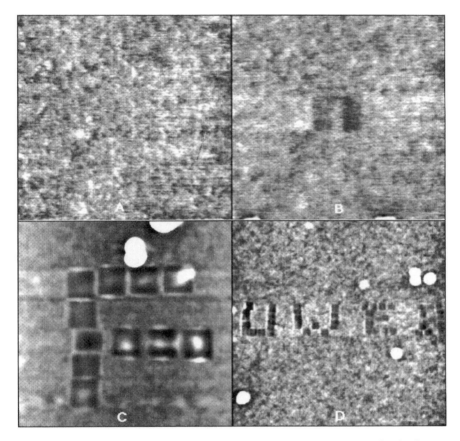

FIGURE 5. Nanolithography progression montage. A soft overlayer on a hard substrate (plasma deposited C_3F_6 on silicon) is etched in patterns of increasing complexity. (**A**) A blank field (3 μm^2, R_a(nm) = 0.47 $\pm$ 0.10) of the C_3F_6 surface. (**B**) A 500 nm^2 box etched for 2 min at a force of $\approx$100 nN and a scan rate of 40 μm/sec. (**C**) Arrangement of 500 nm^2 boxes into the letter F. Each box is $\approx$1.4 nm deep, while the total letter size is 2.6 μm. (**D**) Arrangement of 200 nm^2 boxes (1–2 nm deep) into a series of letters spelling the acronym UWEB.[28]

arranging spots of erosion into recognizable shapes, letters, or even words, can be produced. FIGURE 5 illustrates this progression.

The resolution of such lithographic techniques is limited by the width of the AFM tip, on the order of 5–50nm. This size scale represents approximately an order of magnitude improvement over conventional optical methods. However, as shown in FIGURE 5, the etch spots can display some positional drift, due to the material properties of the sample positioner, commonly a piezoelectric crystal. Such crystals exhibit non-linearities in their behavior such as creep and hysteresis that effectively limit the resolution of the nanolithography to a scale much greater than the tip size. Development of improved tip-sample positioning systems is an area of active research. The possibilities of biological nanolithography with the AFM have been illustrated with Langmuir Blodgett (LB) films transferred to solid surfaces. By scanning the films at forces >50nN, a number of groups have shown the AFM can erode such films, monolayer by monolayer, in discrete patterns.[25,26] Recently, Mazzola and Fodor displayed the ability to remove a patterned array of streptavidin from a biotinylated surface by scanning at high forces.[27] These studies illustrate the possibility of creating a biological surface architecture using the AFM to carve a surface pattern of both controlled lateral dimension and depth. Arrangement of such patterns may make it possible to expose specific chemical groups in a well defined surface array. In this way, a biomaterial surface could be engineered to present specific chemistry with a spatial orientation that directs a biological response. Much like FIGURE 5, where boxes are arranged to communicate an idea, UWEB, a surface might be engineered to communicate a biological idea to the cell leading to cytokine release or cell surface receptor expression.

RECOGNITION MICROSCOPY

If a set of force curves is taken at each pixel as the tip scans over a surface, a three-dimensional image is generated where each pixel contains force spectral content. Images can then be generated with contrast dependent upon which part of the force spectrum is used. If specific interactions occurred, these events could be coded as bright or dark regions in the image. This type of imaging can be performed in practice by rastering the surface under a functionalized tip and monitoring the resulting forces as the separation distance is held constant. Alternately, the additional force may be detected as a torsion of the AFM cantilever, termed lateral force microscopy (LFM).[29–31] When the image created has contrast that is generated not by a differential in height, but by a differential in specific attractive or repulsive force, the image is referred to as a chemical recognition image. As such, each pixel is representative of a particular binding affinity for the functionalized tip by the surface.

This effect has been demonstrated with DNA base pair interactions.[32] DNA bases were self-assembled on both gold coated tips and gold surfaces. Of all 16 possible combinations, only the interaction of complementary base pairs resulted in ordered images (FIG. 6). From force curve analyses, it was found that the specific hydrogen bonding interaction between adenine-thymine bases was ≈54pN. The image created by the DNA base pair interactions suggests the possiblility of sequencing DNA with specific recognition events. Recently, the ability to image linearly stretched DNA and measure the interaction forces between single stranded oligonucleotides with the AFM has been demonstrated.[33,34] Therefore it may be possible to generate an image where the contrast arises from the specific interactions between an oligonucleotide functionalized tip, and linearly stretched single strand DNA on the surface. Such an image could reflect the presence of a mutated codon, or reveal a directed insertion to correct a defect.

However, recognition imaging is certainly not limited to DNA interactions. As shown in the above section, tips may be functionalized with many types of molecules. Chemically sensitive images have been obtained from hydrophilic tips and micropatterned surfaces.[35] Commercially available bio-functionalized tips are available with antibodies, biotin, and other biomolecules.[36] Thus, for example, it may be possible to image a cell surface with specific recognition events, to follow the kinetic course of cell surface receptor expression, or perhaps measure the binding affinity of tips functionalized with novel therapeutic proteins.

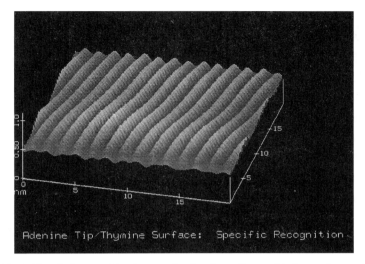

FIGURE 6. Chemical recognition image of a thymine self-assembled monolayer with a tip coated with an adenine self-assembled monolayer. Operating in "constant height" or "force mode," the *y* axis (units of nN) represents repulsive forces between the tip and the sample, and therefore, the darker regions represent attractive forces. Passband filtering of the image power spectral density was applied to sharpen the contrast in the image. The ordered self-assembly rows can be seen, along with the individual base pair interactions, measured at periodicities of 0.95 nm $\times$ 0.34 nm.

SUMMARY

The scanning probe microscopies provide a unique view of biological and biomedical systems at a nanoscale appropriate to appreciate molecular events. The advent of these methods has brought the ability to acquire quantitative information at the molecular level. Given the proliferation of microscopes and associated methods, the probability for important discoveries is high. If tempered with an appreciation for the potential for artifacts, the SPMs may revolutionize our view of biological systems and biomaterials interactions with those systems.

REFERENCES

1. WIESENDANGER, R. 1994. Scanning probe microscopy and spectroscopy: Methods and applications. Cambridge University Press. Cambridge, UK.
2. SARID, D. 1994. Scanning force microscopy: With applications to electric, magnetic, and atomic forces. Oxford University Press. New York.
3. MOU, J., W. SUN, J. YAN, W. S. YANG, C. LIU, Z. ZHAI, Q. XU & Y. XIE. 1991. Underwater scanning tunneling microscopy of organic and biological molecules. J. Vac. Sci. Tech. B **9:** 1566–1569; LINDSAY, S. M., Y. L. LYUBCHENKO, N. J. TAO, Y. Q. LI, P. I. ODEN, J. A. DEROSE & J. PAN. 1993. Scanning tunneling microscopy and atomic force microscopy studies of biomaterials at a liquid solid interface. J. Vac. Sci. Tech. A. **11:** 808–815.
4. LEWIS, K. B. & B. D. RATNER. 1996. Imaging fibrinogen adsorbed on noble metal surfaces

with scanning tunneling microscopy: correlation of images with ESCA, SIMS, and radiolabeling studies. Coll. Surf. B: Biointerfaces. **7:** 259–269. ZHANG, J., Q. CHI, S. DONG & E. WANG. 1994. Ordered arrays of myoglobin adsorbed on the surfactant modified surface by scanning tunneling microscopy. Surf. Sci. **321:** L195–L201. LEE, G., D. F. EVANS, V. ELINGS & R. D. EDSTROM. 1991. Observation of phosphorylase kinase and phosphorylase b at solid-liquid interfaces by scanning tunneling microscopy. J. Vac. Sci. Tech. B **9:** 1236–1241.

5. BOLAND, T. & B. D. RATNER. 1994. Two dimensional assembly of purines and pyrimidines on Au(111). Langmuir **10:** 3845–3852. KANAI, M., T. KAWAI, K. MOTAI, X. D. WANG, T. HASHIZUME & T. SAKURA. 1995. Scanning tunneling microscopy observation of copper-phthalocyanine molecules on Si(100) and Si(111) surfaces. Surf. Sci. Lett. **329:** L619–L623.

6. DUNLAP, D. D. & C. BUSTAMANTE. 1989. Images of single-stranded nucleic acids by scanning tunneling microscopy. Nature **342:** 204–206. YOUNGQUIST, M. G., R. J. DRIS-CALL, T. R. COLEY, W. A. GODDARD & J. D. BALDESCHWIELER. 1991. Scanning tunneling microscopy of DNA: Atom resolved imaging, general observations and possible contrast mechanism. J. Vac. Sci. Tech. B **9:** 1304–1308.

7. Digital Instruments Nanoscope II Scanning Probe Microscope Instruction Manual. Digital Instruments, Inc. 112 Robin Hill Road, Santa Barbara, CA 93117. http://www.di.com

8. BUSTAMANTE, C. & D. KELLER. 1995. Scanning force microscopy in biology. Physics Today **48:** 32–38.

9. MARTIN, Y. & H. K. WICKRAMASINGHE. 1994. Method for imaging sidewalls by atomic force microscopy. Appl. Phys. Lett. **64:** 2498–2500.

10. VESENKA, J., S. MANNE, R. GIBERSON, T. MARSH & E. HENDERSON. 1993. Colloidal gold particles as an incompressible atomic force microscope imaging standard for assessing the compressibility of biomolecules. Biophys. J. **65:** 992–997.

11. VESENKA, J., R. MILLER & E. HENDERSON. 1994. Three-dimensional probe reconstruction for atomic force microscopy. Rev. Sci. Instrum. **65:** 2249–2251.

12. RADMACHER, M., M. FRITZ & P. K. HANSMA. 1995. Imaging soft samples with the atomic force microscope: Gelatin in water and propanol. Biophys. J. **69:** 264–270.

13. MARSHALL, G. W. JR., M. BALOOCH, R. J. TENCH, J. H. KINNEY & S. J. MARSHALL. 1993. Atomic force microscopy of acid effects on dentin. Dent. Mater. **9:** 265–268.

14. CASSINELLI, C. & M. MORRA. 1994. Atomic force microscopy studies of the interaction of a dentin adhesive with hard tooth tissue. J. Biomed. Mater. Res. **28:** 1427–1431.

15. FLORIN, E. L., M. RIEF, H. LEHMANN, M. LUDWIG, C. DORNMAIR, V. T. MOY & H. E. GAUB. 1995. Sensing specific molecular interactions with the atomic force microscope. Biosens. Bioelect. **10:** 895–901.

16. BUTT, H. J. 1991. Measuring electrostatic, van der Waals, and hydration forces in electrolyte solutions with an atomic force microscope. Biophys. J. **60:** 1438–1444.

17. KNAPP, H. F., W. WIEGRABE, M. HEIM, R. ESCHRICH & R. GUCKENBERGER. 1995. Atomic force microscope measurements and manipulation of Langmuir-Blodgett films with modified tips. Biophys. J. **69:** 708–715.

18. NAKAGAWA, T., K. OGAWA & T. KURUMIZAWA. 1994. Atomic force microscope for chemical sensing. J. Vac. Sci. Tech. B **12:** 2215–2218.

19. XU, S. & M. F. ARNSDORF. 1995. Electrostatic force microscope for probing surface charges in aqueous solutions. Proc. Natl. Acad. Sci. USA **92:** 10384–10388.

20. FLORIN, E. L., V. T. MOY & H. E. GAUB. 1994. Adhesion forces between individual ligand receptor pairs. Science **264:** 415–417.

21. LEE, G. U., D. A. KIDWELL & R. J. COLTON. 1994. Sensing discrete streptavidin-biotin interactions with atomic force microscopy. Langmuir **10:** 354–357.

22. CHILKOTI, A., T. BOLAND, B. D. RATNER & P. S. STAYTON. 1995. The relationship between ligand-binding thermodynamics and protein-ligand interaction forces measured by atomic force microscopy. Biophys. J. **69:** 2125–2130.

23. HAN, T., J. M. WILLIAMS & T. P. BEEBE JR. 1995. Chemical bonds studied with functionalized atomic force microscopy tips. Anal. Chim. Acta **307:** 365–376.

24. WILLIAMS, J. M., T. HAN & T. P. BEEBE JR. 1996. Determination of single-bond forces from contact force variances in atomic force microscopy. Langmuir **12:** 1291–1295.

25. GARNAES, J., T. BJORNHOLM & J. A. N. ZASADZINSKI. 1994. Nanoscale lithography on Langmuir-Blodgett films of behinic acid. J. Vac. Sci. Tech. B **12:** 1839–1842.
26. FUJIHARA, M. & H. TAKANO. 1994. Atomic force microscopy and friction force microscopy of Langmuir-Blodgett films for microlithography. J. Vac. Sci. Tech. B **12:** 1860–1865.
27. MAZZOLA, L. & S. P. A. FODOR. 1995. Imaging biomolecule arrays by atomic force microscopy. Biophys. J. **68:** 1653–1660.
28. University of Washington Engineered Biomaterials. http://www.uweb.engr.washington. edu/uweb
29. FUJIHIRA, M. & Y. MORITA. 1994. Atomic force microscopy and friction force microscopy of chemically modified surfaces. J. Vac. Sci. Tech. B. **12:** 1609–1613.
30. FRISBIE, C. D., L. F. ROZSNYAI, A. NOY, M. S. WRIGHTON & C. M. LIEBER. 1994. Functional group imaging by chemical force microscopy. Science. **265:** 2071–2074. WILBUR, J., H. A. BIEBUYCK, J. C. MACDONALD & G. M. WHITESIDES. 1995. Scanning force microscopies can image patterned self assembled monolayers. Langmuir **11:** 825–831. NOY, A., C. D. FRISBIE, L. F. ROZSNYAI, M. S. WRIGHTON & C. M. LIEBER. 1995. Chemical force microscopy: Exploiting chemically-modified tips to quantify adhesion, friction, and functional group distributions in molecular assemblies. J. Am. Chem. Soc. **117:** 7943–7951.
31. GREEN, J.-B. D., M. T. MCDERMOTT, M. D. PORTER & L. M. SIPERKO. 1995. Nanometer-scale mapping of chemically distinct domains at well-defined organic interfaces using frictional force microscopy. J. Phys. Chem. **99:** 10960–10965.
32. BOLAND, T. & B. D. RATNER. 1995. Direct measurement of hydrogen bonding in DNA nucleotide bases by atomic force microscopy. Proc. Natl. Acad. Sci. USA **92:** 5297–5301.
33. HU, J., M. WANG, H.-U. G. WEIER, P. FRANTZ, W. KOLBE, D. F. OGLETREE & M. SALMERON. 1996. Imaging of single extended DNA molecules on flat (aminopropyl)-triethoxysilane-mica by atomic force microscopy. Langmuir **12:** 1697–1700.
34. LEE, G. U., L. A. CHRISEY & R. J. COLTON. 1994. Direct measurement of the forces between complementary strands of DNA. Science **266:** 771–773.
35. AKARI, S., D. HORN, H. KELLER & W. SCHREPP. 1995. Chemical imaging by scanning force microscopy. Adv. Mater. **7:** 549–551.
36. BioForce Laboratory, 112 Robin Hill Road, Santa Barbara, CA 93117. http://www. bioforcelab.com

XPS and SIMS Studies of Surfaces Important in Biofilm Formation

Three Case Studies

BONNIE J. TYLER[a]

Department of Chemical Engineering and
Center for Biofilm Engineering[b]
Montana State University
Bozeman, Montana 59717

Although the importance of biofilms in medicine, industry and the environment is well established, the initial adhesion events that lead to biofilm formation are still poorly understood. It is known that a layer of biopolymers adsorbs rapidly to most surfaces and forms a conditioning film when they are placed in an aqueous environment. In the human body, this conditioning film consists primarily of plasma proteins. Cells then adhere either specifically to the adsorbed biopolymers or non-specifically to the surface or to the conditioning film. In an implanted medical device the cells may be endogenous to the human body (platelets, macrophages, fibroblasts, osteoblasts, endothelial cells, *etc.*) or they may be invading bacteria or fungi. In either case, the behavior of these adherent cells is critical to the long term patency of the implanted device.

The processes leading to cell adhesion are poorly understood in part because the chemistry and structure of 1) the material surface, 2) the biopolymer conditioning film, and 3) the cell surface are often poorly understood. X-ray Photoelectron Spectroscopy (XPS) and Secondary-Ion Mass Spectroscopy (SIMS) can be used to investigate all three of these contributors to the cell-adhesion process. In this paper three case studies will be presented to illustrate how XPS and SIMS can be used to investigate synthetic polymer surfaces, to characterize molecular interactions between adsorbed biomolecules and polymer surfaces, and to probe molecules on cell surfaces.

The first case study presented is a 1992 study of the surface chemistry of a commercial medical grade polyurethane.[1] XPS and SIMS are well established as accurate techniques for probing polymer surfaces so the objective in presenting this case study is not to illustrate the efficacy of XPS and SIMS but to demonstrate the importance of doing accurate surface analysis even when using a standard polymer.

The use of XPS and SIMS to study protein adhesion is far less established, but recent studies have demonstrated their potential in this field. The second case study is an investigation of mussel adhesive protein adsorption on hydrophobic polymers published in 1996.[2-4] The objective in presenting this case study is to demonstrate the effectiveness of XPS and SIMS for studying conditioning films.

The final case study presented is a SIMS and XPS investigation of four strains of *Streptococcus salivarius.* Although XPS studies of cell surfaces were published almost a decade ago,[5] the use of SIMS to study cell surfaces is in its infancy. This

[a] Tel: (406) 994-6853; Fax: (406) 994-5308; E-mail: bonnie_t@erc.montana.edu
[b] A National Science Foundation Engineering Research Center.

case study is a work in progress and is presented to suggest possibilities for using SIMS as a powerful biological tool.

CASE STUDY ONE

Surface Characterization of a Commercial Medical Grade Polyetherurethane[1]

Segmented polyurethanes have been used in a wide variety of clinical devices including the total artificial heart, pacemakers, and breast augmentation implants. The mechanical properties and soft tissue compatibility of these polymers has lead to their widespread use as biomaterials. The surface region of polyurethanes, important in the biological response to the polymer, often differs from the bulk of the polymer. Processing of the polyurethane, degree of phase segregation, low molecular weight fragments, additives, and contaminants can all contribute to the polymer surface characteristics. The need to determine the surface characteristics of the polymers and to assure reproducible surface properties is critical for producing successful implants.

Biomer is a polyetherurethaneurea and it is thought to be manufactured from poly(tetramethylene oxide) (PTMO), methylene-*bis* phenyl-diisocyanate, and ethylene diamine.[6] Researchers from the University of Utah and 3M have also observed evidence of the additives BHT, santo white powder, and poly(diisopropylaminoethyl methacrylate) (DPA-EMA) in some Biomer lots.[6,7] Some lots investigated at the University of Utah contained large fractions of the poly(diisopropylaminoethyl methacrylate) while others contained none.

Both the bulk and surface properties of two lots of Biomer, lot BSP067 (1982) and lot BSUA001(1987) were studied. Bulk chemistry of the two lots was analyzed using transmission infrared spectroscopy and gel permeation chromatography. The surfaces of the two lots were analyzed using ESCA and Static SIMS.[1]

Although infrared studies did not reveal differences in the bulk chemistry of the two Biomer lots, XPS and static SIMS studies revealed significant differences in the surface chemistry. Detail from the XPS spectra of the lot BSP067 is shown in FIGURE 1. Lot BSP067 shows a significant contribution from ether moieties while this contribution is nearly absent in lot BSUA001 (FIG. 2). The binding energies of the C1s, N1s, and O1s peaks in lot BSUA001 suggest the presence of esters and amines at the surface rather than the ethers and urethanes observed in lot BSP. Depth profiles calculated from angle-resolved XPS data (FIG. 3) show that the outer 20Å of lot BSP067 is enriched with polyether. In contrast, there is no polyether present in the outer 20Å region of lot BSUA001. Positive ion SIMS spectra of these surfaces confirm the XPS results and allow us to identify the exact chemistry of the polymer surfaces. The major peaks in the SIMS spectra from lot BSP067 at 73, 71, and 73 m/z are indicative of the PTMO soft segment. Peaks from the hard segment are not seen. The major peaks in the SIMS spectra from lot BSUA001 at 128, 114, and 44 m/z are indicative of diisopropylaminoethyl methacrylate (DPA-EMA). Neither hard nor soft segment polyetherurethane peaks could be found in this spectra. The SIMS spectra also showed peaks from the additives Santowhite powder and BHT suggesting that they are also enriched at the surface.

Both the angle-dependent ESCA and SIMS showed a total absence of the ether, urethane and urea moieties in the upper 20Å of lot BSUA. The magnitude of the surface activity of the additive is striking and is comparable to that noted for a *bis*-stearamide extrusion lubricant used in Pellethane™ polyurethanes.[8] The DPA-EMA additive, however, could not be removed by extraction with any common solvent

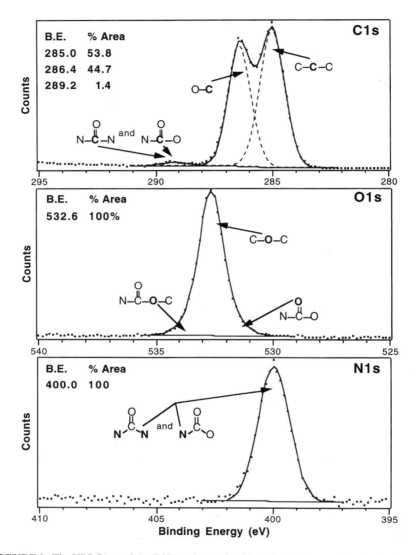

FIGURE 1. The XPS C1s peak for BSP can be resolved into three component peaks: hydrocarbon (285 eV), ether (286.4 eV) and amide (289.2 eV). The XPS N1s peak for BSP consists of a Gaussian peak at 400 eV. The XPS O1s peak for lot BSP has been fit with one 65% Gaussian peak at 532.6 eV. Ether linkages are the principal contributor to this peak. Contributions from the amide oxygens are too small to be accurately resolved.

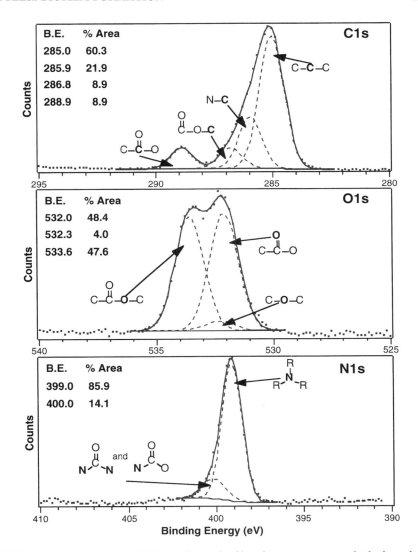

FIGURE 2. The XPS C1s for BSUA can be resolved into four component peaks: hydrocarbon (285 eV), amine (285.9 eV), and esters (286.8 eV and 288.9 eV). The N1s for BSUA can be resolved into two peaks: amine (399 eV) and amide (400 eV). The O1s peak for lot BSUA can be resolved into three peaks: two ester peaks (532.0 eV and 533.6 eV) and an ether peak (532.3 eV).

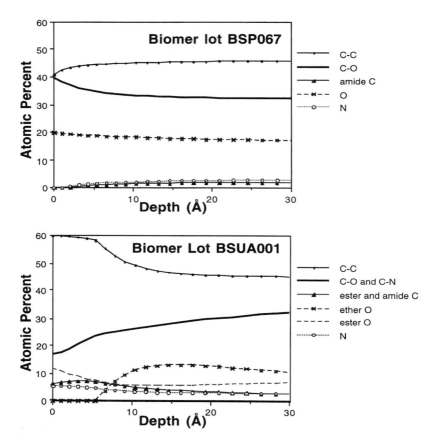

FIGURE 3. Concentration depth profiles calculated from angle dependent XPS data show the two lots have opposite trends in the surface region. Polyether functionalities are enriched in the upper 5Å–10Å of lot BSP but are completely absent in the upper 5Å–10Å of lot BSUA.

or by precipitation in methanol. In contrast, lot BSP, which did not contain the DPA-EMA additive, showed surface characteristics common for polyurethanes, including enrichment of the polyether in the surface region.

These results of this study emphasize the importance of surface sensitive analysis methods for determination of polymer surface chemistry and for the manufacture of polymers with reproducible surface properties. This study has also yielded new information about the nature of PEU surfaces. Our results indicate that both low and high molecular weight additives can significantly modify the surface character of a PEU.

In the past, concerns with additives in biomaterials have centered on their leachability and toxicity. This study suggests that the surface activity of non-leachable additives may be equally important. Because the biological response to a material is dependent on surface structure, there is reason to believe that the

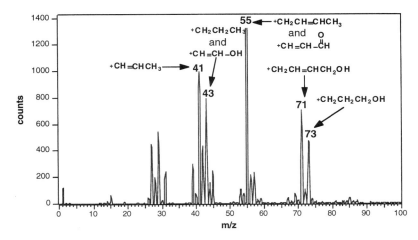

FIGURE 4. The positive ion SIMS for lot BSP contains peaks characteristic of PTMO, MDI, and an antioxidant. The negative ion SIMS for lot BSP shows only a few low m/z fragments.

additives may play a role in determining the biocompatibility of these polymers. Much controversy already exists in the literature relating to the biological interactions of Biomer. The existence of two lots differing in surface chemistry may help to explain this controversy.

Hundreds of papers have been published discussing the biological interactions of Biomer. Rarely has the lot number been specified and in most cases detailed

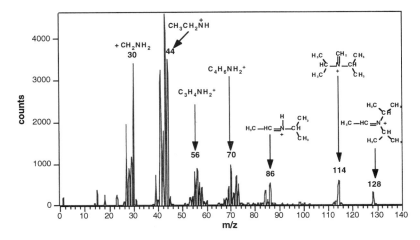

FIGURE 5. The positive ion SIMS for lot BSUA contains peaks for the DPA-EMA additive. Characteristic ions for PTMO and MDI are absent. The negative ion SIMS for lot BSUA contains methacrylate backbone peaks and peaks for the diisopropylamino ethyl side chain.

surface analysis was not performed. All of these studies must be viewed with some caution, since Biomer from different lots may have vastly different surface compositions. In fact, although no chlorine or silicon was observed in these two lots, these components have been observed by us and others at the surface of some Biomer samples. The results of this study emphasize the importance of accurate surface characterization even when using a standard commercial polymer.

CASE STUDY TWO

Investigation of Mussel Adhesive Protein Adsorption on Polystyrene and Poly(octadecylmethacrylate) Using Angle-dependent XPS, AFM, and SIMS[2-4]

The marine mussel, *Mytilus edulis,* is able to adhere tenaciously to virtually any solid surface in sea water by means of bissel thread. Mussel Adhesive Proteins (MAP) are a cocktail obtained from *M. edulis* that is believed to contain the adhesive component of the bissus. MAP contains *M. edulis* foot proteins one and two (MeFP-1 and MeFP-2) in equal quantities. MeFP-1 has a well characterized structure consisting of repeating hexa- and deca-peptide motifs with very little secondary structure.[2] Both MeFP-1 and MeFP-2 contain novel amino acids including dihydroxyphenyl-L-alanine (L-DOPA) and 4- and 3 mono and di-transhydroxyproline. It is believed that these functional groups may confer an adhesive character to the proteins but the nature of these protein-surface interactions has not been proven. The goal of this work was to identify the chemical interactions between MAP and two hydrophobic polymer surfaces, polystyrene (PS) and polyoctadecylmethacrylate (POMA).

Purified MAP was obtained from Swedish Bioscience Laboratory. PS and POMA (from Aldrich) were spin cast onto optically smooth, silanized germanium from 1.5% (W/V) solution in toluene and dried for 24 hours before protein adsorption. MAP was allowed to adsorb onto the polymer surfaces from a 50 μg/ml solution at pH 8.0 for 1 hour and then rinsed in pH 8.0 solution for 3 min at a flow rate of 100 ml/min. The surfaces were analyzed with AFM, angle-resolved XPS, ATR-FTIR and SIMS.

Angle-resolved XPS studies were performed both on dried samples and hydrated samples at liquid nitrogen temperature. Results of the angle-resolved XPS studies

TABLE 1. XPS Atomic Concentration of MAP Adsorbed to PS and POMA, Dehydrated at Room Temperature[2]

Sample	Take-off Angle	Sampling Depth	Atomic Percent		
			C	O	N
MAP	80	84.3	80.07	13.88	6.05
adsorbed to	35	49.1	78.67	14.02	7.31
polystyrene	22	32.1	74.92	16.90	8.18
	15	22.2	74.14	17.57	8.29
MAP	80	84.3	88.66	10.02	1.32
adsorbed to	35	49.1	88.10	10.87	1.03
POMA	22	32.1	90.25	8.54	1.21
	15	22.2	91.30	7.60	1.09

TABLE 2. XPS Atomic Concentration as Determined by XPS of MAP Adsorbed to PS and POMA, Hydrated at LN$_2$ Temperature[3]

Sample	Take-off Angle	Sampling Depth	Atomic Percent		
			C	O	N
MAP	80	84.3	79.21	14.46	6.33
adsorbed to	35	49.1	74.78	16.15	9.08
polystyrene	22	32.1	68.73	19.41	11.85
	10	22.2	66.95	20.01	13.04
MAP	80	84.3	79.10	16.55	4.34
adsorbed to	35	49.1	79.76	15.61	4.63
POMA	22	32.1	77.69	17.00	5.31
	15	22.2	77.41	16.68	5.92

are shown in TABLES 1 and 2. Take-off angles are measured from the surface. Although ATR-FTIR results suggest approximately equal amounts of protein on both surfaces, XPS results show consistently higher nitrogen content on the MAP/PS styrene surface. The nitrogen content on the MAP/PS surface increases at glancing take-off angle (lower sampling depth) but the nitrogen content on the POMA/PS surface remains nearly constant as the take-off angle is varied.

The data in TABLES 1 and 2 suggest that the adsorbed MAP on POMA is patchy with protein islands greater than the XPS sampling depth. The MAP on PS forms

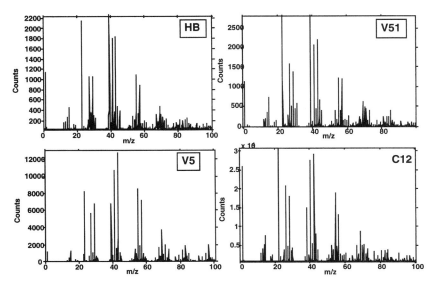

FIGURE 6. Low mass region of positive SIMS spectra for four strains of *S. salivarius*. Peaks are indicative of proteins, sugars, and hydrocarbons on the surface.

a thinner more contiguous film. When the samples are analyzed hydrated, more nitrogen is seen on both samples. Trends with take-off angle are similar to those for the dehydrated samples. The hydrated film suggests both films are more contiguous when hydrated.

AFM studies of hydrated and dehydrated samples confirm the XPS data. The AFM images of the MAP on POMA show a fibrous network on the surface. The surface is very heterogeneous with large fiber like structure up to 19 nm in height and 179 nm in width with some as long as 2.4 μm. The MAP/PS surface showed closely packed, round, repeating structures averaging 9.48 nm in height and 33.02 nm in width.[2,3]

At a pH of 8, the catechol functionality on the L-DOPA can undergo a spontaneous reverse dismutation to the o-quinone that is capable of interacting through a quinhydron charge-transfer complex. This reaction, which is catalyzed in the marine mussel, allows fiber formation in the MAP similar to those seen on the POMA surface. No fibers were seen on the polystyrene surface.[2] We hypothesize that protein orients its aromatic residues (L-DOPA and tyrosine) toward the polystyrene surface to maximize pi-pi interactions with the surface. This pi-pi bonding with the surface prevents the formation of the quinhydron charge-transfer complex. The pi-pi bonding also causes the protein layer to be more tightly bound to the surface so that the film remains nearly contiguous even when dehydrated.

SIMS analysis of the surfaces also supports this hypothesis.[4] Polyaminoacid fragments from the deca-peptide sequence are seen on both surfaces. On the POMA surface the predominant polypeptide seen contains L-DOPA showing that the aromatic groups are present in the upper 20Å. On the PS surface tyrosine and L-DOPA are not seen suggesting that they are oriented toward the polymer surface.[4]

This case study demonstrates that the functional groups present on PS and POMA polymer surfaces will influence MAP-MAP and MAP-surface interactions. The study emphasizes complimentary nature of XPS, AFM, and SIMS.

CASE STUDY THREE

SIMS Studies of Four Strains of Streptococcus salivarius

The outermost surface of baterial cells plays a crucial role in bacterial adhesion phenomena. The chemical composition and structural arrangement of the cells surface is extremely complex due to the presence of a large variety of chemical components and surface appendages of different lengths. Gram positive bacteria have a well defined, rigid cell wall consisting of a 15 to 30 nm thick peptidoglycan layer which commonly supports a layer of proteinaceous surface appendages which can vary in length from 50 to 400 nm.[9]

The gram positive *S. salivarius* strains used in this study were obtained, freeze dried courtesy of H. J. Busscher and H. C. van der Mei.[5] The four strains studied include *S. salivarius* HB and three mutants (V5, V51, and C12) that show an increasing loss of the proteinaceous fibrillar layer. The surfaces of the four strains have been extensively characterized for antigenic composition, presence or absence of surface appendages,[10] the relative amounts of lipo(teichoic acid)/teichoic acid exposed at the surface, the surface free energy,[11] adhesive behavior,[12] infrared spectrum,[13] and zeta potentials.[5] The elemental composition of the surface of the freeze-dried cells has been published by van der Mei *et al.*[5] The objective of this work is to determine the utility of SIMS for measuring these cell surface properties.

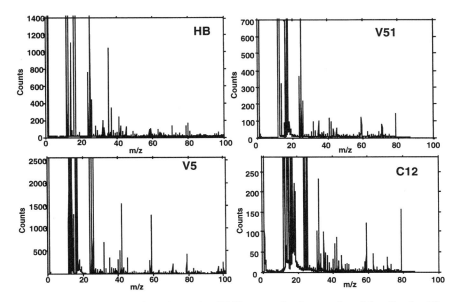

FIGURE 7. Low mass region of negative SIMS spectra for four strains of *S. salivarius*. The peak at 42 (CNO) is characteristic of proteins and the peak at 79 (PO3) is indicative of teichoic acid.

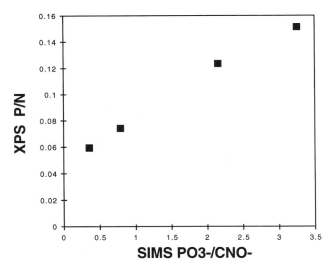

FIGURE 8. The SIMS PO_3^-/CNO^- ratio shows a strong correlation to the XPS P/N ratio.

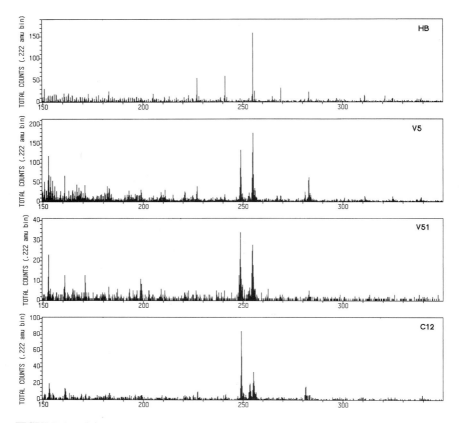

FIGURE 9. High mass region of the negative SIMS spectra of four strains of *S. salivarius*. Peaks at 255 m/z and 161 m/z are indicative of teichoic acid.

SIMS spectra of the freeze-dried cells were collected on an PHI/Evans TRIFT Time of Flight Secondary Ion Mass Spectrometer with a Cs Ion source. In all cases, the total ion dose was kept below 10^{12} ions/cm² to insure that the static limit was not exceeded. In the low mass region of the positive ion spectra (FIG. 6) peaks for sodium, potassium, calcium and clusters of organic ions can be identified. The spectra indicate the presence of proteins, hydrocarbons, and carbohydrates. Although differences in the peak intensity ratio's for the different strains can be observed, simple correlations between these data and known surface characteristics of the cells have not yet been identified. The low mass region of the negative ion spectra are shown in FIGURE 7. Key peaks can be seen at 42 m/z (CNO^-) indicative of protein and 79 m/z (PO_3^-) indicative of the teichoic acid cell wall. FIGURE 8 shows the SIMS PO_3^-/CNO^- peak ratio plotted against XPS N/P ratio measured by van der Mei *et al.*[5] The correlation is excellent.

The high mass region of the negative ion spectra shown in FIGURE 9 for all the cell strains shows peaks at 255 m/z and 161 m/z that are indicative of teichoic

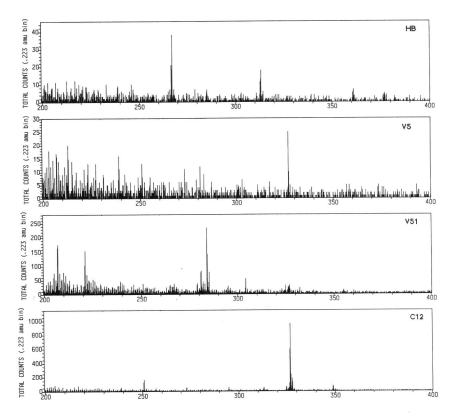

FIGURE 10. High mass region of the positive SIMS spectra of four strains of *S. salivarius*. The peaks show distinctive differences between the four strains. The peak at 327 m/z seen on the mutant strains is absent in the parent HB strain.

acid. Peaks at 249 m/z and 155 m/z are present only on the mutant strains. FIGURE 10 shows the high mass region of the positive ion spectra from the four strains. Only the mutant strains show a peak at 327 m/z. Obvious differences between the spectra suggest distinct molecular species on the surface of each strain.

These preliminary results demonstrate that SIMS is sensitive to cell surface differences in the four strains of *S. salivarius*. A simple correlation between the SIMS spectra and XPS results has been identified and teichoic acid fragments are evident on the cell surfaces. These initial results indicate great promise for probing cell surface chemistry with SIMS. Future work will include expanding the data set by including SIMS spectra from other cells characterized by van der Mei,[5,11-13] exploration of multivariate correlations between the SIMS data sets and other measured surface properties, analysis of model compounds to aid in the assignment of SIMS fragments, and analysis of frozen hydrated cells.

SUMMARY

Although the importance of cell adhesion to synthetic surfaces is well established, a detailed description of the molecular interactions important in adhesion still eludes researchers. In order to fully understand the adhesion events that lead to biofilm formation on synthetic materials it is necessary to have an accurate understanding of the synthetic material surface, to understand the composition and orientation of biopolymers that adsorb to the material, and to understand the surface chemistry of cells that ultimately adhere. The simplest of these three surfaces, the synthetic material, commonly presents a profound level of complexity and presents a wide variety of chemical functional groups in many orientations at the surface. The conditioning film surface and cell surface show yet greater levels of complexity. The three case studies presented here demonstrate that XPS and SIMS are valuable techniques for studying all three of these surfaces. They are not only capable of providing an accurate analysis of the synthetic polymer surface but they are also sensitive to the composition and orientation of biomolecules. The potential for rapid characterization of cell surfaces with SIMS demonstrated in the final case study suggests that intelligent application of these techniques may ultimately aid in answering the elusive question of how cells adhere to synthetic surfaces.

REFERENCES

1. TYLER, B. J., B. D. RATNER D. G. CASTNER & D. BRIGGS. 1992.
2. BATY, A. M., P. A. SUCI, B. J. TYLER & G. G. GEESEY. 1996. J. Colloid Interface Sci. **177:** 307–315.
3. BATY, A. M. 1995. Master's Thesis, Montana State University.
4. SCHAMBERGER, P. C., A. M. BATY, B. FROLAND, B. J. TYLER, G. G. GEESEY, P. J. MCKEOWN & L. E. DAVIS. 1995. Surfaces and Biomaterials, Sept.
5. VAN DER MEI, H. C., A. J. LEONARD, A. H. WEERKAMP P. G. ROUXHET & H. J. BUSSCHER. J. Bacteriol. **170:** 2462–2466.
6. BELISLE, J., S. K. MAIER & J. A. TUCKER. 1990. J. Biomed. Mater. Res. **24:** 1585–1598.
7. RICHARDS, J. M., W. H. MCCLENNEN & H. L. C. MEUZELAAR. 1990. J. Appl. Polym. Sci. **40:** 1–12.
8. RATNER, B. D. 1983. In Physicochemical Aspects of Polymer Surfaces, vol. 2. Plenum Publishing Corp. New York, p. 969.
9. HANDLEY, P. S., P. I. CARTER & J. FIELDING. 1984. J. Bacteriol. **157:** 64–72.
10. WEERKAMP, A. H., P. S. HANDLEY, A. BAARS & J. W. SLOT. 1987. J. Bacteriol. **165:** 746–755.
11. VAN DER MEI, H. C., A. J. LEONARD, A. H. WEERKAMP P. G. ROUXHET & H. J. BUSSCHER. 1982. Colloids and Surfaces **32:** 297–305.
12. VAN DER MEI, H. C., A. H. WEERKAMP & H. J. BUSSCHER. 1987. J. Microbiol. Meth. **6:** 277–287.
13. VAN DER MEI, H. C., J. NOORDMANS & H. J. BUSSCHER. 1989. Biochim. Biophys. Acta **991:** 395–398.

Bacterial Infection of Biomaterials

Experimental Protocol for *in Vitro* Adhesion Studies[a]

JAMES D. BRYERS[b] AND SARA HENDRICKS

Department of Chemical Engineering and
The Center For Biofilm Engineering[c]
Montana State University
Bozeman, Montana 59717

Modern medical and surgical therapy is predicated on the use of catheters and endoprosthestic implants. Patients faced with death or disability are now routinely restored to health because of artificial organs, organ supplements, ventricular assist devices, and assorted endoprostheses. The production of biomaterials in the U.S. is a \$400 million per year industry. It is estimated that over 5 million artificial or prosthetic parts are implanted per annum in the United States alone.[1] However, over half of hospital-acquired infections are associated with implants or indwelling medical devices; with the case-to-fatality ratio of these infections ranging between 5–60%.[1,2] Bacterial infections by adherent bacteria have been observed[1] on prosthetic heart valves (valve endocarditis), cardiac pacemakers, vascular prostheses, intravascular catheters, cerebrospinal fluid shunts, orthopedic implants, urinary catheters, ocular prostheses and contact lenses, and intrauterine contraceptive devices (IUCDs).

The body reacts to prosthetic implants by coating them with a film comprising various proteins (*e.g.*, fibronectin, laminin, fibrin, collagen, immunoglobulins) some or all of which can serve as binding ligands to the receptors of colonizing bacteria. Bacteria, transported to the substratum by either molecular diffusion or convective transport, can adhere by either a nonspecific adhesion mechanism (governed by electrostatic forces acting between the cell and surface) or a specific adhesion binding reaction. Certain cell surface molecules, termed "receptors" can bind to specific molecules, termed "ligands," found on the substratum. Once attached to the substratum, bacteria can produce copious amounts of extracellular mucopolysaccharides[3,4] that bind divalent cations, forming a tenacious matrix of extracellular polymers.[5] These bacterial polymers can mix with those of other species, polymers of host cells, or blood platelets to form a mixed-cell line biofilm that is highly resistant to rigorous antibiotic challenges.[6-8] Dankert *et al.*[1] and Jacques *et al.*[9]

[a] The authors would like to thank both the National Science Foundation (BES-94 104 29 and EEC-89 07 039) and the Engineering Foundation for their financial and intellectual support of this effort.
[b] Address correspondence to Dr. Bryers at The Center for Biomaterials, The University of Connecticut, Farmington, CT 06030-1615. Tel: (860) 679-7568; Fax: (860) 679-1370; E-mail: JBryers@nso2.uchc.edu
[c] A National Science Foundation Engineering Research Center.

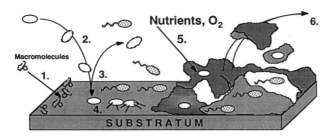

FIGURE 1. Processes governing biofilm formation. Numbered processes defined in text.

provide excellent reviews of the bacterial infections associated with a myriad of indwelling biomedical devices.

Processes Governing Bacterial Biofilm Formation: A Process Analysis

Microbial cells (predominantly bacteria) and their extracellular polymers associated with a substratum are called *biofilms*.[10,11] Bacterial attachment, biofilm formation and persistence are governed by a complex set of physical, chemical, and biological processes all acting simultaneously. The reader is directed to a number of excellent review articles[10–13] that provide substantially more detail on each process and on the overall biofilm formation phenomenon.

As shown in FIGURE 1, development of a bacterial biofilm comprises the following fundamental processes: 1) substratum pre-conditioning by adsorption of fluid phase organic molecules; bacterial cell deposition to the conditioned substratum; 2) cell transport to the surface; 3) cell desorption; 4) cell adhesion to the substratum; 5) bacterial metabolism (cell substrate conversion; cell growth and replication; extracellular exopolymer production; cell starvation, death, lysis); and 6) biofilm removal (cell and biofilm detachment; biofilm sloughing). Naturally, the relative influence of each process is dependent upon the specific system, the prevailing environmental conditions, and slow biological changes throughout the lifetime of the biofilm.

Simple unstructured models of biofilm formation can be written. Biofilm formation is assumed to occur on surfaces exposed to a well mixed bulk fluid phase; thus, tacitly neglecting any spatial heterogeneity in the bulk liquid. Any mass transfer limitations in the bulk liquid will only complicate the already difficult task of determining the kinetics of a heterogeneous reaction. Suspended biomass in the bulk liquid arises owing either to cell growth and replication or to detachment of biofilm material. Planktonic cells leave the liquid phase by either the effluent liquid leaving the reactor volume or by cell deposition onto the reactor surfaces. A single sterile growth limiting substrate, S, enters the reactor where it is consumed by either the suspended or biofilm-bound cells. Any reasonable measure of both biofilm and suspended cell concentrations is acceptable (cell number, biomass dry weight, biomass organic carbon). However, to complete the material balances over the entire system, one most know the stoichiometric relationship between changes in the suspended and attached cell concentrations due to growth and the limiting substrate utilized.

FIGURE 2. Progression of both liquid phase and surface parameters during mixed culture biofilm formation in a completely mixed rotating annular reactor operated at a dilution rate well in excess of the culture maximum growth rate.[15] Lines represent predictions of a computer simulation of an unstructured model.

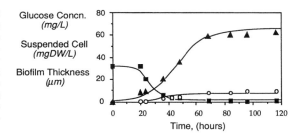

Based on these assumptions, material balances for both the suspended cell biomass and single growth limiting substrate can be written as equations **1** and **2**,

Suspended biomass balance:
$$VdX/dt = -FX + R_{gs}V + R_{det}A - R_{dep}A \tag{1}$$

Limiting substrate balance:
$$VdS/dt = F(S_{in} - S) - [R_{gs}V/Y_{X/S}] - [R_{gb}A/Y_{B/S}] \tag{2}$$

where X = suspended cell biomass (M/L^3), S = limiting substrate concentration (M/L^3), V = reactor volume (L^3), R_{gs} = rate of suspended cell growth ($M/T-L^3$); R_{det} = rate of biofilm detachment ($M/T-L^2$); R_{dep} = net rate of bacterial cell deposition at a substratum ($M/T-L^2$); R_{gb} = rate of adherent cell growth ($M/T-L^2$); $Y_{X/S}$ = yield coefficient for suspended cells (M_x/M_s), $Y_{B/S}$ = yield coefficient for biofilm mass (M_x/M_s), and A = reactor area (L^2). Rate expressions for the remaining process rates (R_{gs}, R_{det}, R_{dep}, R_{gb}) have been defined by Bryers and Characklis[14] with several depending directly on changing biofilm amount, limiting substrate and suspended biomass concentration.

Biofilm net accumulation can be described by equation **3**,

$$\textit{Biofilm net accumulation}: A[dB/dt = R_{dep} + R_{gb} - R_{det}] \tag{3}$$

where B = concentration of adherent bacterial cells or biofilm amount (M/L^2).

Since rate expressions for both planktonic and biofilm growth are non-linear saturation kinetic functions of the instantaneous substrate concentration and first order functions of X and B, respectively, equations **1–3** are coupled, non-linear ordinary differential equations that require either simultaneous numerical integration (for the transient situation) or simultaneous algebraic solution under conditions of steady-state (*i.e.*, dS/dt, dX/dt, and $dB/dt = 0$). Numerous biofilm accumulation studies have been carried out that can be mathematically described by the above set of equations, as shown in FIGURE 2. Should the reactor be operated at a hydraulic residence time shorter than the generation time of the cells, then one can assume the term $[R_{gs}V]$ is negligible; however, the corresponding term in equation **2** representing suspended cell substrate metabolism $[R_{gs}V/Y_{X/S}]$ cannot be disregarded unless in the specific system it is determined small compared to the other terms or substrate is not supplied.

In a simple bacterial adhesion study, experiments can be carried out without exogenous substrate, thus the R_g terms in equations **1–3** could be ignored. Thus, equation **3** becomes,

$$dB/dt = R_{dep} - R_{det} \qquad (4)$$

and is valid for as long as adherent bacterial replication is zero.

Bacterial Adhesion to Biomaterials: "What's Wrong with This Experiment?"

Unfortunately most, if not all, studies on cell adhesion carried out in the biomaterials literature fail to recognize that the total number of cells attached to a surface at any given time is the net result of not only cell adhesion but also cell desorption and cell replication. Substratum chemistry variations or environmental changes (flow velocity, nutrient conditions, *etc.*) may influence adhesion processes or growth of adherent cells but not detachment, or vice versa, thus making any correlations of net accumulation to the varied parameters difficult at best. Consequently, only a limited number of studies provide data that can be extrapolated with confidence to system conditions that mimic indwelling prosthetic devices.

Over a 6 year period from 1990–1996, a total of 134 cell "adhesion studies" reported in the biomaterials literature (*i.e.*, J. Biomed. Mater. Res.; Biomaterials; J. Med. Microbiol.), almost 91% were carried out as batch reactors, under stagnant fluid conditions, with no assessment of the time-dependent fluid chemical conditions. Consider a typical "adhesion study." Suppose one wishes to assess a new material pre-treatment for its ability to prevent cell adhesion and subsequent infection. Typically, samples of both a material control and the treated material will be exposed to one or more bacterial species. These bacteria will be cultivated in shake-flask batch cultures, using trypticase soy broth or brain heart infusion media to a pre-set point in their growth; typically mid- to late-exponential growth phase. Cells are then centrifuged, separated from the used culture media, washed several times in buffered saline solution, and retained for use as an inoculum for the "adhesion study." The material samples are placed in individual petri dishes, a solution of fresh media at approximately 15 g/L used to cover the material, and the bacterial concentrate above used to inoculate the solution. At some pre-set time period, the material sample is withdrawn, washed a number of times with saline buffer, and the adherent cells determined. Example of the results of such an adhesion study are shown in FIGURE 3A and replotted versus time in 3B; no citation is provided out of courtesy to the authors.

Consider the number of experimental flaws inherent to the above experiment, in light of the discussion of biofilm formation processes above. Assume that the goal in this study is to determine the effects of PEO pre-treatment on bacterial "adhesion." First, the biomaterials were submerged in nutrient broth at a concentration of 15 g/L and open to the atmosphere so that one can expect cell growth to occur within the fluid phase once inoculated. Consequently, the biomaterial will be exposed to time-dependent conditions of fluid nutrient and suspended cell concentration. Any cells attaching to the surface will also grow in this luxuriant environment so that changes in adherent cell numbers would be due not only to cell adhesion but also to cells desorbing and cells replicating. Hydrodynamic conditions, if any, are ill-defined at best and cell movement to and from the surface could be by either sedimentation, diffusion for non-motile, by motility for flagellated bacteria. Consequently, any "adhesion kinetics" could be transport limited and resultant data in reality would reflect the kinetics of these other slower processes.

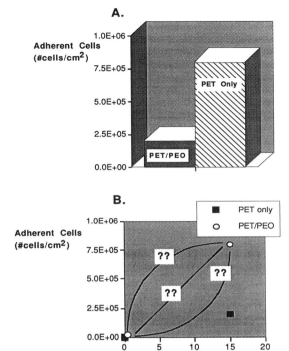

FIGURE 3. A and **B**. Original data (**A**) and time course rendition (**B**) of data for *Pseudomonas aeruginosa* exposed to PET and PEO-treated PET biomaterial samples submerged in quiescent petri dishes filled with 15 g/L trypticase soy broth.

Differences in adherent cell numbers between the two biomaterials could be due to the effects of PEO on cell adhesion but they could also be the result of PEO effects on either adherent bacterial desorption or PEO effects on adherent cell growth. Given that data were collected at only one time point, no kinetic information is possible. Other subtle flaws include: a) use of stock lab cultures as bacterial sources versus clinical isolates; the former cells often losing much of their surface adhesion structures upon repeated passages, b) washing the cells of the inoculum which also removes critically important surface adhesion structures, and c) destructive sampling and washing of biomaterials which can dislodge adherent cells biasing results.

EXPERIMENTAL PROTOCOL FOR BACTERIAL ADHESION TO BIOMATERIALS: BEST PRACTICES

Biofilm Reactor Systems Prerequisites

Irrespective of the application or study objective, a biofilm experimental system must contain certain critical components: a) the biofilm study reactor itself (where the surface accumulation of cells and biofilm will be studied) and b) the environmental support system which controls the experimental conditions (*e.g.*, temperature, flow velocity, nutrient concentrations, pH). Owing to the possibilities of mass transfer limitations of dissolved nutrients and particulates (*i.e.*, the bacteria) to the target surface, we only recommend those experimental systems that create a flow of the bulk fluid phase; otherwise, instead of truly determining bacterial adhesion kinetics, your data will erroneously reflect cell sedimentation rates or surface growth rate limitations. Flow of the bulk liquid in a biofilm experiment can be mandated for several overlapping reasons: to study biofilm accumulation either a) as a function of fluid velocity or shear stress, b) as a function of a nutritional limitation or kinetic parameter (nutrients or growth rate) in a simulated flow environment, or c) as a means of eliminating any potential mass transfer rate limitations.

The experimental laboratory system operating *in vitro* should have the ability to control or vary a number of experimental parameters as summarized in TABLE 1. Control of experimental parameters is the luxury of *in vitro* laboratory systems. While certain parameters may not be controlled in field studies or *in vivo* situations, the reactor system should at least provide for their determination.

Diagnostic Methods

The diagnostic tools and experimental systems employed to study bacterial attachment and biofilm formation processes depend to large extent upon the scope of the specific problem. In a biomaterials context, most studies are interested in bacterial cell adhesion (although as shown oftentimes the conditions are such that cell replication is inadvertently promoted) and thus are only interested in analyzing the dynamics of early adhesion-desorption events (eq. **4**) and relating those dynamics to properties of the substratum. Other studies (*e.g.*, antibiotic efficacy against established biofilms, interaction between an established biofilm and host phagocytic cells) may require techniques that analyze such dynamics spatially within a biofilm. Here, we will review briefly the methods available to sample and analyze bacterial attachment and biofilm formation processes.

Invasive Sampling

Detection of biofilms often requires direct sampling and removal of a finite quantity of attached material from a reactor surface for a number of destructive analytical procedures that measure overall biofilm amount (cell mass or biofilm thickness), a component of the biofilm structure (biofilm carbon, cell number, biofilm protein), or biofilm cell activity (ATP, dehydrogenase activity, active DNA synthesis). Reactor designs to provide access for destructive sampling involve remov-

TABLE 1. Experimental Variables

Chemical Parameters	Physical Parameters	Biological Parameters
Substrate type	Temperature	Microorganism type
Substrate concentration	Fluid shear stress	Culture type (mixed vs. pure)
pH	Heat flux	Suspended cell concentration
Inorganic ions	Surface composition	Antagonist organisms
Dissolved oxygen	Surface texture	
Microbial inhibitors	Fluid residence time	

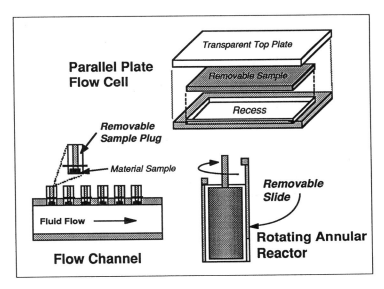

FIGURE 4. Examples of different types of removable reactor test surfaces.

able sections of substratum; some of which are quite arcane, other rather ingenious. However, all destructive sampling devices have some impact on the construction of the reactor. Examples of three different removable sample techniques are presented in FIGURE 4.

Almost any parameter determined by any molecular (ATP, DNA, total protein, specific enzyme, oligonucleotide probes), cytochemical (acridine orange, DAPI, Hoechst stains) or immunofluorescent staining, or cellular activity (CTC, INT, plate counting) technique that has been applied to planktonic (freely suspended) cells can be used to quantifying changes in cell concentrations on a substratum. Note: sample acquisition is itself a "system invasive" process and the subsequent analytical techniques are all sample destructive. Another drawback to destructive analyses is that the parameter value determined represents an average over the entire sample, which ignores any spatial variations in that parameter that may exist.

Non-invasive Diagnostics

The "holy grail" of biofilm researchers is an analytical method that causes as little disturbance to the biofilm and the reactor operation as possible. Regrettably, most parameters of interest in cell adhesion and biofilm accumulation require destructive sampling and analyses.

True non-invasive diagnostics of biofilm accumulation, amount, and biofilm-cell reactivity are limited to relatively few sophisticated techniques. The simplest of these techniques is on-line microscopy that places the biofilm reactor within the viewing field of a microscope. This technique requires a reactor dimension compatible with the microscope; preferably a flat reactor surface on which to focus and

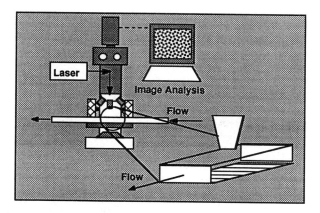

FIGURE 5. On-line surveillance of bacterial cell adhesion using conventional light or confocal laser scanning microscopy under flowing fluid conditions.

obviously a reactor that is transparent. Microscopic observation of adherent cells can be quantified and preserved by use of video recorders or image analyzer systems that digitize observed images and saves those images on a computer for future numerical interpretations (FIG. 5).

For about ten years, confocal scanning laser microscopy (CSLM) has been a tool in the biological sciences. CSLM use confocal apertures or "pinholes" to create a thin (0.4 μm) depth-of-field which eliminates out-of-focus light. Laser light sources provide the intense, highly coherent, collimated light necessary to penetrate thick specimens. The laser light is used to excite fluorophores, either those intrinsic (chlorophyll) to the sample or selected chemical or immunological stains intentionally applied to the sample. Resultant fluorescence is detected by a photomultiplier and a digital image collected. Using a computer-manipulated stage, optical sections in a three-dimensional grid can be collected. This allows for the first time the ability to digitally locate cells on a substratum or within a biofilm, non-invasively.[16] Fluorochromes are available that can be used to localize and measure intracellular and extracellular conditions in three dimensions within living biofilms. Camper *et al.*[17] report developing an image analysis software that has been used to collect images of bacterial adhesion patterns from the CSLM, digitize those images, then superimpose those images onto similar digitized images collected from any one of a number of other analytical instruments (*e.g.*, X-ray photoelectron spectroscopy, atomic force microscopy, Time-of-Flight Secondary Ion Mass Spectroscopy); all images collected at the same location on the substratum. Use of these latter surface chemical analytical instruments (XPS and TOF-SIMS) for biomaterials diagnostics will be detailed by other contributions in this volume.

Another technique that has been used to collect, non-invasively, information on the molecular chemistry of cell adhesion is Attenuated Total Reflectance (ATR) waveguides integrated within flow cells coupled with Fourier Transform Infrared Spectroscopy (FT-IR). Atoms and groups of atoms within a molecule vibrate with a characteristic frequency and will absorb light at these frequencies. Light containing infra-red frequencies can be focused on a molecule and the amount of light absorbed measured as a function of frequency. Specific IR absorptions can thus be assigned to particular bonds and alterations in these bonds due to changes in local environment can be assessed from resultant spectral details. Recent increases in the capability of FT-IRs and the focusing of the IR wave within specific crystal waveguides (germanium or zinc selenide crystals) allows one to establish a standing IR evanescent wave at the surface of the crystal. Fourier transform signal processing and multiple scanning allows aqueous samples to be processed where the IR spectra of molecules directly adjacent to the waveguide can be collected. In biological systems the IR absorbance of water must be subtracted via computer manipulations to provide the IR spectra of molecules accumulating at the crystal surface. The effective depth of penetration for the evanescent IR wave is a function of crystal material and the wavenumber but ranges around 0.3–0.7 μm, thus providing spectra that reflect those chemical species directly adjacent to the surface.

ATR/FT-IR has been used to study the effects of protein conditioning films on alginate adsorption to the germanium surface.[18] Alginate adsorbed in greater quantities to protein-coated ATR crystals than to uncoated ones. For the development of biofilms on ATR crystals, the resultant spectrum is the integral of all biomolecules on the surface and over the entire surface. Bremer and Geesey[19] report the chemical changes that occur, after inoculating with a microbial culture, at a germanium ATR crystal situated within a flow cell as detected by FT-IR. Spectral intensities representing various bonds within proteins (amide I at 1645 cm^{-1}; amide II at 1550 cm^{-1}) and polysaccharide (C-O stretches at 1058 cm^{-1}) are seen to accumulate with time indicating the feasibility of the ATR/FT-IR system to detect biofilm formation (FIG. 6). Since the IR wave can only penetrate less than 1 μm into the biofilm, the reported increases in absorbance intensities most likely

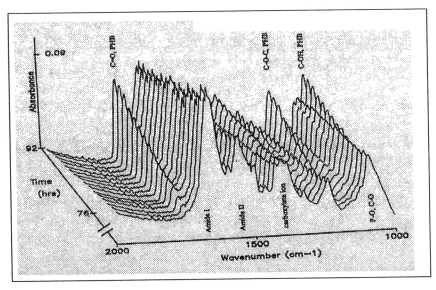

FIGURE 6. Three-dimensional plot of time-dependent ATR-FT-IR spectra showing characteristic protein, polysaccharide, and poly-β-hydroxybutyrate production at a surface of a germanium crystal.[21]

indicate increases in cell surface coverage of the crystal and not increases in biofilm thickness. A plot of attached cells per area versus the increases in area under the amide I peak was generated to estimate a lower limit of detection by FT-IR of ~5 × 10^5 cells/cm^2. In a medical application, ATR/FT-IR was used to follow the penetration of an antibiotic (100 μg/mL ciprofloxacin) into the IR wave region underneath a *Pseudomonas aeruginosa* biofilm.[20] Transport of the antibiotic was monitored using the IR bands at 1303 and 1270 cm^{-1}.

Most of the on-line, non-invasive techniques above are carried out within parallel plate flow cells that are most often constant in cross-sectional area down the entire length of the channel. One alternative design, an intentional expansion in channel width, can be employed to affect turbulence and controlled flow separation in the channel. The main advantage of a parallel plate flow cell is that on-line, non-invasive microscopic observations of cell adhesion at an inner surface can be carried out continuously on the microscope stage (FIG. 5). The reader must be aware, that although rectangular flow cells can subject attaching bacterial cells to either laminar or turbulent flow conditions, with known surface velocities and shear stresses, calculation of the Reynolds Number and surface shear stresses are different for rectangular versus circular cross-sections. A specific volumetric flow rate applied to a circular tube will not establish the same fluid velocity, Reynolds Number, or shear stresses in a rectangular duct.

To create flow separation (*i.e.*, turbulence) in a rectangular flow cell while still at a low flow velocity, a variable cross-sectional area can be employed. To study endothelial cell responses to complex flows, one can simulate regions of flow separation observed *in vivo* using a conventional parallel plate flow chamber modified to produce an asymmetric sudden expansion . The asymmetric sudden expansion flow path is created using a medical grade silicone rubber gasket inserted between the two plates. Thickness of the gasket sets the expansion. At the gasket edge the wall shear stress is zero and its magnitude increases with increasing distance from the gasket edge until a maximum is reached. Then, the shear stress declines, passing through zero at the separation point, until it reaches its final value downstream. The size of the recirculation zone, which represents the distance from the gasket edge to the point at which the wall shear stress is zero, depends upon the Reynolds Number and the expansion ratio. In general, for a given expansion ratio, the size of the recirculation zone increases linearly with Reynolds Number until a critical Reynolds Number is reached and additional recirculation eddies appear.[22,23]

SUMMARY

Some of the more common reactor systems and novel diagnostic tools employed in the study of bacterial cell adhesion and biofilm formation have been described. Sampling and experimental requirements are shown to greatly influence the design and construction of a biofilm reactor. As analytical techniques evolve, the capability to non-invasively follow the development of biofilms and to assess the attached cell reactivity has increased. Both non-invasive and invasive diagnostic methods affect the type and design of biofilm flow reactor with both types of analyses providing complementary information on biofilm processes. To correctly interpret the contribution of a specific rate process to the net accumulation of cells at a substratum, one requires a reactor system devoid of any mass transfer limitations and a process analysis approach to allow for the correct collection and analysis of data.

REFERENCES

1. DANKERT, J., A. H. HOGT & J. FEIJEN. 1986. *In* CRC Critical Reviews in Biocompatibility **2(3):** 219–301.
2. STAMM, W. E. 1978. Ann. Intern. Med. **89:** 764.
3. APPLEGATE, D. H. & J. D. BRYERS. 1991. Biotechnol. Bioeng. **37:** 17–25.
4. DAVIES, D. G., A. M. CHAKRABARTY & G. G. GEESEY. 1993. Appl. Environ. Microbiol. **59:** 1181–1186.
5. COSTERTON, J. W., R. T. IRVIN & K. J. CHENG. 1981. Ann. Rev. Microbiol. **35:** 299–324.
6. MILLS, J., L. PULLIAM, L. DULL, J. MARZOUK, W. WILSON & J. W. COSTERTON. Infect. Immun. **43:** 359–367.
7. NICKEL, J. C., J. HEATON, A. MORALES & J. W. COSTERTON. 1986. J. Urol. **135:** 586–588.
8. BROWN, M. R. W., D. G. ALLISON & P. GILBERT. 1988. Antimicrob. Chemother. **22:** 777–780.
9. JACQUES, M., T. J. MARRIE & J. W. COSTERTON. 1987. Microb. Ecol. **13:** 173–191.
10. CHARACKLIS, W. G. & K. C. MARSHALL. 1990. Biofilms. J. Wiley & Sons. New York.
11. CHARACKLIS, W. G. & P. A. WILDERER, Eds. 1989. Structure and Function of Biofilms. Dahlem Conference Life Science Research Report Nr. 46. J. Wiley & Sons. Berlin.
12. BRYERS, J. D. 1988. *In* Physiological Models in Microbiology, Vol. II. M. J. Bazin & J. I. Prosser, Eds.: 1091. CRC Press. Boca Raton, FL.
13. MARSHALL, K. C., Ed. 1984. Microbial Adhesion and Aggregation. Dahlem Conference Life Science Research Report Nr. 31. Springer-Verlag. Berlin.
14. BRYERS, J. D. & W. G. CHARACKLIS. 1996. *In* Biofilms—Science and Technology. Kluwer Academic Publishers. The Netherlands, pp. 221–237.
15. TRULEAR, M. G. 1983. Cellular Reproduction and Extracellular Polymer Formation in the Development of Biofilms. Ph.D. Dissertation, Montana State University, Bozeman, MT.
16. BRELJE, T. C., M. W. WESSENDORF & R. L. SORENSON. 1993. Methods in Cell Biol. **38:** 97–181.
17. CAMPER, A. C., M. A. HAMILTON, K. R. JOHNSON & P. STOODLEY, G. J. HARKIN & D. S. DALY. 1994. Ultrapure Water **11:** 26–35.
18. ISHIDA, K. P. & P. R. GRIFFITHS. 1993. J. Colloid Interface Sci. **160:** 190–200.
19. BREMER, P. J. & G. G. GEESEY. 1991. Biofouling **3:** 89–100.
20. SUCI, P. A., M. W. MITTLEMAN, F. P. YU & G. G. GEESEY. Antimicrob. Agents Chemother. **38:** 2127–2133.
21. NIVENS, D. E., R. J. PALMER & D. C. WHITE. 1995. J. Industrial Microbiol. **15:** 263–276.
22. ARMALY, B. F., F. DURST, J. C. F. PEREIRA & B. SCHONUNG. 1983. J. Fluid Mech. **127:** 473–496.
23. MACAGNO, E. O. & T. K. HUNG. 1967. J. Fluid Mech. **28:** 43.

Fibrinogen-dependent Adherence of Macrophages to Surfaces Coated with Poly(ethylene oxide)/Poly(propylene oxide) Triblock Copolymers[a]

STEPHEN M. O'CONNOR,[b,d] SAMANTHA J. PATUTO,[c]
STEVIN H. GEHRKE,[b] AND GREGORY S. RETZINGER[c]

[b]Department of Chemical Engineering
[c]Department of Pathology and Laboratory Medicine
University of Cincinnati
Cincinnati, Ohio 45221

Implanted polymeric materials frequently elicit an inflammatory response character-ized by the accumulation of both proteins and macrophages. Since the adsorption of proteins to an implant is immediate, inflammatory cells likely never make contact with the material itself; rather they interact with the adsorbed proteins. The proteins that predominate in this adsorbed layer include fibrinogen, albumin and immuno-globulins.[1]

Fibrinogen, which plays a central role in blood coagulation, collects at sites of inflammation. Implanted materials to which fibrinogen adsorbs also attract large numbers of macrophages.[2] Importantly, macrophages themselves bind fibrinogen.[3] Whether this binding is receptor-mediated or not, it indicates interaction between macrophages and fibrinogen, supporting the notion that coagulation and inflamma-tion are intimately related.[3]

Tissue macrophages and their precursor cells, monocytes, are part of the mono-nuclear phagocyte system (MPS). A major function of these phagocytes is to dispose of bacteria and damaged or dying cells.[1,4] Phagocytosis involves the attachment of particles to the cell surface, ingestion of particles by the cell, and digestion of the particles within the cell. The capture of foreign particles by cells of the MPS as well as the focal localization of those cells is believed to be mediated by adsorbed plasma proteins.[5,6] Clearly, much about inflammation could be learned from studying the interactions of fibrinogen, macrophages and surfaces.

In this work, microscopic polystyrene-divinylbenzene beads coated with selected members of a series of $PEO_\alpha PPO_\beta PEO_\alpha$ copolymers were used to examine the interactions of monocytes/macrophages with surfaces. These particular triblock copolymers were chosen for this study because by simply changing the ratio of their PEO and PPO segment lengths, the amphiphilic character of the surface to which they are adsorbed could be altered. Some of these copolymers are adjuvants, pro-moting cellular accumulation and inflammation[7,8]; others are innocuous.[6,9–11]

[a] This work was supported by a Research Challenge Grant from the University of Cincinnati to G.S.R. and S.H.G., a Whitaker Foundation fellowship to S.M.O. provided through the Ohio Center for Cardiovascular Biomaterials, and by a grant to G.S.R. from the Ohio Affiliate of the American Heart Association.

[d] Author to whom correspondence should be addressed.

THP-1 cells were also used for our studies. These cells resemble human monocytes in morphology, secretory products, and the expression of oncogenes, membrane antigens and genes involved in lipid metabolism.[12]

Herein we identify differences in the adherence of THP-1 cells to beads coated with well-defined triblock copolymers. Our results demonstrate that chemically similar but physicochemically dissimilar surfaces can elicit very different adhesive responses. We propose that the different responses relate to differences in the interactions of the surfaces with fibrin(ogen).

MATERIALS AND METHODS

Reagents and Chemicals

Triblock copolymers (Pluronic® polyols) of the form $PEO_\alpha PPO_\beta PEO_\alpha$ were used as received from BASF Corporation (Parsippany, NJ). The nomenclature, molecular weight, composition and hydrophile-lipophile balance (HLB) of the copolymers used for this study are given in TABLE 1. By intention, the number of propylene ether subunits comprising the PPO segment of the molecules of this study was either 56 or 69. Human fibrinogen, Grade L, from American Diagnostica (Greenwich, CT) was desalted by gel filtration chromatography using as matrix material Sephadex G-25 (Pharmacia, Uppsala, Sweden) and as eluent 0.01 M Tris-HCl, pH 7.40. The salt-free fibrinogen was divided into aliquots which were stored at -20°C until use. Before use, a frozen aliquot of fibrinogen solution was first thawed to room temperature, diluted to a desired concentration using an appropriate buffered salt solution, and then heated to 37°C to dissolve any residual cryoprecipitate. The fibrinogen concentration of stock solutions was determined using the molar absorptivity of the protein at 280 nm, 5.12×10^5 L $\cdot$ mol^{-1} $\cdot$ cm^{-1}. As necessary, fibrinogen was labeled uniformly using Na^{125}I from Amersham (Arlington Heights, IL) and IODO-GEN from Pierce Chemical (Rockford, IL) according to an established procedure.[13] Fatty acid-free bovine serum albumin (BSA) was from ICN (Cleveland, OH). Polystyrene-divinylbenzene beads of diameter 6.4 ± 1.9 μm and beads of diameter 25.7 ± 10.0 μm were from Seradyn (Indianapolis, IN). Prior to coating them with a surfactant and/or protein, beads were first washed and lyophilized as described elsewhere.[14] Water was deionized and then distilled using an all-glass apparatus. THP-1 cells were from the American Type Culture Collection

TABLE 1. $PEO_\alpha PPO_\beta PEO_\alpha$ Triblock Copolymers

Copolymer	Molecular Weight	HLB[a]	α[b]	β[c]
F108	14600	27	129	56
F127	12600	22	97	69
P105	6500	15	37	56
P104	5900	13	31	56
P123	5750	8	20	69
L121	4400	0.5	5	69
L101	3800	1	7	56

[a] Hydrophile-lipophile balance
[b] Number of ethylene oxide monomer units in a PEO block.
[c] Number of propylene oxide monomer units in a PPO block.

(Rockville, MD). They were cultured in routine fashion at 37°C in 5% CO_2. For this purpose, a serum-free culture medium, AIM-V, was used (Gibco BRL, Grand Island, NY).

Coating Beads with Triblock Copolymers

Using low energy sonication (55 Hz, < 0.32 watt $\cdot$ cm^{-2}), a 25.0 mg sample of dry beads was dispersed in 5.0 ml of water containing a copolymer at a concentration of 1.0 mg $\cdot$ ml^{-1}. Most coatings were performed using water that had been pre-equilibrated to room temperature. Owing to their limited solubility at room temperature, however, L101 and L121 were dissolved and coated on beads using water at 4°C. Copolymer-coated beads were pelleted by centrifugation at 1500 $\times$ g for 3.0 min., and the corresponding supernatant was discarded. Beads were then washed three times using a fresh 5.0 ml aliquot of water and a brief pulse, 10 s, of low energy sonication.

Coating Beads with Proteins

Samples containing 25.0 mg of either copolymer-free beads or beads that had been coated with a copolymer as described above were dispersed using brief, 10–30 s, low energy sonication in buffered aqueous medium containing protein. The protein-containing medium was 5.0 ml of either 0.02 M Tris-HCl, pH 7.40, containing 2.0 mg $\cdot$ ml^{-1} of ^{125}I-fibrinogen or unlabeled fibrinogen, or 0.02 M Tris-HCl containing 1.0 mg $\cdot$ ml^{-1} bovine serum albumin. To facilitate the dispersion of dry, copolymer-free beads in protein-containing media, such beads were first "wetted" using 2.0 ml of water:ethanol, 9:1 (v/v), and then rinsed with an equal volume of water. After being dispersed in a protein-containing medium, beads were pelleted by centrifugation at 1500 $\times$ g for 3.0 min. They were subsequently washed three times using 5.0 ml of water.

Cell Adhesion Studies

Beads (25.7 $\pm$ 10.0 μm) that had been coated with various materials were dispersed in AIM-V medium, and aliquots of these dispersions, each containing 330 beads, were added to wells of a 24-well tissue culture plate (Costar, Cambridge, MA). One hundred thousand freshly harvested THP-1 cells suspended in fresh culture medium were then added to the wells so that the total volume of culture medium in each well was 1.0 ml. Using a rotary shaker, plates containing the bead-cell mixtures were rotated at ~60 rpm for 2.0 h at room temperature. During this period, the cells on the plates were occasionally inspected using an inverted microscope. After this time, the number of beads associated with cells was quantitated. For this purpose, we determined microscopically the number of cells that had adhered to beads in a field representative of the surface of a given well. The first 60 solitary beads encountered in a representative field served as the population sample.

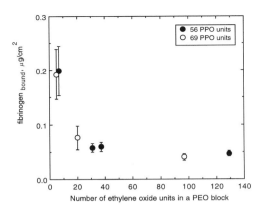

FIGURE 1. Adsorption of fibrinogen to copolymer-coated polystyrene-divinylbenzene beads (6.4 ± 1.9 μm). The surface coverage of fibrinogen on beads coated with PEO$_\alpha$PPO$_\beta$PEO$_\alpha$ copolymers decreases as the PEO segment length increases. Fibrinogen surface coverage on uncoated beads is 0.49 μg · cm^{-2}.

RESULTS AND DISCUSSION

Adsorption of Fibrinogen onto Triblock Copolymer–Coated Beads

The binding of fibrinogen onto copolymer-coated beads was first quantified. As shown in FIGURE 1, the amount of ^{125}I-fibrinogen that binds to beads decreases as the PEO segment length, thus HLB, of the coating increases. The surface concentration of fibrinogen on unmodified beads is 0.49 μg · cm^{-2}.[15] All of the copolymers inhibit substantially the binding of fibrinogen to the hydrophobic beads. Of the copolymer-coated beads, those coated with the copolymers having the shortest PEO chains, L101 and L121, bind the most fibrinogen, but still less than 50% of that which binds to copolymer-free beads. The more hydrophilic molecules which have longer PEO chains, F108 and F127, bind the least amount of fibrinogen—only about 10% of the saturation coverage of fibrinogen on copolymer-free beads.

Adherence of THP-1 Cells to Beads

After 2.0 h, the adherence of THP-1 cells to beads pre-coated with the copolymers and either fibrinogen or bovine serum albumin was quantified. Representative examples of the interaction of THP-1 cells with copolymer-modified beads are given in FIGURE 2. In FIGURE 2A is shown an example of the typical interaction of cells with a bead pre-coated with a hydrophobic copolymer (L101) and fibrinogen. FIGURE 2B shows the typical interaction of cells with a bead pre-coated with a hydrophilic copolymer (F108) and fibrinogen.

We found first that only very few THP-1 cells adhered to beads coated with any of the copolymers and albumin as compared to beads coated with any of the copolymers and fibrinogen (FIGURE 3). The figure shows the arithmetic mean of cells bound per bead with each copolymer/protein/cell system. All of the albumin-coated surfaces bound less than one cell per bead. All of the fibrinogen-coated beads, whether pre-coated with copolymer or not, bound more cells than albumin-coated beads. For copolymer-coated beads, the number of adherent cells correlates with the surface concentration of fibrinogen. The number of adherent cells is greatest for beads coated with fibrinogen and the most hydrophobic copolymers.

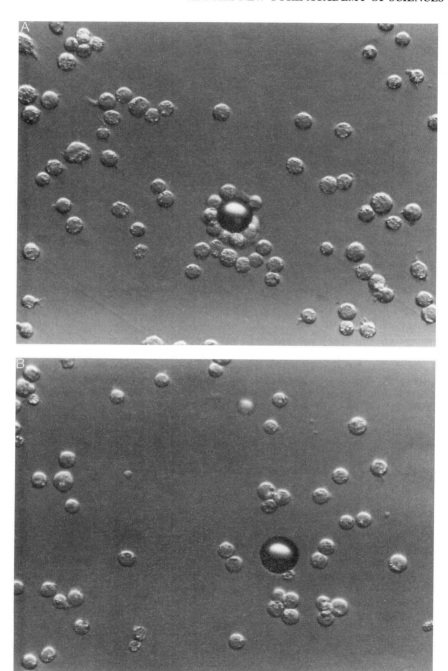

FIGURE 2. Adherence of THP-1 cells to copolymer-coated, fibrinogen-treated, polystyrene-divinylbenzene beads (25.7 ± 10.0 μm). **A**: Bead coated with L101. **B**: Bead coated with F108.

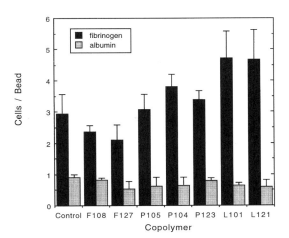

FIGURE 3. Macrophage binding to polystyrene-divinylbenzene beads (25.7 ± 10.0 μm). Beads were coated with the copolymers and either fibrinogen or albumin. Copolymer-free beads were used as controls. The results are reported as the mean ± SEM. N = 60. For beads coated with fibrinogen, only L101, L121 and P104 are significantly different from control for $p \leq 0.05$ by the Mann-Whitney rank sum test.

DISCUSSION

Our interest in $PEO_\alpha PPO_\beta PEO_\alpha$ triblock copolymers was prompted by a desire to understand how surfaces influence cellular adhesion and inflammation. Our results indicate that the adhesion of inflammatory cells to surfaces coated with the copolymers correlates with the amount of adsorbed fibrinogen. However, surfaces modified with the most hydrophobic of the copolymers bind much less fibrinogen than copolymer-free beads, yet the number of cells that adhere to the former surface is greater than the number of cells that adhere to the latter surface. All available evidence indicates that resident amphiphiles influence the orientation and/or conformation of adsorbed fibrin(ogen) and, consequently, the biological processivity of the bound adhesive protein.[15] It appears that the adsorption process exposes and/or masks certain reactive sites, rendering fibrin(ogen) more or less susceptible to proteolysis and polymerization. We hypothesize that the low HLB surfactants may act as inflammatory agents by facilitating fibrin(ogen)-dependent cellular adhesion. Presently, we are using enzymatic probes and epitope mapping to identify changes that occur in fibrinogen structure following adsorption of the protein to various surfactant-coated surfaces.

SUMMARY

The role of fibrinogen in the adherence of macrophages to polymer surfaces was studied using a human cell line (THP-1 cells) and polystyrene-divinylbenzene beads coated with poly(ethylene oxide)/poly(propylene oxide) copolymers of the form $PEO_\alpha PPO_\beta PEO_\alpha$. The amphiphilic character of the surface of the beads was varied using a series of copolymers with constant PPO core lengths but different PEO segments. Fibrinogen-dependent adherence of monocytes/macrophages to the modified beads was then assessed.

The adherence of THP-1 cells to copolymer-coated beads correlates well with the amount of fibrinogen bound to the beads. Those beads coated with the most hydrophobic surfactant molecules bound the most fibrinogen and the most cells. On these surfaces, the concentration of fibrinogen was less than half that of the protein on unmodified beads. Despite the lower amount of bound fibrinogen, the number of adherent cells was 37% greater than the number of adherent cells on fibrinogen-coated, copolymer-free beads. Beads coated with the most hydrophilic surfactants bound just 10% the amount of fibrinogen bound to unmodified beads. On these surfaces, the number of adherent cells was decreased by ~25% with respect to the number of cells bound to beads coated with fibrinogen alone. We propose that the hydrophobic surfactant molecules may act as inflammatory agents by facilitating fibrinogen-dependent cellular adhesion.

REFERENCES

1. RYAN, G. B. & G. MAJNO, Eds. 1977. Inflammation. The Upjohn Co. Kalamazoo, MI.
2. TANG, L. & J. W. EATON. 1995. Inflammatory responses to biomaterials. Am. J. Clin. Pathol. **103:** 466–471.
3. ALTIERI, D. C., P. M. MANNUCCI & A. M. CAPITANIO. 1986. Binding of fibrinogen to human monocytes. J. Clin. Invest. **78:** 968–976.
4. GRIFFIN, F. M. 1982. Mononuclear cell phagocytic mechanisms and host defense. *In* Advances in Host Defense Mechanisms, vol. 1, Phagocytic Cells. J. I. Gallin & A. S. Fauci, Eds.: 33. Raven Press. New York.
5. O'MULLANE, J. E., C. J. DAVISON, K. PETRAK & E. TOMLINSON. 1988. Adsorption of fibrinogen on to polystyrene latex coated with the non-ionic surfactant, poloxamer 338. Biomaterials **9:** 203–204.
6. ILLUM, L., L. O. JACOBSEN, R. H. MULLER, E. MAK & S. S. DAVIS. 1987. Surface characteristics and the interaction of colloidal particles with mouse peritoneal macrophages. Biomaterials **8:** 113–117.
7. HUNTER, R. L., J. MCNICHOLL & A. A. LAL. 1994. Mechanisms of action of nonionic block copolymer adjuvants. AIDS Res. Human Retroviruses **10(Supp. 2):** S95–S98.
8. HUNTER, R. L., F. STRICKLAND & F. KÉZDY. 1981. The adjuvant activity of nonionic block polymer surfactants I. The role of hydrophile-lipophile balance. J. Immunol. **127:** 1244–1250.
9. MOGHIMI, S. M., I. S. MUIR, L. ILLUM, S. S. DAVIS & V. KOLB-BACHOFEN. 1993. Coating particles with a block co-polymer (poloxamine 908) suppresses opsonization but permits the activity of dysopsonins in the serum. Biochim. Biophys. Acta **1179:** 157–165.
10. TAN, J. S., D. E. BUTTERFIELD, C. L. VOYCHECK, K. D. CALDWELL & J. T. LI. 1993. Surface modification of nanoparticles by PEO/PPO block copolymers to minimize interactions with blood components and prolong blood circulation in rats. Biomaterials **14:** 823–833.
11. WALTROUS-PELTIER, N., J. UHL, V. STEEL, L. BROPHY & E. MERISKO-LEVERSIDGE. 1992. Direct suppression of phagocytosis by amphiphatic polymeric surfactants. Pharm. Res. **9:** 1177–1183.
12. AUWERX, J. 1991. The human leukemia cell line, THP-1: A multifaceted model for the study of monocyte-macrophage differentiation. Experientia **47:** 22–30.
13. FRAKER, P. J. & J. C. SPECK. 1978. Protein and cell membrane iodinations with a sparingly soluble chloroamide, 1,3,4,6-tetrachloro-3a,6a-diphrenylglycoluril. Biochem. Biophys. Res. Commun. **80:** 849–857.
14. RETZINGER, G. S. & M. C. MCGINNIS. 1990. A turbimetric method for measuring fibrin formation and fibrinolysis at solid-liquid interfaces. Anal. Biochem. **186:** 169–178.
15. COOK, B. C. & G. S. RETZINGER. 1994. Lipid microenvironment influences the processivity of adsorbed fibrin(ogen): Enzymatic processing and adhesivity of the bound protein. J. Coll. Interface Sci. **162:** 171–181.

Effect of External Oxygen Mass Transfer Resistances on Viability of Immunoisolated Tissue[a]

EFSTATHIOS S. AVGOUSTINIATOS[b]
AND CLARK K. COLTON[c]

Department of Chemical Engineering
Massachusetts Institute of Technology
Cambridge, Massachusetts 02139-4307

Transplantation of cells or tissues with differentiated functions has promise in treatment of human disease, but the need for immunosuppressive drugs may have serious side effects.[1,2] One approach to minimizing or eliminating immunosuppression is immunoisolation[3] of the transplanted tissue by a semipermeable membrane to protect it from immune rejection, thereby creating an implantable biohybrid artificial organ.[4–10] The membrane protects the transplanted tissue from components of both the cellular and humoral immune response but permits passage of the secreted product. At the same time, the transport properties of the graft tissue, membrane, and surrounding host tissue must permit sufficient supply of nutrients and oxygen, as well as the removal of metabolic waste products, by diffusion from or to the nearest blood supply.

The cells may be encapsulated at a high tissue-like density, or they may be dispersed in the form of individual cells or cell aggregates (*e.g.*, islets of Langerhans) in an extracellular gel matrix such as agar, alginate, or chitosan. High density culture, if attainable, is advantageous because it minimizes the size of the implanted device. The amount of tissue required for transplantation in an immunoisolation device is determined by the secretion rate of the desired agent per cell and the amount of the active agent required by the body;[9] it ranges from 10^6 to more than 10^9 cells and depends upon the specific medical application.[11] The complexity and difficulty of all aspects of the problem increases with the volume of implanted tissue required. Thus, it is not surprising that some central nervous system applications, which require the least amount of transplanted tissue,[11] are the first to advance to clinical testing.[8]

MAINTENANCE OF CELL VIABILITY AND FUNCTION

Maintenance of cell viability and function is essential and, in the absence of immune rejection, is limited by the supply of nutrients and oxygen. Oxygen diffusion

[a] This study was supported in part by NIH Grant No. 1 R43 DK51909-01.
[b] Tel: (617) 253-6483; Fax: (617) 252-1651; E-mail: eavgoust@alum.mit.edu
[c] Author to whom correspondence should be addressed: Prof. Clark K. Colton, Room 66-452; Department of Chemical Engineering, MIT, 77 Massachusetts Avenue, Cambridge, MA 02139-4307; Tel: (617) 253-4585; Fax: (617) 252-1651; E-mail: ckcolton@mit.edu

limitations in tissue *in vivo* are far more severe than for glucose.[12] The requirements of specific tissues for other small molecules and for macromolecules are poorly understood or have not yet been quantified; transport limitations for large molecules are highly dependent upon immunoisolation membrane properties, whereas oxygen supply limitations are always serious and are the focus of this paper. If the local oxygen concentration drops to sufficiently low levels, the cells will die. Hypoxia at levels high enough to keep cells alive can nonetheless have deleterious effects on cell functions that require high cellular ATP concentrations, for example, ATP-dependent insulin secretion.[13]

Oxygen supply to encapsulated cells depends in a complicated way upon a variety of factors, including 1) the site of implantation and the local oxygen partial pressure P in the blood, 2) the spatial distribution of host blood vessels in the vicinity of the implant surface, 3) the oxygen permeability of the membrane or encapsulant, 4) the oxygen consumption rate of the encapsulated cells, 5) the geometrical characteristics of the implant device, and 6), the tissue density and spatial arrangement of the encapsulated cells or tissues. The original concept of a biohybrid artificial organ,[9] and the design which has received the most extensive study in large animals, is an intravascular arteriovenous shunt in the form of a semipermeable membrane tube through which arterial blood flows and on the outside of which the implanted tissue is contained in a housing. This approach provides the best oxygen supply ($P = 100$ mm Hg) but suffers from the need to break the cardiovascular system and may be limited to only a small fraction of patients. One alternative is an extravascular device in the form of a planar or cylindrical diffusion chamber implanted, for example, in subcutaneous tissue or intraperitoneally. Such devices are exposed to the mean P of the microvasculature, about 40 mm Hg. Implantation in soft tissue is further disadvantaged if a foreign body response occurs, producing an avascular layer adjacent to the membrane typically on the order of 100-μm thick. This fibrotic tissue increases the distance between blood vessels and implant, and the fibroblasts in that layer consume oxygen. Recently, there has been reported[14] discovery of a class of microporous membranes that induce neovascularization at the material-tissue interface. The angiogenic process takes 2–3 weeks[15] for completion, and the vascular structures remain indefinitely. By bringing blood vessels close to the implant, oxygen delivery is improved. Another alternative for an extravascular implant is spherical microcapsules implanted, for example, in the peritoneal space. The spherical geometry is advantageous from the standpoint of mass transfer.

Despite encouraging results with various tissues and applications,[8,9] the problem of oxygen transport limitations is one of the major hurdles that remain. The maximum P (about 40 mm Hg) available for extravascular devices limits the thickness of viable tissue that can be supported. In a previous article[11] we mathematically analyzed the effect of oxygen supply limitations on the design of immunoisolation devices. We estimated the maximum viable (non-anoxic) tissue thickness that can be supported subject to three limitations in our model: 1) Oxygen consumption rate was assumed to follow zero-order kinetics. Use of Michaelis-Menten kinetics with an accurate value for the critical (minimum necessary) oxygen partial pressure for tissue viability P_C would lead to larger thickness estimates. 2) The increase in the oxygen solubility α and diffusivity D in the encapsulated tissue/gel matrix composite with increasing matrix volume fraction ε was ignored. Inclusion of this phenomenon would also increase the thickness estimates. 3) The presence of external mass transfer resistances (which would decrease thickness estimates) was ignored. This effect can be substantial, especially for the slab geometry.[9] In this paper we address the latter two issues, focussing especially on the external mass transfer resistances resulting from the presence of immunoisolation membranes and sur-rounding host tissue, while retaining the assumption of zero-order kinetics, which allows an analytical treatment of the problem. We also allow for a value of P_C different from zero.

MATHEMATICAL ANALYSIS

We consider steady state oxygen transport and consumption by tissue immunoi-solated in three idealized geometries: 1) a planar diffusion chamber in which a slab of tissue of uniform half-thickness L_1 is confined between two parallel membranes; 2) a cylindrical diffusion chamber in which tissue is confined within a tubular membrane of uniform internal radius R_1; and 3) a spherical microcapsule containing spherical tissue of radius R_1. The implanted tissue/matrix compartment is assumed to be surrounded by a total of $n - 1$ layers comprised of membranes and host tissue. The overall membrane structure is composed of some number of different membrane layers, each with unique permeability properties. The membrane layer adjacent to the tissue/matrix composite is acellular; the membrane layers further away may be infiltrated by cells; the cells in the ith layer consume oxygen at their own unique rate V_i assumed to be independent of local oxygen partial pressure. Outside of the membrane layers there are a number of host tissue layers arranged in series, each again with its own characteristic permeability and oxygen consumption properties, assumed independent of local oxygen partial pressure. Each layer is treated mathematically in the same way, and each is assumed to have the same shape as the implanted device (planar, cylindrical, or spherical). In each layer i we assume that the tissue is homogeneously distributed with an average tissue volume fraction $1 - \varepsilon_i$, where ε_i is the non-tissue void fraction associated, for example, with extracellular matrix or the membrane material in which cells are dispersed. The case of $\varepsilon_1 = 0$ corresponds to a high-density tissue-like arrangement of trans-planted cells, where the subscript 1 denotes the viable tissue/matrix layer.

A specific example of immunoisolated tissue surrounded by two membrane layers and one host tissue layer adjacent to the outer membrane layer in a planar configuration is shown schematically in FIGURE 1. Layer 0 is the necrotic core and is the layer closest to the center of symmetry; layer 1 is the viable transplanted tissue/gel matrix composite; layer 2 is an acellular membrane; layer 3 is a second membrane layer, in this case infiltrated by host cells; and layer 4 is a fibrotic layer comprised of host cells and extracellular matrix. Examples representing subsets of this geometry will be examined in detail later in this paper. FIGURE 1 is presented at this point to help the reader follow the mathematical analysis developed below which is kept in its most general form.

If there is no tissue in the immunoisolation device or membrane layers, the value of P throughout the device equilibrates with that of the surrounding tissue. Implanted tissue in layer 1 consumes oxygen that must be supplied by diffusion, thereby inducing a drop in P through the layer. The oxygen consumption requires a sufficient flux of oxygen N_{S1} over the entire surface $S1$ of layer 1 at its interface with the acellular membrane. This flux, in combination with the mass transfer resistances (and any additional oxygen consumption) of the external layers, induces additional drops in P between the external oxygen partial pressure P_{ext} of the nearest blood supply and P_{S1}. This problem is substantially more complex than analysis of just the implanted tissue alone because the total external P drop, $P_{ext} - P_{S1}$, depends upon the oxygen consumption rate of layer 1, which itself depends upon the amount of viable tissue, which in turn depends upon P_{S1}.

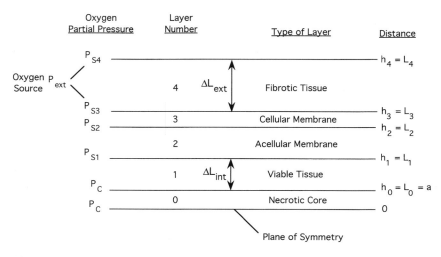

FIGURE 1. Schematic representation of planar immunoisolation device. Half of the device, lying on one side of the plane of symmetry, is shown. Distance parameter h is applicable to all geometries; L applies to slabs.

The species conservation equation in general notation applicable to every geometry that describes steady-state diffusion and reaction of oxygen in layer i is

$$D_i \nabla^2 c_i = V_i \qquad (1)$$

where D_i is the effective diffusion coefficient of oxygen through layer i and ∇^2 is the Laplacian operator (the second derivative of concentration with respect to one spatial direction, since each geometry is symmetric about a plane, line, or point). The concentration of oxygen c_i is linearly related to the oxygen partial pressure P_i by

$$c_i = \alpha_i P_i \qquad (2)$$

where α_i is the Bunsen solubility coefficient of oxygen in layer i. V_i is the intrinsic reaction velocity or rate of oxygen consumption per unit volume of layer i. A simplified but reasonable representation of the dependence of oxygen consumption rate on oxygen concentration is given by Michaelis-Menten kinetics,

$$V_i = Vmax_i(1 - \varepsilon_i)\frac{c_i}{Km_i + c_i} \qquad (3)$$

where $Vmax_i$ is the maximum consumption rate per unit volume of tissue in layer i, and Km_i is the respective Michaelis-Menten constant. At low concentrations where $c_i \ll Km_i$, the reaction rate is first order in c_i,

$$V_i = Vmax_i(1 - \varepsilon_i)\frac{c_i}{Km_i} \qquad (4)$$

whereas at high concentration where $c_i \gg Km_i$, the reaction rate is zero order in c_i,

$$V_i = Vmax_i(1 - \varepsilon_i) \tag{5}$$

These equations must be solved simultaneously for all layers $i = 1, 2, \ldots, n$ subject to $2n$ boundary conditions. In this general formulation, we include in the center of the tissue/matrix compartment the presence of a necrotic core (dead tissue) which forms when $P = P_C$, the oxygen partial pressure at which cells die. At the necrotic core/viable tissue interface, there is no net oxygen flux because of lack of an oxygen source or sink inside the necrotic core,

$$\text{at } z = a = h_0, \quad \frac{dc_1}{dz} = 0 \tag{6}$$

where the distance variable z is equal to x (distance from center of a slab) or r (radial distance from center of a cylinder or sphere) and a is the half-thickness of the necrotic core (same as h_0). For the case where $P_1 > P_C$ at $z = 0$, a necrotic core does not develop ($a = 0$). Under these conditions, the same boundary condition, Equation 6, applies at $z = 0$ because of symmetry. We take the oxygen partial pressure to be specified as P_{ext} at the external surface of the outermost layer n where the oxygen source lies,

$$\text{at } z = h_n, P_n = P_{Sn} = P_{ext} \tag{7}$$

where the subscript S denotes a value at the external surface of any given layer. At each one of the $n - 1$ interfaces between adjacent layers, the oxygen partial pressure in each layer is the same

$$\text{at } z = h_i, \quad P_i = P_{Si} = P_{i+1} \tag{8}$$

and the oxygen flux in each layer is also the same,

$$\text{at } z = h_i, \quad (D\alpha)_i \frac{dP_i}{dz} = (D\alpha)_{i+1} \frac{dP_{i+1}}{dz} \tag{9}$$

If the full nonlinear Michaelis-Menten expression is used, solution of Equations 1–3, and 6–9 requires numerical methods. For oxygen partial pressures at the outer surface of the viable tissue ($z = h_1$) substantially higher than Km (about 0.44 mm Hg at 37°C[16]), and for values of P_C between 0.1 and 0.3 mm Hg,[17] the difference between the thickness of the necrotic core and of the viable tissue layer predicted by the two kinetics expressions (zero-order and Michaelis-Menten) is not very large.[11] By replacing Equation 3 with Equation 5 for zero-order kinetics, the problem can be solved analytically. In the resulting set of equations, there is one parameter, the half-thickness of the anoxic core a, that is unknown. In the viable part of the tissue/matrix compartment (layer 1), P_1 decreases from $P_1 = P_{S1}$ at $z = h_1$ to $P_1 = P_c$ at $z = a$. For $z \leq a$ (layer 0), the tissue is necrotic, and $P_0 = P_C$. The solutions for the partial pressure profile in the region $a \leq z \leq h_1$, as well as the value of a in each geometry in terms of P_{S1}, are as follows:

Slab

$$\left(\frac{P}{P_S}\right)_1 = 1 - \left(\frac{VL^2}{2\alpha DP_S}\right)_1 \left[1 - \left(\frac{x}{L_1}\right)^2 - 2\left(\frac{a}{L_1}\right)\left(1 - \frac{x}{L_1}\right)\right] \tag{10}$$

$$\frac{a}{L_1} = 1 - \left[\frac{2\alpha D(P_S - P_C)}{VL^2}\right]_1^{1/2} \tag{11}$$

Cylinder

$$\left(\frac{P}{P_S}\right)_1 = 1 - \left(\frac{VR^2}{4\alpha DP_S}\right)_1 \left[1 - \left(\frac{r}{R_1}\right)^2 - 2\left(\frac{a}{R_1}\right)^2 \ln\left(\frac{R_1}{r}\right)\right] \tag{12}$$

a is obtained by implicit solution of

$$\left(\frac{a}{R_1}\right)^2 \left[1 + 2\ln\left(\frac{R_1}{a}\right)\right] = 1 - \left[\frac{4\alpha D(P_S - P_C)}{VR^2}\right]_1 \tag{13}$$

Sphere

$$\left(\frac{P}{P_S}\right)_1 = 1 - \left(\frac{VR^2}{6\alpha DP_S}\right)_1 \left[1 - \left(\frac{r}{R_1}\right)^2 - 2\left(\frac{a}{R_1}\right)^3\left(\frac{R_1}{r} - 1\right)\right] \tag{14}$$

$$\frac{a}{R_1} = \frac{1}{2} + \cos\left(\frac{\omega + 4\pi}{3}\right) \tag{15}$$

where

$$\omega = \arccos\left\{-1 + \left[\frac{12\alpha D(P_S - P_C)}{VR^2}\right]_1\right\} \qquad 0 \le \omega \le \pi \tag{16}$$

The quantity

$$\phi^2 = \left[\frac{Vh^2}{\alpha D(P_S - P_C)}\right]_1 \tag{17}$$

that appears in these equations is the square of a dimensionless parameter ϕ called the Thiele modulus which is a measure of the rate of oxygen consumption relative to the rate of oxygen diffusion in the tissue/matrix compartment.

To calculate the size of the necrotic core from Equations **11**, **13**, and **15–16**, one must calculate P_{S1},

$$P_{S1} = P_{ext} - \sum_{i=2}^{n} (\Delta P_i) \tag{18}$$

where

$$\Delta P_i = P_{Si} - P_{Si-1} \tag{19}$$

is the oxygen partial pressure drop through layer i. By solving Equation **1** in layer i, subject to boundary conditions **6–9**, ΔP_i can be calculated for each of the three geometries:

Slab

$$\Delta P_i = \frac{1}{(\alpha D)_i}\left\{V_i\frac{(L_i - L_{i-1})^2}{2} + (L_i - L_{i-1})\sum_{j=1}^{i-1}[V_j(L_j - L_{j-1})]\right\} \tag{20}$$

Cylinder

$$\Delta P_i = \frac{1}{2(\alpha D)_i} \left\{ V_i \left[\frac{R_i^2 - R_{i-1}^2}{2} - R_{i-1}^2 \ln\left(\frac{R_i}{R_{i-1}}\right) \right] \right.$$

$$\left. + \ln\left(\frac{R_i}{R_{i-1}}\right) \sum_{j=1}^{i-1} [V_j(R_j^2 - R_{j-1}^2)] \right\} \tag{21}$$

Sphere

$$\Delta P_i = \frac{1}{3(\alpha D)_i} \left\{ V_i \left[\frac{R_i^2 - R_{i-1}^2}{2} - R_{i-1}^2 \left(1 - \frac{R_{i-1}}{R_i}\right) \right] \right.$$

$$\left. + \left(\frac{1}{R_{i-1}} - \frac{1}{R_i}\right) \sum_{j=1}^{i-1} [V_j(R_j^3 - R_{j-1}^3)] \right\} \tag{22}$$

In Equations **20–22**, the terms involving V_i correspond to the partial pressure drop in layer i caused by consumption inside layer i itself, while the terms involving V_j, $j = 1, \ldots, i - 1$, correspond to the sum of the components of pressure drop in layer i caused by the consumption in other layers located closer to the center of symmetry.

For the case of a slab, each of these latter terms has the form $[\Delta L_i/(\alpha D)_i][V_j \Delta L_j]$, where $\Delta L_i = L_i - L_{i-1}$ and $\Delta L_j = L_j - L_{j-1}$. The first term in brackets is the mass transfer resistance of the ith layer, and the second term is the portion of the oxygen mass transfer flux out of the ith layer that is required to support the viable tissue in the jth layer. Thus, the summation expression in Equation **20** is the oxygen flux exiting from the ith layer that meets the oxygen consumption needs of the tissue in all of the layers closer to the center of symmetry. Analogous terms are similarly present in Equations **21** and **22**.

Equations **18–22** provide a solution for P_{S1} involving $h_0 = a$, the necrotic core half-thickness, which is the parameter whose value is to be determined from Equations **11**, **13**, and **15–16**. An iterative procedure is required to solve for a, involving an initial guess for a, explicit calculation of P_{S1} from Equations **18–22**, and then calculation of a new value for a from Equations **11**, **13**, and **15–16**. This last calculation of a is explicit for slabs, implicit for cylinders, and implicit for spheres (or explicit solution of a cubic equation). This procedure is repeated until the current and new values of a converge.

The calculational effort required can be reduced by means of the following observation. Because the cells in the membranes and surrounding host tissue respire at a rate independent of local oxygen partial pressure, the oxygen partial pressure drop caused by oxygen consumption in these external layers is not affected by phenomena in the tissue/matrix compartment, including the development of a necrotic core. Thus, we can isolate from Equations **20–22** the terms of the total pressure drop associated with oxygen consumption in the external layers which do not depend on the half-thickness of the anoxic core a; in this way the iterative procedure described above can be simplified, or even eliminated, as shown below. The pressure drop in all layers caused by consumption in layer i, denoted ΔP_{Vi}, can be calculated by collecting from Equations **20–22** those terms that depend on V_i. The results for each of the three geometries are as follows:

Slab

$$\Delta P_{Vi} = V_i \left\{ \frac{1}{(\alpha D)_i} \frac{(L_i - L_{i-1})^2}{2} + (L_i - L_{i-1}) \sum_{j=i+1}^{n} \left[\frac{L_j - L_{j-1}}{(\alpha D)_j} \right] \right\} \tag{23}$$

Cylinder

$$\Delta P_{Vi} = V_i \left\{ \frac{1}{2(\alpha D)_i} \left[\frac{R_i^2 - R_{i-1}^2}{2} - R_{i-1}^2 \ln\left(\frac{R_i}{R_{i-1}} \right) \right] \right. \tag{24}$$

$$\left. + \frac{R_i^2 - R_{i-1}^2}{2} \sum_{j=i+1}^{n} \left[\frac{\ln\left(\dfrac{R_j}{R_{j-1}} \right)}{(\alpha D)_j} \right] \right\}$$

Sphere

$$\Delta P_{Vi} = V_i \left\{ \frac{1}{3(\alpha D)_i} \left[\frac{R_i^2 - R_{i-1}^2}{2} - R_{i-1}^2 \left(1 - \frac{R_{i-1}}{R_i} \right) \right] \right. \tag{25}$$

$$\left. + \frac{R_i^3 - R_{i-1}^3}{3} \sum_{j=i+1}^{n} \left[\frac{\dfrac{1}{R_{j-1}} - \dfrac{1}{R_j}}{(\alpha D)_j} \right] \right\}$$

In Equations 23–25, the terms involving $(\alpha D)_i$ correspond to the pressure drop caused by consumption in layer i which occurs inside layer i itself, while the terms involving $(\alpha D)_j$, $j = i + 1, \ldots, n$ correspond to the sum of the components of pressure drop caused by consumption in layer i which occur in other layers located closer to the oxygen source.

In terms of the above formulation, a necrotic core develops when $P_0 = P_{s0} = P_C$, and

$$P_{ext} - \sum_{i=1}^{n} (\Delta P_{Vi}) = P_C \tag{26}$$

The sum of the oxygen partial pressure drops in all layers induced by the layer of viable transplanted tissue (layer 1) is obtained by rearranging Equation 26:

$$\Delta P_{V1} = P_{ext} - \sum_{i=2}^{n} (\Delta P_{Vi}) - P_C \tag{27}$$

ΔP_{V1} is the maximum available pressure drop ($P_{ext} - P_C$) minus the sum of the pressure drops in the external layers associated with oxygen consumption in the external layers. It therefore represents the actual maximum available value for the sum of the pressure drop due to oxygen consumption in layer 1 plus the pressure drops in the external layers induced by oxygen consumption in layer 1. ΔP_{V1} is independent of the properties of the transplanted tissue (except for P_C) and can be calculated using Equation 27 and one of Equations 23–25 to calculate ΔP_{Vi}, $i = 2, \ldots, n$, thereby leading to a simpler equation containing the unknown half-thickness of the necrotic core a.

These results in dimensionless form are formulated in terms of a modified Thiele modulus ϕ_m, defined by

$$\phi_m^2 = \left(\frac{Vh^2}{\alpha D}\right)_1 \frac{1}{\Delta P_{V1}} \tag{28}$$

and a dimensionless length ξ,

$$\xi = \frac{h_0}{h_1} = \frac{a}{h_1} \tag{29}$$

ξ can be expressed (explicitly or implicitly) in terms of ϕ_m and one additional parameter A, which is a function of the permeabilities and thicknesses of the various layers. The results for the three geometries, obtaining by combining Equations **23**, **24**, or **25**, and **27**, are as follows:

Slab

$$\frac{1}{\phi_m^2} = \frac{(1 - \xi)^2 + 2(1 - \xi)A}{2} \tag{30}$$

$$\xi = (1 + A) - \left(\frac{2}{\phi_m^2} + A^2\right)^{1/2} \tag{31}$$

where

$$A = \left(\frac{\alpha D}{L}\right)_1 \sum_{j=2}^{n} \left[\frac{L_j - L_{j-1}}{(\alpha D)_j}\right] \tag{32}$$

Cylinder

$$\frac{1}{\phi_m^2} = \frac{1 - \xi^2(1 + 2\ln\xi) + 2(1 - \xi^2)A}{4} \tag{33}$$

where

$$A = (\alpha D)_1 \sum_{j=2}^{n} \left[\frac{\ln\left(\dfrac{R_j}{R_{j-1}}\right)}{(\alpha D)_j}\right] \tag{34}$$

Sphere

$$\frac{1}{\phi_m^2} = \frac{(2\xi^3 - 3\xi^2 + 1) + 2(1 - \xi^3)A}{6} \tag{35}$$

where

$$A = (\alpha D R)_1 \sum_{j=2}^{n} \left[\frac{\dfrac{1}{R_{j-1}} - \dfrac{1}{R_j}}{(\alpha D)_j}\right] \tag{36}$$

The dimensionless parameter A is related to the inverse of a Biot number Bi. The

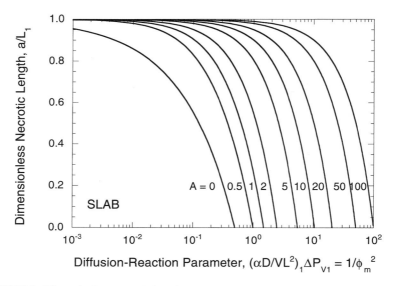

FIGURE 2. Dimensionless necrotic length a/L_1 for a slab as a function of a diffusion-reaction parameter $(\alpha D/VL^2)_1 \Delta P_{V1} = 1/\phi_m^2$.

Biot number is the ratio of the internal diffusive mass transfer resistance (layer 1) to the total external (sum of layers 2 to n) diffusive mass transfer resistance. When $\xi \neq 0$, the precise relationships are

Slab

$$A = \frac{1}{Bi}(1 - \xi) \tag{37}$$

Cylinder

$$A = \frac{1}{Bi}\ln\left(\frac{1}{\xi}\right) \tag{38}$$

Sphere

$$A = \frac{1}{Bi}\left(\frac{1}{\xi} - 1\right) \tag{39}$$

In contrast to A, Bi can be calculated only after ξ is evaluated. When the oxygen source is adjacent to the tissue/matrix composite, then the external resistance and the external oxygen consumption are zero, $A = 0$, and Equations 30–31, 33, and 35 reduce to Equations 11, 13, and 15–16. In analogy with the previous calculation procedure, the solution for ξ is explicit for slabs, Equation 31, implicit for cylinders, Equation 33, and implicit for spheres, Equation 35 (or explicit solution of a cubic equation). However, the additional iteration in the solution for a (or ξ) required in the previous calculation procedure is no longer needed. FIGURES 2–4 are plots

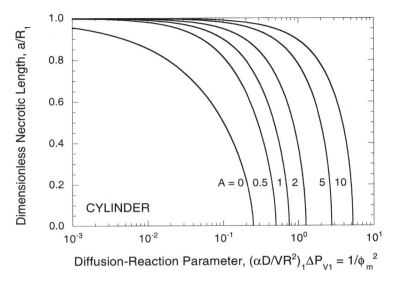

FIGURE 3. Dimensionless necrotic length a/R_1 for a cylinder as a function of a diffusion-reaction parameter $(\alpha D/VR^2)_1 \Delta P_{V1} = 1/\phi_m^2$.

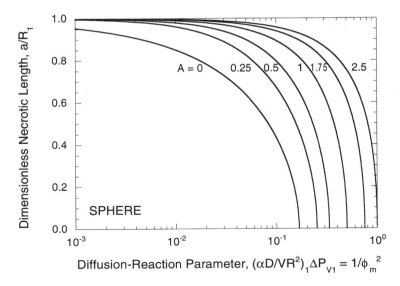

FIGURE 4. Dimensionless necrotic length a/R_1 for a sphere as a function of a diffusion-reaction parameter $(\alpha D/VR^2)_1 \Delta P_{V1} = 1/\phi_m^2$.

of ξ as a function of $1/\phi_m^2$ for various values of the parameter A for each geometry. The different ranges of A plotted in each figure are based upon estimates of physically reasonable bounds on permeability and geometric parameters.

To recapitulate the approach presented above, we want to estimate the thickness of the viable tissue,

$$\Delta h_{int} = h_1 - h_0 = (1 - \xi)h_1 \qquad (40)$$

given the actual internal half-thickness of the device, h_1. We refer to h_1 as "half-thickness" because the other half, which is mathematically identical, lies on the other side of the center of symmetry, but we refer to Δh_{int} as "thickness" because it can be physically separated by dead tissue from its mirror image. To determine Δh_{int}, we calculate $1/\phi_m^2$ using Equations **23**, **24**, or **25**, **27**, and **28**, A from Equations **32**, **34**, or **36**, ξ from Equations **30–31**, **33**, or **35**, and Δh_{int} from Equation **40**.

Once ξ (and therefore h_0 as well) is known, the required oxygen flux N_{S1} through the interface between the viable tissue/matrix compartment and the acellular membrane can be calculated from

$$N_{S1} = \left(V\frac{Volume}{Area}\right)_1 = Vmax(1 - \varepsilon_1)\frac{h_1^m - h_0^m}{m\,h_1^{m-1}} \qquad (41)$$

and the volume fraction F of tissue that is viable from

$$F = 1 - \xi^m \qquad (42)$$

where m equals 1 for slabs, 2 for cylinders, and 3 for spheres.

Although it may be possible for a biohybrid artificial pancreas to perform beneficially while having a core of dead tissue, it is desirable to prevent or minimize the loss of viability of any of the immunoisolated tissue for several reasons. First, cell lysis may be associated with release of wastes and deleterious agents, such as proteolytic enzymes, which serve to enlarge the region of dead cells beyond that attributable solely to low oxygen partial pressure. Secondly, antigenic proteins or protein fragments released from dying cells (especially xenogeneic tissue) may be able to diffuse through the immunoisolation membrane, thereby eliciting a humoral immune response. A sufficiently high density of antigen release from the device may also induce a local cellular response in the immediate vicinity of the device, thereby substantially increasing the external oxygen consumption rate and further depleting the oxygen available for supporting the internal implanted tissue.[9]

The maximum thickness of tissue which can be supported without causing a dead tissue core, under the assumption of zero-order kinetics for the oxygen consumption rate, can be calculated from Equations **28**, **30**, **33**, and **35** by setting ξ equal to zero (and using L'Hôpital's rule for the case of a cylinder) to obtain

$$\text{for } h_0 = 0, \qquad \frac{1}{\phi_m^2} = \frac{1 + 2A}{2m} \qquad (43)$$

and

$$\Delta h_{int} = (h_1 - h_0)_{max} = h_1 = \left[\left(\frac{\alpha D}{V}\right)_1 \Delta P_{V1}\frac{2m}{1 + 2A}\right]^{1/2} \qquad (44)$$

where m equals 1 for slabs, 2 for cylinders, and 3 for spheres. The trend of increasing maximum viable half-thickness from slab to cylinder to sphere is consistent with the trends we previously noted for the case of no external diffusion resistance.[11]

Because A is a function of h_1, Equation **44** must be solved iteratively for cylinders and spheres. Alternatively, a cubic equation can be solved for spheres. For slabs, Equation **44** is a quadratic equation in terms of $h_1 = L_1$ that can be easily solved analytically. An alternative solution for slabs is based on recognizing that the absence of curvature in the planar geometry renders the presence of a necrotic core mathematically immaterial. That is, the maximum thickness of the viable layer in the absence of a necrotic core is the same as the thickness of the viable layer in the presence of a necrotic core of arbitrary size. Therefore, we can choose an arbitrary value for L_1, with the only requirement that it be large enough to guarantee the presence of a necrotic core, calculate ξ from Equation **31**, and calculate the thickness of the viable layer ΔL_{int} from Equation **40**. The reader can easily verify the independence of ΔL_{int} from L_1 by substituting Equations **28** and **32** into Equation **31** and solving for $(1 - \xi)L_1$. A similar treatment is not possible for the cylindrical or spherical geometries where the size of the necrotic core affects the curvature of layer 1, and $(1 - \xi)R_1 = R_1 - R_0$ depends on the value of R_1.

EXAMPLES

In this section we will illustrate the use of the mathematical analysis in four examples, each of which is a subset of the arrangement schematically depicted in FIGURE 1. Islet tissue is homogeneously distributed in a slab ($i = 1$) of 2% Ca-alginate gel matrix with a tissue density of either 100% ($1 - \varepsilon_1 = 1$) in examples 1 and 3, or 10% ($1 - \varepsilon_1 = 0.1$) in examples 2 and 4. The tissue is immunoisolated from the host tissue by means of either a single-layer, cell-retentive, non-vascularizing membrane ($i = 2$) in examples 1 and 2, or, in examples 3 and 4, a composite membrane consisting of two layers[9] comprised of the same single-layer membrane ($i = 2$) laminated to an outer vascularizing membrane ($i = 3$). In all examples we will consider conditions at long times after implantation at which the host response to the implant has reached quasi-steady state. For the examples with a vascularizing outer membrane (3 and 4), we assume that the transplanted tissue has been able to survive the potentially severe diffusional limitations that may be present immediately following device implantation, *e.g.*, by implanting a device devoid of tissue, waiting until the neovascularization process has completed, and then injecting the tissue/gel matrix composite through a port.[9,15,18]

The single-layer membrane ($i = 2$) is a 30-μm thick,[19] 0.45 μm hydrophilic PTFE Biopore (Millipore) membrane which protects the transplant from invasion by host immune cells. We take the membrane void fraction to be 0.65[19] and assume it is occupied by extracellular fluid with properties equal to those of water at 37°C, $\alpha = 1.27 \times 10^{-9}$ mol/cm³ · mm Hg, $D = 2.70 \times 10^{-5}$ cm²/s, and permeability 3.43×10^{-14} mol/(cm · mm Hg · s) at 37°C.[16] In the examples with the composite membrane (3 and 4), layer 2 is bonded to a 15-μm thick[19] outer vascularizing membrane (layer 3) designated 5 μm expanded PTFE (Gore) that allows penetration of host cells without flattening on the interior membrane surfaces, thereby inducing growth of blood vessels[9,15] at the outer membrane surface ($S3$). The void fraction is taken to be 0.85[19] in layer 3 and is assumed to be occupied by extracellular fluid (80% of total volume) with permeability equal to that of water (as in layer 2) and infiltrating cells (5% of total volume). The volume fraction of infiltrating cells was estimated from photomicrographs of 8-μm pore diameter vascularizing membranes implanted for 329 days.[15]

We assume that the oxygen partial pressure of the microvasculature is 40 mm Hg, and that this value is uniformly available at the outer surface of the vascularizing membrane. Thus, $P_{S3} = P_{ext} = 40$ mm Hg. In the examples with the single-layer, non-vascularizing membrane, there is an avascular fibrotic host tissue layer ($i = 4$) between the membrane and the nearest blood vessels. Although the vascularizing membrane layer is absent in these examples, we will refer to the fibrotic tissue as layer 4 and let layer 3 have zero thickness for consistency. The thickness and cellularity of the fibrotic capsule change with post-implantation time. For example, at day 21 and with a 0.22-μm pore diameter membrane, there is a 75-μm thick avascular fibrotic layer containing about 30% volume fraction cells (fibroblasts), as estimated from a photomicrograph.[15] At longer times, the fibrotic capsule thickness is about 100 μm with about 5–10% cells.[20] For a mature fibrotic response, we assume $\Delta L_{ext} = L_4 - L_2 = 100$ μm and $1 - \varepsilon_4 = 0.1$. Assuming uniformity of oxygen partial pressure at the edge of the fibrotic layer ($S4$), the outer boundary condition becomes $P_{S4} = P_{ext} = 40$ mm Hg.

We arbitrarily chose the value of 250 μm for L_1 so that there is sufficient distance for P to drop to P_C in all four examples, in which case layer 1 thickness ΔL_{int} is also the maximum possible tissue/gel matrix half-thickness in the absence of necrosis.

For the critical oxygen partial pressure we take from the literature[17] $P_{S0} = P_C = 0.1$ mm Hg. The exact value of P_C is of minor importance in this analysis with zero-order kinetics, but it could be very important under certain conditions if Michaelis-Menten kinetics are used.[11,21]

Tissue parameter values at 37°C are taken as follows. Reported oxygen consumption rates of fibroblasts vary widely. We use an average of $V = 3.2$ (± 1.1) $\times$ 10^{-8} mol/cm$^3 \cdot$ s,[22–25] a value essentially identical to that for islet tissue, $V = 3.2$ (± 0.8) $\times$ 10^{-8} mol/cm$^3 \cdot$ s, under high glucose concentration (300 mg/dl).[16,21] The oxygen diffusivity in connective tissue is about 50% of that in water,[26] about the same as that for islet tissue, $D = 1.3$ (± 0.2) $\times$ 10^{-5} cm^2/s.[21] We assume that the oxygen diffusivity and solubility for the cells inside the vascularizing membrane and in the fibrotic capsule, as well as for the connective tissue in the fibrotic capsule, are the same as for islet tissue. We use an average oxygen solubility of $\alpha = 1.0 \times$ 10^{-9} mol/cm$^3 \cdot$ mm Hg[16] from literature values for various tissues.

To calculate the effective permeability $(\alpha D)_{eff} = (\alpha D)_i$ in each layer i, we use the Maxwell relationship[27]

$$\frac{(\alpha D)_{eff}}{(\alpha D)_c} = \frac{2 - 2\theta + \rho(1 + 2\theta)}{2 + \theta + \rho(1 - \theta)} \tag{45}$$

where

$$\rho = \frac{(\alpha D)_d}{(\alpha D)_c} \tag{46}$$

Subscripts c and d refer to continuous and dispersed phases, respectively, and θ is the volume fraction of the dispersed phase. When more than 2 phases are present in a layer, Equation **45** is used in sequential steps. In layer 1, $(\alpha D)_{eff}$ in a 2% Ca-alginate matrix, calculated from Equation **45** with $\theta = 0.02$ and $\rho = 0$, is reduced 3% relative to its value in water, which is in good agreement with literature data.[28–31] Then, the matrix is treated as the continuous phase and the tissue as the dispersed phase. In layer 2 the membrane material is treated as the dispersed phase with zero permeability. In layer 3, cells are first considered to be the dispersed phase in an extracellular liquid continuous phase, and then the membrane material is considered

TABLE 1. Values of Independent and Dependent Parameters and Dimensionless Groups in Examples

Parameters	Examples 1 Fibrotic $1 - \varepsilon_1 = 1$	2 Fibrotic $1 - \varepsilon_1 = 0.1$	3 Vascularized $1 - \varepsilon_1 = 1$	4 Vascularized $1 - \varepsilon_1 = 0.1$
$L_3 - L_2$ (μm)	0	0	15	15
$L_4 - L_3 = \Delta L_{ext}$	100	100	0	0
V_1 (10⁻⁸ mol/cm³ · s)	3.2	0.32	3.2	0.32
V_3	—	—	0.16	0.16
V_4	0.32	0.32	—	—
$(\alpha D)_1$ (10⁻¹⁴ mol/ cm · mm Hg · s)	1.3	3.1	1.3	3.1
$(\alpha D)_2$	1.9	1.9	1.9	1.9
$(\alpha D)_3$	—	—	2.6	2.6
$(\alpha D)_4$	1.3	1.3	—	—
ϕ_m	7.5	1.5	6.2	1.3
$1/\phi_m^2$	0.018	0.42	0.026	0.61
A	0.48	1.1	0.11	0.27
ξ	0.96	0.67	0.86	0.13
L_0	241	169	215	32
$L_1 - L_0 = \Delta L_{int}$	9.0	81	35	218
$\Delta L_{int}(1 - \varepsilon_1)$	9.0	8.1	35	21.8
ϕ	39	4.3	10	1.6
$1/\phi^2$	6.4 × 10⁻⁴	0.053	0.010	0.38
Bi	0.074	0.28	1.3	3.3
P_{S1} (mm Hg)	1.1	3.5	15	25
N_{S1} (10⁻¹¹ mol/cm² · s)	2.9	2.6	11	7.0
N_{S3}	—	—	12	7.2
N_{S4}	6.1	5.8	—	—

For all examples, $P_{ext} = 40$ mm Hg, $P_C = 0.1$ mm Hg, $L_1 = 250$ μm, $L_2 - L_1 = 30$ μm.

the dispersed phase in the composite continuous phase. In layer 4, the cells are treated as the dispersed phase in a continuous phase of connective tissue. Equation **45** was developed for the case of spheres dispersed in a continuous phase and gives only approximate estimates of permeability for the membranes which are better modeled as fibrous media. Given information for the fiber radius and orientation in each membrane, one could calculate more accurately the effective diffusivity of oxygen in these layers.[32–35]

For all four examples, the values of independent parameters associated with the thickness, oxygen consumption, and permeability of each layer, as well as dimensionless groups ϕ_m and A, are listed in TABLE 1, followed by the values of parameters and dimensionless groups derived from the solution.

FIGURE 5A is a plot of the viable tissue layer thickness ΔL_{int} versus the fibrotic tissue layer thickness ΔL_{ext} for several values of $1 - \varepsilon_1$. Figure 5B is a similar plot except that the ordinate is the equivalent thickness of high density tissue $\Delta L_{int}(1 - \varepsilon_1)$, or volume of tissue per unit area. $\Delta L_{int}(1 - \varepsilon_1)$ is the volume/area of compacted tissue which would remain if all the gel matrix is removed. In both figures, the results for $\Delta L_{ext} = 100$ μm and $1 - \varepsilon_1 = 1$ and 0.1 correspond to examples 1 and 2, respectively. The results for $\Delta L_{ext} = 0$ and $1 - \varepsilon_1 = 1$ and 0.1

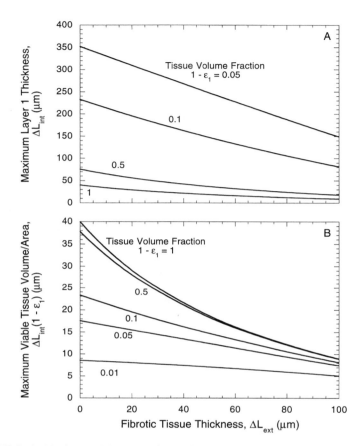

FIGURE 5. A: Maximum viable tissue (layer 1) thickness ΔL_{int} as a function of the fibrotic tissue (layer 4) thickness ΔL_{ext} for different values of $1 - \varepsilon_1$. Parameters are the same as for examples 1 and 2, except for the variations in ΔL_{ext} and $1 - \varepsilon_1$. **B:** Maximum viable tissue volume per unit area $\Delta L_{int}(1 - \varepsilon_1)$ as a function of the fibrotic tissue (layer 4) thickness ΔL_{ext}. Same conditions as for **(A)**.

differ slightly from examples 3 and 4 because there is no vascularizing membrane (layer 3) present for the results in FIGURE 5.

TABLES 2–5 contain the individual partial pressure drop components in the form of a matrix arranged in two ways. Each term ΔP_{ij} in row i and column j is the partial pressure drop in layer j induced by oxygen consumption in layer i. Dashes indicate ΔP_{ij} $(i > j)$ that do not exist, based on the geometry of the problem. The rightmost column contains the total partial pressure drop ΔP_{Vi} (summed through all layers) induced by oxygen consumption in layer i. The sum of the terms in each column j is the total partial pressure drop ΔP_j through layer j induced by oxygen consumption in all layers. The totals each way add up to $P_{ext} - P_C = 39.9$ mm Hg. For example, in TABLE 2, $\Delta P_{14} = 22.1$ mm Hg is the drop across the fibrotic layer

TABLE 2. ΔP Components (mm Hg): Example 1 (fibrotic, $1 - \varepsilon_1 = 1$)

		Layer posing diffusive resistance (j)				
		1	2	4	Total	
Layer	1	1.0	4.5	22.1	27.6	
consuming	2	—	0	0	0	ΔP_{Vi}
oxygen (i)	4	—	—	12.3	12.3	
	Total	1.0	4.5	34.4	39.9	
			ΔP_j			

TABLE 3. ΔP Components (mm Hg): Example 2 (fibrotic, $1 - \varepsilon_1 = 0.1$)

		Layer posing diffusive resistance (j)				
		1	2	4	Total	
Layer	1	3.4	4.1	20.0	27.6	
consuming	2	—	0	0	0	ΔP_{Vi}
oxygen (i)	4	—	—	12.3	12.3	
	Total	3.4	4.1	32.3	39.9	
			ΔP_j			

TABLE 4. ΔP Components (mm Hg): Example 3 (vascularized, $1 - \varepsilon_1 = 1$)

		Layer posing diffusive resistance (j)				
		1	2	3	Total	
Layer	1	15.4	17.9	6.6	39.8	
consuming	2	—	0	0	0	ΔP_{Vi}
oxygen (i)	3	—	—	0.1	0.1	
	Total	15.4	17.9	6.6	39.9	
			ΔP_j			

TABLE 5. ΔP Components (mm Hg): Example 4 (fibrotic, $1 - \varepsilon_1 = 0.1$)

		\multicolumn{4}{c}{Layer posing diffusive resistance (j)}	
		1	2	3	Total	
Layer	1	24.7	11.0	4.0	39.8	
consuming	2	—	0	0	0	ΔP_{Vi}
oxygen (i)	3	—	—	0.1	0.1	
	Total	24.7	11.0	4.1	39.9	
		\multicolumn{4}{c}{ΔP_j}	

induced by oxygen consumption in layer 1, $\Delta P_{44} = 12.3$ mm Hg is the drop across the fibrotic layer induced by oxygen consumption within that layer itself, and $\Delta P_4 = 34.4$ mm Hg is the total partial pressure drop across the fibrotic layer. These results identify the dominant contributions to the total ΔP which provides guidance for improving device design and performance.

FIGURES 6 and 7 contain profiles of oxygen partial pressure as a function of the distance x from the center of the symmetry for examples 1–4. The profiles for values of x between any two interfaces were obtained by solving Equation **1** within all layers (equations not presented). In FIGURE 6, layer 3 is absent.

The differences between the fibrotic (examples 1 and 2) and the vascularized (examples 3 and 4) situations are dramatic. In example 1, the thickness of the viable tissue layer ΔL_{int} is just 9 μm, while in example 3 it is about 35 μm. In examples 2 and 4, the respective thicknesses are about 81 and 218 μm. This demonstrates the critical importance of neovascularization at the membrane/host tissue interface. The differences between the fibrotic and the vascularized examples can be explained in various ways. We begin with simple physical concepts. The maximum oxygen partial pressure driving force available for supporting the implanted tissue is $P_{ext} - P_C = 39.9$ mm Hg. When a fibrotic layer is present (examples 1 and 2), oxygen consumption by cells in layer 4 depletes the oxygen and causes a partial pressure drop, $\Delta P_{44} = 12.3$ mm Hg, thereby reducing the available driving force to $\Delta P_{V1} = 27.6$ mm Hg. This value is then divided up between the various layers in proportion to their relative diffusive oxygen mass transfer resistances. This is apparent by writing Equation **23** for example 1 as

$$\text{Layer} \qquad 1 \qquad\qquad 2 \qquad\qquad 4$$

$$\Delta P_{V1} = V_1(L_1 - L_0) \left[\frac{1}{2} \frac{(L_1 - L_0)}{(\alpha D)_1} + \frac{(L_2 - L_1)}{(\alpha D)_2} + \frac{(L_4 - L_2)}{(\alpha D)_4} \right] \qquad \textbf{(47)}$$

$V_1(L_1 - L_0)$ is the oxygen flux (oxygen consumption rate per unit area) required to support the tissue in layer 1, and each term in the brackets is the mass transfer resistance of its respective layer. The factor of 1/2 for layer 1 reflects the oxygen consumption that occurs in that layer. Direct substitution of parameter values for example 1 from TABLE 1, without conversion of length units, leads to 3.5, 15.8, and 76.9, for layers 1, 2, and 4, respectively, in units of 10^{14} μm · cm · mm Hg/mol · s, with a total of 96.2. The fraction of the total resistance represented by each layer

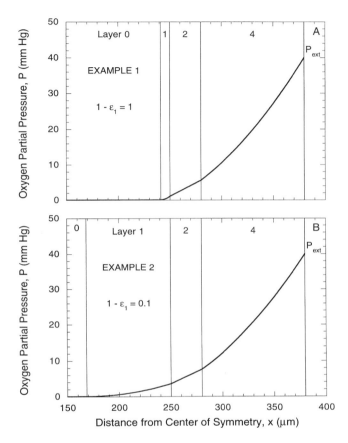

FIGURE 6. Oxygen partial pressure as a function of distance from the center plane of a slab (layers 0 and 1) with half-thickness 250 μm, immunoisolated by a single-layer non-vascularizing membrane (layer 2). The membrane is surrounded by fibrotic host tissue (layer 4) exposed at its surface to P_{S4} = 40 mm Hg. **A:** Volume fraction of transplanted tissue in layer 1, $1 - \varepsilon_1$ = 1, example 1. **B:** Volume fraction of transplanted tissue in layer 1, $1 - \varepsilon_1$ = 0.1, example 2. Most of layer 0, throughout which $P = P_C$, is not shown.

is then 0.036, 0.164, and 0.799 for layers 1, 2, and 4, respectively. Multiplication of these fractions by 27.6 leads to the values of ΔP_{ij} in row 1 of TABLE 2. Of the remaining 5.5 mm Hg external pressure drop outside of the fibrotic layer, ΔP_{12} = 4.5 mm Hg is used up across the cell retentive membrane (layer 2), leaving only $\Delta P_{11} = P_{S1} - P_C$ = 1.0 mm Hg to support the implanted tissue. Thus, the oxygen consumption by cells in the fibrotic layer and its high mass transfer resistance relative to the other layers combine to use up about 86% of the maximum driving force, thereby effectively starving the implanted tissue of oxygen.

When a vascularizing membrane is added (examples 3 and 4), blood vessels are brought close to its outer surface, and the effects of the fibrotic layer are eliminated.

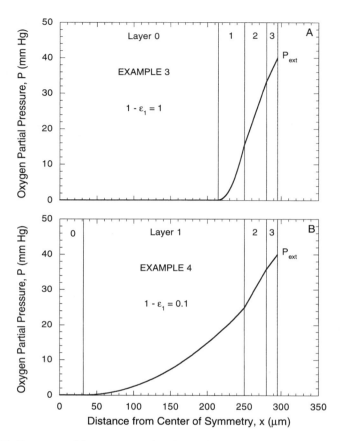

FIGURE 7. Oxygen partial pressure as a function of distance from the center plane of a slab (layers 0 and 1) with half-thickness 250 μm, immunoisolated by a composite vascularizing membrane (layers 2 and 3) exposed at its surface to $P_{S3} = 40$ mm Hg. **A:** Volume fraction of transplanted tissue in layer 1, $1 - \varepsilon_1 = 1$, example 3. **B:** Volume fraction of transplanted tissue in layer 1, $1 - \varepsilon_1 = 0.1$, example 4.

Oxygen consumption by cells in layer 3 is negligible, so that $\Delta P_{V1} \simeq P_{ext} - P_C$. The relative mass transfer resistance of layer 3 is small. That of layer 2 is now more important, and $\Delta P_{12} = 17.9$ mm Hg is substantial. Nonetheless, there is a large increase in ΔP_{11} to 15.4 mm Hg (example 3) which is associated with a fourfold increase in ΔL_{int} to 35.4 μm (about 71 μm thickness of viable tissue in the entire device).

These trends are reflected in the values of the dimensionless groups and other parameters. For example, in shifting from a fibrotic layer to a vascularized interface, $1/\phi_m^2$ increases modestly as a result of increased ΔP_{V1}, and A decreases fourfold, both of which tend to decrease ξ (FIG. 2) and increase ΔL_{int}. Bi increases 17-fold (example 3), reflecting a change from dominant limitations by the external mass transfer resistance to a situation where external and internal resistances are comparable. The Thiele modulus decreases about fourfold, reflecting the increase in $P_{S1} - P_C$, but the large values of ϕ in both cases are consistent with a rate of oxygen consumption that is large with respect to the rate of oxygen diffusion in layer 1. The increase in oxygen flux N_{S1} directly parallels the increase in ΔL_{int}.

As tissue volume fraction $1 - \varepsilon_1$ in layer 1 decreases (FIG. 5), ξ decreases and ΔL_{int} increases markedly. This trend reflects the competing effects of 1) increased permeability $(\alpha D)_1$ and lower V_1, leading to markedly decreased ϕ_m and ϕ (which decrease ξ and increase ΔL_{int}), and 2) increased A which has the opposite effect. Because of the extreme decrease in ξ and concomitant increase in ΔL_{int}, Bi also increases, reflecting the relative increase in the internal mass transfer resistance as ΔL_{int} increases. Although ΔL_{int} increases with decreasing $1 - \varepsilon_1$, the equivalent tissue thickness $\Delta L_{int}(1 - \varepsilon_1)$ does not. Between $1 - \varepsilon_1 = 1$ and 0.5, $\Delta L_{int}(1 - \varepsilon_1)$ is insensitive to $1 - \varepsilon_1$; however, it decreases substantially as $1 - \varepsilon_1$ decreases to low values. Thus, there is no improvement to be gained in the equivalent thickness of viable tissue by decreasing tissue volume fraction, at least for the case of homogeneously distributed tissue in a slab. However, because a larger fraction of the tissue is exposed to very low P in the high density limit, there may be some benefit from the standpoint of overall tissue function (e.g., insulin secretion) which deteriorates at low P.

CONCLUDING REMARKS

In this article we have analyzed the effects of external mass transfer resistances and oxygen consumption in the external layers surrounding immunoisolated tissue with the assumption of zero-order kinetics for the oxygen consumption rate. We derived relationships that allow the prediction of the maximum supportable viable thickness for different device geometries. Through example calculations for a slab geometry, we showed the detrimental effects of an oxygen-consuming host fibrotic tissue layer surrounding the device and the necessity of inducing vascularization close to the outer membrane surface.

A limitation in our mathematical model is the assumption of zero-order oxygen consumption kinetics by the transplanted tissue. Use of Michaelis-Menten kinetics, which more accurately describes oxygen consumption rate, would lead to decreasing oxygen consumption rate as oxygen partial pressure decreases, thereby producing larger estimates of the viable tissue thickness. An accurate estimate of P_C is much more important in conjunction with the use of Michaelis-Menten kinetics than with zero-order kinetics, because use of the former leads to oxygen profile predictions that are flatter as P drops below the Michaelis-Menten constant Km and towards P_C. Development of models using the nonlinear Michaelis-Menten kinetics, which requires numerical solution, is planned for a subsequent study.

REFERENCES

1. KAHAN, B. D. 1989. Cyclosporine. N. Engl. J. Med. **321:** 1725–1738.
2. FUNG, J. J., M. ALESSIANI & K. ABU-ELMAGD. 1991. Adverse effects associated with the use of FK 506. Transplant. Proc. **23:** 1305–1308.
3. SCHARP, D. W., N. S. MASON & R. E. SPARKS. 1984. Islet immunoisolation: The use of hybrid artificial organs to prevent islet tissue rejection. World J. Surg. **8:** 221–229.

4. COLTON, C. K. & E. S. AVGOUSTINIATOS. 1991. Bioengineering in development of the hybrid artificial pancreas. ASME J. Biomech. Eng. **113:** 152–170.
5. BELLAMKONDA, R. & P. AEBISCHER. 1994. Review: Tissue engineering in the nervous system. Biotech. Bioeng. **43:** 543–554.
6. LYSAGHT, M. J., B. FRYDEL, D. EMERICH & S. WINN. 1994. Recent progress in immunoisolated cell therapy. J. Cellular Biochem. **56:** 196–203.
7. MIKOS, A. G., M. G. PAPADAKI, S. KOUVROUKOGLOU, S. L. ISGHANG & R. C. C. THOMPSON. 1994. Mini-review: Islet transplantation to create a bioartificial pancreas. Biotech. Bioeng. **43:** 673–677.
8. AEBISCHER, P. & M. J. LYSAGHT. 1995. Immunoisolation and cellular xenotransplantation. Xeno **3:** 43–48.
9. COLTON, C. K. 1995. Implantable biohybrid artificial organs. Cell Transplant. **4:** 415–436.
10. LANZA, R. P. & W. L. CHICK. 1995. Encapsulated cell transplantation. Transplant. Rev. **9:** 217–230.
11. AVGOUSTINIATOS, E. S. & C. K. COLTON. 1997. Design considerations in immunoisolation. *In* Principles of Tissue Engineering. R. P. Lanza, R. Langer & W. L. Chick, Eds. : 333–346. R. G. Landes. Austin, TX.
12. TANNOCK, I. F. 1972. Oxygen diffusion and the distribution of cellular radiosensitivity in tumors. Brit. J. Radiol. **45:** 515–524.
13. DIONNE, K. E., C. K. COLTON & M. L. YARMUSH. 1993. Effect of hypoxia on insulin secretion by isolated rat and canine islets of Langerhans. Diabetes **42:** 12–21.
14. BRAUKER, J. H., V. E. CARR-BRENDEL, L. A. MARTINSON, J. CRUDELE, W. D. JOHNSTON & R. C. JOHNSON. 1995. Neovascularization of synthetic membranes directed by membrane microarchitecture. J. Biomed. Mat. Res. **29:** 1517–1524.
15. PADERA, R. F. & C. K. COLTON. 1996. Time course of membrane microarchitecture-driven neovascularization. Biomaterials **17:** 277–284.
16. DIONNE, K. E. 1989. Effect of hypoxia on insulin secretion and viability of pancreatic tissue. Ph.D. Thesis. Massachusetts Institute of Technology, Cambridge, MA.
17. ANUNDI, I. & H. DE GROOT. 1989. Hypoxic liver cell death: Critical Po$_2$ and dependence of viability on glycolysis. Am. J. Physiol. **257:** G58-G64.
18. JOHNSON, R. C., V. CARR-BRENDEL, L. MARTINSON, S. NEUENFELDT, S. YOUNG, C. VERGOTH, D. HODGETT, D. MARYANOV, S. JACOBS, R. HILL, T. J. THOMAS & J. BRAUKER. 1994 An organoid structure for the implantation of genetically engineered cells and pancreatic islets [abstract]. Cell Transplant. **3:** 221.
19. NEUENFELDT, S. (Baxter Healthcare). 1996. Personal communication.
20. BRAUKER, J. H. (Baxter Healthcare). 1996. Personal communication.
21. AVGOUSTINIATOS E. S. 1997. Oxygen diffusion limitations in the bioartificial pancreas. Ph.D. Thesis. Massachusetts Institute of Technology, Cambridge, MA.
22. HOFFNER, S. E. S., R. W. J. MEREDITH & R. B. KEMP. 1985. Estimation of heat production by cultured cells in suspension using semi-automated flow microcalorimetry. Cytobios **42:** 71–80.
23. ROBINSON, B. H., J. WARD, P. GOODYER & A. BAUDET. 1986. Respiratory chain defects in the mitochondria of cultured skin fibroblasts from three patients with lacticacidemia. J. Clin. Invest. **77:** 1422–1427.
24. AYMARD, C., M. MALGAT, J.-P. MAZAT & J. KOENIG. 1993. Effect of the mutation *muscular dysgenesis* on the mitochondria metabolism of fibroblasts *in vitro.* C.R. Acad. Sci. Paris, Life Sciences **316:** 529–532.
25. KUNZ, D., C. LULEY, S. FRITZ, R. BOHNENSACK, K. WINKLER, W. S. KUNZ & C.-W. WALLESCH. 1995. Oxygraphic evaluation of mitochondrial function in digitonin-permeabilized mononuclear cells and cultured skin fibroblasts of patients with chronic progressive external ophthalmoplegia. Biochem. Molec. Med. **54:** 105–111.
26. GRODZINSKY, A. (Massachusetts Institute of Technology). 1997. Personal communication.
27. MAXWELL, J. C. 1881. A Treatise on Electricity and Magnetism, Vol. 1, p. 440. Clarendon Press. London, UK.
28. PRESTON, B. N. & J. McK. SNOWDEN. 1972. Model connective tissue systems: The effect of proteoglycans on the diffusional behavior of small non-electrolytes and microions. Biopolymers **11:** 1627–1643.

29. TANAKA, H., M. MATSUMURA & I. A. VELIKY. 1984. Diffusion characteristics of substrates in Ca-alginate gel beads. Biotech. Bioeng. **26:** 53–58.

30. MERCHANT, F. J. A., A. MARGARITIS, J. B. WALLACE & A. VARDANIS. 1987. A novel technique for measuring solute diffusivities in entrapment matrices used in immobilization. Biotech. Bioeng. **30:** 936–945.

31. KUROSAWA, H., M. MATSUMURA & H. TANAKA. 1989. Oxygen diffusivity in gel beads containing viable cells. Biotech. Bioeng. **34:** 926–932.

32. OGSTON, A. G., B. N. PRESTON & J. D. WELLS. 1973. On the transport of compact particles through solutions of chain polymers. Proc. R. Soc. Lond. A. **333:** 297–316.

33. PERRINS, W. T., D. R. MCKENZIE & R. C. MCPHEDRAN. 1979. Transport properties of regular arrays of cylinders. Proc. R. Soc. Lond. A. **369:** 207–225.

34. JOHANSSON, L. & J.-E. LÖFROTH. 1993. Diffusion and interaction in gels and solutions. 4. Hard sphere Brownian dynamics simulations. J. Chem. Phys. **98:** 7471–7479.

35. JOHNSON, E. M., D. A. BERK, R. K. JAIN & W. M. DEEN. 1996. Hindered diffusion in agarose gels: Test of the effective medium model. Biophys. J. **70:** 1017–1026.

Controlled Drug Release from Self-Catalyzed Poly(Ortho Esters)

STEVEN Y. NG, THIERRY VANDAMME,
MICHELLE S. TAYLOR, AND JORGE HELLER

Advanced Polymer Systems
3696 Haven Avenue
Redwood City, California 94063

Poly(ortho esters) are a versatile family of biodegradable polymers that have been under development since the early 1970s, and three distinct families, shown in SCHEME 1, have been described. Comprehensive reviews of poly(ortho esters) prepared prior to 1992 have been published.[1,2]

To date, the most successful polymer is that derived from the reaction between a diol and a diketene acetal, shown in SCHEME 2, using the diketene acetal 3,9-diethylidene-2,4,8,10-tetraoxaspiro [5.5] undecane.

Even though poly(ortho esters) contain a hydrolytically labile ortho ester group, they are very stable even when exposed to a neutral aqueous environment. This stability is due to the highly hydrophobic nature of these polymers that have a saturated water-vapor sorption ranging between 0.3 and 0.75 w/w, depending on whether the material is in the glassy or rubbery state.[3] FIGURE 1 shows weight loss as a function of time for a polymer prepared from 1,6-hexanediol and 3,9-dimethylene-2,4,8,10-tetraoxaspiro [5.5] undecane.

To achieve useful rates of polymer hydrolysis, it is necessary to use small amounts of acidic excipients that are physically incorporated into the polymer.[4] Then, the rate of hydrolysis can be manipulated by varying the pKa and/or concentration of the acidic excipient. Although a number of different acidic excipients have been used with poly(ortho esters), good results can be achieved by using suberic acid.

A schematic depiction of the catalyzed erosion process is shown in FIGURE 2. According to this process, when a device containing physically dispersed drug and excipient (suberic acid) is placed in an aqueous environment, water will gradually diffuse into the device and dissolve the excipient in the surface layers, where the lowered pH will accelerate the rate of hydrolysis. This process has been analyzed in terms of the movement of two fronts, an eroding front, F_1 and a hydration front F_2.[5] When the movement of these two front is synchronized, surface erosion is obtained. When the rate of movement of F_2 is higher than F_1, bulk erosion is observed.

Although use of excipients represents a useful means of controlling the rate of polymer erosion, diffusion of the excipient from the polymer is a serious problem that not only complicates kinetics of drug release, but more importantly, eventually leads to an excipient-depleted polymer that will remain in the tissues for a significant length of time. This residual polymer has been referred to as "ghosts" and its formation has been mathematically modeled.[6,7]

In order to eliminate complications inherent in using a low molecular weight excipient, the use of macromolecular excipients could be considered. However, a better approach is to incorporate into the polymer backbone a short segment that readily hydrolyzes to an acidic product which then acts as the acidic excipient and catalyzes the hydrolysis of ortho ester linkages in the polymer. Then, by controlling

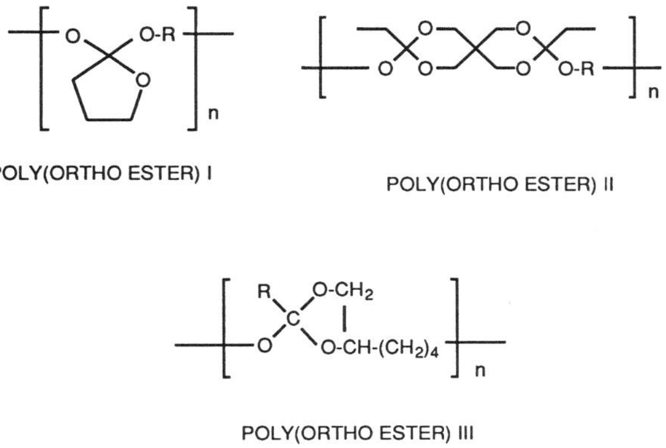

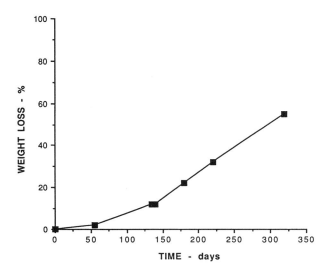

SCHEME 1

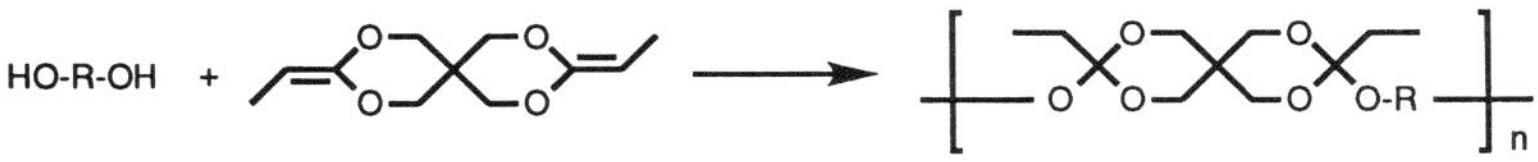

SCHEME 2

FIGURE 1. Weight loss as a function of time for a polymer prepared from 3,9-dimethylene-2,4,8,10-tetraoxaspiro [5.5] undecane and 1,6-hexanediol. 0.05 M phosphate buffer, pH 7.4, 37°C. (Reprinted with permission from ref. 8, Copyright 1997, American Chemical Society.)

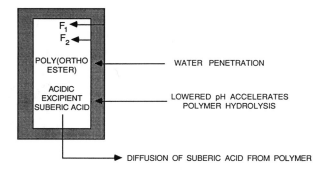

FIGURE 2. Schematic representation of erosion of a poly(ortho ester) containing dispersed suberic acid. F_1 is movement of eroding front, F_2 is movement of hydration front.

the amount of such a segment in the polymer, the rate of erosion can be accurately controlled without complications arising from excipient diffusion.

We have found that a useful segment is a glycolic acid dimer and in this manuscript we describe polymer synthesis and some initial drug release studies. A more detailed synthesis of this, and related materials has been described.[8]

EXPERIMENTAL SECTION

Materials

Triethylene Glycol Glycolide

In a dry-box, 15.07 g (100 mmoles) of triethylene glycol and 11.06 g (100 mmoles) of glycolide were weighed into a 50 ml flask. The flask was sealed with a rubber septum and heated overnight at 180°C in an oil bath. The resulting material was not purified and was used directly in the polymerization reaction.

trans-Cyclohexanedimethanol Glycolide

In a dry-box, 22.18g (154 mmoles) of *trans*-cyclohexanedimethanol and 17.86 g (154 mmoles) of glycolide were weighed into a 50 ml flask. The flask was sealed with a rubber septum and heated overnight at 180°C in an oil bath. The resulting material was not purified and was used directly in the polymerization reaction.

n-Decanediol Glycolide

In a dry-box, 15.0g (86 mmoles) of *n*-decanediol and 9.98 g (86 mmoles) of glycolide were weighed into a 50 ml flask. The flask was sealed with a rubber septum and heated overnight at 180°C in an oil bath. The resulting material was not purified and was used directly in the polymerization reaction.

Polymerization

Under anhydrous conditions 13.515 g (90 mmoles) of triethylene glycol and 2.663 g (10 mmoles) of the triethylene glycol monoglycolide described above were weighed into a 250 ml flask and the mixture dissolved in 50 ml of tetrahydrofuran. Then 19.103 g (90 mmoles) of 3,9-diethylidene-2,4,8,10-tetraoxaspiro [5.5] undecane were added. After the exothermic reaction subsided, the solution was first concentrated on a roto-evaporator and the remaining solvent removed in a vacuum oven at 40°C.

Polymer Characterization

Molecular weights were determined by Gel Permeation Chromatography (GPC) using tetrahydrofuran as the solvent, polystyrene molecular weight standards and a Turbochrome software package. Melting temperatures were determined by using a melting stage apparatus.

Preparation of Drug-containing Devices

Solid devices were fabricated by first dissolving 1.8 g of polymer in approximately 5 ml of tetrahydrofuran and then adding 0.2 g of drug. The mixture was vigorously stirred and then transferred to a teflon pan and dried under vacuum at approximately 40°C. The dry mixture was then transferred to a dye, heated to 65°C, maintained at 20,000 psi for 5 min. and cooled to room temperature. Disks weighing approximately 22 mg were cut from the films with a heated circular punch. For ointment-like polymers, 10 wt% drug was mixed into the polymer at, or slightly above room temperature, using a mortar and pestle.

Determination of Erosion and Drug Release Rates

Weighed polymer samples were incubated at 37°C in pH 7.4, 0.05M phosphate buffer and at selected time intervals, samples were removed and dried to constant weight for mass loss determination.

Drug release kinetics were conducted in triplicate in 0.05 M phosphate buffer in sealed test tubes maintained at 37°C under gentle agitation using an American Rotator V apparatus. At preselected intervals, an aliquot of solution was removed and replaced with fresh buffer. The drug concentration in the solution was determined by UV spectrophotometry at 264 nm for 5-fluorouracil and 495 nm for FITC-labeled bovine serum albumin. Solid devices were placed in dialysis bags which were mechanically moved up and down in a test tube with 25 ml of buffer. The dialysis bags were permeable up to a molecular weight of 8000 kD. For ointment like materials, approximately 100 mg was weighed into a small polyethylene cap which was then placed in a test tube with buffer.

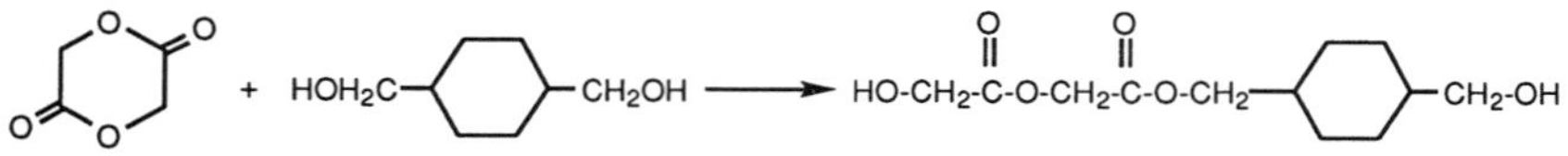

SCHEME 3

RESULTS AND DISCUSSION

Polymer Hydrolysis

To prepare polymers that contain a hydrolytically labile segment, a monomer containing a glycolide dimer is first prepared as shown for *trans*-cyclohexanedimethanol in SCHEME 3.

A polymer using *trans*-cyclohexanedimethanol glycolide and *trans*-cyclohexanedimethanol is then prepared as shown in SCHEME 4. Varying the relative proportions of the two diols controls the amount of glycolic acid dimer in the polymer.

Because this polymer contains glycolic acid dimer segments which, unlike poly(ortho ester) segments, are not stable at pH 7.4 and 37°C, when placed in an aqueous environment, the glycolic acid dimer segments will hydrolyze to generate glycolic acid which will catalyze hydrolysis of the ortho ester linkages in the polymer backbone. The hydrolysis is shown in SCHEME 5.

Erosion of a polymer based on *trans*-cyclohexanedimethanol and *trans*-cyclohexanedimethanol glycolide, as a function of glycolic acid dimer segment concentration, is shown in FIGURE 3. Clearly, incorporation of glycolic acid dimer segments into the polymer not only results in a significant improvement in erosion kinetics which now proceed by close to zero order kinetics to completion, but also allow an accurate control over erosion rate.

FIGURE 4 shows weight loss and changes in number average molecular weight as a function of time for a 50/50 copolymer of *trans*-cyclohexanedimethanol glycolide and *trans*-cyclohexanedimethanol. The points represent weights of remaining polymer and molecular weights of the remaining polymer. There is a slight induction

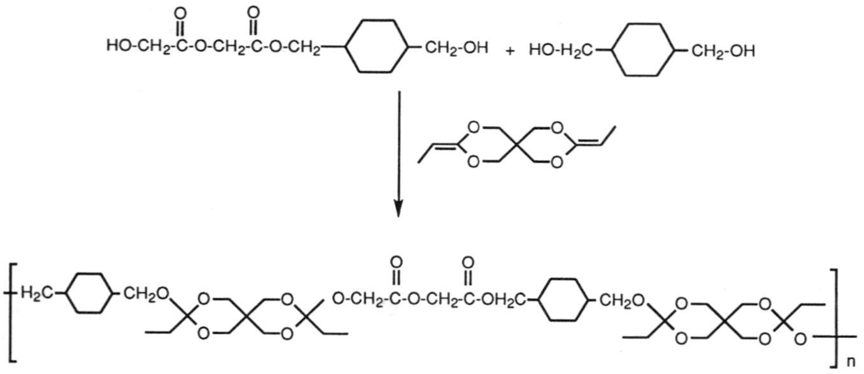

SCHEME 4

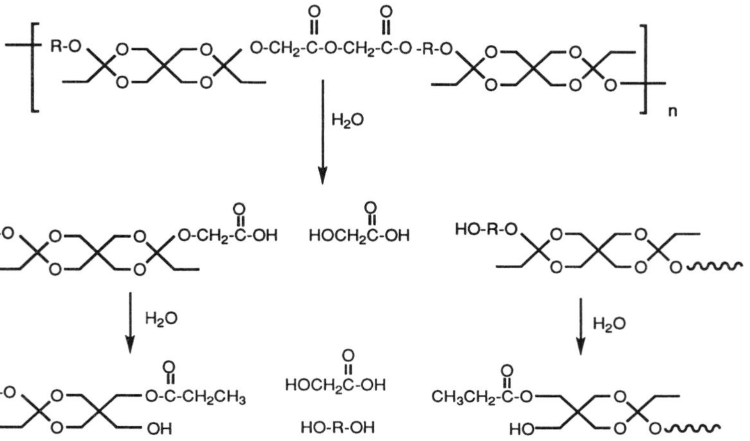

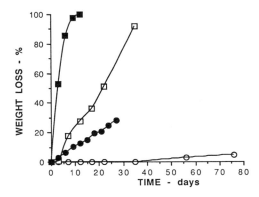

SCHEME 5

time of about two days where no weight loss, nor molecular weight decrease is detected, after which the molecular weight decreases steadily until about day 20, after which it remains relatively constant at about one half of the original value. Rate of weight loss remains relatively constant throughout the entire study carried out over 60 days.

In view of the relatively high concentration of glycolic acid dimer segments in the polymer backbone, it is clear that these segment hydrolyze gradually since rapid hydrolysis of all segments would result in a cleavage of the backbone at the glycolic acid dimer segments with a consequent decrease of polymer molecular weight to a value of about 350. Thus, the linearity of weight loss and the slow changes in molecular weights are consistent with a process that occurs predominantly in the surface layers of the device with a gradual production of glycolic acid. At this point the discontinuity in the rate of molecular weight change that occurs at day 20 is not understood.

FIGURE 3. Weight loss as a function of poly(glycolic acid) dimer content for a polymer prepared from 3,9-diethylidene - 2,4,8,10 - tetraoxaspiro [5.5] undecane, *trans*-cyclohexanedimethanol glycolide (tCDM/Gly) and *trans*-cyclohexanedimethanol (tCDM). 25/75 tCDM-tCDM/Gly (■), 50/50 tCDM-CDM/Gly (□), 25/75 tCDM-tCDM/Gly (●), 90/10 tCDM-tCDM/Gly (○). 0.05 M phosphate buffer, pH 7.4, 37°C. (Reprinted with permission from ref. 8, Copyright 1997, American Chemical Society.)

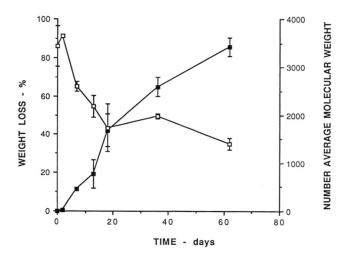

FIGURE 4. Weight loss (■) and changes in number average molecular weight (□) as a function of time for a polymer prepared from 3,9-diethylidene-2,4,8,10-tetraoxaspiro [5.5] undecane and a 50/50 mixture of *trans*-cyclohexanedimethanol glycolide and *trans*-cyclohex-anedimethanol. 0.05 M phosphate buffer, pH 7.4, 37°C. (Reprinted with permission from ref. 8, Copyright 1997, American Chemical Society.)

Polymer Physical Properties

The usefulness of a drug delivery system not only depends on an ability to control erosion rate and drug release kinetics, but also depends on an ability to vary mechanical properties so that devices that have physical properties tailored to a specific application can be prepared.

By varying the nature of the diols used in the synthesis, it is possible to prepare materials that are solids, or at room temperature are semisolids that can either be fluid enough so that they can be injected, or that soften at temperatures below 45°C. Such materials can be warmed and injected, but at body temperature become so viscous that no deformation takes place, even when pressure is applied.

The availability of polymers that at room temperature are fluid, ointment-like materials, or that can be converted to such materials by gentle heating, offers significant benefits for the delivery of sensitive therapeutic agents such as peptides and proteins because such materials can be incorporated by a simple mixing proce-dure in the absence of solvents, and at temperatures low enough so that no loss of protein activity would be expected. Further, delivery systems can be fabricated without any exposure of the protein to water. Although not yet verified, such delivery devices should be able to deliver peptides and proteins without loss of activity.

The polymer shown in SCHEME 4 is a solid material, but by using the triethylene glycol glycolide/triethylene glycol monomer pair, shown in SCHEME 6, it is possible to prepare materials that at the body temperature of 37°C are extremely viscous materials that do not flow even when pressure is applied, but at temperatures no higher than about 45°C are fluids that can be injected with a hypodermic syringe. TABLE 1 shows the effect of monomer ratios on softening temperatures.

$$\underset{\text{O}}{\overset{\text{O}}{\parallel}} \quad \underset{\text{O}}{\overset{\text{O}}{\parallel}}$$

HO-CH₂C-O-CH₂-C-O-(CH₂CH₂O)₃-H   HO-(CH₂CH₂O)₃-H

SCHEME 6

TABLE 1. Softening Points of Poly(Ortho Esters) Prepared from Triethylene Glycol Monoglycolide (TEG/GLY) and Triethylene Glycol (TEG)

TEG/GLY	TEG	Softening Point (°C)
100	0	35
50	50	40
10	90	45

By using the decanediol glycolide/decanediol monomer pair shown in SCHEME 7, materials can be prepared that at room temperature are ointment-like semisolids.

Drug Release Studies

Because one of the more important applications of bioerodible polymers is in the treatment of cancer where a bioerodible device containing an antineoplastic agent is used to deliver the agent systemically, or where the implant is located at the site from which a tumor has been excised, studies with devices containing 5-fluorouracil (5-FU) have been carried out. 5-FU release from a polymer constructed from *trans*-cyclohexanedimethanol glycolide and *trans*-cyclohexanedimethanol, used at varying ratios is shown in FIGURE 5.

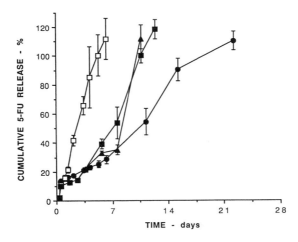

FIGURE 5. 5-Fluorouracil (5-FU) release from a polymer prepared from 3,9-diethylidene-2,4,8,10-tetraoxaspiro [5.5] undecane, *trans*-cyclohexanedimethanol glycolide (tCDM/Gly) and *trans*-cyclohexanedimethanol (tCDM) as a function of diol ratios. (□) 75/25 tCDM-CDM/Gly, (■) 80/20 tCDM-tCDM/Gly, (▲) 85/15 tCDM-tCDM/Gly, (●) 90/10 tCDM-CDM/Gly. 0.05 M phosphate buffer, pH 7.4, 37°C. Drug loading 10 wt%.

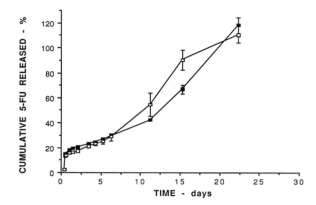

FIGURE 6. Release of 5-fluorouracil (5-FU) from a polymer prepared from 3,9-diethylidene-2,4,8,10-tetraoxaspiro [5.5] undecane, a 10/90 mixture of *trans*-cyclohexanedimethanol glycolide and *trans*-cyclohexanedimethanol (■) and a 10/90 mixture of hexanediol glycolide and hexanediol (□). 0.05 M phosphate buffer, pH 7.4, 37°C. Drug loading 10 wt%.

These data show that excellent linear release has been achieved. Most importantly, when all drug has been delivered, only traces of polymer remain. Further, rate of release can be controlled by the concentration of the glycolic acid dimer segment in the polymer. Although devices containing 15 and 20 wt% of monomer with a glycolic acid dimer segment erode at about the same rate, release rates of one, two and three weeks have been achieved. These are therapeutically useful release rates.

FIGURE 6 compares 5-FU release from two polymers prepared using the same amount of *trans*-cyclohexanedimethanol glycolide, and either *trans*-cyclohexanedimethanol or 1,6-hexanediol, another hydrophobic diol. The effect is minimal, confirming that with hydrophobic polymers, the dominant factor determining release kinetics is the concentration of the glycolic acid dimer segment in the polymer.

As already mentioned, an important application for these polymers is the delivery of peptides and proteins, because they offer the potential for delivering these agents without loss of activity. FIGURE 7 shows results of two experiments, where release of bovine serum albumin (BSA) and 5-FU from polymers prepared using triethylene glycol glycolide and triethylene glycol, at a 50/50 molar ratio was determined. This particular polymer is an example of a material that at body temperature is a nondeformable semisolid, but at 42°C is fluid enough so that it can be injected. BSA and 5-FU were incorporated by mixing these materials into the warm polymer. It is interesting to note that both 5-FU, a small, water soluble molecule and BSA, a 60 kD water soluble macromolecule are delivered at about the same rate, suggesting that the dominant mode of drug release is erosion and not diffusion.

FIGURE 8 shows release of BSA from a polymer prepared from a 95/5 molar ratio of *n*-decanediol glycolide and *n*-decanediol, shown in SCHEME 7. This particular material has an ointment-like consistency at room temperature. The results show that the protein is released at excellent zero order kinetics, even though the material has an ointment-like consistency. Thus, diffusional release is minimal and release is again predominantly controlled by polymer erosion. As with all systems studied, virtually no polymer remains when drug delivery has been completed.

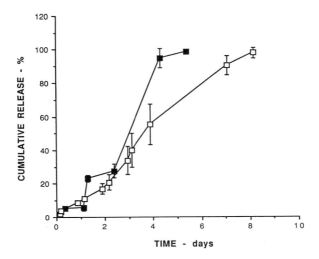

FIGURE 7. Release of 5-fluorouracil (5-FU) (■) and FITC-labeled bovine serum albumn (BSA) (□) from a polymer prepared from 3,9-diethylidene-2,4,8,10-tetraoxaspiro [5.5] undecane and a 50/50 mixture of triethylene glycol glycolide and triethylene glycol. 0.05 M phosphate buffer, pH 7.4, 37°C. Drug loading 10 wt%.

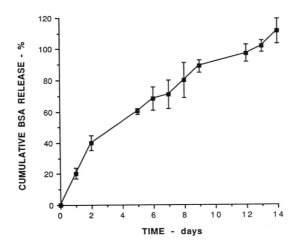

FIGURE 8. Release of FITC-labeled bovine serum albumn (BSA) from a polymer prepared from 3,9-diethylidene-2,4,8,10-tetraoxaspiro [5.5] undecane and a 5/95 mixture of decane-diol glycolide and decanediol. 0.05 M phosphate buffer, pH 7.4, 37°C. Drug loading 10 wt%.

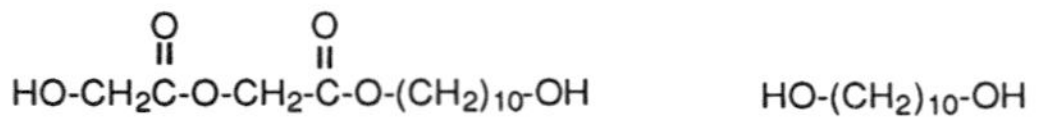

$$\underset{\text{HO-CH}_2\text{C-O-CH}_2\text{C-O-(CH}_2)_{10}\text{-OH}}{\overset{\displaystyle O \qquad O}{\overset{\displaystyle \| \qquad \|}{}}} \qquad \text{HO-(CH}_2)_{10}\text{-OH}$$

SCHEME 7

CONCLUSIONS

Incorporating varying amounts of glycolic acid dimer segments into a poly(ortho ester) allows excellent control over the rate of erosion and concomitant drug release without complications arising from diffusion of an acidic excipient from the polymer. Further, drug release from this new family of polymers is constant and polymer erosion is reasonably well synchronized with drug depletion. By using flexible monomers, it is possible to prepare materials into which sensitive therapeutic agents such as proteins and antigens can be incorporated under conditions sufficiently benign so that no loss of activity would be expected. Of particular interest are materials that at body temperature are extremely viscous semisolids that do not deform even under significant shear-forces, but at temperatures close to and below about 45°C are sufficiently fluid so that they can be injected.

REFERENCES

1. HELLER, J. 1993. Poly(ortho esters) Adv. Pol. Sci. **107:** 41–92.
2. HELLER, J. 1990. Development of poly(ortho esters): A historical overview. Biomaterials **11:** 659–665.
3. NGUYEN, T. H., K. J. HIMMELSTEIN & T. HIGUCHI. 1985. Some equilibrium and kinetic aspects of water sorption in poly(ortho esters) Int. J. Pharm. **25:** 1–12.
4. HELLER, J. 1986. Control of polymer surface erosion by the use of excipients. *In* Polymers in Medicine II, E. Chielini, P. Giusti, C. Migliaresi & L. Nicolais, Eds.: 357–368. Plenum Press. New York.
5. HELLER, J. 1985. Controlled drug release from poly(ortho esters)—A surface eroding polymer J. Controlled Release **2:** 167–177.
6. THOMBRE, A. G. & K. J. HIMMELSTEIN. 1985. A simultaneous transport-reaction model for controlled drug delivery from catalyzed bioerodible polymer matrices. AICH J. **31:** 759–766.
7. JOSHI, A., K. & J. HIMMELSTEIN. 1991. Dynamics of controlled release from bioerodible matrices J. Controlled Release **15:** 95–104.
8. NG, S. Y., T. VANDAMME, M. S. TAYLOR & J. HELLER. 1997. Macromolecules. **30:** 770–772.

Factors Determining
Hydrogel Permeability

STEVIN H. GEHRKE,[a] JOHN P. FISHER,[b]
MARIA PALASIS,[c] AND MEGHAN E. LUND[d]

Department of Chemical Engineering
University of Cincinnati
Cincinnati, Ohio 45221-0171

HYDROGELS

Hydrogels are water-swollen networks of biological, synthetic, or semi-synthetic polymers.[1,2] In contrast to polymer solutions, the polymer chains in hydrogels are crosslinked, either chemically or physically. Since the polymer chains are held together by crosslinks, hydrogels behave like solids rather than liquids, despite containing at least 20 and often over 90% water by weight. Thus hydrogels exhibit elastic responses to stress rather than the viscoelastic responses of uncrosslinked polymer solutions of equivalent composition.

The most significant property of a gel is its equilibrium degree of swelling (Q), the amount of water absorbed by the gel, expressed as the ratio of swollen gel volume (or mass) to dry gel volume (or mass). The high water content of gels makes them soft, rubbery, hydrophilic materials, which enhances biocompatibility owing to reduced mechanical irritation and minimized interfacial tension. Their permeability to water and solutes can be readily adjusted by varying the crosslinker concentration at synthesis or copolymerizing with more hydrophilic or more hydrophobic monomers.[1]

Hydrogels have many technological uses, both medical and non-medical.[1-7] Owing to their often good biocompatibility and easily adjustable permeability, they have been used in a range of biomedical applications including contact lenses, diapers, soft and hard tissue prostheses, bioartificial organs, and others.[3,6,8] The most intensively studied biomedical application for hydrogels is as vehicles for the delivery of pharmaceuticals. Hydrogels can be used to release drugs slowly over time, protect drugs from degrading environments, or to trigger release in response to a wide variety of chemical and physical stimuli.[1,3,6,9] In these gel applications, it is often the transport of solutes through the gel which determines the performance of the resulting product.

[a] Author to whom correspondence should be addressed: Department of Chemical Engineering, Mail Location 0171, University of Cincinnati, Cincinnati, OH 45221-0171; Tel: (513) 556-2766; Fax: (513) 556-3473: E-mail: sgehrke@alpha.che.uc.edu

[b] Tel: (513)-556-2761; Fax: (513) 556-3473; E-mail: jfisher@uceng.uc.edu

[c] Current address: Dr. Maria Palasis, Boston Scientific Corporation, One Boston Scientific Place, Natick, MA 01760-1537; Tel: (508) 650-8329; Fax: (513)-650-8937; E-mail: palasism@bsci.com

[d] Current address: Ms. Meghan E. Lund, Bayer Corporation, 356 Three Rivers Parkway, Addyston, OH 45001; Tel: (513) 467-2415; E-mail: Meghan-E.Lund.B@bayer.com

Hydrogels are especially attractive for the delivery of peptide or protein-drugs (*e.g.*, therapeutic proteins like amylase, used to treat pancreatitis) because they can provide a hydrophilic environment for the protein and thus help preserve its activity.[10,11] Most therapeutic proteins are vulnerable to the proteases in the digestive tract and also have difficulty crossing the skin and other barrier membranes. Implantable drug release systems are viable alternatives for delivering therapeutic proteins.[12,13] Recently, pH-sensitive gels (gels which swell and shrink in response to changes in pH) based on poly(*N*-isopropylacrylamide) have been proposed for enteric drug delivery and studied for the release of amylase.[14] At gastric pH (1.4) the gel is collapsed and negligible release was observed. At enteric pH (6.8–7.4) the gel swells extensively, permitting sustained release within the intestines.

The actual development and commercialization of drug delivery devices is complicated. Effective treatment of disease using delivery devices requires an understanding of how drugs diffuse through polymer matrices and tissues as a function of the physico-chemical properties of both drug and matrix. Furthermore, most published studies have been made isolated from living systems and therefore in the absence of any stringent delivery requirements or effects of extraneous substances. Actual drug therapy with drug delivery devices is complicated by the presence of chemical species naturally present in the body and the presence of biological barriers. The rate of drug release is most often limited by the diffusion out of the polymer. But a recent study by Saltzman and Radomsky concerning the diffusion and elimination of drugs released from polymers to brain tissue determined that the rate of release may also depend on interactions between drug molecules and the tissue surrounding an implant.[15] Penetration enhancers have been incorporated into transdermal delivery devices in order to reduce the barrier resistance of the stratum corneum, allowing drugs to reach living tissues at a greater rate.[16,17] These penetration enhancers can increase the partitioning of drug into the tissue, which increases permeability.

Many of the issues critical to performance of hydrogel-based drug delivery systems are also operative in the many bioartificial organ designs which use hydrogels as membranes, coatings, capsules and the like. In fact, the permeability performance requirements are even more stringent for most bioartificial organs than for drug delivery systems. First of all, the number of dissolved species whose permeability must be controlled is so much greater in the function of a bioartificial organ. These species cover almost the entire molecular spectrum in terms of molecular size, conformation, and solubility—from oxygen to glucose to immunoglobulins to cells! Secondly, permeation of these diverse species must be controlled both into *and* out of the hydrogel. Thirdly, while most controlled drug delivery systems are for temporary use, most bioartificial organs are for long term, chronic treatment, so permeation characteristics of the latter must be stable over longer periods of time. Finally, the consequences of device failure in the case of most bioartificial organs would be much more serious and difficult to correct than for most drug delivery systems. Thus understanding hydrogel permeability in detail is perhaps more important and complex in bioartificial organs than in any other application of hydrogels.

PERMEABILITY

Hydrogels, owing to their high water contents, provide environments for biomolecules and cells comparable to biological tissues. Many types of hydrogels display good biocompatibility and their permeabilities can be adjusted over very broad ranges. As a result, hydrogels prove useful in a variety of bioartificial organs. It is frequently assumed and often observed that there is a direct relationship between gel swelling and solute permeability;[18,19] specifically, as the swelling of the gel is reduced (*i.e.*, as the water content of the gel declines), the mobility of solutes becomes restricted owing to a smaller average pore size of the gel network. This picture is the basis for an assumption of the existence of a molecular weight cutoff (MWCO) for a particular gel, and the assumption that reducing the swelling degree of the gel, typically by increasing crosslinking of the network, will necessarily result in a reduced MWCO for the hydrogel. However, this simplified picture will hold only if the polymer network is inert and if the means of reducing water content results in uniform reduction in the average mesh size of the gel. But, the network frequently is *not* inert with respect to the diffusing species, and hydrogel networks are *not* generally uniform. Thus the relationship between permeability and gel swelling can be complex. Understanding this relationship is best begun by rigorously defining permeability.

Permeability has been defined in different ways depending upon context, but most typically as the product of a transport property, the diffusion coefficient D_i, and a thermodynamic property, the partition coefficient K_i. This definition arises most directly from the equation for steady state flux of solute 'i' across a membrane from a donor phase to a receptor phase:[20]

$$j_i = \frac{K_i D_i}{L}(C_{di} - C_{ri}) \tag{1a}$$

or:

$$j_i = \frac{P_i}{L}(C_{di} - C_{ri}) \tag{1b}$$

where: j_i = flux of solute 'i' (mol/cm²s);

C_{di} = concentration of solute 'i' in donor phase (mol/cm³);

C_{ri} = concentration of solute 'i' in receptor phase (mol/cm³);

C_{gi} = concentration of solute 'i' in the gel membrane (mol/cm³);

C_{si} = concentration of solute 'i' in solution (mol/cm³);

D_i = diffusion coefficient of solute 'i' (cm²/s);

K_i = partition coefficient of solute 'i' (dimensionless);

    = C_{gi}/C_{si};

P_i = permeability of solute 'i' (cm²/s);

    = $K_i D_i$;

L = membrane thickness (cm).

This equation assumes concentration-independent diffusion and partition coefficients, so that D_i and K_i do not vary from one side of the membrane to the other. An alternative definition of permeability is $P_i' = K_i D_i/L = P_i/L$, but this definition is less desirable because it makes the value of permeability dependent upon the specific physical configuration at hand. Sometimes the concentrations in the gel phase and the solution phase are defined in different concentration units; in this situation K_i will not be dimensionless and the dimensions of P_i will be something other than (length)^2/time. This is most commonly encountered in devices where the gel is in contact with a gas phase, such as a soft contact lens where oxygen permeability is the critical performance parameter.[21] The value of permeability can be readily extracted from a single membrane permeation experiment at steady state; unsteady state measurements can also yield permeability.[20,22] Values of D_i and K_i can also be extracted from these experiments. But since D_i and K_i are, respectively, transport and equilibrium (thermodynamic) properties, they can also be measured independently in separate experiments. D_i is often measured at unsteady-state and K_i at equilibrium.[1,20,22,23]

Understanding and manipulating permeability of a hydrogel requires understanding how the presence of the gel network alters the transport and thermodynamic properties of the system. The diffusion coefficient is defined as the proportionality constant between flux 'j_i' and concentration gradient (dC_i/dz):

$$j_i = -D_i \left(\frac{dC_i}{dz} \right) \tag{2}$$

This equation is known as Fick's First Law, as written in one dimensional form for diffusion along the z-coordinate. The negative sign is included to make D_i a positive quantity since solutes normally diffuse down the concentration gradient from high to low concentration. For solutes in water, the value of D_i depends primarily upon molecular weight, and varies from values on the order of 10^{-5} cm^2/s for simple organic compounds and dissolved gases (*e.g.*, 2.10×10^{-5} cm^2/s for oxygen and 1.06×10^{-5} cm^2/s for glycine) to values on the order 10^{-7} cm^2/s for proteins (*e.g.*, 6.9×10^{-7} cm^2/s for hemoglobin and 2.0×10^{-7} cm^2/s for fibrinogen).[20] Diffusion coefficients of solutes are reduced from the free solution values within a gel, from a negligible reduction within a highly swollen gel, to effective immobilization within a gel of low water content. In gels commonly used for bioartificial organs, the diffusivity can be reduced as little as a few percent to as much as one or two orders of magnitude or more, depending primarily upon the size of the molecule and the water content of the gel. This is discussed in greater detail in later sections of this review.

In contrast to the influence of the gel network upon the diffusion coefficient, which is invariably to reduce the value of D_i in the gel, thermodynamic interactions between the network and the solute can lead to either decreases or increases of the solute concentration within the gel with respect to surrounding solution, and thus K_i can be either greater than or less than one. Often the network is assumed to exclude solutes owing to steric hindrance, but attractive interactions between solutes and the gel (*e.g.*, hydrophobic interactions) may also exist. While the minimum value of K_i is zero (which occurs when no solute is within the gel, so $C_{gi} = 0$), there is no maximum value of K_i. In fact, K_i is often observed to be much greater than one, indicating the presence of attractive interactions between the solute and the gel.[2,23] Particularly in the presence of biospecific interactions or attractive electrostatic interactions, K_i may well have values in the thousands, thus leading to significant increases in the values of permeability. These influences on K_i are discussed later.

Finally, another aspect of gel permeability to consider is the inherent heterogeneity of gel networks. Although the polymer chains which comprise the solid portion

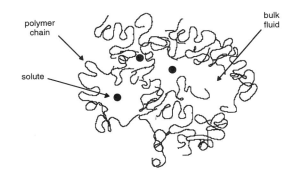

FIGURE 1. Solute diffusion may occur by different mechanisms at different rates in low polymer density and high polymer density regions. Such heterogeneity of hydrogel microstructure typically develops during network formation, as discussed in the text.

of the gel are often conceived of as being uniformly distributed throughout the volume of the gel, gels typically have heterogeneous microstructures. In fact, Silberberg believes that essentially all gels (especially those formed at concentrations of less than approximately 15% polymer, which is typical for hydrogels) necessarily will be formed with low and high density regions, whether the gel is crosslinked chemically, by radiation, or through physical interactions.[24] Basically, the argument is that heterogeneity is the consequence of the fact that formation of a crosslink thereby fixes a region of polymer concentration higher than that of the bulk. This enhances the probability that further crosslinking will occur within this region of high polymer concentration, leading to development of a crosslinked "microgel." Only as reactive sites within the microgel become depleted, do neighboring microgels connect with one another to form the macroscopic gel. But the volumes between microgel clusters are of lower crosslink density than volumes within the microgels.[25] Another source of heterogeneity in gels arises from the fact that the crosslinked network formed may have a lower solubility than the precursor compounds. Thus as the network forms, it may undergo phase separation, further amplifying the microgel effect described above.[26,27] If the change in solubility is sufficiently great to cause precipitation of the network, microporous sponge-like gels are formed.[28-31]

The heterogeneity of hydrogel networks has been confirmed in numerous experimental studies, particularly for polyacrylamide and related gels. Heterogeneity has been demonstrated with small angle neutron scattering (SANS), quasi elastic light scattering (QELS), scanning electron microscopy (SEM), and measurements of solvent permeability.[24,32-35] The effects of gel heterogeneity on permeation is difficult to determine, however, because permeation can occur by different modes through both high and low density regions of the gel, and these modes usually cannot be distinguished in conventional membrane permeation experiments. Knowledge of gel heterogeneity brings up the question of where within the gel the solute is diffusing. It is believed that diffusion in gels generally occurs in the bulk fluid region, as illustrated in FIGURE 1. However, a solute which demonstrates a strong affinity for the gel would interact with the polymer chains as it diffuses. In fact, multiple modes for solute diffusion in gels have been observed.[36-39] The practical significance of this heterogeneity on bioartificial organ performance has not been examined to the best of our knowledge.

Solute diffusion in gels may also be influenced by the nature of water within the gel, as discussed later in detail. It has been stated that understanding the nature of water in polymers is needed to understand solute transport in these systems.[8,40] Water in polymers is considered to be either bound to the polymer (or structured around it) or free (bulk water). Sarbolouki suggested that solute transport does not occur through membranes which contain only bound water in the absence of specific interactions.[41] Several gel researchers have adopted this idea although this effect has not been clearly demonstrated in gel systems.[36,42]

In the remainder of this paper, hydrogel permeability will be examined in view of the factors which affect the partition and diffusion coefficients of solutes with a hydrogel.

PARTITION COEFFICIENTS OF SOLUTES IN GELS

Factors Influencing Solute Partitioning in Hydrogels

When a solution is brought into contact with a gel, the solute will distribute between the bulk solution phase and the gel until the chemical potential of the solute is equal in both phases. The partitioning will depend on the chemical properties (*e.g.*, polarity) of both the solute and gel as well as the physical properties (*e.g.*, size, shape) of each.[43-45] Partitioning is characterized by the partition coefficient, K_i, defined as the ratio at equilibrium of the solute concentration in the gel to that in the external solution. A value of $K_i > 1$ means the solute prefers the gel, $K_i < 1$ indicates the solute prefers the bulk solution and for $K_i = 1$ the solute has no preference.

The partitioning of a solute between a solution and a gel depends upon several interactions. If these interactions are independent of one another, they can be separated into individual partition coefficients that give an overall partition coefficient in the following manner:

$$\ln K_i = \ln K_{i,o} + \ln K_{i,el} + \ln K_{i,hphob} + \ln K_{i,biosp} + \ln K_{i,size} + \ln K_{i,conf} \qquad (3)$$

where *el, hphob, biosp, size,* and *conf,* signify electrical potential, hydrophobic, biospecific affinity, size and conformational effects, respectively.[23,43,44] Any other interactions such as polymer concentration and molecular weight or hydrogen bonding are lumped into the $K_{i,o}$ term. van der Waals forces are sometimes included in the hydrophobic terms, otherwise they are assigned to the $K_{i,o}$ term. Electrostatic interactions are significant only in polyelectrolyte gels with charged solutes, and when they are present they are substantial: charged solutes will be attracted to an oppositely charged network (ion exchange) and excluded from a similarly charged network (Donnan ion exclusion).[46,47] Hydrophobic interactions are important for nonpolar solutes in gels with hydrophobic regions. Biospecific interactions are highly specific interactions between sites on the solute and ligands attached to the gel matrix (these interactions normally must be deliberately built into the solute-gel system). Alterations in the conformation of a protein solute which exposes surfaces different from the native conformation can change the way the solute partitions—this is described by the $K_{i,conf}$ term. Size effects result from the physical aspects of the solute-gel system: the size and shape of the solute and the size of the gel matrix pores. The two main interactions examined in this paper are size exclusion and hydrophobic interaction; electrostatics are only briefly reviewed, as these phenomena are treated in depth in standard references on ion exchange.[47]

Ideal Size Exclusion

The simplest case of solute partitioning occurs when there are no specific solute-gel interactions. The partition coefficient is then determined by the size exclusion term ($K_{i,size}$) only; this is the "ideal" case. Qualitatively, partitioning due to size exclusion is straightforward: as the solute size increases or the gel pore dimensions decrease, the solute becomes increasingly excluded. While diverse models exist in the literature, size exclusion is generally recognized as an entropic phenomenon. Solutes have fewer orientations available (lower entropy) in the gel relative to the free solution due to restrictions imposed upon the solute by the polymer chains. As a result, solutes tend not to enter the gel, even if they are not physically obstructed (*i.e.*, too large to penetrate the gel mesh). A solute's orientational freedom decreases as its size approaches that of the gel mesh. Thus, solute entropy in a gel decreases with increasing solute size resulting in increased exclusion from the gel. For ideal size exclusion, the partition coefficient is between zero and one ($0 < K_i < 1$). This effect is directly related to the equilibrium degree of swelling of the gel, Q, since Q is directly proportional to the polymer volume fraction, ϕ_p, ($Q = 1/\phi_p$), and it is assumed that the mesh size increases as the polymer volume fraction decreases. The limit of $K_i = 1$ will be reached only if the concentration of the solute in the gel is defined per unit volume of solution within the gel, since the gel network itself occupies a specific volume that is inaccessible to the solute. Thus, the partition coefficient is expected to increase as Q increases, asymptotically approaching 1.

Models for Ideal Size Exclusion

Ideal size exclusion models describe the steric partitioning of solutes into the pores of a gel network and assume that the gel polymer is inert and that no non-steric solute-gel interactions exist. However, the presence of the other interactions in a system can increase the solute partitioning such that K_i becomes greater than one. Therefore, if a partition coefficient greater than one is observed then it can be concluded that attractive interactions are present. The reverse is not true; a partition coefficient less than one does not necessarily signify ideal size exclusion. Although the solute is excluded, attractive interactions still can be present to some extent. The repulsive Donnan effect could also contribute to the exclusion of even very small ions. The most common phenomenon that contributes to deviations from ideal size exclusion in nonionic gels is hydrophobicity, as a nonpolar solute will preferentially interact with the hydrophobic regions of the gel, resulting in enhanced solute sorption.[45]

Several theoretical models have been developed for predicting K_i when only steric interactions between the solute and the gel phase are present. Hussain *et al.*[48] recently reviewed the development of these geometric models. A common assumption made in size exclusion models is that the gel is inert and that no solute-gel interactions exist. The classic theory by Ogston was developed for a sphere in a three dimensional array of randomly oriented straight fibers of zero thickness.[49] Giddings *et al.* developed an exclusion theory which predicts that for solutes in a gel, the partition coefficient is directly proportional to $\exp(-M_i^\alpha)$, where M_i is the solute molecular weight and α is the solute geometry factor (1/3 for spheres, 1/2 for random coils, 1 for rigid rods).[50] Many size exclusion models lack network-specific parameters, and therefore necessarily predict that partitioning will be the same in gels with the same degree of swelling, regardless of the type of gel. However, the model developed by Schnitzer for the ideal size exclusion of spherical solutes from a randomly oriented network of fibers includes a variable to account for structural differences in gel materials, the polymer fiber radius (r_f).[51] Still, this parameter is a significant oversimplification of actual gel structure (see earlier discussion of gel heterogeneity). Significant efforts to accurately model size exclusion continue, chiefly in the context of chromatography; a number of recent modeling efforts are collected in the book edited by Potschka and Dubin.[52]

Experimental work has shown that, in general, size exclusion models are of limited use in predicting the separation of solutes by size using size exclusion chromatography.[48] Some error may be attributed to the geometric simplifications made about the solute-gel system. The solutes are usually modeled as spheres, rods or flexible random coils. There is an even wider range of models to describe pores in gels. Statistical models avoid defining specific pore geometries altogether. Common approaches are to model gels as concentrated solutions of rigid rods, randomly intersecting planes or solids with cylindrical cavities.[48,52,53] It is more likely, however, that non-steric interactions present in solute-gel systems, such as electrostatic and hydrophobic interactions, are the causes of any substantial deviations from ideal size exclusion behavior, especially for proteins.[54] These non-steric interactions are usually a strong function of solvent conditions, such as ionic strength and pH, which makes them especially hard to predict.

Nonetheless, to understand the nature of the size exclusion phenomenon it is instructive to examine the predictions of a size exclusion theory. We have found the model developed by Schnitzer to be readily adapted to hydrogels.[2,23,39,45] Modeling the gel network as cylindrical fibers oriented randomly in space, Schnitzer derives the following relationship for the partition coefficient K_i:[51]

$$K_i = \exp\left(-v_e^\circ\right) \exp\left\{ \frac{v_e^\circ\left[1 - \left(\frac{r_m}{r_f}\right)^2\right]}{(1 - v_e^\circ)} \right\}; \qquad (4)$$

where: r_f = network fiber radius;

r_i = solute radius;

r_m = volume exclusion radius, $r_f + r_i$;

v_e° = excluded volume.

The excluded volume of the gel network is $\pi r_f^2 l$ where 'l' is the fiber length per unit volume. In the absence of information about 'l', the excluded volume v_e° can be approximated as the polymer volume fraction (ϕ_p) of the gel, which in turn is the inverse of the equilibrium degree of swelling by $\phi_p = 1/Q$. FIGURE 2 shows theoretical predictions made using this model. Most notable is the predicted absence of distinct molecular weight cutoffs, regardless of solute size or swelling degree (this qualitative result is obtained from essentially all models of size exclusion).

Hydrophobic Interactions

Kauzmann introduced the concept of hydrophobic interactions in 1959 to describe the tendency of nonpolar solutes to adhere to each other in aqueous solutions.[55] Hydrophobic interactions are the most common cause of deviation from ideal size exclusion in nonionic gels.[4] Unfortunately, simply *defining* the exact nature of hydrophobic interactions, much less modeling them, is challenging.[56–58] The molecular basis for hydrophobic interaction has been investigated and discussed extensively by many people.[56–65] Janado has recently reviewed several of the proposed concepts.[57]

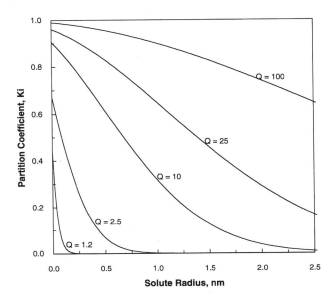

FIGURE 2. Predicted partition coefficients for ideal size exclusion as a function of solute radius and the volume degree of swelling (Q) of gels. Sharp molecular weight cutoffs (MWCO's) are not predicted for size exclusion from gels (curves are calculated using the theory of Schnitzer, assuming a network fiber radius of 0.45 nm, the value for dextran gels[51]).

The hydrophobic effect has been treated within the framework of statistical thermodynamics.[66] Sinanoglu and co-workers derived a cavity theory which describes the energetics of solute behavior in solution in terms of macroscopic properties (*e.g.*, surface tension, solute size).[67] Horvath and co-workers adapted this theory to account for the role of salts in the retention of proteins in reversed phase and hydrophobic affinity chromatography.[60,68,69] It is generally accepted that hydrophobic interactions strengthen with increasing temperature though the rate of increase decreases with temperature.[70,71] However, the relationship between temperature and hydrophobic interactions is complex and dependent on the solute and gels involved.[72]

It is difficult to quantify the effects of solute-gel interactions or predict partition coefficients from hydrophobic interaction theory. Thus an empirical measure of the hydrophobic character of drugs is commonly used, the octanol/water partition coefficient, $K_{o/w}$. This parameter is available for a wide variety of drugs.[73] A solute with a large octanol/water partition coefficient will be only sparingly soluble in water and likely to associate with hydrophobic regions in gels. Thus it is expected that hydrophobic interactions will be most significant for drugs with high values of $K_{o/w}$ in gels which are either of low water content or composed of both hydrophobic and hydrophilic segments.

In most cases, solute partitioning of hydrophilic solutes in very hydrophilic gels like dextran (Sephadex®) shows only small deviations from ideal size exclusion behavior. However, hydrophobic interactions between the solute and gel may dominate partitioning for hydrophobic solutes (those with large $K_{o/w}$), causing large deviations from size exclusion. For example, a partition coefficient greater than one hundred was reported for progesterone in a poly(hydroxyalkyl methacrylate) hydrogel film.[37] Kim *et al.* studied permeation in poly(2-hydroxyethyl methacrylate) (PHEMA) membranes, a relatively hydrophobic hydrogel widely used in biomedical applications.[42] Partition coefficients much greater than one (20 to 235) were reported for the hydrophobic solutes. Partition coefficients for the hydrophilic solutes were two to three orders of magnitude less than those for the hydrophobic solutes, indicating that hydrophobic interactions were less important in determining the partitioning of hydrophilic solutes. There are several other solute-gel systems that have been studied where partition coefficients measured greater than one were attributed to hydrophobic effects.[18,23,39,45,74] For example, Palasis and Gehrke measured partitioning of various drugs in poly(N-isopropylacrylamide) (PNIPAAm) gels as a function of temperature, solute hydrophobicity, and salt type (structure forming or structure breaking).[45] The systems could be manipulated to produce partition coefficients over 250. Overall, the variations in K_i observed were consistent with the concept of hydrophobic interaction.

Electrostatic Interactions

Electrostatic interactions dominate the partitioning behavior of charged solutes in polyelectrolyte gels. When solutes carry the *opposite* charge of the network, and the same charge as the network's counter-ions, substantial sorption of the solute can occur via exchange of the ionic solute for the counter-ions. Depending upon the ionic equilibrium constants, the partition coefficient for ion exchange can be extremely high. When solutes carry the *same* charge as the polymer network, Donnan ion exclusion causes solutes to be excluded from the gel, so that the partition coefficient of the ionic solute is less than one. If no other specific solute-gel interactions are present, for 1 : 1 electrolytes the partition coefficient for excluded ions can be determined from the free solution concentration (C_{si}) and the concentration of fixed charges on the gel network (C_{gel}) by the following relationship:[75]

$$C_{gel} = C_{si}\left(\frac{1}{K_i} - K_i\right) \qquad (5)$$

The analysis of these electrostatic phenomena is well-developed in the ion exchange literature.[47,62]

Concentration Dependence of Partition Coefficients

In the case of ideal size exclusion, solute partitioning is independent of solution concentration except at extremely high concentrations where solutes occupy a significant percentage of the total volume of the system. However, since hydrophobic and electrostatic interactions are (often complex) functions of concentration, solute partition coefficients in systems with such interactions may show a significant concentration dependence (*e.g.*, Eq. **5** above).[39] Observation of concentration-dependent partition coefficient is a strong indication of the presence of interactions other than ideal size exclusion.

DIFFUSION IN GELS

A diffusion coefficient is not a property of the solute itself; rather it is a transport coefficient that applies to a given system relative to a given reference frame for the motion. Different choices of reference velocity, which can be defined relative to the center of mass, center of moles, or center of volume of the system, can lead to differences in values of diffusion coefficients.[20] For a simple two-component system like a solution of a solute in a solvent, there is a single binary diffusion coefficient that applies to both the solute and the solvent (since movement of the solute induces movement of the solvent). For a n-component system, the total number of diffusion coefficients involved is equal to $(n-1)^2$.[20] Treatment of multicomponent diffusion is complex.[76] Fortunately, multicomponent effects are usually negligible in biological systems, and thus the diffusion of each solute can be considered as binary diffusion of the solute in water.[20] Another concern is to recognize that different techniques used to measure solute diffusion coefficients yield different kinds of diffusion coefficients. In the next section, the difference between mutual diffusion and self-diffusion is described. Later, experimental methods of measuring D_i are described.

Mutual and Self-Diffusion Coefficients

Self-diffusion is the result of thermally-induced random walk processes (Brownian motion) experienced by molecules in the absence of an applied external driving force. In an isotropic system, the mean square displacement $\langle r^2 \rangle$ of a Brownian particle as a function of time is given by the Einstein relation:

$$\langle r^2 \rangle = 6D_{si}t \tag{6}$$

where: t = time;

D_{si} = self-diffusion coefficient of species 'i.'

In contrast, under the influence of a concentration gradient, the diffusion process is characterized by the mutual diffusion coefficient, D_i. This is the proportionality constant defined by Fick's law in Equation **2** and used prior to this section. Mutual diffusion describes the relaxation of a gradient in the *total* concentration, whereas the self-diffusion coefficient describes the mean square displacement of individual particles.[77] The mutual and self-diffusion coefficients are equal in the limit of infinite dilution, where the concentration gradient is equal to zero.[78] It has been shown that the mutual diffusion coefficient could be reasonably predicted from the experimental values of the self-diffusion coefficient and the activity coefficient of species 'i' with the following relation:[79]

$$D_i \approx D_{si}\left(1 + \frac{\partial \gamma_i}{\partial x_i}\right) \tag{7}$$

where: D_i = mutual diffusion coefficient of species 'i;'

γ_i = activity coefficient of species 'i;'

x_i = mole fraction of species 'i.'

Factors Affecting Diffusion in Hydrogels

The diffusive motion of molecules in gels is reduced relative to their mobility in solution.[80] This phenomenon is known as "hindered" or "restricted" diffusion and has been demonstrated in several systems with well-defined pores, such as mica membranes with adsorbed polymers and porous glass.[81-85] Several factors can contribute to the reduction in the mobility of solutes in gel networks.[86] These factors can be classified as either chemical or frictional effects.[87] The chemical effect is a result of attractive forces between the solute and gel matrix which reduces solute mobility. Frictional effects include physical size exclusion, hydrodynamics, and solvent structuring. Probably the most obvious frictional effect is physical exclusion. A solute can be obstructed by the presence of an impermeable, slowly moving polymer chain, which thereby increases the solute's effective path length for diffusion. Hydrodynamic friction is the resistance of fluid flow in the proximity of the polymer-solvent interface which creates a drag force on the diffusing molecules. Increased hydrodynamic friction has been said to have a dominant role in the hindered diffusion of solutes in gels.[86,88] Finally, interactions between the solvent and polymer matrix increase the local viscosity of the solvent; this is also known as "solvent structuring."[89] Tanigushi and Horigome state that the water in the vicinity of the polymer (bound water) can be structured around the polymer and therefore be unable to contribute to the transport of solutes, while the bulk water is highly mobile and can solvate the solutes.[90] But investigating the causes of hindered diffusion in gels is difficult using macroscopic diffusion measurements since the various factors which affect diffusion cannot be directly isolated.

Water Mobility in Gels

The state of water in biopolymers and synthetic polymers has been a highly controversial topic in science for some time. Originally, water in these systems was assumed to be much like bulk water. But it was shown that some of the water molecules in protein solutions and cell suspensions interact strongly with the protein molecules.[40] Thus these water molecules are restricted in their motion compared to the water molecules in bulk water. This type of water has been commonly referred to as "bound" water. Other terms which are used include "ordered," "structured," "ice-like," and "non-freezing." Bound water has also been determined to exist in synthetic polymers and polymer gels.[8,91-94] Up to four distinguishably different types of water have been said to exist in some gels.[90] Berendsen summarized the most common definitions of bound water that have been used in the literature, as follows:[95]

a) water that is retained after a defined drying procedure;
b) water that fills the first monolayer, as assumed in certain theoretical interpretations of the adsorption isotherm;
c) water which is not available for the solvation of certain solutes;
d) water that does not freeze at a sharp transition temperature (*i.e.*, the normal freezing point);
e) water that gives no orientational contribution to the dielectric constant at high frequencies, indicating that it is not free to rotate with respect to the macromolecule to which it is attached;
f) water that moves with a macromolecule in sedimentation, diffusion, or viscosity experiments, thereby increasing the hydrodynamic size of the macromolecule;
g) water that shows a slower rate of rotation as measured by magnetic resonance relaxation;
h) water that shows a slower rate of self-diffusion;

i) water that is shown by X-ray or neutron diffraction to occupy regular molecular positions with respect to a macromolecule in a crystal;

j) water that deviates from the normal liquid in density, as determined by light scattering or small-angle X-ray diffraction;

k) water that can be shown by infrared or Raman spectroscopy to be engaged in hydrogen bonding to a macromolecule.

Since each of these definitions are based on experiments which measure different things and therefore yield different results, it is important to note the technique used to determine the states of water in a system and the definition of each state.

Some researchers have separated the water in gels into several different classes based on differences in the mobility of the water molecules. Roorda *et al.* did not detect separate classes of water in poly(hydroxyethyl methacrylate) (PHEMA) gels using differential scanning calorimetry (DSC).[96,97] Rather, they believed that there was an incomplete crystallization of water in the gels to which they attributed to the low diffusion coefficient of the water in the glassy gel and not to a "bound" character of the water. On the other hand, Quinn *et al.* detected three different classes of water in PHEMA and also in poly(N-vinyl pyrrolidone-co-methyl methacrylate) copolymer gels, by nuclear magnetic relaxation (NMR) and DSC techniques.[91,92] By determining nuclear magnetic spin-spin relaxation times, (T_2) they isolated mobile bulk-like water and two types of bound or non-freezable water, one more tightly bound than the other ("bound" and "intermediate" or "interfacial" water, respectively). In their work, DSC did not differentiate between bound and intermediate water. Nuclear magnetic relaxation was used to identify two populations of water molecules in collagen networks.[59] One population was determined to be essentially free water molecules, rotating isotropically, and the other population specifically bound to the network exhibiting anisotropic rotation. However, Hoeve proposed that this "bound" water is actually made up of water molecules which form the maximum number of hydrogen bonds with the collagen and with each other and that all these water molecules diffuse in a liquid-like fashion but that none of them rotate isotropically.[59] Various classes of water molecules in hydrated polymers can be distinguished by their different behavior on a time scale which is long compared to the characteristic times for individual molecular motions.[45] Therefore, the time resolution of the measuring method will determine if these molecules are seen as separate classes. Nuclear magnetic relaxation and dielectric relaxation have been used to distinguish such classes.

Despite the fact that researchers disagree on the "bound" water terminology used and on what exactly the water molecules are doing in these systems, they do agree that water in polymers, biological or synthetic, can have properties which are not typical of bulk water and thus alter solute diffusion in gels. In this paper, the bound/bulk water terminology is used simply to differentiate between water molecules with varying mobilities in gels due to water/network interactions.

Pore and Partition Mechanisms

Predicting diffusion coefficients in hydrogels can also be complicated by other factors besides water structuring which affect solute mobility but are difficult to quantify. One is that hydrogels do not have well-defined pores which are constant in size or location as do solid porous materials. Solute transport in hydrogels has been described as occurring by one of two mechanisms: a pore mechanism and a partition mechanism.[36,38,42] The pore mechanism assumes the solute permeates the polymer by diffusion through the bulk water phase of the swollen polymer while the polymer is assumed to be inert. This mechanism is affected by the relative size of the solute to a hypothetical network "pore." The partition mechanism is said to involve solute dissolution into the polymer structure. Thus, this mechanism is strongly dependent on the chemical properties of both the solute and the polymer. Solutes which have a strong affinity for the gel (as indicated by partition coefficients greater than one) could be expected to diffuse via the partition mechanism. These two mechanisms are the limiting cases; in reality, both may occur to some extent, although one may dominate.[98] However reasonable these ideas, the generality of this hypothesis has not been proven conclusively due to the difficulty in isolating the mechanisms of diffusion from one another.

Kim and co-workers worked to separate the mechanisms of solute diffusion in PHEMA gels.[42] They defined two domains which comprised the gel: domain A consisting of polymer, bound water, and interfacial water and domain B which includes only bulk water (they defined bound water as that strongly associated with the polymer, probably hydrogen-bonded to hydrophilic groups on the polymer, and interfacial water as that associated with hydrophobic interactions between polymer segments). The partition mechanism is assumed to take place in domain A and the pore mechanism in domain B. Thus, they represent the total permeability, P_T, as follows:

$$P_T = P_A + P_B \tag{8}$$

where: P_A = solute permeability in the A domains;

   P_B = solute permeability in the B domains.

The permeabilities are defined as the product of the diffusion coefficient and the partition coefficient in each specific domain. They used this model to interpret values of permeabilities obtained for several hydrophobic steroids by time-lag membrane diffusion experiments in both uncrosslinked PHEMA and in PHEMA crosslinked with ethylene glycol dimethacrylate. Using this model, their calculated values of D_B turned out to be an order of magnitude smaller than those they determined for similarly-sized hydrophilic solutes.

Models for Diffusion in Hydrogels

A variety of models varying widely in utility and complexity have appeared in the literature over the past several decades. Mackie and Meares developed a stochastic theory using a liquid lattice model which accounts for the obstruction effect of the polymer network on solute diffusion.[99] Assuming the polymer blocked a fraction of sites, they derived the following expression:

$$\frac{D_{gi}}{D_i} = \left(\frac{1 - \phi_p}{1 + \phi_p}\right)^2 \tag{9}$$

where: D_{gi} = diffusion coefficient in the gel of solute 'i';

   D_i = diffusion coefficient in solution of solute 'i';

   ϕ_p = polymer volume fraction;

   $= Q^{-1}$;

Q = volume swelling degree of the gel.

This equation was derived assuming that diffusion of a solute (equal in size to a polymer segment) was restricted to the sites unoccupied by the polymer. An allowance was made for the existence of the polymer as chains and occasional crosslinks by assuming one half of the nearest neighbor sites in the same plane as the solute are occupied by adjacent links of the same polymer chain. It is evident from the above relation that D_{gi}/D_i is a constant value irrespective of the diffusing solute and gel. The theory has correlated an observed reduction in the diffusion coefficients of small organic molecules in water swollen cellulose gels.[100] Another empirical equation which can be used to estimate diffusion coefficients of solutes in gels is:[101]

$$\frac{D_{gi}}{D_i} = \exp\left(\frac{-(5 + 10^{-4}\,M_i)}{q}\right) \tag{10}$$

where: M_i = molecular weight of solute 'i';

   q = mass swelling degree of the gel.

Other empirical and theoretical correlations are reviewed by Peppas and Lustig.[102]
   However, the most successful and widely used model describing solute diffusion in hydrated polymers is the theory by Yasuda *et al.*[103] It is more complex than the previous correlations yet is still readily applied. They adapted the theory originally developed by Cohen and Turnbull[104] for molecular transport in liquids to transport in water swollen polymers. The relation is as follows:

$$\frac{D_{gi}}{D_i} = P_{gi} \exp\left(\frac{-Y_i}{Q-1}\right) \tag{11}$$

where: P_{gi} = sieving factor of the gel for solute 'i';

   Q = volume degree of swelling;

   $Y_i = \gamma V_i^*/V_{f,w}$;

   γ = geometric correction factor for the overlap of free volume,

      a value between 1/2 and 1;

   V_i^* = characteristic volume of solute 'i';

   $V_{f,w}$ = free volume of the water.

The theory assumes that the molecule moves only within the free volume of the water-filled regions of the polymer. A diffusive motion is assumed to occur if the molecule attains sufficient energy to overcome the forces holding it to its neighbors and an empty site is available into which the molecule can jump. Thus the appropriate volume for the solute is the cross-sectional area times its jump length:[102,103,105]

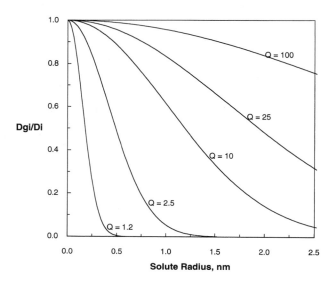

FIGURE 3. Predicted reduction in diffusivity of solute 'i' in a gel (D_{gi}) from the free solution value (D_i) as a function of solute radius and the volume degree of swelling (Q) of gels. Sharp molecular weight cutoffs (MWCO's) are not predicted (curves are calculated using the theory of Yasuda *et al.*[108] and a value of 1.4 nm^{-2} for the lumped parameter Y, the value determined from the data of Peppas and Reinhart[105]).

$$V_i^* = \pi r_i^2 \lambda_i \qquad \qquad (12)$$

where: r_i = hydrodynamic radius of solute 'i';

    λ_i = solute jump length of solute 'i'.

Significantly, the theory assumes an absence of any interactions between the gel network and the solute beyond steric hindrance. Steric hindrance is accounted for by the sieving factor which represents the probability of a solute moving unobstructed through the network. For all but very large solutes (above roughly 60,000 Daltons), the sieving factor can be taken as unity,[103] although theories have been developed for larger solutes which take into account solute sieving by the network.[103,106] The degree of swelling accounts for the reduction in total available volume for solute diffusion due to the presence of the polymer. This theory has been widely used in correlating solute diffusion data in swollen gels (*e.g.*, refs. 18,38,45,46). Although the linear dependence between log D_{gi} and $1/(Q\text{-}1)$ of Equation **12** has been frequently observed, the value of D_i extracted from this theory is often lower than the true value of D_i, due to boundary layer resistance which cannot be entirely eliminated.

    Because of the difficulty in evaluating γ and λ_i, the theory is more useful for correlating experimental data than for making *a priori* predictions. However, to observe the functional form of this equation, theoretical predictions of Equation **12** as a function of solute size are presented in FIGURE 3, assuming that the lumped parameter $Y_i = \gamma \lambda_i / V_{f,w}$ has a value of 1.4 nm^{-2} (based on data in Figure 1 in Peppas and Reinhart[105]), independent of solute size. The important points made by this figure are that the functional form of this theory is similar to that of size exclusion theory and again, that a sharp molecular weight cut-off is not predicted.

Deviations from Diffusion Models

The theories just described essentially assume the network is simply a physical obstruction and neglect all the influences of the gel network on solute diffusion. However, the physical exclusion (steric) effect alone cannot explain values of diffusion coefficients obtained in a number of systems which are much lower than expected.[86,88] Researchers have attributed such unusually low solute diffusion coefficients (from 10 to 80% of the free solution diffusivity) to a variety of different factors. For instance, Kou and Amidon attribute a low phenylpropanolamine diffusivity in swollen poly(HEMA-co-MA) gels to an interaction between the solute and the network.[107] Similarly, Brown and Chitumbo claim the low diffusivity of ethylene glycol and crown [15-5] ether in cellulose gels is due to weak interactive forces between the solute and the gel matrix.[89] Leloup and Colonna attribute the same behavior for bovine serum albumin in amylose gels to hydrodynamic friction between the solute and matrix.[108] Claeys and Arnold claim that the reduction in the rotational diffusion of cyclic guanosine 5'-monophosphate in polyacrylamide and agarose gels with increasing polymer concentration is due to increased hydrodynamic friction.[88] They exclude the possibility of interactions between the probe molecule and gel matrix, although this conflicts with the study of Haggerty *et al.* which demonstrate the existence of both hydrogen-bonding forces and hydrophobic interactions in polyacrylamide gels.[109] Brown and Chitumbo also attributed a reduction in the mobility of various solutes in cellulose and polyacrylamide gels to water structuring around the polymer.[89] Some studies have attributed low measured diffusion coefficients to experimental artifacts, especially boundary layer resistances during sorption or membrane time-lag experiments.[110,111]

In contrast to the cases of lower-than-expected values of diffusion coefficients cited above, for a series of PNIPAAm gels with different swelling degrees, Palasis has observed diffusion coefficients in gels higher than expected based on the Yasuda *et al.* theory.[39,45] This was interpreted as the consequence of heterogeneity of the gel network, meaning that the actual effective mesh sizes of the network are larger than assumed by the theory. The effect of heterogeneity on solute permeation is an area in need of further study.

It is evident from the above studies that the observed reduction in solute diffusivity in gels may occur due to factors other than simple obstruction, as assumed by the theories reviewed in the previous section. Generally, these factors have been difficult to isolate and confirm under the experimental conditions used. Consequently, there is no readily applied quantitative theory available for *a priori* prediction of solute diffusion in hydrogels generally. Thus experimental measurements of permeability are essential when designing bioartificial organs; such techniques are outlined in the next section.

EXPERIMENTAL MEASUREMENT OF PERMEABILITY

Understanding of the nature of permeability for a gel/solute system is best achieved by examining the diffusion and partition coefficients separately. Typical values of D_i for solutes in swollen gels range from 10^{-5} cm^2/s to 10^{-8} cm^2/s (or lower for very large proteins or nucleic acid polymers, especially in gels of low swelling degrees). K_i is always found to be greater than 0 for solutes in gels, and will be less than 1 if the only gel/solute interactions that exist are steric ones, though attractive interactions can cause K_i to become much greater than 1. Techniques for the measurement of the permeability of gels to solutes can be categorized as microscopic or macroscopic.

Microscopic techniques observe molecular movements and commonly yield self-diffusion coefficients. Some of these techniques are even able to distinguish among different modes of molecular motion within a gel. For example, pulsed-gradient spin echo NMR (PGSE-NMR) measures the rate of molecular reorientation which result from shifts in an applied magnetic field. In addition to providing self-diffusion coefficients, PGSE-NMR can also be used to distinguish particular modes of diffusional motion, yielding translational and rotational diffusion coefficients. Dynamic light scattering techniques have also been used for the measurement of self-diffusion coefficients. Examples include quasi-elastic light scattering (QELS),[112,113] which measures the decay in the correlation of a scattered light pattern, and forced Rayleigh scattering (FRS).[114] These have been frequently applied to solutions of macromolecules. Another useful technique (having some elements in common with macroscopic techniques) is Fluorescence Recovery After Photobleaching (FRAP), which measures the rate of solute movement into a laser-bleached spot in solution.[115] FRAP is notably useful in that it can distinguish between diffusive and convective motion. It has been particularly useful in examining biological transport in cells. Since most microscopic methods monitor diffusive motion on a molecular level, the measured diffusion coefficients are not complicated by boundary layer resistances. But these methods require costly equipment and can be difficult to master.[20] Furthermore, they do not normally yield partition coefficients, although they can provide information about whether non-steric interactions exist and if they are significant.

Macroscopic techniques are routinely used to measure mutual diffusion coefficients. The most common experiments are membrane permeation and sorption/desorption.[1] These experiments are easier to perform than the microscopic methods and require only inexpensive equipment. Furthermore, they often provide permeability, diffusivity and partition coefficient all in the same experiment. Since these are more likely to be used by scientists developing bioartificial organs than the microscopic techniques, the macroscopic techniques will be reviewed here in further detail. However, it is important to note that while the experiments are not difficult to understand or perform, experimental artifacts can distort the results. These are discussed at the end of this section.

Membrane Permeation Experiments

Membrane permeation experiments are performed using a diffusion cell, which consists of two reservoirs separated by a membrane. The donor reservoir is filled with a solution of known concentration; the receiver reservoir is filled with a pure solvent or buffer. The concentration in one or both of the reservoirs is then measured over time as the solute permeates the membrane. The appropriate mathematical analysis of the problem depends upon the boundary conditions most convenient to maintain experimentally. There are two common situations: 1) constant concentrations maintained in the donor and receptor reservoirs or 2) a steadily decreasing donor cell concentration (C_{di}) and a steadily rising receptor cell concentration (C_{ri}) as the reservoirs approach equilibrium with one another. The analysis of the former situation is often referred to as the "time-lag" model and the latter as the "pseudo-steady state" model. The mathematical analyses presented below for both of these boundary conditions assume that D_i, K_i and thus P_i are constant and independent of concentration.

The time lag model assumes the following: the donor side of the membrane is held at a constant concentration, the receiver is held at zero concentration, and the membrane is initially at zero concentration.[22] The total amount of the diffusing solute 'm_i' that has passed through the membrane varies with time according to the following relation:

$$\frac{m_i}{LC_{gi}} = \frac{D_i t}{L^2} - \frac{1}{6} - \frac{2}{\pi^2} \sum_{n=1}^{\infty} \frac{(-1)^n}{n^2} \exp\left(\frac{-D_i t}{L^2} n^2 \pi^2\right) \tag{13}$$

where: C_{gi} = the concentration of solute 'i' on the gel side of the donor solution/gel interface. At steady state, which is reached when $D_i t/L^2 > 0.45$, the exponential terms of the equation can be ignored and the equation reduces to:

$$m_i = \frac{D_i C_{gi}}{L}\left(t - \frac{L^2}{6D_i}\right) \tag{14a}$$

Since the interfacial concentration C_{gi} cannot be measured, rather than using this equation, Equation **14b** is used, in which C_{gi} has been replaced by the measured donor cell concentration C_{di}, via the definitions of the partition coefficient and permeability ($D_i C_{gi} = D_i K_i C_{di} = P_i C_{di}$):

$$m_i = \frac{P_i C_{di}}{L}\left(t - \frac{L^2}{6D_i}\right) \tag{14b}$$

A plot of 'm_i' versus time from this limiting equation is a straight line with a time-axis intercept of $L^2/6D_i$, from which D_i is calculated, and a slope of $P_i C_{di}/L$, from which permeability is obtained. K_i is then calculated from the definition of permeability as $K_i = P_i/D_i$. Since the boundary conditions assume constant concentrations, the donor cell volume should be much greater than the receiver, and the receiver solution should be periodically replaced with solute-free solution as its concentration rises. If the solute is not removed from the receiver side, as is more common experimental practice, the time lag model can be applied only within the time window where $D_i t/L^2 > 0.45$ and $(C_{di} - C_{ri})/(C_{di,0} - C_{ri,0}) = \Delta C_t/\Delta C_0 \approx 1$ (the subscripts 't' and '0' indicate the cell concentrations at times 't' and $t = 0$). An example is shown in FIGURE 4, where data was used up to $\Delta C_t/\Delta C_0 = 0.9$.

The pseudo-steady state model, as presented by Cussler,[20] assumes that the donor side is filled with a solution of higher solute concentration than the receiver side and that the flux across the membrane quickly reaches a pseudo-steady state, when there is a linear concentration profile across the membrane. Under these conditions, the following equation is derived:

$$\left(\frac{C_{di} - C_{ri}}{C_{di,o} - C_{ri,o}}\right) = \exp(-P_i \beta t) \tag{15}$$

where: $C_{di,0}$ = concentration of solute 'i' on the donor side at $t = 0$;

$C_{ri,0}$ = concentration of solute 'i' on the receiver side at $t = 0$;

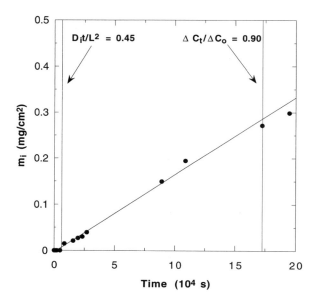

FIGURE 4. Time-lag data analysis for the diffusion of FITC-dextran (4400 Da) through a swollen hydroxypropyl cellulose hydrogel membrane ($Q = 10.5$) at 25°C. Using the fifth ($D_i t/L^2 = 0.43$) through thirteenth ($\Delta C/\Delta C_o = 0.90$) data points, the following values were calculated: $P_i = 6.2 \times 10^{-8}$ cm²/s, $D_i = 9.1 \times 10^{-8}$ cm²/s, and $K_i = 0.68$.

C_{di} = concentration of solute 'i' on the donor side at time t;

C_{ri} = concentration of solute 'i' on the receiver at time t;

β = diffusion cell constant;

$\quad = (A/L)(V_r^{-1} + V_d^{-1})$

A = membrane area;

V_d = donor reservoir volume;

V_r = receptor reservoir volume.

From this equation, the permeability of the gel is readily obtained from the slope of a plot of $-\ln(\Delta C_t/\Delta C_0)$ versus time, as shown in FIGURE 5. This analysis will be valid for data obtained for $D_i t/L^2 > 0.45$, as long as the relaxation time of the membrane is much less than that of the cells.[20]

The difference in solute flux as a function of time predicted by the two models is given in FIGURE 6. The time-lag model explicitly considers the time required to load the membrane with solute and for steady state to be established. Since the concentrations on each side of the membrane are maintained at constant values, the experiment reaches a true steady state. In contrast, the flux under the conditions of the pseudo-steady state slowly but steadily declines from the initial, maximum

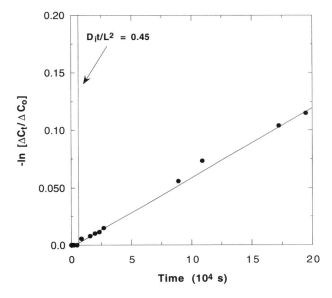

FIGURE 5. Pseudo-steady state data analysis for the diffusion of FITC-dextran (4400 Da) through a swollen hydroxypropyl cellulose hydrogel membrane (Q = 10.5) at 25°C. For the same experiment as in FIGURE 4, but using all data points after the fifth one ($D_i t/L^2 = 0.43$), yields $P_i = 5.8 \times 10^{-8}$ cm^2/s, within 7% of that calculated with the time-lag model. Even closer agreement between the models is not uncommon.

value as the two sides of the cell move toward equilibrium with one another; the time required to load the membrane is neglected by the model. There are advantages and disadvantages to both models. The time-lag model yields P_i, D_i, and K_i values in a single experiment, while the pseudo-steady state model yields only P_i. Thus use of the pseudo-steady state model requires a separate equilibrium sorption experiment to measure K_i, and thus obtain D_i from P_i. However, the error in the intercept of the time-lag model is often quite large and thus may yield highly inaccurate values of D_i. In these cases, equilibrium sorption experiments to obtain K_i still must be performed; then D_i is calculated from the permeability rather than from the time-axis intercept. In practice, the pseudo-steady state boundary conditions are easier to maintain experimentally. It is possible to apply both models to the same experiment, although they will apply over different time ranges; as shown by comparison of FIGURES 4 and 5, which plot the same data. In most cases the models yield similar if not identical values for gel permeability as shown by comparison of these figures. However, discrepancies can occur since different data sets are used, and the severity of the different assumptions made in deriving the equations or applying them to the data may differ from experiment to experiment.

Sorption/Desorption Experiments

Frequently it is difficult to synthesize the gels as membranes; they are often quite fragile, difficult to mount in the diffusion cell, and the experiments may be

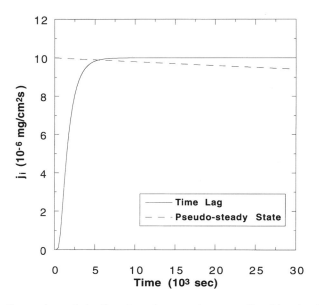

FIGURE 6. Comparison of the flux through a membrane predicted by the time-lag and pseudo-steady state models. Parameters used were $D_i = 1.0 \times 10^{-6}$ cm^2/s, $K_i = 1.0$, L = 0.1 cm, $C_{di} = 1.0$ mg/ml, $C_{ri} = 0$ mg/ml and $V_d = V_r = 10$ ml.

compromised by leaks and tears. Particularly in these cases, measurement of the rate of solute sorption or desorption by gels is a good alternative to membrane permeation experiments. An unsteady-state *sorption* experiment measures the change in solution concentration with time as a gel absorbs solute. An unsteady-state *desorption* experiment measures the change in solution concentration as a gel loaded with a solute releases its solute into the solution. The technique can be applied to any gel sample of uniform geometry—flat sheet, sphere, or cylinder. A cylindrical geometry is often the most convenient to synthesize and to keep immersed in a small volume of solution (thus ensuring a measurable concentration change in the solution over the course of the experiment). From the rate of change in concentration, the diffusion coefficient is obtained, and from the equilibrium solute concentration, K_i is obtained. The only difficult aspect of the experimental design is to keep the solution well-stirred, minimizing the boundary layer resistance.

The sorption experiment can be modeled with the exact solution for the diffusion of a solute into a cylinder of infinite length immersed in a well-stirred solution of finite volume:[22]

$$\frac{M_t}{M_\infty} = 1 - \sum_{n=1}^{\infty} \left[\left(\frac{4\alpha(1 + \alpha)}{4 + 4\alpha + \alpha^2 q_n^2} \right) \exp\left(\frac{-D_i t q_n^2}{r^2} \right) \right] \qquad (16)$$

where   r = radius of the cylinder;

α = (volume of solution/volume of gel)/K_i;

q_n = positive, non zero roots of $\alpha q_n J_0(q_n) + 2J_1(q_n) = 0$.

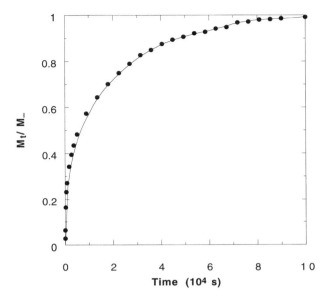

FIGURE 7. Diffusion of acetaminophen (152 D) into a poly(N-isopropylacrylamide) hydrogel cylinder at 35°C (Q = 1.6). The following values were calculated from a least-squares fit to the exact solution of Fick's Law for this situation: $P = 2.5 \times 10^{-7}$ cm^2/s, $D = 3.8 \times 10^{-8}$ cm^2/s and K = 6.6. The curve drawn is the theoretical curve predicted with these parameters.

The diffusion coefficient is extracted from the exact solution with a non-linear least squares curve fit of the experimental data as shown in FIGURE 7 (a linearized limiting case of this equation which simplifies extraction of D_i from sorption data is also available[1,116]). The partition coefficient is determined using the initial and equilibrium data points. Permeability is then calculated from its definition: $P_i = K_i D_i$. This experiment should yield the same values as the membrane permeation experiment as long as no sorption occurs into "dead end" pores, which is highly unlikely in swollen gels.

Experimental Complications

Discrepancies between values of D_i, K_i and P_i obtained by the different unsteady state, steady state, and equilibrium experiments have been found. In part this can be due to the concentration-dependence of D_i and K_i. All of the analyses presented here assume constant D_i and K_i, but each experiment causes different changes in concentration over the course of the experiment. Such deviations are not likely to be significant enough to distort qualitative trends (in the absence of something like concentration-dependent aggregation, which could cause major variations in D_i or K_i). But it may be advisable to perform experiments under conditions which most closely match conditions of the application, all other considerations being equal.

A number of complications may arise with these macroscopic methods which do not usually arise in the microscopic methods. The most significant is the presence of external mass transfer resistance. Imperfect mixing of solution near the surface of the membrane (which is often idealized as an unstirred boundary layer) slows the overall rate of mass transfer across the membrane relative to what it would be if the membrane provided the only resistance to mass transfer. Therefore, if boundary layer resistance on each side of the membrane is not considered, the apparent diffusion coefficient obtained from the data analysis will be smaller than the true value of D_i in the gel itself. Thus both reservoirs must be well-stirred to minimize this boundary layer resistance (mass transfer resistance arising from poor mixing at the surface can be estimated qualitatively by testing whether an increased stirring rate notably increases the permeation rate). The actual degree of boundary layer resistance can be quantified with a series of experiments with membranes of different thicknesses; from this data, contributions to mass transfer resistance from solution and from the membrane can be separated.[117] Another problem is that to obtain measurable concentration differences, large concentration gradients are often imposed. The diffusion coefficient obtained will then be a complex average of the concentration gradient within the gel (which changes with time in unsteady state experiments). Ideally, it would be best to run multiple experiments with similar concentrations on each side of the membrane, to obtain D_i, K_i, and P_i as functions of concentration, but this is often not practical nor feasible. Fortunately, in the absence of concentration-dependent interactions like aggregation, assumption of concentration independence is often reasonable for dilute solutions. Finally, a variety of practical problems may arise when trying to carry out these experiments. For example, experiments using large solutes or gels with low water content can take days, even weeks to obtain sufficient data for analysis; consequently, problems such as the evaporative loss of solvent, degradation of the gel or the solutes may be introduced.

SUMMARY

Developing hydrogel membranes and coatings of appropriate permeability characteristics is key to the success of a number bioartificial organ technologies. Key principles relevant to the design and application of hydrogels for such applications were reviewed. The first key point is that permeability is a function of both transport and thermodynamic properties, the diffusion coefficient and partition coefficient, respectively, and that these parameters can be evaluated separately. Although the aspect of partitioning often emphasized is size exclusion, this review points out that many other relevant interactions come into play, especially hydrophobic and electrostatic interactions, and that these phenomena can dominate size exclusion. Similarly, while the diffusion coefficient also is strongly dependent upon size, other interactions can also cause diffusivity to deviate from theories which consider only solute size and gel swelling. For example, the heterogeneity of hydrogel networks can result in permeabilities that fail to decline as much as might be anticipated if networks were uniform.

ACKNOWLEDGMENTS

Portions of this paper were adapted from the theses of Meghan E. Lund and Maria Palasis (references 23 and 39).

REFERENCES

1. GEHRKE, S. H. & P. I. LEE. 1988. Hydrogels for drug delivery systems. *In* Specialized Drug Delivery Systems: Manufacturing and Production Technology. P. Tyle, Ed.: 333–392. Marcel Dekker. New York.
2. GEHRKE, S. H. 1993. Synthesis, equilibrium swelling, kinetics, permeability and applications of environmentally responsive gels. *In* Responsive Gels: Volume Transitions II. Advances in Polymer Science Series. K. Dusek, Ed. **110:** 81–144. Springer-Verlag. Heidelberg.
3. PEPPAS, N. A. 1987. *In* Hydrogels in Medicine and Pharmacy, vol. 3, Properties and Applications. N. A. Peppas, Ed. CRC Press. Boca Raton, FL.
4. MIKES, O. 1988. High-performance Liquid Chromatography of Biopolymers and Biooligomers. Elsevier. Amsterdam.
5. GEHRKE, S. H., G. P. ANDREWS & E. L. CUSSLER. 1986. Chemical aspects of gel extraction. Chem. Eng. Sci. **41:** 2153–2160.
6. HOFFMAN, A. S. 1987. Applications of thermally reversible polymers and hydrogels in therapeutics and diagnostics. J. Controlled Release **6:** 297–305.
7. BRANNON-PEPPAS, L. & R. HARLAND, EDS. 1990. Absorbent polymer technology. Elsevier. Amsterdam.
8. PEDLEY, D. G. & B. J. TIGHE. 1979. Water binding properties of hydrogel polymers for reverse osmosis and related applications. British Polym. J. **11:** 130.
9. BAKER, R. 1987. Controlled release of biologically active agents. John Wiley & Sons. New York.
10. GEHRKE, S. H., L. UHDEN & M. SCHILLER. 1995. Enhanced loading and activity retention in hydrogel delivery systems. Proceed. Intern. Symp. Control. Rel. Bioact. Mater. **22:** 145–146.
11. RAO, K. P. & R. JEYANTHI. 1991. Controlled peptide delivery: Current status and future prospects. Indian J. Chem. **30B:** 107–117.
12. CARUANA, C. M. 1992. Chemical engineering: Key component to advanced drug delivery systems. Chem. Eng. Prog. **88**(Dec): 12–16.
13. PEPPAS, N. A. & R. LANGER. 1994. New challenges in biomaterials. Science **263:** 1715–1729.
14. DONG, L. C., Q. YAN & A. S. HOFFMAN. 1992. Controlled release of amylase from a thermal and pH-sensitive, macroporous hydrogel. J. Controlled Release **19:** 171–177.
15. SALTZMAN, W. M. & M. L. RADOMSKY. 1991. Drug released from polymers: Diffusion and elimination in brain tissue. Chem. Eng. Sci. **46:** 2429–2444.
16. BARRY, B. W. 1991. Lipid-protein-partitioning theory of skin penetration enhancement. J. Controlled Release **15:** 237–248.
17. DOMB, A., G. W. R. DAVIDSON III & L. M. SANDERS. 1990. Diffusion of peptides through hydrogel membranes. J. Controlled Release **14:** 133–144.
18. FEIL, H., Y. H. BAE, J. FEIJEN & S. W. KIM. 1991. Molecular separation by thermosensitive hydrogel membranes. J. Membr. Sci. **64:** 283–294.
19. BAE, Y. H., T. OKANO & S. W. KIM. 1991. "On-off" thermocontrol of solute transport. II. Solute release from thermosensitive hydrogels. Pharmaceutical Res. **8:** 624–628.
20. CUSSLER, E. L. 1984. Diffusion: Mass Transfer in Fluid Systems. Cambridge University Press. Cambridge.
21. TIGHE, B. J. 1987. Hydrogels as contact lens materials. *In* Hydrogels in Medicine and Pharmacy, vol. 3, Properties and Applications. N. A. Peppas, Ed. **3:** 53–82. CRC Press. Boca Raton, FL.
22. CRANK, J. 1975. The Mathematics of Diffusion, 2nd edit. Oxford University Press. London.
23. LUND, M. 1996. Solute partitioning in hydrogels. M.S. Thesis. University of Cincinnati. Cincinnati, Ohio.
24. SILBERBERG, A. 1992. Gel structural heterogeneity, gel permeability, and mechanical response. *In* Polyelectrolyte Gels. ACS Symposium Series. R. Harland & R. K. Prud'homme, Eds. **480:** 146–158. American Chemical Society. Washington D.C.
25. ZHU, S. & A. HAMIELEC. 1992. Kinetics of polymeric network synthesis via free-radical

mechanisms—Polymerization and polymer modification. Makromol. Chem., Macromol. Symp. **63**: 135–182.

26. DUSEK, K. 1971. Inhomogeneities induced by crosslinking in the course of crosslinking copolymerization. *In* Polymer Networks: Structural and Mechanical Properties. A. J. Chompff, Ed.: 245–260. Plenum Press. New York.

27. SEDLACEK, B. & C. KONAK. 1982. Temperature-induced microsyneresis in swollen polymer gels. J. Colloid. Interf. Sci. **90**: 60–70.

28. GEHRKE, S. H., M. PALASIS & M. K. AKHTAR. 1992. Synthesis of poly(N-isopropylacrylamide) gels of reproducible quality. Polym. Int. **29**: 29–36.

29. KABRA, B. G. & S. H. GEHRKE. 1991. Synthesis of fast response, temperature sensitive poly(N-isopropylacrylamide) gel. Polym. Commun. **32**: 322–323.

30. KABRA, B. G. & S. H. GEHRKE. 1994. Rate limiting steps for solvent sorption and desorption by microporous stimuli-sensitive absorbent gels. *In* Superabsorbent Polymers: Science and Technology. ACS Symposium Series. F. L. Buchholz & N. A. Peppas, Eds. **573**: 76–87. American Chemical Society. Washington D.C.

31. KABRA, B. G., S. H. GEHRKE & R. SPONTAK. 1997. Microporous, responsive hydroxypropyl cellulose gels. I: Synthesis and Microstructure. Macromolecules. In press.

32. WEISS, N., T. VAN VLIET & A. SILBERBERG. 1981. Influence of polymerization initiation rate on permeability of aqueous polyacrylamide gels. J. Polym. Sci. Polym. Phys. Ed. **19**: 1505–1512.

33. WEISS, N. & A. SILBERBERG. 1977. Inhomogeneity of polyacrylamide gel structure from permeability and viscoelasticity. British Polym. J. **9**: 144–150.

34. WEISS, N., T. VAN VLIET & A. SILBERBERG. 1979. Permeability of heterogeneous gels. J. Polym. Sci. Polym. Phys. Ed. **17**: 2229–2240.

35. SHIBAYAMA, M. & T. TANAKA. 1993. Phase transition and related phenomena of polymer gels. *In* Responsive Gels: Volume transitions I. Advances in Polymer Science Series. K. Dusek, Ed. **109**: 1–62. Springer-Verlag. Heidelberg.

36. PARK, T. G. & A. S. HOFFMAN. 1991. Immobilization of *Arthrobacter simplex* in thermally reversible hydrogels: Effect of gel hydrophobicity on steroid conversion. Biotech. Prog. **7**: 383–390.

37. ZENTNER, G. M., J. R. CARDINAL, J. FEIJEN & S. Z. SONG. 1979. Progestin permeation through polymer membranes IV: Mechanism of steroid permeation and functional group contribution to diffusion through hydrogel films. J. Pharm. Sci. **68**: 970–975.

38. GILBERT, D. L., T. OKANO, T. MIYATA & S. W. KIM. 1988. Macromolecular diffusion through collagen membranes. Int. J. Pharm. **47**: 79–88.

39. PALASIS, M. 1994. The influence of interactions on the diffusion of solutes in responsive gels. Ph.D. Thesis. University of Cincinnati. Cincinnati, OH.

40. JAMES, T. L. 1975. Nuclear magnetic resonance in biochemistry. Academic Press. New York.

41. SARBOLOUSKI, M. N. 1973. Probing the state of absorbed water by diffusion technique. J. Appl. Polym. Sci. **17**: 2407–2414.

42. KIM, S. W., J. R. CARDINAL, S. WISNIEWSKI & G. M. ZENTNER. 1980. Solute permeation through hydrogel membranes: Hydrophilic vs. hydrophobic solutes. *In* Water in Polymers. ACS Symposium Series. S. P. Rowland, Ed. **127**: 347–359. American Chemical Society. Washington D.C.

43. WALTER, H., D. E. BROOKS & D. FISHER. 1985. Partitioning in Aqueous Two-Phase Systems. Academic Press. New York.

44. ALBERTSSON, P. A. 1986. Partition of cell particles and macromolecules, 3rd edit. Wiley-Interscience. New York.

45. PALASIS, M. & S. H. GEHRKE. 1992. Permeability of responsive poly(N-isopropylacrylamide) gel to solutes. J. Controlled Release **18**: 1–12.

46. GEHRKE, S. H. & E. L. CUSSLER. 1989. Mass transfer in pH-sensitive hydrogels. Chem. Eng. Sci. **44**: 559–566.

47. HELFFERICH, F. 1962. Ion exchange. McGraw-Hill. New York.

48. HUSSAIN, S., M. S. MEHTA, J. I. KAPLAN & P. L. DUBIN. 1991. Experimental evaluation of conflicting models for size exclusion chromatography. Anal. Chem. **63**: 1132–1138.

49. OGSTON, A. G. 1958. The spaces in a uniform random suspension of fibers. Trans. Far. Soc. **54:** 1754–1757.
50. GIDDINGS, J. C., E. KUCERA, C. P. RUSSELL & M. N. MYERS. 1968. Statistical theory for the equilibrium distribution of rigid molecules in inert porous networks. Exclusion chromatography. J. Phys. Chem. **72:** 4397–4408.
51. SCHNITZER, J. E. 1988. Analysis of steric partition behavior of molecules in membranes using statistical physics. Biophys. J. **54:** 1065–1076.
52. POTSCHKA, M. & P. L. DUBIN, Eds. 1996. Strategies in size exclusion chromatography. ACS Symposium Series. **635.** American Chemical Society. Washington D.C.
53. RIGHETTI, P. G. 1981. On the pore size and shape of hydrophilic gels for electrophoretic analysis. *In* Electrophoresis '81. Walter de Gruyter & Co. Berlin.
54. DUBIN, P. L. & J. M. PRINCIPI. 1989. Optimization of size exclusion separation of proteins on superose columns. J. Chrom. **479:** 159–164.
55. KAUZMANN, W. 1959. Some factors in the interpretation of protein denaturation. Adv. Protein Chem. **14:** 1–63
56. DUBIN, P. L. & J. M. PRINCIPI. 1989. Hydrophobicity parameter of aqueous size exclusion chromatography gels. Anal. Chem. **61:** 780–781.
57. JANADO, M. 1988. Partitioning: Hydrophobic interactions. *In* Aqueous Size Exclusion Chromatography. P. L. Dubin, Ed. Elsevier. Amsterdam.
58. CHRISTENSON, H. K., P. M. CLAESSON & J. L. PARKER. 1992. Hydrophobic attraction: A reexamination of electrolyte effects. J. Phys. Chem. **96:** 6725–6728.
59. HOEVE, C. A. J. 1980. *In* Water in polymers. ACS Symposium Series. S. P. Rowland, Ed. **127:** 135–146. American Chemical Society. Washington D.C.
60. HORVATH, C., W. MELANDER & I. MOLNAR. 1976. Solvophobic interactions in liquid chromatography with nonpolar stationary phases. J. Chromatogr. **125:** 129–156.
61. RUCKENSTEIN, E. & V. LESINS. 1988. Classification of liquid chromatographic methods based on the interaction forces: The niche of potential barrier chromatography. *In* Downstream Processing: Equipment and Techniques. A. Mizrahi, Ed.: 246–312. Alan R. Liss, Inc. New York.
62. SCOPES, R. K. 1987. Protein purification: Principles and practice, 2nd. edit. Springer-Verlag. New York.
63. FAUSNAUGH, J. L., L. A. KENNEDY & F. E. REGNIER. 1984. Comparison of hydrophobic-interaction and reversed-phase chromatography of proteins. J. Chromatogr. **317:** 141–155.
64. BYWATER, R. P. & N. V. B. MARSDEN. 1988. *In* Chromatography: Fundamentals and Applications of Chromatographic and Electrophoretic Methods. Part A. E. Heftmann, Ed. Elsevier. Amsterdam.
65. TANFORD, C. 1973. The Hydrophobic Effect. J. Wiley & Sons. New York.
66. NEMETHY, G. & H. A. SCHERAGA. 1962. Structure of water and hydrophobic bonding proteins. I. A model for the thermodynamic properties of liquid water. J. Chem. Phys. **36:** 3382–3400.
67. SINANOGLU, O. 1968. Solvent effects on molecular associations. *In* Molecular Associations in Biology. B. Pullman, Ed.: 427–445. Academic Press. New York.
68. HORVATH, C. & W. MELANDER. 1977. Liquid chromatography with hydrocarbonaceous bonded phases; Theory and practice of reversed phase chromatography. J Chromatogr. Sci. **15:** 393–404.
69. MELANDER, W. R., D. CORRADINI & C. HORVATH. 1984. Salt-mediated retention of proteins in hydrophobic-interaction chromatography. J. Chromatogr. **317:** 67–85.
70. SEIPKE, G., H. MULLNER & U. GRAU. 1986. HPLC of proteins. Angew. Chem. Int. Ed. Engl. **25:** 530–548.
71. BEN-NAIM, A. 1980. Hydrophobic interactions. Plenum Press. New York.
72. GOHEEN, S. C. & S. C. ENGELHORN. 1984. Hydrophobic interaction high performance liquid chromatography of proteins. J. Chrom. **317:** 55–65.
73. YALKOWSKY, S. H., S. C. VALVANI & T. J. ROSEMAN. 1983. Solubility and partitioning VI: Octanol-water partition coefficients. J. Pharm. Sci. **72:** 866–870.
74. SASSI, A. P., H. W. BLANCH & J. M. PRAUSNITZ. 1992. Crosslinked gels as water

absorbents in separations. *In* Polymer Applications for Biotechnology. D. S. Soane, Ed. Prentice Hall. New York.

75. HARSH, D. C. & S. H. GEHRKE. 1990. Characterization of ionic water absorbent polymers: Determination of ionic content and effective crosslink density. *In* Absorbent Polymer Technology. L. Brannon-Peppas & R. S. Harland, Eds.: 103–124. Elsevier. Amsterdam.

76. CUSSLER, E. L. 1976. Multicomponent diffusion. Elsevier. Amsterdam.

77. SCHOEN M. & C. HOHEISEL. 1984. The mutual diffusion coefficient D_{12} in binary liquid mixtures. Molecular dynamics calculations based on Lennard-Jones (12-6) potentials. I. The method of determination. Molec. Phys. **52:** 33–56.

78. SCALETTAR, B. A., J. R. ABNEY & J. C. OWICKI. 1988. Theoretical comparison of the self diffusion and mutual diffusion of interacting membrane proteins. Proc. Natl. Acad. Sci. USA **85:** 6726–6730.

79. GIBBS, S. J., E. N. LIGHTFOOT & T. W. ROOT. 1992. Protein diffusion in porous gel filtration chromatography media studied by pulsed field gradient NMR spectroscopy. J. Phys. Chem. **96:** 7458–7462.

80. TONG, J. & J. L. ANDERSON. 1996 Partitioning and diffusion of proteins and linear polymers in polyacrylamide gels. Biophys. J. **70:** 1505–1513.

81. SATTERFIELD, C. N., C. K. COLTON & W. H. PITCHER, JR. 1973. Restricted diffusion in liquids within fine pores. AIChE J. **19:** 628–635.

82. BALTUS, R. E. 1989. Partition coefficients of rigid, planar multisubunit complexes in cylindrical pores. Macromolecules **22:** 1775–1779.

83. DEEN, W. M. 1987. Hindered transport of large molecules in liquid-filled pores. AIChE J. **33:** 1409–1425.

84. ADAMSKI, R. P. & J. L. ANDERSON. 1987. Configurational effects on polystyrene rejection from microporous membranes. J. Polym. Sci. Part B. Polym. Phys. **25:** 765–775.

85. COLTON, C. K., C. N. SATTERFIELD & C. J. LAI. 1975. Diffusion and partitioning of macromolecules within finely porous glass. AIChE J. **21:** 289–298.

86. MUHR, A. H. & J. M. V. BLANSHARD. 1982. Diffusion in gels. Polymer **23:** 1012–1026.

87. JOHANSSON, L., U. SKANTZE & J. E. LOFROTH. 1991. Diffusion and interaction in gels and solutions. 2. Experimental results on the obstruction effect. Macromolecules **24:** 6019–6023.

88. CLAEYS, I. L. & F. H. ARNOLD. 1989. Nuclear magnetic relaxation study of hindered rotational diffusion in gels. AIChE J. **35:** 335–338.

89. BROWN, W. & K. CHITUMBO. 1975. Solute diffusion in hydrated polymer networks. J. Chem. Soc. Farad. Trans. I **71:** 1–11.

90. TANIGUSHI, Y. & S. HORIGOME. 1975. The states of water in cellulose acetate membranes. J. Appl. Poly. Sci. **19:** 2743–2748.

91. QUINN, F. X., E. KAMPFF, G. SMYTH & V. J. MCBRIERTY. 1988. Water in hydrogels. 1. A study of water in poly(n-vinyl-2-pyrrolidone/methyl methacrylate) copolymer. Macromolecules **21:** 3191–3198.

92. SMYTH, G., F. X. QUINN & V. J. MCBRIERTY. 1988. Water in hydrogels. 2. A study of water in poly(hydroxyethyl methacrylate). Macromolecules **21:** 3198–3204.

93. QUINN, F.X., V. J. MCBRIERTY, A. C. WILSON & G. D. FRIENDS. 1990. Water in hydrogels. 3. Poly(hydroxyethylmethacrylate)/saline solution systems. Macromolecules **23:** 4576–4581.

94. MCBRIERTY, V. J., F. X. QUINN, C. KEELY, A. C. WILSON & G. D. FRIENDS. 1992. Water in hydrogels. 4. Poly(N-vinyl-2-pyrrolidinone-methyl-methacrylate)/saline systems. Macromolecules **25:** 4281–4284.

95. BERENDSEN, H. J. C. 1975. *In* Water: A Comprehensive Treatise. F. Franks, Ed. **5**. Plenum Press. New York.

96. ROORDA, W. E., J. A. BOUWSTRA, M. A. DE VRIES, H. E. JUNGINGER, J. DE BLEYSER & J. C. LEYTE. 1987. Hydrogels as elastic solutions. Proceed. 14th Inter. Symp. Contr. Rel. Bioact. Mat. **14:** 146–147.

97. ROORDA, W. E., J. A. BOUWSTRA, M. A. DE VRIES, H. E. JUNGINGER, J. DE BLEYSER & J. C. LEYTE. 1988. Elastic solutions of polymer in water. Proceed. 15th Inter. Symp. Contr. Rel. Bioact. Mat. **15:** 258–259.

98. ZENTNER, G. M., J. R. CARDINAL & S. W. KIM. 1978. Progestin permeation through polymer membrane II: Diffusion studies on hydrogel membranes. J. Pharm. Sci. **67:** 1352–1355.

99. MACKIE, J. S. & P. MEARES. 1955. The diffusion of electrolytes in a cation-exchange resin membrane. I. Theoretical. Proc. Roy. Soc. Lond. A **232:** 498–509.

100. NYSTROM, B., M. E. MOSELEY, W. BROWN & J. ROOTS. 1981. Molecular motion of small molecules in cellulose gels studied by NMR. J. Appl. Polym. Sci. **26:** 3385–3394.

101. DAVIS, B. K. 1974. Diffusion in polymer gel implants. Proc. Natl. Acad. Sci. USA **71:** 3120–3123.

102. PEPPAS, N. A. & S. R. LUSTIG. 1986. Solute diffusion in hydrophilic network structures. *In* Hydrogels in Medicine and Pharmacy. Vol. I. Fundamentals. N. A. Peppas, Ed. **1:** 57–83. CRC Press. Boca Raton, FL.

103. YASUDA, H., A. PETERLIN, C. K. COLTON, K. A. SMITH & E. W. MERRILL. 1969. Permeability of solutes through hydrated polymer membranes. Part III. Die Makromol. Chem. **126:** 177–186.

104. COHEN, M. H. & D. TURNBULL. 1959. Molecular transport in liquids and glasses. J. Chem. Phys. **31:** 1164–1169.

105. PEPPAS, N. A. & C. T. REINHART. 1983. Solute diffusion in swollen membranes. Part I. A new theory. J. Membr. Sci. **15:** 275–287.

106. LUSTIG, S. R. & N. A. PEPPAS. 1988. Solute diffusion in swollen membranes. IX. Scaling laws for solute diffusion in gels. J. Appl. Polym. Sci. **36:** 735–747.

107. KOU, J. H. & G. L. AMIDON. 1990. Release of phenylpropanolamine from dynamically swelling poly(hydroxyethyl methacrylate-co-methacrylic acid) hydrogels. Poly. Mat. Sci. Eng. **63:** 158–162.

108. LELOUP, V. M., P. RING & P. COLONNA. 1990. Studies on probe diffusion and accessibility in amylose gels. Macromolecules **23:** 862–886.

109. HAGGERTY, L., J. H. SUGARMAN & R. K. PRUD'HOMME. 1988. Diffusion of polymers through polyacrylamide gels. Polymer **29:** 1058–1063.

110. GRIMSHAW, P. E., A. J. GRODZINSKY, M. L. YARMUSH & D. M. YARMUSH. 1990. Selective augmentation of macromolecular transport in gels by electrodiffusion and electrokinetics. Chem. Eng. Sci. **45:** 2917–2920.

111. DONG, L. C., A. S. HOFFMAN & Q. YAN. 1994. Dextran permeation through poly(N-isopropylacrylamide) hydrogels. J. Biomater. Sci. Polymer Edn. **5:** 473–484.

112. BLOOMFIELD, V. A. & T. K. LIM. 1978. Quasi-elastic laser light scattering. *In* Methods in Enzymology. S. N. Timashef & C. H. W. Hirs, Eds. **48:** 415–421. Academic Press. New York.

113. SELLEN, D. B. 1986. The diffusion of compact macromolecules within hydrogels. Br. Polym. J. **18:** 28–31.

114. WESSON, J. A., H. TAKEZOE, H. YU & S. P. CHEN. 1982. Dye diffusion in swollen gels by forced Rayleigh scattering. J. Appl. Phys. **53:** 6513–6519.

115. WARE, B. R. 1984. Fluorescence photobleaching recovery. American Lab. **April:** 16–28.

116. LEE, P. I. 1983. *In* Controlled Release of Bioactive Materials. R. W. Baker, Ed.: 135–153. Academic Press. New York.

117. HWANG, S. T., T. E. S. TANG & K. KAMMERMEYER 1971. Transport of dissolved oxygen through silicon rubber membrane. J. Macromol. Sci.-Phys. **B5:** 1–10.

Permeability Assessment of Capsules for Islet Transplantation[a]

ALVIN C. POWERS,[b,c,e] MARCELA BRISSOVÁ,[d]
IGOR LACÍK,[d] A. V. ANILKUMAR,[d]
KEIVAN SHAHROKHI,[b] AND TAYLOR G. WANG[d]

[b]Division of Endocrinology
Department of Medicine
Vanderbilt University
Nashville, Tennessee, 37232

[c]Department of Veterans Affairs Medical Center
Nashville, Tennessee 37232

[d]Center for Microgravity Research
Vanderbilt University School of Engineering
Nashville, Tennessee 37235

The principle of immunoisolation, that hormone- or protein-secreting cells could be enclosed in a semi-permeable membrane which would protect cells from immune attack yet allow influx of molecules important for cell function/survival and efflux of desired cellular products, has great potential to treat a variety of human diseases via cell transplantation.[1-6] Immunoisolation may allow transplantation of cells without the need for immunosuppression and the transplantation of cells from non-human species (xenograft). The permeability of immunoisolation devices must balance two potentially conflicting requirements.[1-3,5,7,8] First, cells enclosed within the device must receive biologic molecules necessary for viability and normal function.[1,7,9-12] In addition, to low molecular weight molecules (amino acids, ions, glucose, etc.), most cells require interaction with an incompletely defined array of growth factors such as transferrin and IGF-I. The second requirement regarding permeability is that destructive components of the immune system should be prevented from entering the immunoisolation device. Cells of the immune system such as lymphocytes and macrophages are easily excluded by all immunoisolation devices, but many soluble products of the immune system such as immunoglobulins, complement proteins, cytokines, and nitric oxide may also be cytotoxic to immunoisolated cells. However, these soluble immune products span a wide range of molecular sizes and the product(s) responsible for the immune-mediated cytotoxicity of immunoisolated cells are not known.[13-18] Further confounding the selection of an optimal permeability is that the factors responsible for immune toxicity to islets may differ depending on whether the immune process is an allograft reaction, an xenograft

[a] These studies were supported by a grant from NASA ("Encapsulation of Living Cells"), grants from the Department of Veterans Affairs Research Service, the Vanderbilt School of Engineering and the Vanderbilt Diabetes Research and Training Center (NIH DK20593).

[e] Author to whom correspondence should be addressed: Endocrinology, 715 MRB II, Vanderbilt University, Nashville, TN 37232; Tel: (615) 936-1653; Fax (615) 936-1667; E-mail: Powersac@ctrvax.Vanderbilt.edu

reaction, or a recurrence of the autoimmune process that originally caused insulin-dependent diabetes mellitus.

While permeability optimization is clearly important for all types of immunoisolation devices, the desired permeability is not known. This limitation stems partly from deficits in knowledge about which molecules should be allowed to traverse the semi-permeable membrane and which molecules should be excluded and also partly from experimental obstacles that have prevented a systematic study of permeability. In addition, prior approaches have not defined the true permeability of membranes, but only a molecular weight cut-off to a single solute. In an effort to determine the optimal permeability of immunoisolation devices, we have created a series of capsules that differ only by their permeability and have carefully quantified their permeability using two complementary methods.

RESULTS AND DISCUSSION

Development of a New Capsule with Adjustable Features

Our cell encapsulation team has developed a new capsule that has several advantages over currently available systems.[19] This new capsule is formed by complexation of oppositely charged polyelectrolytes: sodium alginate (SA), cellulose sulfate (CS) and poly(methylene-co-guanidine) (PMCG) in the presence of Ca^{2+} and Na^+ ions.[19,20] These capsules have markedly improved mechanical strength compared with the widely used alginate/poly(L-lysine) capsules.[19,20] This encapsulation system also provides the flexibility to independently adjust other capsule parameters such as membrane thickness, diameter, but more importantly, pore size of the capsular membrane. The newly designed capsule is a result of simultaneous interaction of multiple components and the structure of the capsular membrane can be viewed as a fibrous network consisting of segments with different length. Capsule permeability has been altered by changing: i) polyanion concentration, ii) polycation composition, and iii) additional treatment of the capsules with secondary polycation. Using this methodology,[19,21] a series of capsules with different permeabilities has been created and characterized (see TABLE 1).

Theoretical Considerations in Measuring Capsule Permeability

The ability of a solute to diffuse across a semi-permeable membrane of an immunoisolation device depends on the membrane pore size, size and shape of the

TABLE 1. Series of Capsules that Span a Range of Exclusion Limits

Capsule Number	Dextran Molecular Weight (Daltons)	Viscosity Radius R_η (nm)	Protein Molecular Weight (Daltons)
1	230,000	11.7	1,770,000
2	120,000	8.5	750,000
3	44,000	5.1	200,000
4	19,000	3.4	67,000
5	13,800	2.9	44,000
6	3,200	1.4	6,500

This table adapted from reference 21.

solute molecules, and electrostatic/hydrophobic interactions between the membrane and the solute. Another important consideration is the ability of some proteins to combine monomer units into larger associates (dimers, trimers).

Permeability of immunoisolation devices has been measured either by indirect measurements of solute entry or by detection of solute inside immunoisolation devices.[8,22,23] Most permeability studies have been performed with microcapsules.[24–33] Measurements of capsule permeability have been conducted with either individual capsules using confocal[34] or fluorescence microscopy[31] or with a batch of capsules using UV spectrophotometry[32,35] and HPLC[36] to detect a decrease/increase of the solute concentration in surrounding medium. Test solutes used in prior studies have been either proteins or dextrans (labeled or unlabeled). The most detailed permeability measurements have been performed with alginate/poly-L-lysine/alginate capsules, but the reported permeabilities of essentially the same capsule by different laboratories are rather contradictory. This disagreement likely arises from a lack of standardization of test solutes and measuring techniques and minor differences in encapsulation procedure. Traditionally, the permeability of immunoisolation devices is characterized by so-called molecular weight cut-off, meaning the lowest molecular weight of solute excluded by the membrane. This type of characterization is inadequate since what membrane pores actually "see" is not solute molecular weight but its shape and size, which determine solute conformation. Another disadvantage of prior measurements is that the "exclusion limit" or molecular weight cut-off of the capsular membrane has been based on its impermeability to one or just a few selected solutes, usually bovine serum albumin or IgG. The result is not the true permeability of the membrane, but rather an upper limit based on a single solute. In addition, such approaches are not capable of addressing whether the membrane also excludes solutes smaller in size than the test solute. Valid comparisons between studies, or comparisons between different immunoisolation devices, are not possible because of differences in test solutes and methods to measure permeability. For example, one cannot compare the molecular weight cut-off determined with dextrans measured by microscopy and the molecular weight cut-off determined by UV spectrophotometry of a single protein.

Another confounding variable in the assessment of permeability is the poor correlation between molecular weight and size of various solutes. For example, some studies have used a solute with a hard sphere conformation (globular protein) while other studies have used a solute with a flexible coil conformation (polysaccharides like dextrans). FIGURE 1 shows how viscosity radius (R_η) of different solutes varies with their molecular weight.[37] In the case of polysaccharides, the macromolecular dimension increases monotonously with molecular weight of solute, while in the case of proteins, the data exhibit scatter around the best fit curve (up to 17% of R_η) suggesting that even proteins with substantially different molecular weight may assemble into the structures of the same size.[21,37] Thus, the molecular weight cut-off determined with one solute may be markedly different than the result with another solute (even though the solutes have the same molecular weight).

Measurement and Control of Capsule Permeability

The ideal assessment of permeability should consider both the physical size of the protein (its macromolecular dimensions, not its molecular weight) and chemical interactions between the membrane and the protein. Our approach to permeability assessment of immunoisolation membranes is: i) measure pore size of capsular membrane using solutes which have known physical dimensions and which do not

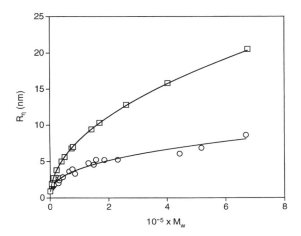

FIGURE 1. Viscosity radius vs. molecular weight. The relationship between the viscosity radius (R_η) and the molecular weight of dextrans ($\triangle$) and globular proteins ($\bigcirc$) was calculated as described.[37] (This figure was adapted from Analytical Biochemistry[37] with permission.)

exhibit electrostatic/hydrophobic interactions with the membrane; ii) correlate such measurements to the physical size of biologically relevant proteins; iii) determine capsule permeability to biologically relevant proteins.

Evaluation of Capsule Permeability by Size Exclusion Chromatography

Size exclusion chromatography (SEC) of capsules allows one to test capsule permeability to a homologous series of solutes over a reasonably wide range of molecular sizes.[38,39] In SEC, solute molecules are partitioned according to their macromolecular dimensions between eluant in the interstitial volume and stagnant liquid phase and the eluant within the capsules, which comprise the column packing.[38,39] We have adapted SEC to determine the permeability of capsules to a dextrans which span a range of molecular sizes (TABLE 1).[21,37] In order to compare the membrane exclusion limit defined by dextrans with that for proteins, we converted the dextran molecular weight to its viscosity radius R_η. Using the protein molecular weight and viscosity radius R_η relationship in FIGURE 1, the molecular weight for globular proteins with the same R_η as the dextran standards was derived (TABLE 1). There is a major difference between the exclusion limit defined with dextran standards and the predicted molecular weight of globular proteins. This difference is quite notable in the molecular weight range for most common cellular proteins (5 kD to 200 kD).

New Methodology to Measure Influx/Efflux of Biologically Relevant Proteins

SEC with dextran molecular weight standards allows one to estimate the apparent pore size of the capsular membrane based on the known size of the solute molecules. But the relevant molecules for the concept of immunoisolation are proteins, not dextrans. However, to utilize SEC for the study of proteins becomes more difficult because proteins differ in conformation, in the ability to self-associate or aggregate, and in their charge/hydrophobic interaction with the tested membrane.

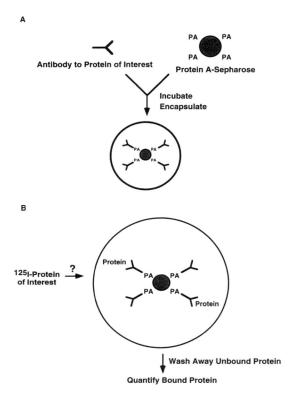

FIGURE 2. New method for measuring entry of proteins into capsules. **A**: Either a monoclonal antibody or a polyclonal antibody directed at the protein of interest is incubated with protein A-sepharose (PAS) to allow antibody binding via the Fc region. The PAS-antibody complex is encapsulated as usual. **B**: The encapsulated PAS-antibody complex is incubated with a tracer amount of the iodinated protein of interest ($\sim$10,000 cpm) for selected intervals. After washing, the amount of iodinated protein bound by the PAS-antibody complex is quantified in a gamma counter. Unencapsulated PAS and empty capsules serve as positive and negative controls, respectively.

New methodology which allows measurement of influx of biologically relevant proteins at physiologic concentrations has been developed (FIG. 2).[21] Protein A sepharose (PAS) is incubated with either a polyclonal or monoclonal antibody raised against the protein of interest. The PAS-antibody complex is then encapsulated. Following incubation with the radiolabeled protein of interest, the capsules are washed and protein entry into the capsule is quantified. The only requirements for this technique are an antibody against the protein of interest and the ability to radiolabel the protein. Thus, the permeability to a wide range of proteins can be assessed. Other advantages of this method compared to prior techniques are: 1) the permeability of any protein possibly important for immunoisolation can be tested; 2) the radiolabeled protein is present at low concentration (1 ng/mL) which is the physiologic range for most proteins; 3) a series of proteins with a range of

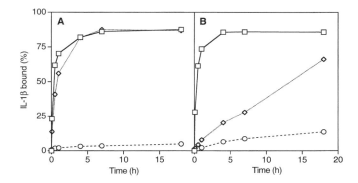

FIGURE 3. IL-1 entry into capsules of different permeability. The time course of IL-1β entry into capsule with 230 kD exclusion limit (**A**) or 3.2 kD exclusion limit (**B**) is shown. For each panel, the binding to free PAS ($\square$), encapsulated PAS ($\diamond$), and empty capsules ($\bigcirc$) is shown. (This figure was reproduced from Journal of Biomedical Materials Research[21] with permission.)

molecular weights can be used; 4) the technique is easily adapted to any immunoisolation device.

The permeability of two proteins, interleukin-1β (IL-1β) and IgG, has been assessed with the series of capsules in TABLE 1.[21] The time course of IL-1β binding is very similar for free and encapsulated PAS/antibody complex in the capsule with the largest exclusion limit (capsule with a 230 kD exclusion limit; capsule 1 in TABLE 1) (FIG. 3). However, IL-1β entry was significantly delayed (but not completely prevented) in a capsule with the lowest exclusion limit (capsule with a 3.2 kD exclusion limit; capsule 6 in TABLE 1) (FIG. 3). The biologic importance of this observation is not clear.

Similar studies were performed to assess entry of IgG into capsules of two different permeabilities as defined by SEC studies with dextrans.[21] IgG was easily able to enter capsules with the 230 kD exclusion limit (capsule 1 in TABLE 1). In contrast, entry of IgG was reduced when the exclusion limit was lowered to 44 kD (capsule 3 in TABLE 1). As shown in TABLE 1, the exclusion limit of 44 kD (defined with dextrans) is quite close to the predicted molecular size of IgG (5.2 nm). These results indicate the excellent correlation of measurements with the PAS system and SEC.

Function of Islets Enclosed in Capsules with Different Exclusion Limit

Using two capsules with different exclusion limits (230 and 120 kD), glucose-stimulated insulin secretion by encapsulated islets did not differ in a cell perifusion system (FIG. 4).[21] Glucose-stimulated insulin secretion of encapsulated islets was well-preserved in both capsules, but there was a slight delay in the insulin secretory peak in comparison with unencapsulated islets. The importance of this delay in insulin secretion *in vivo* is not clear.

Future Directions

We hypothesize that an optimal permeability for immunoisolation devices exists and that use of this permeability will enhance islet function and survival and mini-

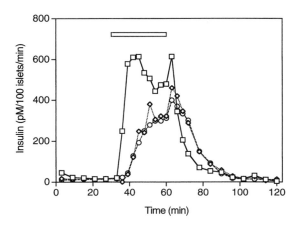

FIGURE 4. Insulin secretion by encapsulated islets. Insulin secretion by encapsulated rat islets was evaluated in a perifusion apparatus as described (19). Following a baseline perifusion with 2 mM glucose, either free islets or encapsulated islets were stimulated with 20 mM glucose + 0.045 mM IBMX (*bar at top*). The capsules with an exclusion limit of 230 kD (○) and 120 kD (◇) based on dextran exclusion measurements were compared to free islets (□). (This figure was reproduced from Journal of Biomedical Materials Research[21] with permission.)

mize the immune reaction to transplanted islets. This series of capsules will allow a systematic examination of permeability (as a function of pore size), while all other experimental variables such as type of immunoisolation device, cell type, and transplantation conditions are held constant. Information about the optimal membrane pore size from our studies, integrated with information about optimal surface chemistry, should be useful in the design of a variety of immunoisolation devices.

SUMMARY

Despite considerable progress in the development of immunoisolation devices, the optimal permeability of such devices is not known. This limitation stems partly from deficits in knowledge about which molecules should be allowed to traverse the semipermeable membrane and which molecules should be excluded, and also partly from experimental obstacles that have prevented a systematic study of permeability. To determine the optimal permeability of immunoisolation devices, we have created a series of microcapsules (800 μM diameter) that span a broad range of molecular exclusion limits yet are identical in wall thickness and chemical composition. Capsule permeability was precisely defined by two complementary methods— size exclusion chromatography (SEC) and a newly developed methodology to assess permeability of biologically relevant proteins. The entry of interleukin-1β-^{125}I was significantly delayed, but not prevented, when the capsule exclusion limit was decreased from 230 kD to 3.2 kD, as determined by SEC with dextran standards. The influx of IgG was as predicted, based on the viscosity radius R_η of IgG and the capsule exclusion limit defined by SEC. Glucose-stimulated insulin secretion by encapsulated pancreatic islets did not differ as capsule permeability was decreased from a molecular exclusion limit of 230 kD to 120 kD. These studies should assist in the design of immunoisolation devices by defining the permeability optimal for cell function and also should be applicable to any cell type or immunoisolation device.

REFERENCES

1. COLTON, C. K. & E. S. AVGOUSTINIATOS. 1991. Bioengineering in development of the hybrid artifical pancreas. J. Biomech. Eng. **113:** 152–170.
2. LANZA, R. P., S. J. SULLIVAN & W. L. CHICK. 1992. Islet transplantation with immunoisolation. Diabetes **41:** 1503–1510.
3. CHANG, T. M. 1992. Hybrid artificial cells: microencapsulation of living cells. ASAIO J. **38:** 128–130.
4. MAKI, T., C. J. MULLON, B. A. SOLOMON & A. P. MONACO. 1995. Novel delivery of pancreatic islet cells to treat insulin-dependent diabetes mellitus [Review]. Clin. Pharmacokinetics **28:** 471–482.
5. REACH, G. 1994. Bioartificial pancreas. Transplant. Proc. **26:** 397–398.
6. LANZA, R. P., J. L. HAYES & W. L. CHICK. 1996. Encapsulated cell technology. Nature Biotechnol. **14:** 1107–1111.
7. COLTON, C. K. 1994. Engineering issues in islet immunoisolation. *In* Immunoisolation of Pancreatic Islets. R. P. Lanza & W. L. Chick, Eds.: 13–20. Austin, TX. R. G. Landes Company.
8. GOOSEN, M. F. A. 1994. Fundamentals of microencapsulation. *In* Immunoisolation of Pancreatic Islets. R. P. Lanza & W. L. Chick, Eds.: 21–44. Austin, TX. R. G. Landes Company.
9. BODZIONY, J. 1992. Bioartificial endocrine pancreas: Foreign-body reaction and effectiveness of diffusional transport of insulin and oxygen after long-term implantation of hollow fibers into rats. Res. Exp. Med. **192:** 305–316.
10. SCHREZENMEIR, J., J. KIRCHGESSNER, L. GERO, L. A. KUNZ, J. BEYER & W. MUELLER-KLIESER. 1994. Effect of microencapsulation on oxygen distribution in islet organs. Transplantation **57:** 1308–1314.
11. KUHTREIBER, W. M., R. P. LANZA, A. M. BEYER, K. S. KIRKLAND & W. L. CHICK. 1993. Relationship between insulin secretion and oxygen tension in hybrid diffusion chambers. ASAIO J. **39:** M247–M251.
12. DIONNE, K. E., C. K. COLTON & M. L. YARMUSH. 1993. Effects of hypoxia on insulin secretion by isolated rat and canine islets of Langerhans. Diabetes **42:** 12–21.
13. WEBER, C., J. AYRES-PRICE, M. COSTANZO, A. BECKER & A. STALL. 1994. NOD mouse peritoneal cellular response to poly-L-lysine-alginate microencapsulated rat islets. Transplant. Proc. **26:** 1116–1119.
14. HEALD, K. A., T. R. JAY & R. DOWNING. 1994. Assessment of the reproducibility of alginate encapsulation of pancreatic islets using the MTT colorimetric assay. Cell Transplant. **3:** 333–337.
15. WEBER, C. J., S. ZABINSKI, T. KOSCHITZKY, L. WICKER, R. RAJOTTE, V. D'AGATI, L. PETERSON, J. NORTON, K. REEMTSMA. 1990. The role of CD4+ helper T cells in the destruction of microencapsulated islet xenografts in nod mice. Transplantation **49:** 396–404.
16. WIJSMAN, J., P. ATKISON, R. MAZAHERI, B. GARCIA, T. PAUL, J. VOSE, G. O'SHEA & C. STILLER. 1992. Histological and immunopathological analysis of recovered encapsulated allogeneic islets from transplanted diabetic BB/W rats. Transplantation **54:** 588–592.
17. WEBER, C., V. D'AGATI, L. WARD, M. COSTANZO, R. RAJOTTE & K. REEMTSMA. 1993. Humoral reaction to microencapsulated rat, canine, and porcine islet xenografts in spontaneously diabetic NOD mice. Transplant. Proc. **25:** 462–463.
18. WEBER, C. J. & K. REEMTSMA. 1994. Microencapsulation in small animals—xenografts. *In* Immunoisolation of Pancreatic Islets. R. P. Lanza & W. L. Chick, Eds.: 59–80. Austin, TX. R. G. Landes Company.
19. WANG, T. G., I. LACIK, M. BRISSOVA, A. PROKOP, D. HUNKELER, A. V. ANILKUMAR, R. GREEN, K. SHAHROKI & A. C. POWERS. 1997. An encapsulation system for the immunoisolation of pancreatic islets. Nature Biotechnol. **15:** 358–362.
20. LACIK, I., M. BRISSOVA, A. V. ANILKUMAR, A. C. POWERS & T. G. WANG. 1997. New capsule with tailored properties for the encapsulation of living cells. J. Biomed. Mater. Res. In press.

21. BRISSOVA, M., I. LACIK, A. C. POWERS, A. V. ANILKUMAR & T. G. WANG. 1997. Control and measurement of permeability for design of microcapsule cell delivery system. J. Biomed. Mater. Res. In press.

22. VANDENBOSSCHE, G. M., P. VAN OOSTVELDT & J. P. REMON. 1991. A fluorescence method for the determination of the molecular weight cut-off of alginate-polylysine microcapsules. J. Pharm. & Pharmacol. **43**: 275–277.

23. CROOKS, C. A., J. A. DOUGLAS, R. L. BROUGHTON & M. V. SEFTON. 1990. Microencapsulation of mammalian cells in a HEMA-MMA copolymer: Effects on capsule morphology and permeability. J. Biomed. Mater. Res. **24**: 1241–1262.

24. ZONDERVAN, G. J., H. J. HOPPEN, A. J. PENNINGS, W. FRITSCHY, G. WOLTERS & R. VAN SCHILFGAARDE. 1992. Design of a polyurethane membrane for the encapsulation of islets of Langerhans. Biomaterials **13**: 136–144.

25. KESSLER, L., M. APRAHAMIAN, M. KEIPES, C. DAMGE, M. PINGET & D. POINSOT. 1992. Diffusion properties of an artificial membrane used for Langerhans islets encapsulation: An in vitro test. Biomaterials **13**: 44–49.

26. GROHN, P., G. KLOCK, J. SCHMITT, U. ZIMMERMANN, A. HORCHER, R. G. BRETZEL, B. J. HERING, D. BRANDHORST, H. BRANDHORST, T. ZEKORN et al. 1994. Large-scale production of Ba(2+)-alginate-coated islets of Langerhans for immunoisolation. Exp. Clin. Endocrinol. **102**: 380–387.

27. KESSLER, L., M. PINGET, M. APRAHAMIAN, P. DEJARDIN & C. DAMGE. 1991. In vitro and in vivo studies of the properties of an artificial membrane for pancreatic islet encapsulation. Horm. Metab. Res. **23**: 312–317.

28. SAWHNEY, A. S. & J. A. HUBBELL. 1992. Poly(ethylene oxide)-graft-poly(L-lysine) copolymers to enhance the biocompatibility of poly(L-lysine)-alginate microcapsule membranes. Biomaterials **13**: 863–870.

29. FRITSCHY, W. M., G. H. WOLTERS & R. VAN SCHILFGAARDE. 1991. Effect of alginate-polylysine-alginate microencapsulation on in vitro insulin release from rat pancreatic islets. Diabetes **40**: 37–43.

30. CLAYTON, H. A., N. J. LONDON, P. S. COLLOBY, P. R. BELL & R. F. JAMES. 1991. The effect of capsule composition on the biocompatibility of alginate-poly-l-lysine capsules. J. Microencapsulation **8**: 221–233.

31. HALLE, J. P., S. BOURASSA, F. A. LEBLOND, S. CHEVALIER, M. BEAUDRY, A. CHAPDELAINE, S. COUSINEAU, J. SAINTONGE & J. F. YALE. 1993. Protection of islets of Langerhans from antibodies by microencapsulation with alginate-poly-L-lysine membranes. Transplantation **55**: 350–354.

32. GOOSEN, M. F. A., G. O'SHEA, H. M. GHARAPETIAN, S. CHOU & A. M. SUN. 1985. Optimization of microencapsulation parameters: Semipermeable microcapsules as a bioartificial pancreas. Biotechnol. Bioeng. **27**: 146–150.

33. LACY, P. E., O. D. HEGRE. A. GERASIMIDI-VAZEOU, F. T. GENTILE & K. E. DIONNE. 1991. Maintenance of normoglycemia in diabetic mice by subcutaneous xenografts of encapsulated islets. Science **254**: 1782–1784.

34. VANDENBOSSCHE, G. M. R., P. VAN OSTVELDT, J. DEMEESTER & J.-P. REMON. 1993. The molecular weight cut-off of microcapsules is determined by the reaction between alginate and polylysine. Biotechnol. Bioeng. **42**: 381–386.

35. KING, G. A., A. J. DAUGULIS, P. FAULKNER & M. F. A GOOSEN. 1987. Alginate-polylysine microcapsules of controlled membrane molecular weight cutoff for mammalian cell culture engineering. Biotechnol. Prog. **3**: 231–240.

36. COROMILI, V. & T. M. CHANG. 1993. Polydisperse dextran as a diffusing test solute to study the membrane permeability of alginate polylysine microcapsules. Biomater. Artificial Cells Immobilization Biotechnol. **21**: 427–444.

37. BRISSOVA, M., M. PETRO, I. LACIK, A. C. POWERS & T. G. WANG. 1996. Evaluation of microcapsule permeability via inverse size exclusion chromatography. Anal. Biochem. **242**: 104–111.

38. JERABEK, K., A. REVILLON & E. PUCCILLI. 1993. Pore structure characterization of organic-inorganic materials by inverse size exclusion chromatography. Chromatographia **36**: 259–262.

39. KLEIN, J., J. STOCK & K. D. VORLOP. 1983. Pore size and properties of spherical Ca-alginate biocatalysis. Eur. J. Appl. Microbiol. Biotechnol. **18**: 86–91.

Modulation of Surface and Bulk Properties of Biomedical Polymers

K. J. L. BURG,[a,e] J. M. ALLAN,[b,c] S. L. ROWETON,[d]
AND S. W. SHALABY[b,c]

[a]Department of General Surgery Research
Carolinas Medical Center
Charlotte, North Carolina 28232-2861

[b]Department of Bioengineering
Clemson University
Clemson, South Carolina 29634-0905

[c]Poly-Med Inc.
Center for Applied Technology
Westinghouse Road
Pendleton, South Carolina 29670

[d]Institute of Materials Science
University of Connecticut,
Storrs, Connecticut 06269-3136

Polymers have the distinct advantage over the traditional metallic biomaterials that their properties may be readily adjusted and customized by relatively simple processing changes. Each individual polymeric material has a large range of potential characteristics that may be explored by process modulation. Indeed, it is this adaptability coupled with the rather recent incorporation of polymeric materials into biomedical devices that presents many opportunities for research in polymer processing and characterization. This paper attempts to overview specific examples of surface and bulk property modulation of biomedical polymers that have been the subjects of several research projects at Clemson University over the past few years. The discussion addresses the molecular orientation of a nonabsorbable system and an absorbable system, the formation of absorbable and nonabsorbable microporous systems, two surface chemical activation methods for a nonabsorbable system, and self-reinforcement of a nonabsorbable system. The underlying motivation for all six studies is the enhancement of polymeric properties to better suit a particular biomedical application. The properties addressed are the mechanical qualities, the degradation characteristics, and the cellular affinity to the system. These qualities are integral to the biocompatibility and longevity of the system.

[e] Author to whom correspondence should be addressed: Department of General Surgery Research, Cannon Research Building, Room 406, Carolinas Medical Center, P.O. Box 32861, Charlotte, NC 28232-2861; Tel: (704) 355-7449; Fax: (704) 355-8832; E-mail: kburg@ carolinas.org

ORIENTATION

Orientation of the molecular chains may be used to enhance the mechanical integrity of a polymeric device and therefore widen the scope of device application. These features are attained in a simple manner that more complicated alternatives such as self-reinforcement cannot achieve.[1,2] Polydioxanone, for example, is an absorbable material which is used commonly in wound repair in its compliant, low modulus, monofilament suture form. Upon orientation, however, the material acquires a substantially higher modulus, allowing for its use as pins in orthopedic hard tissue applications.[3] This orientation process is applicable to both nonabsorbable and absorbable systems. Orientation of an absorbable system may additionally change the degradation pattern and therefore potentially influence the tissue reaction extent and duration. Orientation may therefore be considered to modulate both the surface and bulk properties.

Ultrahigh molecular weight polyethylene (UHMWPE) is a simple, biostable system which may be readily manipulated mechanically. The limitations of this material in high shear stress, bending, and torquing biomedical applications demand additional requirements such as metal backing, cross-linking, or reinforcement.[4-9] As these solutions are not always adequate, the use of molecular orientation was studied. It was found[10] that application of a solid-state compression method[11] to UHMWPE can greatly improve the tensile strength and modulus of an UHMWPE film (TABLE 1). Further analyses showed that, at a given temperature, the modulus may be compression ratio dependent. Solid-state compression may eliminate, or at least reduce, delamination that can occur during the standard tensile drawing technique, while achieving comparable advantageous properties. Orientation may be exploited to increase the modulus and decrease creep,[12] critical to such biomedical applications as acetabular cup design.

It was postulated that the molecular orientation of an absorbable film will not only change the mechanical features of the device, but it will also affect the degradation profile of the material after exposure to an aqueous solution.[13,14] Results of comparative studies have verified this postulate using poly-l-lactide films (PLLA) with a twofold compression ratio. It was found, by both optical and chemical analysis, that the oriented material degrades in a more gradual fashion beginning at the more disordered exterior. The nonoriented material, in contrast, tends to degrade preferentially from the interior, which could conceptually result in a sudden, potentially detrimental, delayed release of acidic material into the surrounding tissue. The concept of degradation profile manipulation has great significance in the optimization of several absorbable applications, including drug delivery devices, fracture fixation plates or rods, as well as defect repair patches. In addition, the enhancement of mechanical features of the absorbable device may contribute to the success of load bearing absorbable implants, a currently limited application for this inherently weaker group of polymers.

TABLE 1. Representative Tensile Properties of $70 \times 15 \times 1.5$ mm Films[a]

T (°C)	Compression Ratio	Yield Strength (MPa)	Modulus (MPa)
Control	1.0	24.4 ± 0.6	484 ± 44
115	2.0	87.7 ± 26.9	1063 ± 53
115	3.4	117.4 ± 16	1183 ± 14

[a] Averages ± 95% confidence limits, based on a sample size of five.

MICROPOROSITY

Polymeric foams are advantageous in that their topography may be designed to induce cellular ingrowth and tissue repair that is not typically encouraged with a solid substrate. Microporous structures are common in nonmedical applications, *e.g.*, the packaging industry; however, the advent of tissue engineering has promoted the investigation of new, reproducible foam processing methods specifically for biomedical applications.[15-17] This introduces a new realm of considerations, including the processing sensitivity of the absorbable materials as well as the histocompatibility requirements which demand a relatively pure product. The following research[18] addressed a crystallization-induced microphase separation (CIMS) technique which may be readily adapted to address both absorbable and nonabsorbable, continuous, thermoplastic foam processes.

Polyethylene (PE), polypropylene (PP), nylon 6 (N-6), nylon 12 (N-12), and polycaprolactone (PCL) were all successfully treated using CIMS, which employs the use of a readily sublimable and/or leachable, low melting temperature, solid solvent. It was ascertained, through a battery of characterization analyses, that consistent, continuous, open-cell structures were formed. Furthermore, no residual solvent was detected by gas chromatography/mass spectroscopy. Such structures may be useful as templates in orthopedic applications or as surfaces for the *in vitro* development of cell culture technique. Several criteria were set regarding efficacy of the CIMS method, at least two of which must be met in order for effective foam formation to occur: 1) the solvent must promote rapid, facile polymer dissolution; 2) the solvent must be crystallizable, with a melting temperature above $25°C$; 3) the solvent must be capable of participating in solid-solid phase separation; 4) the solvent must be amenable to a broad range of cooling schemes; 5) the solvent must not promote polymer degradation; and 6) the polymer/solvent system must be readily molded, cast, and extruded.

Poly-*p*-dioxanone (PD) and two types of ε-caprolactone/glycolide (CL/G) copolymers were similarly, successfully treated using CIMS. These cases resulted in the formation of continuous, open-cell structures. The pore size was controlled by the manipulation of processing conditions; sizes from 10 microns to 200 microns were successfully achieved in this manner. Furthermore, the processing conditions could be manipulated in order to achieve a range of morphologies and a controlled pore size distribution. Most critical to the absorbable materials, it was determined through solution viscosity that the CIMS process did not affect the molecular weight of the material. A typical example of an absorbable polymer foam structure produced from CIMS is shown in FIGURE 1. Absorbable foams are showing great promise as scaffolds and constructs in the rapidly expanding research area of tissue engineering.

SURFACE ACTIVATION

Surface conductivity and chemical activation are material properties that find use in applications such as orthopedics, where the interfacial interaction between bone and implant is a critical issue. This encompasses fixation and the ability of the material to interlock with its surrounding bony environment since these criteria will dictate the mechanical stability and therefore healing capacity at the implant site. Fixation will depend not only upon the morphology of the surface but also on its chemical reactivity and composition. Surface phosphonylation adds phosphonate

FIGURE 1. Scanning electron micrograph of typical caprolactone-glycolide copolymer.

groups to the surface which can participate in the formation of hydroxyapatite. The phosphonate moieties can further contribute to the organized formation of electrically conductive surfaces. Both systems, surface conductive and phosphonylated substrates, are therefore relevant to bone regeneration.[19–22]

UHMWPE is an ideal test material for surface phosphonylation. A phosphonylated surface effectively offers a binding surface for calcium ions and therefore bony deposition, thus allowing interfacial interlocking between bone and implant. The addition of phosphonate is more stable than alternatives such as phosphate. Research[23,24] showed that surface phosphonylation of UHMWPE may be achieved by covalently binding phosphonate groups to the surface carbon chains (FIG. 2)

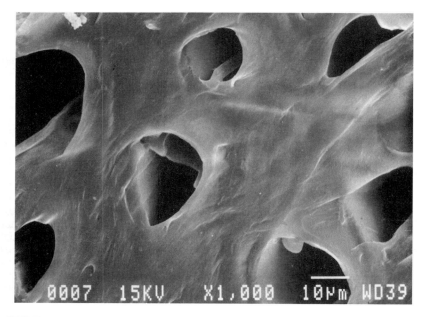

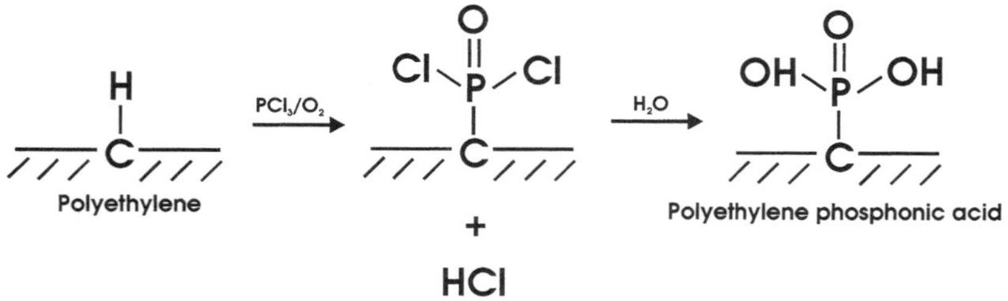

FIGURE 2. Surface phosphonylation of polyethylene.

and that there is an optimal, controllable reaction time with which to maximize the surface integrity. A comparison study[25] was run between phosphonylated groups and phosphonylated groups with ionically bound calcium. The study demonstrated that there was no difference between the affinity of phosphonylated and calcium pretreated phosphonylated samples to calcium from surrounding solution and that the concentration of calcium in the surrounding solution did not affect the amount of calcium bound by the surfaces. Most importantly, the study showed that surface phosphonylation of the UHMWPE was achieved and that the surfaces would induce the formation of calcium phosphate. Such surfaces will have great potential in many biomedical applications.

UHMWPE is also an ideal test material for surface conductivity. Research[26] has shown that surface conducting phosphonylated UHMWPE may be formed by exposure to aqueous pyrrole solution. This processing method is advantageous since it allows an ultrathin surface conducting layer to be deposited upon a preformed biomedical device. The resulting product is hallmarked by the unique structure of the conducting surface. The conducting polymer, polypyrrole, is molecularly bound to the thermoplastic UHMWPE device, which naturally leads to the question of stability and therefore biocompatibility of the surface. Preliminary *in vitro* compatibility studies of UHMWPE compression molded films[27] showed that there are no apparent cytotoxic effects due either to the material or due to leachables. Applications of this technique will be an area of growing interest.

SELF-REINFORCEMENT

One of the most important biomedical applications of UHMWPE is its use as an articulating surface. The major concern in this application is the tendency of the material to creep over several years. In a unique effort to eliminate this problem, studies were conducted on the formation of novel composites of self-reinforced UHMWPE.[9] The studies showed that assemblies of such composites may be achieved: 1) without compromising the orientation of the reinforcing fibers; 2) with the formation of a unique interface between the fiber and the matrix; 3) with the development of unusual transverse strength; 4) with the development of exceptionally high resistance to creep. This form of UHMWPE is extremely desirable for use in articulating surfaces exposed to high loading.

SUMMARY

The surface and bulk modulation of polymeric biomedical devices allows the full range of material properties to be exercised as demanded by custom applications. Polymeric biomaterials are finding greater use as relatively inert and even transient options and so therefore will require thorough processing analyses and the transfer of technology from nonbiomedical applications to the biomedical industry.

REFERENCES

1. WARD, I. M. 1993. Plastics Rubber and Composites Processing and Applications **19(1):** 7.
2. TUNC, D. C. & B. JADHAV. 1985. Polymer Preprints **29:** 383.

3. BHATIA, S., S. W. SHALABY, D. L. POWERS, R. L. LANCASTER & R. L. FERGUSON. 1994. J. Biomater. Sci. Polymer Edn. **6(5):** 435.
4. ROSE, R. M., A. CRUGROLA, M. REIS, W. R. CIMINO, I. PAUL & E. L. RADIN. 1990. Clin. Orthop. **145:** 277.
5. ROSE, R. M., I. PAUL & E. L. RADIN. 1980. J. Bone Jt. Surg. Am. Vol. **62A:** 537.
6. DUPLESSIS, T. A., C. J. GROBBELAAR & F. MARAIS. 1977. Rad. Phys. Chem. **9:** 647.
7. FARLING, G. M. & K. GREER. 1980. *In* Mechanical Properties of Biomaterials. G. W. Hastings & D. F. Williams, Eds. John Wiley & Sons. New York.
8. WRIGHT, M., T. FUBAYASHI & A. H. BURSTEIN. 1981. J. Biomed. Mater. Res. **15:** 719.
9. DENG, M. & S. W. SHALABY. 1995. Polymer News **20:** 329.
10. DENG, M. & S. W. SHALABY. 1997. Unidirectional orientation of ultrahigh molecular weight polyethylene using a new solid state process. *In* Transactions of the 22nd Annual Meeting of the Society for Biomaterials. Society for Biomaterials. New Orleans, LA.
11. SHALABY, S. W., R. A. JOHNSON & M. DENG, Inventors; Clemson University, Assignee. 1996. U.S. Patent 5,529,736.
12. DENG, M., R. A. LATOUR, A. A. OGALE & S. W. SHALABY. 1996. *In* Transactions of the Fifth World Biomaterials Congress. Toronto, Ontario, Canada.
13. BURG, K. J. L. & S. W. SHALABY. 1996. Polymer Preprints **37(2):** 759.
14. BURG, K. J. L. 1996. Effect of Orientation on the Physicochemical and Morphological Changes in Absorbing Polylactide Films. Ph.D. dissertation, Clemson University, Clemson, South Carolina.
15. DE PONTI, R., C. TORRICELLI, M. ALESSANDRO & E. LARDINI, Inventors. 1991. International Patent WO 91/09079.
16. WHANG, K., C. H. THOMAS & K. E. HEALY. 1995. Polymer **36(4):** 837.
17. MIKOS, A. G., A. J. THORSEN, L. A. CZERWONKA, Y. BAO, R. LANGER, D. N. WINSLOW & J. P. VACANTI. 1994. Polymer. **35(5):** 1068.
18. ROWETON, S. & S. W. SHALABY. 1996. *In* Transactions of the Fifth World Biomaterials Congress. Toronto, Ontario, Canada.
19. YASUDA, I. 1955. J. Jpn. Orthop. Assoc. **29:** 351.
20. BASSETT, C. A. L., R. J. PAWLUCK & R. O. BECKER. 1964. Nature **204:** 652.
21. KAMEGAI, A., M. MORI & S. INUE. 1990. J. Cranio. Max. Fac. Surg. **18:** 813.
22. LINDSEY, R. W., J. GROBMAN, R. E. LOGGON, M. PANJOBI & G. E. FRIEDLAENDER. 1987. Clin. Orthop. Rel. Res. **222:** 275.
23. SHALABY, S. W. & S. MCCAIG, Inventors; Clemson University, Assignee. 1996. U.S. Patent 5,491,198.
24. CAMPBELL, C. E., M. A. RUSSELL, J. S. HUDSON, A. F. VON RECUM & S. W. SHALABY. 1996. *In* Transactions of the Fifth World Biomaterials Congress. Toronto, Ontario, Canada.
25. CAMPBELL, C. E., A. M. NELSON, J. S. HUDSON, A. F. VON RECUM & S. W. SHALABY. 1996. *In* Transactions of the Fifth World Biomaterials Congress. Toronto, Ontario, Canada.
26. ALLAN, J. 1993. The Molecular Binding of Inherently Conducting Polymers to Thermoplastic Substrates. M.S. Thesis, Clemson University, Clemson, South Carolina.
27. ALLAN, J., F. J. PEARCE, R. V. GREGORY, T. VAN KOOTEN & S. W. SHALABY. 1996. *In* Transactions of the Fifth World Biomaterials Congress. Toronto, Ontario, Canada.

Purification of Polymers Used for Fabrication of an Immunoisolation Barrier[a]

ALES PROKOP[b] AND TAYLOR G. WANG[c]

[b]Department of Chemical Engineering
[c]The Center for Microgravity Research and Applications
School of Engineering
Vanderbilt University
Nashville, Tennessee 37232

Immunoisolation by means of capsules based on alginate as a matrix offers a very promising strategy to overcome the host immune response that is observed when implanting xenografts. Experiments in animal models have shown that after implantation of alginate-based capsules, loaded with xenografts (cells), foreign-body reactions occur, leading to a formation of a thick extracapsular layer of fibrotic and other cells, physically blocking diffusion in and out of capsules and suffocating the embedded xenografts.[1] Besides alginates, may other polymers (or their mixtures) are used to produce capsules for the same purpose. Many commercially available polymers, contain, however, impurities which exhibit adverse biological activities and thus contribute to a failure of a xenograftic implant. These impurities are of several kinds, such as monomers, catalysts, initiators, *etc.*, which are present in synthetically derived polymers. These impurities can be mostly removed via dialysis because of their small molecular size. Synthetic polymers, however, are better avoided, if possible, unless they mimic natural components of living cells and of their environment. Pyrogens represent the second kind of impurities. They belong to a group of natural compounds of certain gram-negative bacteria (cell wall) and cause a temperature rise when injected intravenously (hence they were called pyrogens). Chemically, they are represented by a variety of complex lipopolysaccharides (LPS) with highly hydrophobic character.[2] The third group (mitogens) is a rather less defined group of organic compounds which activate many cell types (including lymphocytes, fibroblasts, *etc.*). Their activation leads to cell proliferation and to subsequent production of lymphokines (cytokines), involved in the end in inflammatory reactions and implant rejection, if mitogens contaminate polymers used to manufacture such implants. This paper deals with removal of the second and third group of polymer contaminants, namely the pyrogens and mitogens.

The removal of the above substances is not a simple procedure. Both groups of impurities are present in traces in the polymers used but elicit powerful biological responses. Both result from contaminants present in the initial raw material as well as due to polymer processing steps. As most of these polymers are extracted and isolated from natural sources (*e.g.*, seaweeds), the starting material is mostly heavily contaminated, unless an axenic or pure culture is used initially (algae, microbial cells). Zimmermann *et al.*[3] and Klock *et al.*[4] have suggested the use of electrophoresis

[a] The financial support from NASA is greatly acknowledged (NASA #NAGW-1707 "Encapsulation of Living Cells").

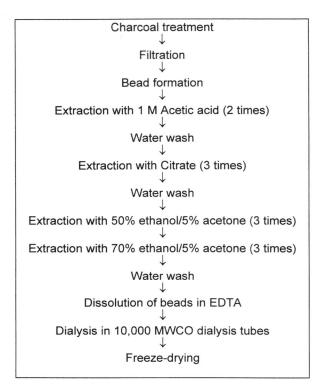

Charcoal treatment
↓
Filtration
↓
Bead formation
↓
Extraction with 1 M Acetic acid (2 times)
↓
Water wash
↓
Extraction with Citrate (3 times)
↓
Water wash
↓
Extraction with 50% ethanol/5% acetone (3 times)
↓
Extraction with 70% ethanol/5% acetone (3 times)
↓
Water wash
↓
Dissolution of beads in EDTA
↓
Dialysis in 10,000 MWCO dialysis tubes
↓
Freeze-drying

FIGURE 1. Summary of extractive purification procedure by Klock *et al.*[4] as applied to alginates.

to separate and remove the above contaminants. The size and charge of chemical species involved serves as a basis for polymer purification. However, such processing is only feasible at a lab scale and at a low-gravity environment and does not represent an economic way of purifying these polymers. The same authors have also suggested a multistep chemical extraction procedure for purification of alginate. This method makes use of a gelling capability of alginate. Specifically, small gelled barium alginate beads are successively chemically treated to remove impurities. The advantages of using beads is that they can be easily separated by sedimentation from an extracting agent. Before the barium alginate beads are made, alginate solution is treated with an active carbon (charcoal) and filtered through a microfiltration device to remove the suspended matter. Beads are then produced and treated successively using the following steps (FIG. 1): a) three extractions for 14 h in 1 M acetic acid (pH 2.3) with water wash in between; b) three extractions for 16 h with 50% ethanol (5% acetone) followed by the extractions with 70% ethanol (5% acetone), all interspersed with a water wash (alcohol/acetone step removes partially lipophilic pyrogens); c) dissolution of beads in 0.25 M EDTA solution (pH 10) (by complexing barium and replacing it by sodium ion); and d) dialysis of the polymer solution using 10,000 MWCO dialysis tube, followed by freeze-drying. Klock *et al.*[4] have demonstrated that while pyrogens are removed, mitogens are removed as well or reduced to an acceptable level.

The present work describes and extends the above chemical extraction procedure to other gel forming polymers as well as simplifies it and suggests new steps to achieve the same. Recently, after our extensive screening of polymers for their capability to form capsules with biocompatible end-products,[5] a need for purification of many other polymers other than alginate emerged. New polymer recipes are now available, using new polymers or their blends to generate biocompatible and mechanically stable capsules, suitable for transplantation.[6]

This procedure makes use of the fact that some other polymers can gel in the presence of small ions (cations). Thus kappa and iota carrageenans can make gel beads in the presence of potassium or calcium salts (KCl, CaCl$_2$); gellan in presence of calcium salt (CaCl$_2$). It is important that the gelled beads stay intact almost to the end of the whole chemical extraction procedure, when they are dissolved by a chelating agent. This is not the case for cellulose sulfate and pectin. The procedure described in this paper is used to maintain their beads in the beaded form. This is accomplished by employing gelling cations throughout the extraction procedure, otherwise the beads dissolve.

Next, improvement is based on the use of organic extraction solvents to remove pyrogens. The use of solvents is extended also to nongelling polymers. A combination with chemical extraction method results in the best scenario. For gelling polymers, chemical treatment prior to bead formation, followed by ethanol and chloroform extraction, resulted in superior quality of polymers. For nongelling polymers, a combination of chloroform treatment of a solution was also very good in achieving the desired product quality.

EXPERIMENTAL

Polymers

The following polymers were used: LV Keltone alginate (Kelco/Merck, San Diego, CA), HV Keltone alginate (Kelco), HVCR Keltone alginate (Kelco), Manugel GHB alginate (Kelco), UP LVG alginate (Pronova Biopolymer, Drammen, Norway), UP MVG alginate (Pronova), cellulose sulfate (Janssen Chimica, Geel, Belgium), Gelcarin GP-911 NF kappa carrageenan (FMC Corp., Newark, CT), Gelcarin GP-379 NF iota carrageenan (FMC), kappa carrageenan (Wako Pure Chemical Ind., Richmond, VA), Gelrite deacylated gellan (Kelco), carboxymethylcellulose, medium molecular weight (Sigma, St. Louis, MO) and low-esterified pectin 315 NH ND (Sanofi Bio-Industries, Paris, France).

Chemicals

Ethanol, acetone, chloroform, ethyl ether and phenol were purchased from Sigma.

Other Materials

Polysulfone cartridge (MiniCapsule Filter, 0.22 μm, Gelman, Ann Arbor, MI), Acticlean Etox column (Sepragen, Carlsbad, CA).

Pyrogen Determination

Pyrogen content was determined by a standard gel-clot LAL method (Associates of Cape Cod, Woods Hole, MA) or by a chromogenic LAL method (LAL test kit QCL 1000, Whitaker Bioproducts, Walkersville, MD).

Mitogen Determination

Mitogens were determined in a bioassay. Klock *et al.*[4] used a splenocyte culture coupled with a haemacytometer count or MTT assay. In our case, we used normal rat kidney cells (NRK) followed by a DNA determination to assay their growth. The culture was treated with 10 nM of EDTA/NaOH (pH 11.3) for 20 min at 37°C. This treatment released DNA. The EDTA extract was subjected to a fluorometric DNA assay. A TNE buffer and Hoechst 33258 dye (Polysciences, Warrington, PA) was used to permit DNA determination in the range 10–400 ng/ml. TNE buffer consisted of 2 M NaCl (Fisher), 10 mM Tris/HCl (Sigma) and 1 mM EDTA (Sigma). A TK0100 dedicated minifluorometer (Hoefer Scientific Instruments, San Francisco, CA) was used to measure the fluorescence. Epidermal growth factor (Sigma) was used as a standard mitogen.

RESULTS

Rationale for Polymer Purification

Several disadvantages of Klock's procedure can be noted: 1) the considerable length of the procedure lends itself to the possibility of polymer degradation. Based on our observations, a polymer viscosity is often reduced to some degree (10–30%), supporting this notion; 2) our experience shows that in addition to polymer degradation (lower molecular weight) some chemical extraction steps may lead to polymer modification (*e.g.*, partial esterification of carboxyl groups of alginate chain by ethanol, as detected by NMR; note results are not presented in detail), leading to a nonfunctional behavior of alginate. Our procedure attempts to simplify Klock's procedure in terms of number of steps involved and time (and to extend this procedure to other gelling polymers) and, in addition, incorporates several new steps, namely extraction with organic solvents as well as pyrogen removal by a proprietary ligand coupled to a chromatographic carrier (or by a positively charged cartridge). The latter step also allows for extension to nongelling polymers.

Simplification and Extension of Klock's Procedure

TABLE 1 presents a comparison of original Klock's procedure with some other treatments. Column (1) presents results for Klock's procedure as applied to a particular alginate. The efficiency of pyrogen removal was high. Procedures (2)–(7) are simpler, omitting some steps (and adding some others instead). Discussion on TABLE 1 can be summarized as follows: 1) Klock's extractive procedure yields high purity (high pyrogen removal efficiency) but often to a lower molecular mass product (not documented here); 2) extraction times and number of repetitive steps can be often reduced (not documented); 3) single-step charcoal or chloroform treatment

TABLE 1. Comparison of Klock's Procedure with Other Treatments on Alginates

| | Pyrogen Level in EU/gram Dry Weight | | | | | | |
	1^a	2	3	4	5	6	7
Raw material	32,700	6,400	17,600	15,400	15,600	15,000	15,200
Charcoal							
once	·	·	·	·	·	·	
twice		·					
Filtration	·	·	$·^b$	·	·	·	
Beads/BaCl$_2$	·	·					
Extraction							
A-C-E	·						
Chloroform							·
0.1 N NaOH					·		
Etox column				·			
Dialysis	·	·					
Freeze-drying	·	·	·	·			
Final value	640	$1,920^c$	1,800	3,590	2,050	1,000	2,000
% Removal	98	70	90	77	87	93	88

^{a} HV Keltone, (2)–(7)—HVCR Keltone.
^{b} Polysulfone filter.
^{c} 625 by gel-clot method.

yields satisfactory levels of impurities; 4) "residual" pyrogens (as derived from alkali-treated samples) may be partially due to other polysaccharides present in algae extracts, reactive in the LAL gel-clot detection system (glucans); and 5) glucanase treatment showed (not presented here) that pyrogen "levels" can be further lowered by this enzymatic step. Note, both alkali and enzymatic steps don't represent a practical purification procedure as product is partially destroyed (polysaccharide) or procedure is expensive. They are considered merely as an analytical procedure.

Different organic solvents are often used to isolate LPS from bacteria.[7] It is thus not surprising that chloroform can remove pyrogens. As pyrogens are in part hydrophobic, having a lipid moiety, suitable organic solvent and their mixtures have been tested by us for removal of pyrogens: chloroform and phenol/chloroform/ethyl ether (5/5/8 mixture by volume). Both appear to be effective when applied to dried polymer powder or in a mixture with water. The former method is more advantageous as the removal of solvent is simply by vacuum drying. The use of solvent in a mixture with water is also feasible. However, in some cases, a dispersion is formed, which is difficult to separate.

The original Klock's procedure was then applied to other gelling polymers (polysaccharides gelled by small molecular ionic species, ionotropic gelation): cellulose sulfate (gelled by potassium ions; this is considered a novel observation as there is no literature entry on this subject), kappa and iota carrageenans (by potassium or calcium ions), gelan (by calcium ions), carboxymethylcellulose (CMC) (by aluminum ions) and low-esterified pectin (by calcium ions). TABLE 2 presents some results. It can be concluded that Klock's procedure works with other gelling polymers and purification efficiency is satisfactory. It was surprising to observe very high initial levels of pyrogens in cellulose sulfate (CS) as the starting material for synthesis (cellulose) should be relatively free of pyrogens because of the cellulose processing conditions. This finding could be due to the CS interference in the assay or due to

TABLE 2. Extension of Klock's Procedure to Other Polymers (Example)

| | EU/gram Dry Weight | | |
| | 8 | 9 | 10 |
	Cellulose Sulfate Janssen	kappa-Carrageenan Fluka	Gelrite Gellan Kelco
Raw material	63,000	1,250	2,500
Charcoal			
once	.	.	.
twice	.		
Filtration	.	.	.
Beads	Potassium	Potassium	Calcium
Extraction			
Acetic acid-A	.	.	.
Citrate-C		.	.
Ethanol-E	.	.	.
Dialysis	.	.	.
Freeze-drying	.	.	.
Final value	690	200	250
% Removal	90	84	90

a high pyrogen content in this particular source of CS (no other is available on the market).

A special note is necessary in terms of gelling of CS and low-esterified pectin: the beads are not stable throughout the whole extraction procedure. In order to preserve beads, it was essential to maintain at least 1% (wt) potassium chloride concentration in all chemical extraction steps till the end of purification (for CS) and 0.5% (wt) calcium chloride (for pectate).

TABLE 3 presents pyrogen content in some polymers as measured by us in comparison with some published data. It can be observed that ultra pure alginates are now readily available (since this work was concluded, Kelco has launched an ultra pure product) and that other polymers should be purified, if considered for biomedical applications.

TABLE 4 presents a comparison between pyrogen and mitogen content for two commercial polymers. A Kelco sodium alginate has been purified by a combined chloroform-charcoal treatment and product compared to nonpurified one. Two

TABLE 3. Pyrogen Content in Polymers and Comparison with Published Data (in EU/gram)

		Reference
LV Keltone Algin (Kelco)	6,300	our data
Manugel DPB (Kelco)	99,800	our data
UP LVG Alginate (Pronova)	910	our data
UP MVG Alginate (Pronova)	310	our data
kappa carrageenan (Wako)	3,900	our data
Low-esterified pectin 315 NH ND (SBI)	2,400	our data
Carboxymethylcellulose, medium MW (Sigma)	1,080	our data
Manugel GHB Algin (Kelco)	140,000	Zimmermann et al.[1]

Note that all measurements were made on freeze-dried samples or on samples from a manufacturer and all, perhaps, contain some moisture (around 10%). No correction has been applied.

TABLE 4. Pyrogen and Mitogen Content of Three Commercial Alginate Samples (compared at 1% wt level of polymer)

Sample	Pyrogens EU/ml	Mitogens % Inhibition vs. Control
Purified HV Keltone alginate (Kelco) as above)	22	8
Ultrapure UP LVG alginate (Pronova)	9	8
Nonpurified HV Keltone alginate (Kelco)	327	15

triplicate runs were used for the mitogen assay. In this assay, higher inhibition of a test culture vs. control signifies higher content of mitogens, as observed for nonpurified alginates.

DISCUSSION

Possible mechanisms involved in Klock's purification procedure can be summarized as follows: 1) pyrogen adsorption in the charcoal capillaries of convenient size. Endotoxin removal by charcoal has been documented in the literature.[8,9] We have observed that different charcoals behave differently and it is the relative capillary size to LPS molecular size which may govern the effective pyrogen removal. The LPS aggregation and heterogeneity is another factor; 2) extractive removal of low molecular mass species and polymer breakdown products, as well as their adsorption on charcoal; 3) inactivation and extraction of pyrogens via alkalic[10] and hydrophilic (in case of ethanol) interactions; 4) removal of heavy metals by a chelating agent (citrate); and 5) simultaneous removal of mitogens, a group of low molecular species acting on many cell types.

Additional mechanisms can be ascribed to our extension of Klock's procedure: 6) extractive removal of LPS by organic solvents via hydrophobic interactions; and 7) pyrogen removal by a ligand attached to a sorbent/filter. We have not investigated different chemistries of ligands. Mitzner *et al.*[11] reported on cellulosic beads with immobilized polyethylene ligand and Hanasawa *et al.*[12] on fibrous carrier with coupled polymyxin B. Both ligands exhibit polycationic functionalities. A polymer contamination by a ligand leakage products may be an issue. In our case, we tested a polysulfone filter, exhibiting a stable polycationic surface chemistry and thus devoid of ligand leakage. Nonspecific adsorption of polyanionic polymers may be a problem in this case (as well as with other ligands mentioned above). Although Bommer *et al.*[13] reported on a total capture of LPS in a dialysis system with a closed loop having a polysulfone filter, our data show that some "residual" LPS remains in the polymer solution even after such a filtration step (TABLE 1).

It is well established that some polymers can interfere with the LAL gel-clot method. Among them, notably glucan (laminarin, *etc.*) can give false readings.[14-16] Some residual readings observed after purification by several researchers can thus be explained on the basis of apparent pyrogenicity. Adam *et al.*[17] observed residual pyrogen readings even after multiple detergent aided extractions. Although glucans can interfere in the LAL assay, their pyrogenicity *in vivo* is very small. Glucans can originate from other algae or yeasts while certain algae species are harvested from the sea for polymer extraction and manufacturing. During this process bacterial pyrogens and mitogens can contaminate the product because of the raw material used and because of nonaseptic manipulation of the product.

The following techniques have been developed: 1) a simplified method of purification of gelling polymers by chemical extraction, particularly suitable for alginates, carrageenans, gelan, pectin and cellulose sulfate; 2) a method of chemical purification of cellulose sulfate and pectin, featuring the presence of low molecular gelling ions throughout the extractive procedure; 3) a method of purification of gelling and nongelling polymers by means of chloroform extraction of dry polymers, followed by a chemical treatment of their solutions; and 4) "residual" pyrogens may be an analytical artifact due to other interfering polymers.

A simple calculation of safety limits for the assumed device is presented in the APPENDIX.

SUMMARY

A multistep extraction procedure has been tested for purification of natural and semi-synthetic polymers used for fabrication of an immunoisolation barrier for implanting animal cells. This procedure, originally described by Klock et al. for alginates, has been adapted for other gelling polymers to remove pyrogens (endotoxins) and mitogens. Several other steps have also been tested, resulting in a new and simple procedure for polymer purification, giving satisfactory levels of contamination. Endotoxin levels have been quantified by means of chromogenic and gel-clot LAL methods. A simple calculation of the endotoxin permissible levels shows that the quality of purified polymers exceeds FDA specifications for implantable polymers.

ACKNOWLEDGMENTS

Authors appreciate an input of I. Lacik of the analysis of polymer solutions by means of NMR and of S. DiMari in the mitogen assay.

REFERENCES

1. ZIMMERMANN, U. et al. 1992. Production of mitogen-contamination free alginates with variable ratios of mannuronic acid to glucuronic acid by free flow electrophoresis. Electrophoresis 13: 269–274.
2. NOWOTNY, A. 1987. Review of the molecular requirements of endotoxin actions. Revs. Infect. Dis. 9(Suppl. 5): S503–S511.
3. ZIMMERMANN, U. et al., Inventors. 1993. Mitogen-free substance, its preparation and its use. World patent 93116111. Date of application: August 19.
4. KLOCK, G. et al. 1994. Production of purified alginate suitable for use in immunoisolated implantation. Appl. Microbiol. Biotechnol. 40: 638–643.
5. PROKOP, A. et al. 1997. Water soluble polymers for immunoisolation. I. Complex coacervation and cytotoxicity. Advances in Polymer Science. In press.
6. PROKOP, A. et al. 1997. Water soluble polymers for immunoisolation. II. Evaluation of multicomponent systems. Advances in Polymer Science. In press.
7. GLANOS, C. et al. 1969. A new method for the extraction of R lipopolysaccharides. European J. Biochem. 9: 245–249.
8. NOLAN, J. P. et al. 1975. Endotoxin binding by charged and noncharged resins. Proc. Soc. Exptl. Biol. Med. 149: 766–770.

9. PEGUES, A. S. *et al.* 1979. The removal of 14C labelled endotoxin by activated charcoal. Int. J. Artif. Organs **2:** 153–158.
10. SOMLYO, B. *et al.* 1992. Molecular requirements of endotoxin (ET) actions: Changes in the immune adjuvant, the liberating and toxic properties of endotoxin during alkaline hydrolysis. Int. J. Immunopharmac. **14:** 131–142.
11. MITZNER, S. *et al.* 1993. Extracorporeal endotoxin removal by immobilized polyethylene-imine. Artif. Organs **7:** 775–781.
12. HANASAWA, K. *et al.* 1989. New approach to endotoxic and septic shock by means of polymyxin B immobilized fiber. Surg. Gynecol. Obstet. **168:** 323–331.
13. BOMMER, J. *et al.* 1987. No evidence for endotoxin transfer across high flux polysulfone membranes. Clin. Nephrol. **27:** 278–282.
14. MIKAMI, T. *et al.* 1982. Gelation of Limulus amoebocyte lysate by simple polysaccharides. Microbiol. Immunol. **26:** 403–409.
15. IKEMURA, K. *et al.* 1989. False-positive result in Limulus test caused by Limulus amebocyte lysate-reactive material in immunoglubulin products. J. Clin. Microbiol. **27:** 1965–1968.
16. ROSLANSKY, P. F. & T. J. NOWITSKY. 1991. Sensitivity of Limulus amebocyte lysate (LAL) to LAL-reactive glucans. J. Clin. Microbiol. **29:** 2477–2483.
17. ADAM, O. *et al.* 1995. A nondegradative route for the removal of endotoxin from polysaccharides. Analyt. Biochem. **225:** 321–327.
18. Anonymous. 1987. Guideline on validation of the limulus amebocyte lysate test as end-product endotoxin test for human and animal parenteral drugs, biological products, and medical devices. Food and Drug Administration, Rockville, MD.

APPENDIX

Calculation of endotoxin permissible limits

(1) Dosage of encapsulated pancreatic islets per capsule

It is assumed that the number of xenogeneic islets needed for implantation to alleviate the need for insulin is on the average 15,000 islets/kg of human body weight. Assuming body weight of 70 kg on the average, the total requirement is 1.05×10^6 islets per patient. Assuming the loading of 2 islets/capsule and capsule size about 0.7 mm, the volume of one capsule is $\pi \, d^3/6 = 0.18 \, mm^3$ and the total volume of capsules required is $0.18 \times 1.05 \times 1,000/2 = 47$ ml (or grams). Note that the total requirement is very much sensitive to the capsule size.

(2) Limit calculation based on the maximum dose

Endotoxin limit dose allowed by FDA is 5 EU/kg.
5 EU/kg $\times$ 70 kg / 47 ml = 7.4 EU/ml of polymer solution, which is easily attainable. Note that when 7.4 EU/ml is divided by the quantity of a given polymer in the capsule, say 6 mg/ml for alginate, the result is 1.22 EU/mg per dry weight of polymer or 1220 EU/g of dry weight of alginate. Our purified alginate reads 600–3600 EU/g dry weight. Compare this number with the specifications provided for "pyrogen free" UP Pronova alginates: 300–910 EU/g. This clearly shows that our purification procedure, if properly selected, is adequate.

(3) Limit calculation based on device limits

FDA permits 20 EU/device, thus the limit in EU/ml is as follows:
20 EU/device divided by 47 ml/device (one application) = 0.1 EU/ml (or 0.05 EU/ml for one islet per capsule).

Mechanical Characterization of Biomaterials[a]

J. E. SANDERS[b] AND S. G. ZACHARIAH[c]

Department of Bioengineering
University of Washington
Seattle, Washington 98195

Mechanical characterization of biomaterials and its incorporation into biomaterial design can help to prevent the following three and other similar clinical scenarios:

- An artificial ligament after 24 months of use is 9% longer than when implanted, thus it does not stabilize the knee unless the knee is put in excessive flexion;
- A lower-limb amputee using a prosthesis experiences skin breakdown two days after moving to a stairway-access-only second floor apartment;
- In static tissue culture models, cells respond favorably to a cardiac valve implant material but when implanted *in vivo* and put under mechanical stress the valve material is encapsulated and material-tissue anchoring is not achieved.

Though prevention of all three of these cases involves, in part, a need for mechanical characterization of the biomaterials, the fundamental knowledge desired is different for each case. The first case requires an understanding and subsequent design modification to change the material's fatigue properties under long-term continual loading. The second case requires determining stresses and strains in a complex shape (an amputee residual limb) under complex loading conditions and subsequent prosthesis redesign to control those stresses and strains to appropriate levels. The third case requires an understanding of tissue response to mechanical stress and suggests a need for design modifications that encourage material-tissue anchoring under mechanical loading conditions. For each case, mechanical characterization potentially provides critical information into important performance issues as well as a means for evaluation of new designs. In this paper, techniques for mechanical characterization of biomaterials in terms of experimental material testing, computational modeling, and assessing tissue response to mechanical stress and strain are discussed.

EXPERIMENTAL MATERIAL TESTING

A material put under uniaxial tension will deform, and in the case of a soft tissue will typically exhibit a non-linear response (FIG. 1). Biomaterial designers

[a] Funded by the National Institute of Child and Human Development (NIH grant number HD31445) and the Whitaker Foundation.
[b] Department of Bioengineering, Box 357962, Harris 309, University of Washington, Seattle, WA 98195; Tel: (206) 685-8296; Fax: (206) 543-6124; E-mail: sanders@limbs.bioeng.washington.edu
[c] Department of Bioengineering, Box 352255, University of Washington, Seattle, WA 98195; Tel: (206) 685-3488; Fax: (206) 543-6124; E-mail: zach@limbs.bioeng.washington.edu

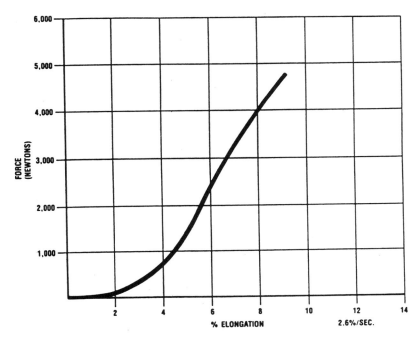

FIGURE 1. A force vs. elongation curve for a Gore-Tex™ expanded PTFE prosthetic liga-ment. The sample was loaded in a tensile testing machine at a strain rate of 2.6% strain per second. The curve is similar to that for normal ligament in that a "toe region" is followed by a stiffer linear segment. (From Bolton & Bruchman.[1])

attempt to match their material response with that of the natural tissue being replaced, paying close attention to the yield and failure levels to make sure the replacement material will tolerate stress levels experienced *in vivo*. This goal has been achieved in many tissues, for example Gore-Tex™ for knee ligaments.[1] How-ever, a much more challenging issue is the long-term mechanical performance of the biomaterial and matching that to the natural tissue. Many biomaterials, for example the artificial ligament shown in FIGURE 2, fatigue over time and undergo plastic deformation. In the case discussed above, if the deformation is excessive the result is a ligament that is then too long for the joint, one that is slack unless the knee is in excessive flexion, making the implant relatively useless. Thus an important utility of mechanical characterization is to identify materials that will potentially be problematic *in vivo* in terms of material properties, failure, and fatigue.

COMPUTATIONAL MODELING: PREDICTING STRESSES AND STRAINS IN COMPLEX SYSTEMS UNDER COMPLEX LOADING CONDITIONS

Experimental mechanical testing is adequate for assessing an implant's mechani-cal response provided the biomaterial experiences *in vivo* loading of magnitudes

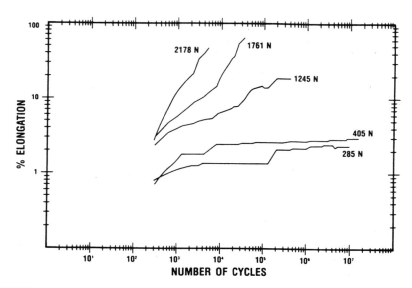

FIGURE 2. Cyclic creep test results of a Gore-Tex expanded PTFE prosthetic ligament. Test samples were loaded at 1 Hz at the force levels shown. Elongation increased more rapidly at the higher force levels than at the lower force levels. (From Bolton & Bruchman.[1])

and directions under which it is tested *in vitro*. However, implanted biomaterials are often subjected to a range of different loading conditions, so many that it quickly becomes too cumbersome to test the materials under all of these conditions. If the materials are linear (exhibit linear stress-strain curves) then results from different loading configuration can be superposed. For example, the strain under simultaneous axial and shear force can be determined by assessing the strains for each load applied separately. However, biological soft tissues and their replacement materials are typically non-linear, making superposition infeasible. Further, while experimental assessment of simply shaped specimens (*e.g.*, dumbbell-shaped samples) is straightforward, most implants are of more complex shape, complicating the mounting, load application, and measurement procedures in testing them.

An approach to predicting stresses and strains in complex shapes and/or non-linear materials is finite element (FE) analysis. The concept of FE analysis is to break up the object of complex shape into a number of small elements of simple shape (*e.g.*, "brick" elements) for which a solution can be determined. A computational analysis is carried out whereby loads and/or displacements are applied to the edges of the model and each element is analyzed by its interaction with nearby elements. Quality of the solution depends on the quality of the elements (*e.g.*, edge angles, aspect ratios), and specialized algorithms for creating element meshes have been created for some applications, for example lower-limb prosthetics.[2] The computational analysis corresponds to the minimization of a potential energy functional. In other words, in a computational sense the stresses and strains in the complex body (in the many finite elements) are determined such that a minimum potential energy in the entire body is achieved.

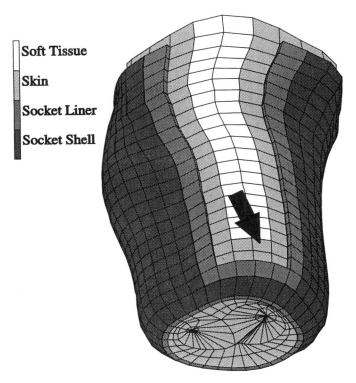

FIGURE 3. Anterior inferior view of a finite element model of a below-knee prosthetic socket and residual limb. Some of the elements on the anterior surface have been removed to show the layers: soft tissue, skin, socket liner, and socket shell. The arrow indicates the anterior distal tibia region of the residual limb.

A strong feature of FE analysis is the capability to determine changes in stresses and strains in a system of materials for different loading situations (boundary conditions) as well as different design shapes (geometries) and materials (material properties). As an example of the capabilities of FE analysis in biomaterials, consider an application in lower-limb prosthetics. The stresses on the residual limb at the interface with the prosthetic socket are determined using FE analysis. The model contains a number of materials including muscle (soft tissue), skin, liner, and socket materials (FIG. 3). In this case a region of skin on the anterior distal tibia is weaker than the surrounding skin (arrow in FIG. 3), as would occur for example if a skin graft or artificial skin were used because of a defect. Results from an analysis of loading during the stance phase of walking, a "typical" condition for which protheses are designed and fit, are shown in FIGURE 4a. Results show a relatively well-distributed normal stress distal to the patellar tendon. Next consider the stress distribution when the force in the lower leg is directed more horizontal and the moment is increased by 40%. This condition would occur when the amputee changed his or her gait style, walking up stairs, for example. The stress distribution on the

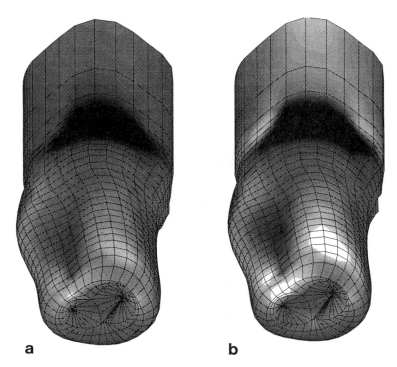

a   b

FIGURE 4. Grayscale maps of pressures on the skin surface, as estimated by finite element analysis (anterior inferior view). White indicates a high pressure and black indicates a low pressure; maximal pressures were approximately 100 kPa. **a:** Pressure estimates under a typical maximal load encountered during normal walking (35% of stance phase). **b:** Pressure estimates under a modified load: the resultant force from case **a** was rotated 20° in the sagittal plane, and the bending moment in the sagittal plane was increased by 40%. Grayscales are the same in both plots. Results show an increase in anterior distal pressures for case **b** compared with case **a**. The model assumed linear, isotropic, homogenous (Hookean) material properties for all elements, and did not permit slip and separation at the interface between the skin and socket liner elements.

residual limb changes, now concentrating stresses at the skin substitute location, an area of weaker tissue (FIG. 4b). Thus the predictions achieved here in this dry lab setting are of potential utility to a prosthesis or biomaterial designer. The designer would modify the interface materials (socket, liner), socket shape, or artificial skin properties so as to reduce the stress in this weak skin region. A strong utility of FE analysis is to predict stresses and strains in systems of materials under conditions the biomaterials were not initially designed for, providing insight before a design is used *in vivo*. It is important to recognize that model results cannot be considered valid until verified against experimental measurement, an area of concentrated research in lower-limb prosthetics[3] and other bioengineering-related disciplines.

Though FE analysis is potentially an extremely useful tool, there are important challenges that currently limit its application and utility in biomaterial design. Current challenges relate mainly to the specification of the material properties for the biomaterials. Soft tissues and their interactions at interfaces with implanted materials are difficult to characterize accurately in a computational sense. Material properties are typically history-dependent, non-linear, exhibit hysteresis, and deform plastically. Cartilage, for example, has been modeled as a biphasic porovisco-elastic material.[4] Such complex characterization may be required to achieve accurate model results for some tissues.

ASSESSING TISSUE RESPONSE TO MECHANICAL STRESS AND STRAIN

Perhaps one of the most fascinating aspects of mechanical characterization of biomaterials that is starting to be capitalized on more extensively is tissue response to mechanical stress and strain. At the cellular level, soft tissues will respond differently according to the load and geometry constraints placed on them. As discussed below, the evidence is building, particularly in the cell biology literature, where only the tissue and not its interaction with implant materials is considered. The challenge for implant designers, however, is to use the biological response to mechanical loading to advantage in design. In other words, biomaterialists can use the cellular-level response capabilities to design more effective tissue-material interfaces for mechanical loading. Below a discussion of some of this literature in the soft tissue area is followed by an example of how the concept of tissue response to load can be fused with other areas of mechanical characterization to enhance biomaterial design.

Regardless of the soft tissue type, there are some commonalties in our current understanding of tissue response to stress. Under stress levels that are high but not of sufficient magnitude to destroy the tissue, in certain cells the biomechanical input is transduced into a biochemical change that ultimately results in a change in gene expression in the cells. Signals are sent from these sensory cells, via cytokines or possibly others means, to effector cells that participate in tissue reorganization to enhance the mechanical stability of the tissue. Once the appropriate reorganization is completed, the tissue enters a state of relative homeostasis, though turnover rates of components, extracellular proteins for example, may still be enhanced compared to the case where no continual stress is applied.

Loading Effects

Most of the studies investigating soft tissue response to load have been conducted in skin, ligaments (and tendons), and cardiac tissue, appropriate because of the biomechanical needs of artificial skin, replacement ligaments, and heart valves and grafts.

Skin and Ligaments

A recently developed model to investigate skin adaptation[5] illustrates the capability of soft tissue remodeling in response to stress. Skin on the hind limb of an anesthetized pig was put under 1 Hz cyclic normal and shear stress for 1 hour/day

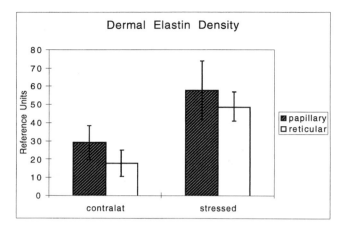

FIGURE 5. Elastin density from a preliminary study on skin adaptation to mechanical stress. In this test animal, elastin density in both the papillary and reticular dermis increased for stressed compared with contralateral control skin.

for 1 month at load levels comparable to those experienced at the stump-socket interface in persons with lower-limb amputations. Preliminary results suggest adaptive changes, particularly in the elastin architecture in the papillary dermis (FIG. 5). Possibly those changes have a role in enhancing epidermal-dermal attachment to strengthen the skin, thus could be important to consider in artificial skin design.

Numerous studies in tissue response to stress have been conducted *in vitro* using collagen gel/fibroblast models. Protein and collagen synthesis, mRNA for procollagen types I, II, and VI, and fibronectin and elastin were all increased in gels bound to a stainless steel ring compared with free floating gels.[6] Fibroblasts cultured within collagen gels contract the gels as a result of cell traction forces on the collagen fibers,[7,8] forces that require a cytoskeleton[9] and are comparable in magnitude to those observed in contracting skin wounds.[9,10] Contractile proteins that cause gel contraction are the same as those responsible for cell locomotion.[11] Ligament equivalents developed by positioning two posts held rigidly apart in a fibroblast/collagen gel culture strengthen over time, occurring through the formation of BAPN-sensitive lysyl oxidase catalyzed crosslinks.[12] Ingber[13] discusses in detail the transduction of force from the extracellular matrix to the cytoskeleton occurring via integrins, suggesting this is a first step leading to global cytoskeletal rearrangements and intracellular mechanotransduction events.

Cardiac Tissue

Perhaps the most extensive body of work on tissue response to stress has to do with cardiovascular applications, tissue response under fluid flow conditions.[14] It has been well-documented that endothelial cells elongate and align with the flow direction (see, *e.g.*, ref. 15). Numerous experimental flow chambers have been assembled, typically with a monolayer of cells attached to the bottom surface such

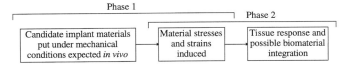

Figure 6. Block diagram illustrating the tissue-biomaterial response to *in vivo* loading as a two-step process. Experimental mechanical testing and computational modeling are effective for investigation of Phase 1. Assessment of tissue response to mechanical stress and strain and incorporation of that information into analytical models can facilitate progress on Phase 2.

that a controlled fluid flows through the channel over the cells. Shear stresses quickly stimulate increases in F-actin filament density[16] and appear to stimulate endothelial cell regeneration in the repair process.[17] Low shear stresses tend to decrease the rate of adherence in neutrophils.[18]

Geometry Effects

Other soft tissue studies demonstrate that it is not only the stress and strain applied to the cells that influence the response, it is also the geometry confining the cells that is important. Brauker[19] in subcutaneous implants in rats found that pore sizes in the range of 0.8 μm to 8.0 μm, large enough to allow host cell penetration, produced a better histological result than materials with pore dimensions outside of this range. Qualitative results using a rabbit animal model suggest better performance (less fibrous encapsulation) of catheter implants through the skin if the catheters are coated with a porous silicone cuff.[20] Thus it is a combination of stress, strain, and geometry that are important mechanical factors in tissue response.

APPLICATION TO BIOMATERIAL DESIGN

Experimental testing and finite element analysis provide means for establishing relationships between the material design and the stresses and strains induced in the material when put under *in vivo* load levels (Phase 1 in Fig. 6). Though tissue response to stress and strain (Phase 2) in soft tissue is at this point most commonly assessed by experimental techniques, by quantifying those changes tissue response can be incorporated into a computational analysis tool, providing an extension of FE analysis and a link between the two phases of the problem. Such combined experimental and analytical models are of utility in biomaterial design because they allow parametric analyses thus insight into which design features should be modified to achieve desired tissue responses.

An example is given below for the case of a porous biomaterial design for a soft-tissue application such as a valve implant or a skin percutaneous anchoring device. The material, a square membrane with nine equally spaced holes, is a rubber-like material (Ogden material[21]) loaded under uniaxial strain conditions. Results (Fig. 7a) show that strains and strain gradients tended to be concentrated at the tops and bottoms of the pores. Under biaxial loading conditions, however, as might

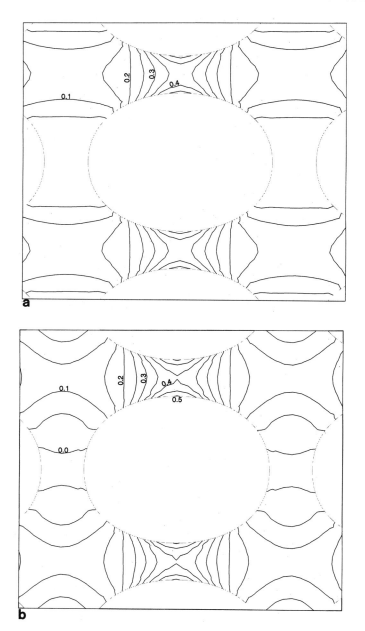

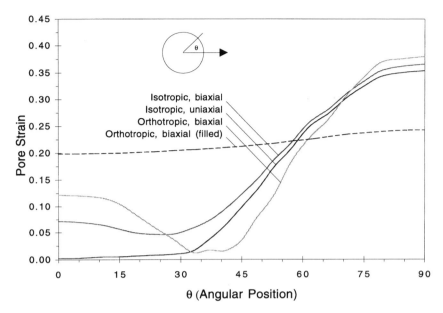

FIGURE 8. Plots of estimated pore surface strain against angular position on a circular pore for different material properties (isotropic, and orthotropic aligned with the direction of stretch), displacement conditions (uniaxial stretch, and laterally constrained biaxial stretch) and pore states (empty, and filled with tissue ingrowth (tissue stiffness is 75% of material stiffness)). Results are from a two-dimensional, plane-stress, finite element model of a porous membrane undergoing 20% stretch assuming linear, homogenous properties for all materials.

be achieved in a heart valve for example, the circumference of the pore increases. Thus maximum pore strain increases ($\sim$10%). Potentially cells at the tissue-material interfaces will be overstressed and die, making the material ineffective. Use of an orthotropic material (stiffer in the transverse than longitudinal direction) helps to reduce the strain in the 30 degree to 70 degree range but at the expense of a higher strain gradient and maximal strain (FIG. 8). However, as shown in FIGURE 8, tissue integration—which can be achieved if pore dimensions are properly controlled[19,20]— can drastically reduce both the maximal strain and strain gradient at the inter-

←

Figure 7. Contour plots of the maximum principal strain around the central pore of a nine-pore porous membrane under 20% stretch, as estimated by two-dimensional, plane-stress, finite element analysis of a square specimen. **a:** Uniaxial stretch: the edges of the specimen parallel to the direction of stretch are left free. The direction of stretch is horizontal. **b:** Laterally constrained biaxial stretch: the edges of specimen parallel to the direction of stretch are prevented from lateral displacement. The model assumed an elastomeric material whose nonlinear large strain behavior was described by a three-term Ogden constitutive relation for incompressible, rubber-like materials.

face. Thus the model suggests that the filled orthotropic material is "safest" in terms of strain distribution at the interface.

FUTURE DIRECTIONS

The combination of experimental testing, analytical modeling, and knowledge of tissue response to load creates a powerful tool for mechanical characterization of biomaterials and one that can be incorporated into biomaterial design. Important areas that need further development include integration of these concepts with material chemical and tissue biochemical characterization as well as material fabrication techniques. Design optimization, which can use results from parametric sensitivity analyses to determine the optimal design parameters to achieve a specified tissue response for example, is also an innovative direction. A systematic approach that integrates these different concepts should prove valuable in future biomaterial design efforts.

SUMMARY

Experimental testing and computational modeling are two useful tools for mechanical characterization of biomaterials, providing insight into material stresses and strains and the possibility of mechanical failure and fatigue. Another interesting issue to consider, however, is tissue response to mechanical stress and strain and incorporation of that knowledge into design to create materials that form mechanically effective tissue-material interfaces *in vivo*. Experimental testing, computational modeling, and tissue response to stress and strain are discussed in the context of enhancing biomaterial design.

REFERENCES

1. BOLTON, C. W. & W. C. BRUCHMAN. 1985. The Gore-Tex™ expanded polytetrafluoroethylene prosthetic ligament. Clin. Orthop. Rel. Res. **196:** 202–213.
2. ZACHARIAH, S. G., J. E. SANDERS & G. TURKIYYAH. 1996. Automated hexahedral mesh generation from biomedical image data: Applications in limb prosthetics. IEEE Trans. Rehab. Eng. **4:** 91–102.
3. ZACHARIAH, S. G. & J. E. SANDERS. 1996. Interface mechanics in lower-limb external prosthetics: A review of finite element models. IEEE Trans. Rehab. Eng. **4:** 288–302.
4. MAK, A. F. 1986. Apparent viscoelastic behavior of articular cartilage—Contributions from intrinsic matrix viscoelasticity and interstitial fluid flow. J. Biomech. Eng. **108:** 123–130.
5. SANDERS, J. E., J. L. GARBINI, J. M. LESCHEN, M. S. ALLEN & J. E. JORGENSEN. 1997. A bi-directional load applicator for the investigation of skin response to mechanical stress. IEEE Trans. Biomed. Eng. **44:** 290–296.
6. LAMBERT, C. A., E. P. SOUDANT, B. V. NUSGENS & C. M. LAPIERE. 1992. Pretranslational regulation of extraacellular matrix macromolecules and collagenase expression in fibroblasts by mechanical forces. Lab. Invest. **66:** 444–451.
7. BELL, E., B. IVARSSON & C. MERRIL. 1979. Production of a tissue-like structure by contraction of collagen lattices by human fibroblasts of different proliferative potential in vitro. Proc. Natl. Acad. Sci. USA **76:** 1274–1278.
8. STOPAK, D. & A. K. HARRIS. 1982. Connective tissue morphogenesis by fibroblast traction. Dev. Biol. **90:** 383–398.

9. KOLODNEY, M. S. & R. B. WYSOLMERSKI. 1992. Isometric contraction by fibroblasts and endothelial cells in culture: A quantitative study. J. Cell Biol. **117:** 73–82.
10. DELVOYE, P., P. WILIQUET, J. L. LEVEQUE, V. NUSGENS & C. M. LAPIERE. 1991. Measurement of mechanical forces generated by skin fibroblasts embedded in the three-dimensional collagen gel. J. Invest. Dermatol. **97:** 898–902.
11. TOMASEK, J. J. 1990. A serum factor promotes the generation of tension by fibroblasts in attached collagen lattices. J. Cell Biol. **111:** 148a.
12. HUANG, D., T. R. CHANG, A. AGGARWAL, R. C. LEE & H. P. EHRLICH. 1993. Mechanisms and dynamics of mechanical strengthening in ligament-equivalent fibroblast-populated collagen matrices. Ann. Biomed. Eng. **21:** 289–305.
13. INGBER, D. E., L. DIKE, L. HANSEN, S. KARP, H. LILEY, A. MANIOTIS, H. McNAMEE, D. MOONEY, G. PLOPPER, J. SIMS & N. WANG. 1994. Cellular tensegrity: Exploring how mechanical changes in the cytoskeleton regulate cell growth, migration, and tissue pattern during morphogenesis. Int. Rev. Cytol. **150:** 173–224.
14. HAYASHI, K., A. KAMIYA & K. ONO, Eds. 1996. Biomechanics: Functional Adaptation and Remodeling. Springer-Verlag. New York.
15. DAVIES, P. F., A. REMUZZI, E. J. GORDON, C. F. DEWEY, JR. & M. A. GIMBRONE, JR. 1986. Turbulent fluid shear stress induced vascular endothelial cell turnover in vitro. Proc. Natl. Acad. Sci. **83:** 2114–2117.
16. OOKAWA, K., M. SATO & N. OHSHIMA. 1992. Changes in the microstructure of cultured porcine aortic endothelial cells in the early stage after applying a fluid-imposed shear stress. J. Biomech. **25:** 1321–1328.
17. ANDO, J. H., H. NOMURA & A. KAMIYA. 1987. The effect of fluid shear stress on the migration and proliferation of cultured endothelial cells. Microvasc. Res. **33:** 62–70.
18. WORTHEN, G. S., L. A. SMEDLEY, M. G. TONNESEN, D. ELLIS, N. F. VOELKEL, J. T. REEVES & P. M. HENSON. 1998. Effects of shear stress on adhesive interaction between eutrophils and cultured endothelial cells. J. Appl. Physiol. **63:** 2031–2041.
19. BRAUKER, J. H., V. E. CARR-BRENDEL, L. A. MARTINSON, J. CRUDELE, W. D. JOHNSON & R. C. JOHNSON. 1995. Neovascularization of synthetic membranes directed by membrane microarchitecture. J. Biomed. Mat. Res. **29:** 1517–1524.
20. SEARE, W. J. 1995. A unique biointegrating porous cuff (Searematrix) which reduces infection and biofilm formation on CAPD catheters. 7th Congress of the International Society for Peritoneal Dialysis, Stockholm, Sweden, June 18–21, 1995.
21. OGDEN, R. W. 1984. Non-Linear Elastic Deformations. Halsted Press. New York.

The Biochip

A New Membrane Bioreactor System for the Cultivation of Animal Cells in Defined Tissue-like Cell Densities[a]

THOMAS SEEWÖSTER,[b] SANDRA WILMSMANN,
ANDREAS WERNER, AND JÜRGEN LEHMANN

Institute of Cell Culture Technology
Faculty of Technical Sciences
University of Bielefeld
D-33501 Bielefeld, Germany

Today mass cell cultivation of mammalian cells enters new fields of innovations, as in the shadow of gene therapy direct medical applications of animal cells and viruses become reality. Especially for the replacement of complex organ functions by tissue-engineering techniques,[1-3] the need for large amounts of defined and active cells is tremendous. For example, to ensure a sufficient metabolic capacity by a treatment with primary hepatocytes for acute liver failures, approximately 20–40% of the native human liver cell mass is required. This is $7.0–14.0 \times 10^{10}$ active cells in total.[4] A standard stirred tank suspension bioreactor with an optimal cell density of 3.0×10^6 cells/ml would have a volume of 20–45 L. As only small blood or plasma volume is available for treatment with a bioartificial liver,[5-9] a large active surface has to be provided by the bioartificial devices to guarantee an efficient exchange of molecules between cells and liquid. Owing to the necessity of a large amount of cells combined with a small liquid volume available from the patient, the development of perfused high cell density systems is demanded.

A suitable model that reflects all these conditions is the three-dimensional structure of glands that show high metabolic activity. Such organs, *e.g.*, the liver, have a laminar structure infiltrated with a large network of vascular capillaries in which each tissue unit has a cell layer thickness of 30–90 μm to ensure an optimal flux of metabolites through the tissue.

Here we report the current state of investigation towards the development of a new culture system based on the native three-dimensional microarchitecture of gland tissues. The main aims are a reproducible free adjustable three-dimensional microarchitecture in the range of 30–90 μm layer thickness, which allows free nutrient flow through the layer. It is expected that in a few years immortalized cells or recombinant cell lines will replace primary cells owing to an economic provision of well-characterized cells. Therefore, a recombinant model cell line was used instead of a primary hepatocyte to investigate the growth and expression behavior at cell-cell contacts in a high cell density situation. Besides the development of a

[a] This work was funded by the European Union (BIO2-CT94-3069) and was additionally supported by a Max-Buchner research fellowship for S.W. (No. 1847).
[b] *Present address*: BASF Bioresearch Corporation, PD Department, 100 Research Drive, Worcester, MA 01605-4314; Tel: (508) 849-2500; Fax: (508) 754-6742; E-mail: seewoet@BBC01.worcester.basf-corp.com

high density culture system itself, the problems regarding a reproducible, standardized long-term provision of a viable cell culture should be solved.

RESULTS AND DISCUSSIONS

A recombinant CHO cell line expressing the humanized anti-lysozyme antibody D1.3 was used as a model cell line. The cell line was already adapted to serum-free conditions, and the optimized culture medium based on a 1:1 mix of DMEM/F12 allows densities in standard batch cultures up to 3.5×10^6 viable cells/ml. Detailed description of medium composition, cell counting, and analysis of metabolites were given previously.[10]

For a continuous provision of viable cell culture, a chemostat process was used, whereby the cell-dependent dilution rate, the main parameter of a chemostat, had to be determined. During several long-term cultivations (50–90 days) the dilution rate was varied to obtain a high viability within the steady-state. A sufficient dilution rate was found at $0.55 \ d^{-1}$ (data not shown) keeping a viability of 98%. Higher dilution rates near the maximum growth rate of $0.8 \ d^{-1}$ led to instability of the culture due to washout effects.

FIGURES 1 and 2 show cross-sections of two models of the high cell density units, the biochip. The model in FIGURE 1 consists of three different components. The cell grid, a platinum-coated metal foil, similar to a shaving blade, defines the cell layer thickness. It can be manufactured exactly by galvanic techniques in 0.01 μm steps. Because of the platinum layer, the metal is biocompatible in a wide range of different oxygen-containing or salt-containing liquids. To form separated cell chambers or metabolic units within the cell grid, two standard commercially available microfiltration membranes were placed on both sides of the metal. Although preliminary screening of different membranes (3 celluloseacetate, 2 cellulose, and 2 polyethersulfone membranes in a pore size range of 0.2–5.0 μm) showed that all

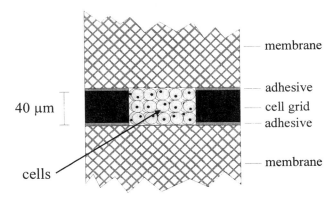

FIGURE 1. Schematic cross-section of one biochip chamber of model 1. Original prototype consists of one cell grid (150 mm diameter) with 7000 chambers, each 1 mm in diameter $\times$ 40 μm. In the available volume of 228 μl a total amount of 9.5×10^7 cells could be packed (packed volume for this cell line is 2.4 μl $\times 10^{-6}$ cells, whereby all cells are viable).

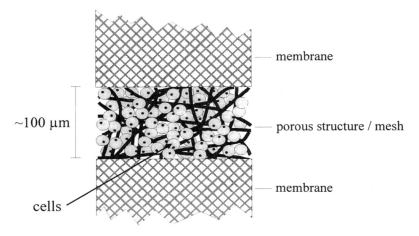

$\sim 100\ \mu m$

cells

FIGURE 2. Schematic cross-section of biochip model 2. Cells were cultivated in a macroporous structure (polysulfone or polyester) that allows for cell adsorption.

membranes are biocompatible and provide a sufficient trans-membrane flux, the celluloseacetate membrane (0.45 μm pore size) was favored, because no cell adsorption was observed on this homogeneous surface. Membrane and metal were stuck together with a biocompatible pressure-sensitive adhesive, commonly used in plasters. Because of the pressure-sensitive characteristics, the adhesive can be used several times. For transferring the cells from the low density pre-culture (chemostat) into the biochip system, the top membrane was removed and a defined amount of cells was placed onto the cell grid. Medium was then slowly removed through the bottom membrane so that the cells were sucked totally into the cell grid. The cell grid was then closed again with the top membrane. In model 2 (FIG. 2) the metal foil of model 1 was replaced by different macroporous membranes (polysulfone or polyester), which allow a good cell adherence. Depending on the manufacturing process these membranes have a thickness of approximately 100 μm. No adhesive was used in this model. The macroporous structure was loaded with cells in a petri-dish. Within one day nearly all cells were attached on the polymer. On account of SEM photos it had been shown that the cell density achievable in model 2 was slightly lower than in model 1. The packed units of both models were placed and fixed in a modified 150 mm membrane holder, normally used for medium filtration, integrated into a conditioning loop and continuously perfused with medium in cross-flow mode. The loop consisted of a standard stirred tank bioreactor equipped with a bubble-free aeration system and several pH, pO_2, and temperature sensors. To provide the highly densed cell package (228 μl) with nutrients, 1.5 L of medium was circulating in the loop with a flow rate of 900 ml/min.

FIGURE 3 shows a cultivation over four days in the biochip model 1 (metal foil). For monitoring the metabolism, glucose, lactate, ammonia and amino acids were measured once a day. The cell concentration was only measured before inoculation of the biochip and afterwards by resuspending all cells of the biochip. The increasing lactate concentration together with the decreasing glucose concentration and additional changes in the amino acid concentrations (data not shown) show that the

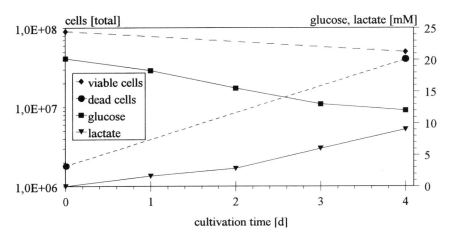

FIGURE 3. Short-term cultivation in the biochip model 1 (metal foil). Cells were counted before and after the run.

cell population is still active, but the viability of the culture decreased from 98% to 56% although no nutrient limitation was observed in the medium loop. Nevertheless, the cells survived these first runs of the new high cell density system. A few problems occurred during the transfer into the biochip due to the manual loading process, but these are not insoluble. Therefore, the inoculation of the biochip system should be more reproducible and reliable, especially for upscaling of the system. Additionally, the adhesive also needs to be stronger to keep the membranes fixed on the cell grid over a long period of peristaltic pressure, and the membrane holder requires optimization to have the smallest dead volume and to ensure an optimal flow.

CONCLUSIONS

The new high cell density system "biochip" has gone successfully through the first tests. It is possible to move cells from a continuous suspension culture system where the cells stay at low densities and show continuous growth into a system where they stay at tissue-like cell densities and are restricted from further growth by space limitations. Owing to a sufficient nutrient supply through that bioartificial structure, a long-term maintenance of cell metabolism seems to be possible.

SUMMARY

Based on the laminar structure of the human liver tissue, a high cell density membrane bioreactor was developed that emulates a cell layer thickness of 40 μm. The "biochip" consists of a platinum-coated metal cell grid covered with two microfiltration membranes to form separate cell chambers of defined volume. Starting with a continuous chemostat process, the viability of a model suspension cell culture could be stabilized at 98%. In a second step these cells were transferred into the biochip system and were cultivated successfully for several days under tissue-like cell densities in a modified membrane holder under cross-flow conditions.

ACKNOWLEDGMENT

We would like to thank the Sartorius AG, Germany, for kind provision of membranes and Mr. H. Brinkmann for excellent manufacturing of the biochip prototypes and the additional equipment.

REFERENCES

1. GALLETTI, P. M. 1991. Organ replacement: A dream come true. *In* Discovering New Worlds in Medicine. R. Johnsson-Hegyeli & A. M. Marmont du Haut Champ, Eds.: 262–277. Farmitalia Carlo Erba. Milan.
2. GALLETTI, P. M. 1992. Bioartificial organs. Artificial Organs **16:** 55–60.
3. COLTON, C. K. 1995. Implantable biohybrid artificial organs. Cell Transplant. **4:** 415–436.
4. KASAI, S. *et al.* 1994. Is the biological artificial liver clinically applicable? A historic review of biological artificial liver support systems. Artificial Organs **18:** 348–354.
5. ROZGA, J. *et al.* 1993. Development of a hybrid bioartificial liver. Ann. Surg. **217:** 502–511.
6. NYBERG, S. L. *et al.* 1993. Evaluation of a hepatocyte-entrapment hollow fiber bioreactor: A potential bioartificial liver. Biotechnol. Bioeng. **41:** 194–203.
7. GERLACH, J. *et al.* 1989. Use of hepatocytes in adhesion and suspension cultures of liver support bio-reactors. Int. J. Artificial Organs **12:** 788–792.
8. BADER, A. *et al.* 1995. Reconstruction of liver tissue in vitro: Geometry of characteristic flat bed, hollow fiber, and spouted bed bioreactor with reference to the in vivo liver. Artificial Organs **19:** 941–950.
9. LI, A. P. *et al.* 1993. Culturing of primary hepatocytes as entrapped aggregates in a packed bed bioreactor: A potential bioartificial liver. In Vitro Cell. Dev. Biol. **29A:** 249–254.
10. SEEWÖSTER, T. & J. LEHMANN. 1995. Influence of targeted asparagine starvation on extra- and intra-cellular amino acid pools of cultivated Chinese hamster ovary cells. Appl. Microbiol. Biotechnol. **44:** 344–350.

Artificial Cells and Bioencapsulation in Bioartificial Organs[a]

THOMAS MING SWI CHANG[b]

*Artificial Cells & Organs Research Centre
Departments of Physiology, Medicine & Biomedical Engineering
Faculty of Medicine
McGill University
Montreal, Quebec, Canada H3G 1Y6*

Modern research on bioartificial organs is based on molecular and cellular approaches. Even before 1972 there were many ways of preparing bioartificial materials. In 1972 an ad hoc committee formulated the term *Immobilization* to cover all the different approaches.[1] This blanket term is subdivided into four main classes: 1) Adsorption; 2) Covalent linkage, 3) Matrix entrapment, and 4) Encapsulation. Since *Immobilization Biotechnology* is a very large area, this paper discusses only one of the four approaches—encapsulation.

The first reports on artificial cells bioencapsulating biologically active material were published by this author as early as 1957[2] and 1964.[3] He showed that it is possible to bioencapsulate hemoglobin, enzymes, proteins, cells, microorganisms, adsorbents, magnetic materials and other biologically active materials (FIG. 1).[1–6] The artificial cells protect the encapsulated biological materials from the extracellular environment. At the same time the enclosed materials continue to act in the intracellular environment. Like biological cells, artificial cells contain biologically active materials. However, artificial cells can contain both biological and synthetic materials. The membranes of artificial cells can also be extensively varied using many different types of synthetic or biological materials. The permeability can be controlled over a wide range. For example, selectively permeable ultrathin synthetic membranes can retain macromolecules like proteins and enzymes. At the same time it allows the rapid diffusion of peptide and smaller molecules. This way, the enclosed material can be retained and separated from undesirable external materials. At the same time, the large surface area and the ultrathin membrane allows permeant substrate and products to diffuse randomly. Ten ml of 20 micron diameter artificial cells have a total surface area of about 20,000 cm². The membrane thickness is 200 ångstroms. As a results, mass transfer of permeant molecules across 10 ml of artificial cells can be 100 times higher than that for a standard hemodialysis machine. Variations in dimensions are also possible. Dimensions depend on the type of use and contents. Microcapsules in the microns diameter range are used for bioencapsulation of enzymes, protein, peptide, microorganisms, organelles, cells and others. Nanocapsules in the nanometer range are best used for enzymes, protein, peptide, antibiotics, and hemoglobin. Artificial red blood cells have been prepared

[a] T.M.S.C. gratefully acknowledges the operating grants and career investigatorship from the Medical Research Council of Canada and the Quebec MESST Virage "Centre of Excellence in Biotechnology" award.
[b] Fax: (514) 398-4983; E-mail: artcell@physio.mcgill.ca; web: http://www.physio,mcgill.ca/artcell

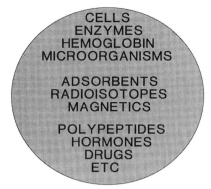

CELLS
ENZYMES
HEMOGLOBIN
MICROORGANISMS

ADSORBENTS
RADIOISOTOPES
MAGNETICS

POLYPEPTIDES
HORMONES
DRUGS
ETC

FIGURE 1. Artificial cells for bioencapsulation of a larger number of biologically active materials for use in biotechnology and medicine. (From Chang.[38] Used with permission of Marcel Dekker Publisher.)

by crosslinking hemoglobin molecules to form polyhemoglobin consisting of 4 to 10 molecules. These possible variations in contents and membrane materials allow for one to have unlimited variations in the properties of artificial cells.[2–11]

CELL ENCAPSULATION

Chang first developed a drop method for the bioencapsulation of cells and proposed its use in cell therapy (FIG. 2).[5,6] "Microencapsulation of intact

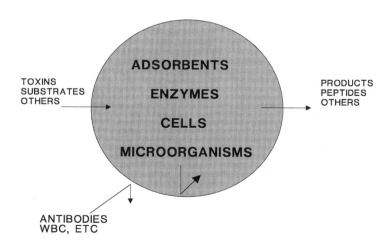

ADSORBENTS

TOXINS
SUBSTRATES
OTHERS

ENZYMES

PRODUCTS
PEPTIDES
OTHERS

CELLS

MICROORGANISMS

ANTIBODIES
WBC, ETC

FIGURE 2. Artificial cells for bioencapsulation in bioartificial organs. The enclosed materials are separated from external antibodies and leukocytes and prevented from immunological rejection. Smaller permeant materials can equilibrate rapidly across the membrane to be acted on by the enclosed material. (From Chang.[38] Used with permission of Marcel Dekker Publisher.)

cells. . . . . the enclosed material might be protected from destruction and from participation in immunological processes, while the enclosing membrane would be permeable to small molecules of specific cellular product which could then enter the general extracelluar compartment of the recipient. . . . . . . The situation is comparable to that of a graft placed in an immunologically favourable site."[5] With increasing interests in biotechnology, many groups are now actively exploring this approach.[9-14] A large amount of work has been reported on using this for bioencapsulation of islets.[10-13] These efforts will be reported on by others in this conference.

Bioencapsulation of Hepatocytes

We have been using bioencapsulated hepatocytes in basic studies to study the feasibilities of encapsulated cells in cell and gene therapy. Typically, hepatocytes were enclosed within alginate-polylysine-alginate (APA) microcapsules of 300 μm mean diameters. Different concentrations can be encapsulated, for example 1.1 mL of microcapsules can contain 15×10^6 hepatocytes.[15-17] The 300 μm diameter microcapsules are flexible. They can be injected using syringes with 18 gauge needles. Permeability of the membrane can be adjusted. Detailed analysis has been carried out using HPLC analysis of a large spectrum of molecular weight dextran.[18] The permeability can be adjusted to have different cut off molecular weight depending on the applications. Thus, for hepatocytes, it can be adjusted to allow albumin to pass through but not immunoglobulin. After isolation from the liver, the percentage of viable hepatocytes as determined by trypan blue stain exclusion was about 80%. After bioencapsulation of hepatocytes the percent of viable cells was 63.40%.[19]

Experimental Cell Therapy in Rats with Fulminant Hepatic Failure

Our earlier studies showed that rats with galactosamine-induced fulminant hepatic failure which received control artificial cells died 66.1 ± 18.6 hours after galactosamine induction.[15] The survival time of the group which received one peritoneal injection of 4.00 ml of microcapsules containing 7.40×10^6 hepatocytes was 117.3 ± 52.7 hours S.D. Paired analysis showed that this is significantly ($p < 0.025$) higher than that of the control group. The total number of hepatocytes injected in this initial study was very small. Later study by another group using higher concentrations of hepatocytes resulted in increase in long-term survival rates.[20]

Experimental Cell Therapy in Gunn Rats—An Animal Model for Human Non-Hemolytic Hyperbilirubinemia (Crigler-Najjar Type I)

We have investigated the use of artificial cells containing hepatocytes as cell therapy to lower bilirubin levels in Gunn rats.[16,17] In the first experiment, 3.5 months old Gunn rats weighing 258 ± 12 grams were used. During the 16-day control period, the serum bilirubin increased at a rate of 0.32 ± 0.07 mg/100 ml per day. This reached 14.00 ± 1.00 mg/100 ml at the end of the control period. Each animal then received an intraperitoneal injection of 1.10 ml of microcapsules containing 15×10^6 viable Wistar rat hepatocytes. Twenty days after implantation of the encapsulated hepatocytes, the serum bilirubin decreased to a level of 6.00 ± 1.00 mg/100 ml. The level remained low 90 days after the implantation. In the second experiment, control groups of Gunn rats were compared to those receiving cell therapy. The bilirubin levels did not decrease in the control group and the group which received control microcapsules contained no hepatocytes. In the group receiving encapsulated hepatocytes there was significant decreases in the plasma bilirubin level. Analysis showed that implanted encapsulated hepatocytes lowered bilirubin by carrying out the function of the liver in the conjugation of bilirubin.[21] Dixit's groups has also carried out extensive studies using these Gunn rats and their results supports our findings. They will be reporting in details on their research.

Immunoisolation of Bioencapsulated Rat Hepatocytes When Implanted into Mice

We also studied the implantation of free or bioencapsulated rat hepatocytes intraperitoneally into 20–22 g male normal CD-1 Swiss mice or CD-1 Swiss mice with galactosamine-induced fulminant hepatic failure (FHF).[19] This is a basic study to see if rat hepatocytes can remain viable and be immunoisolated inside freely floating artificial cells in mice. Therefore, aggregated microcapsules were not analyzed since these hepatocytes do not have good viability under this condition.

As expected, rat hepatocytes implanted into normal CD-1 Swiss mice were rapidly rejected. By the 14th day, there were no intact hepatocytes detected in the mice. Rat hepatocytes after implantation into CD-1 Swiss mice with galactosamine-induced FHF were rejected completely after 4–5 days. In the case of bioencapsulated hepatocytes, not only did they stay viable, there was also a significant increase ($p < 0.001$) in the percentage of viable hepatocytes within the microcapsules after two days of implantation. The percentage of viable cells increased with time so that 29 days after implantation, the viability increased from the original 62% to nearly 100%. There was no significant changes in the total number of hepatocytes in the microcapsules. The viability of encapsulated rat hepatocytes implanted into galactosamine induced FHF mice also increased to nearly 100%.

In conclusion, rat hepatocytes in free floating microcapsules can be immunoisolated. As a result, xenograft of rat hepatocytes are not immunologically rejected in mice. Instead, we have the unexpected findings of improvement in cell viability when followed for up to 29 days.

Hepatocyte-secreted Hepatic Stimulatory Factor Is Retained Inside the Microcapsule Artificial Cells

We found that hepatocytes in the microcapsule secrete factor(s) capable of stimulating liver regeneration.[22] This factor is retained inside the microcapsules after secretion. Sephacryl gel chromatography shows that this factor has a molecular weight of over 110,000 D. The hepatic-stimulating factor accumulating in the microencapsulated hepatocyte suspension, helps to increase the viability and recovery of the membrane integrity of hepatocytes inside the artificial cells.

The Single Major Obstacle to Clinical Use of Cell Encapsulation Is Long-Term Biocompatibility

Basic research using bioencapsulated hepatocytes, islets and other types of cells, shows the feasibility of using bioencapsulation for cell therapy. Further improvements in biocompatibility may allow this approach to be used for cell and gene therapy in human. This is becoming increasingly feasible because of the increasing progress in genetic engineering and molecular biology. The one single major obstacle is to have microcapsules which are so biocompatible that they can function for a sufficient length of time after implantation. Much research on this very important issue is ongoing by many excellent research groups, whose progress is being reported in this volume. We have examined one area in the biocompatibility of microcapsules containing cells as follows.

Procedure Specific for Encapsulating High Concentrations of Smaller Cells Like Hepatocytes or Microorganisms

The general procedure used for alginate-polylysine-alginate cell encapsulation was originally designed for the bioencapsulation of a few islets.[12-14] When this procedure is used to bioencapsulate a high concentration of dispersed cells like hepatocytes or microorganisms, the following problems can occur.[23] Some cells are incorporated into the membrane matrix and some of these cells are also exposed on the surface of the membrane (FIG. 3). When these microcapsules are implanted, the hosts immediately recognize the protruding cells on the surface resulting in acute cell-mediated host immune response and rejection. Even when the cells were integrated into the membrane matrix without protrusion, this resulted in a weak and poorly formed area in the membrane. When these were implanted into mice, macrophage and lymphocytes perforated the capsular membrane and infiltrated the microcapsule at these sites.

To prevent the above problem, we worked out the following approach (FIG. 4), the details of which have been published.[24,25] Very briefly, small calcium alginate gel microspheres containing entrapped cells were first formed. These gel micro-

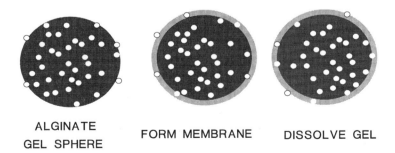

ALGINATE GEL SPHERE   FORM MEMBRANE   DISSOLVE GEL

FIGURE 3. Standard method of cell encapsulation when used for high concentrations of small cells can result in some cells being entrap or exposed on the surface of the membrane. When implanted this can result in membrane weakness and immunorejection. (From Wong & Chang.[23] Used with permission of Marcel Dekker Publisher.)

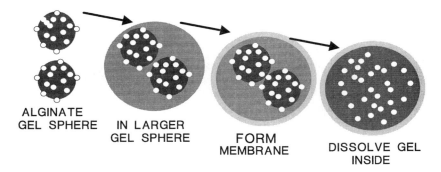

ALGINATE
GEL SPHERE   IN LARGER
              GEL SPHERE   FORM
                                MEMBRANE   DISSOLVE GEL
                                                INSIDE

FIGURE 4. A two-step method has been designed to prevent this problem. (From Wong & Chang.[24] Used with permission of Marcel Dekker Publisher.)

spheres are then resuspended in alginate solution to form larger microspheres. When these smaller microspheres are entrapped within the large microspheres, the larger ones do not have cell extruding on the surface. Thus during membrane formation, there was no cell entrapment in the membrane. Microscopic studies show that the encapsulated cells are not embedded into the membrane matrix.[24,25] Implantation resulted in better immunoisolation.

BIOENCAPSULATION OF GENETICALLY ENGINEERED MICROORGANISMS

Bioencapsulation of Genetically Engineered E. coli *Cells for Urea and Ammonia Removal*

Urea and ammonia removal are needed in kidney failure, liver failure, environmental decontamination, and regeneration of the water supply in space travel. Standard dialysis is effective for terminal renal failure patients, but it is expensive and many countries cannot afford to use dialysis to treat their patients. Many years ago, extensive effort to find an oral approach was not successful. The one major obstacle was the inability to remove the large amount of urea. With the availability of genetically engineered microorganisms, we are studying the use of bioencapsulated genetically engineered *E. coli* DH5 cells containing *K. aerogens* urease gene.[26,27]

Factors in the Bioencapsulation Process

The concentration of alginate is very crucial in the microencapsulation of this genetically microorganism. Our analysis shows that 2.00% (W/V) alginate resulted in well formed microcapsules with the maximum number of encapsulated bacterial cells.[26] We find that an air flow rate of 2.00 L/min is suitable for preparing microcapsules with an average diameter of 500 ± 45 μm diameter. We also analyzed the optimal liquid flow rate.[26] The mechanical strength of the alginate microbeads and APA microcapsules as a function of cell leakage was studied. Results showed that the microencapsulated microorganisms were stable when agitated up to 210 rpm for 7 hours.[26]

Analysis of in Vitro *Efficiency and Stability in the Removal of Urea and Ammonia*

Log phase microencapsulated bacteria lowered 87.89 ± 2.25% of the plasma urea within 20 minutes and 99.99% of urea in 30 minutes. Furthermore, the encapsulated bacteria decrease plasma ammonia concentration from 975 ± 70.15 to 81.15 ± 7.37 μM in 30 minutes.[26] This ammonia removal efficiency of encapsulated bacteria in plasma is not significantly different from that in the aqueous media. One can use encapsulated bacteria prepared by the general procedure for up to three cycles. The urea removal rate is greater in the second and third cycles than in the first. This is probably due to increase in total biomass inside microcapsules with time. There is no leakage of encapsulated bacteria in the first, second and third cycles. We used a single pool model to analyze urea removal efficiency by the encapsulated bacteria. The total fluid compartment was 40 liters with an urea concentration of 100 mg/dl(26). 40.00 ± 8.60 g of APA encapsulated bacteria can remove 87.89 ± 2.25% of the total body urea (40 grams) within 20 minutes and 99.99% in 30 minutes. It requires 388.34 g of oxystarch to remove the same amount of urea under the same conditions. It requires 1212.12 g of microcapsule containing urease-zirconium-phosphate to remove 40 g urea from the total body water. Overall, urea removal efficiency of microencapsulated genetically engineered bacteria is therefore much higher than the best available urea removal systems.

Effectiveness in the Lowering of Systemic Urea Levels in Uremic Rats

Our detailed study has just been reported.[27] The uremic rats are prepared by the surgical removal of one kidney and partial ligation of the other. Blood urea levels in these animals reached uremic levels. Oral administration of microencapsulated *E. coli* DH5 cells once a day resulted in the lowering of the systemic urea level to normal level. This normal level is maintained during the 21 days of daily oral administration. On discontinuation of the oral administration, systemic urea level rapidly returned to its high uremic levels showing that there is no retention of microorganisms in the intestine. Unlike these treated animals, 50% of the control uremic rats receiving control microcapsules died during the 21-day period. Based on this study, calculation shows in a 70 kg patient we only need to give 4 grams of the biomass each day. This is the first time that this is possible. This has therefore solved the major single obstacle of urea removal, the single major problem which has prevented the investigation of oral therapy for terminal renal failure.

Encapsulation of Other Microorganisms

We have also studied the encapsulation of other microorganisms.[28,29] For example we have studied the use of microencapsulated *Pseudomonas pictorum* (ATCC #23328) as another model system because of its ability to degrade cholesterol.[28] In order for lipoprotein-cholesterol macromolecules (50–1000 Å) in plasma to enter the microcapsules we have designed a new method[28] based on open-pore agar to form the microcapsules. These high porosity agar beads stored at 4°C did not show any sign of deterioration. The beads retained its activity even after 9 months of storage. There was no evidence of leakage of the enclosed bacteria. Open pore agar beads were incubated in serum and their cholesterol depletion activity was compared to controls and non-immobilized bacteria. The bacterial action was not significantly different between the immobilized and non-immobilized forms. Bacterial reaction was found to be the limiting step in the overall reaction of immobilized bacteria. Other methods to remove cholesterol (*e.g.*, LDL immunosorbents) are capacity limited. The immobilized microorganism as shown here, has an almost unlimited capacity to deplete cholesterol levels. However, for practical applications, a suitable bacterium with higher rates of cholesterol removal is needed. No doubt this will become available in the future with the help of genetic engineering. Another example is the bioencapsulation of *Erwinia herbicola* for the production of tyrosine.[29] This also has implications for converting phenylalanine to tyrosine in phenylketonuria. Detailed *in vitro* kinetics have been carried out.[29]

OTHER AREAS OF RESEARCH ON ARTIFICIAL CELLS

Bioencapsulation of Bioactive Sorbents

Microencapsulation of bioacitve sorbents is the simplest form of artificial cells which has already been used in routine clinical applications in human for many years. Sorbents like activated charcoal, resins and immunosorbents cannot be used in direct blood perfusion. This is because of particulate embolism and blood cells removal. Sorbents like activated charcoal inside artificial cells no longer caused particulate embolism and blood cells removal.[4,8,9,30,31] Artificial cells with polymer membrane containing adsorbents have been used in hemoperfusion for the routine treatment of patients for many years.[30,31] This includes acute poisoning, high blood aluminum and iron, and supplement to dialysis in kidney failure and in liver failure.[30,31]

Bioencapsulation of Enzymes

Our earlier studies of artificial cells for hereditary enzyme defects includes its successful use for replacement of catalase in acatalasemic mice.[8] It has also been studied for asparagine removal in the treatment of leukemia in animals.[8] The major obstacle was the problem of long-term biocompatibility in implantation. More recently, we found an extensive enterorecirculation of amino acids in the intestine.[32] This allows the use of orally administered artificial enzyme cells to selectively remove specific amino acids from the body, as in phenylketonuria. We also studied the oral administration of artificial cells containing xanthine oxidase.[33] This resulted in decrease in systemic hypoxanthine in a pediatric patient with hypoxanthinuria (Lesch-Nyhan Disease).

Red Blood Cell Substitutes

We reported the use of artificial cells containing hemoglobin as artificial red blood cell substitutes as early as 1957.[2] We extended this to crosslinked hemoglobin in 1964.[3] We then carried out detailed studies.[5,6,8] There was no major interest until the 1980s when problems of HIV in donor blood has resulted in extensive research and developments by many groups.[34–37] Many new developments resulted in cross-linking of hemoglobin from different sources: human hemoglobin, bovine hemoglobin and recombinant hemoglobin,[34–37] A number of these are now in Phase I, Phase II and Phase III clinical trials.[35–37] The second generation of hemoglobin-based blood substitutes based on microencapsulated and nanoencapsulated hemoglobin is being investigated as a more complete red blood cell substitute.[35–37]

SUMMARY

The most common use of artificial cells is for bioencapsulation of biologically active materials. Many combination of materials can be bioencapsulated. The permeability, composition and configurations of artificial cell membrane can be varied using different types of synthetic or biological materials. These possible variations in contents and membranes allow for large variations in the properties and functions of artificial cells.

REFERENCES

1. SUNDARUM, P. V., E. K. PYE, T. M. S. CHANG, V. H. EDWARDS, A. E. HUMPHREY, O. KAPLAN, E. KATCHALSKI, Y. LEVIN, M. D. LILLY, G. MANECKE, K. MOSBACH, A. PATCHORNIK, J. PORATH, H. H. WEETALL & I. B. WINGARD, JR. 1972. Recommendations for standardization of nomenclature in enzyme technology. Biotechnol. Bioeng. **14:** 15–18.
2. CHANG, T. M. S. 1957. Hemoglobin corpuscles. Research Report for Honours Physiology, Medical Library, McGill University. Also reprinted as part of "30th anniversary in Artificial Red Blood Cells Research." J. Biomat. Artificial Cells & Artificial Organs **16:** 1–9, 1988.
3. CHANG, T. M. S. 1964. Semipermeable microcapsules. *Science* **146:** 524–525.
4. CHANG, T. M. S. 1966. Semipermeable aqueous microcapsules ("artificial cells"): With emphasis on experiments in an extracorporeal shunt system. Trans. Am. Soc. Artif. Intern. Organs **12:** 13–19.
5. CHANG, T. M. S. 1965. Semipermeable Aqueous Microcapsules. Ph.D. Thesis, McGill University.
6. CHANG, T. M. S., F. C. MACINTOSH & S. G. MASON. 1966. Semipermeable aqueous microcapsules: I. Preparation and properties. Can. J. Physiol. Pharmacol. **44:** 115–128.
7. CHANG, T. M. S., F. C. MACINTOSH & S. G. MASON. 1971. Encapsulated hydrophilic compositions and methods of making them. Canadian Patent, 873, 815, 1971.
8. CHANG, T. M. S. 1972. Artificial Cells. C. C. Thomas Publisher. Springfield, IL.
9. CHANG, T. M. S. 1991. Artificial Cells. *In* Encyclopedia of Human Biology. R. Dulbecco, Ed. Academic Press. San Diego, CA. **1:** 377–383. (2nd edition in press 1997).
10. CHANG, T. M. S. 1995. Artificial cells with emphasis on bioencapsulation in biotechnology Biotechnol. Annu. Rev. **1:** 267–295.
11. CHANG, T. M. S. & S. PRAKASH. 1997. Artificial cells for bioencapsulation of cells and genetically engineered E. coli. Methods Mol. Biol. **63:** 343–358.
12. LIM, F. & A. M. SUN. 1980. Microencapsulated islets as bioartificial endocrine pancreas. Science **210:** 908–909.
13. GOOSEN, M., Ed. 1992. Fundamentals of Animal Cell Encapsulation and Immobilization. CRC Press. Boca Raton, FL.
14. SOON-SHIONG, P., R. E. HEINTZ, N. MERIDETH, Q. X. YAO, Z. YAO, T. ZHENG, M. MURPHY, M. K. MOLONEY, M. SCHMEHL, M. HARRIS, R. MENDEZ, R. MENDEZ & P. A. SANDFORD. 1994. Insulin independence in a type 1 diabetic patient after encapsulated islet transplantation. Lancet **343:** 950–951.

15. WONG, H. & T. M. S. CHANG. 1986. Bioartificial liver: Implanted artificial cells microencapsulated living hepatocytes increases survival of liver failure rats. Int. J. Artif. Organs 9: 335–346.
16. BRUNI, S. & T. M. S. CHANG. 1989. Hepatocytes immobilized by microencapsulation in artificial cells: Effects on hyperbilirubinemia in Gunn Rats. Biomater. Artif. Cells & Artif. Organs 17: 403–412.
17. BRUNI, S. & T. M. S. CHANG. 1991. Encapsulated hepatocytes for controlling hyperbilirubinemia in Gunn Rats. Int. J. Artificial Organs 14: 239–241.
18. COROMILI, V. & T. M. S. CHANG. 1993. Polydisperse dextran as a diffusing test solute to study the membrane permeability of alginate polylysine microcapsules. Biomater. Artif. Cells Immobilization Biotechnol. 21: 323–335.
19. WONG, H. & T. M. S. CHANG. 1988. The viability and regeneration of artificial cell microencapsulated rat hepatocyte xenograft transplants in mice. Biomater. Artif. Cells Artif. Organs 16: 731–740.
20. DIXIT, V., V. P. GORDON, S. C. PAPPAS & M. M. FISHER. 1989. Increased survival in galactosamine induced fulminant hepatic failure in rats following intraperitoneal transplantation of isolated encapsulated hepatocytes. In Hybrid Artificial Organs. C. Baquey & B. Dupuy, Eds. Colloque ISERM 177: 257–264. Paris, France.
21. BRUNI, S. & T. M. S. CHANG. 1995. Kinetics of UDP-glucuronosyltransferase in bilirubin conjugation by encapsulated hepatocytes for transplantation into Gunn rats. J. Artificial Organs 19: 449–457.
22. KASHANI, S. & T. M. S. CHANG. 1991. Physical chemical characteristics of hepatic stimulatory factor prepared from cell supernatant of hepatocyte cultures. Biomater. Artif. Cells Immobilization Biotechnol. 19: 565–578.
23. WONG, H. & T. M. S. CHANG. 1991. Microencapsulation of cells within alginate poly-L-lysine microcapsules prepared with standard single step drop technique: Histologically identified membrane imperfections and the associated graft rejection. J. Biomater. Artif. Cells Immobilization Biotechnol. 182: 675–686.
24. WONG, H. & T. M. S. CHANG. 1991. A novel two step procedure for immobilizing living cells in microcapsules for improving xenograft survival. Biomater. Artif. Cells Immobilization Biotechnol. 19: 687–698.
25. CHANG, T. M. S. & H. WONG. 1992. A novel method for cell encapsulation in artificial cells. United States Patent No. 5,084,350.
26. PRAKASH, S. & T. M. S. CHANG. 1995. Preparation and in-vitro analysis of microencapsulated genetically engineered E. coli DH5 for urea and ammonia removal. Biotechnol. Bioeng. 46: 621–626.
27. PRAKASH, S. & T. M. S. CHANG. 1996. Microencapsulated genetically engineered live E. coli DH5 cells administered orally to maintain normal plasma urea level in uremic rats. Nature Medicine 2: 883–887.
28. GAROFALO, F. & T. M. S. CHANG. 1991. Effects of mass transfer and reaction kinetics on serum cholesterol depletion rates of free and immobilized Pseudomonas pictorum. Appl. Biochem. Biotechnol. 27: 75–91.
29. LLOYD-GEORGE, I. & T. M. S. CHANG. 1995. Characterization of free and alginate-polylysine-alginate microencapsulated Erwinia herbicola for the conversion of ammonia, pyruvate and phenol into L-tyrosine and L-DOPA J. Bioeng. Biotechnol. 48: 706–714.
30. CHANG, T. M. S. 1975. Microencapsulated adsorbent hemoperfusion for uremia, intoxication and hepatic failure. Kidney Int. 7: S387–S392.
31. WINCHESTER, J. F. 1988. Hemoperfusion. In Replacement of Renal Function by Dialysis. J. F. Maher, Ed.: 439–593. Kluwer Academic Publisher, Boston, MA.
32. CHANG, T. M. S., L. BOURGET & C. LISTER. 1995. New theory of enterorecirculation of amino acids and its use for depleting unwanted amino acids using oral enzyme-artificial cells, as in removing phenylalanine in phenylketonuria. Artif. Cells, Blood Substitutes & Immobilization Biotechnol. 25: 1–23.
33. PALMOUR, R. M., P. GOODYER, T. READE & T. M. S. CHANG. 1989. Microencapsulated xanthine oxidase as experimental therapy in Lesch-Nyhan Disease. Lancet 2(8664): 687–688.

34. CHANG, T. M. S., J. REISS & R. WINSLOW, Eds. 1994. Blood substitutes: General. Special issue. Artif. Cells, Blood Substitutes & Immobilization Biotechnol. **22:** 123–360.
35. CHANG, T. M. S., Ed. 1996. Special abstract issue of the VI International Symposium on Blood Substitutes. Artif. Cells, Blood Substitutes & Immobilization Biotechnol. **24:** 294–466.
36. CHANG, T. M. S., G. GREENBURG & E. TUSCHIDA, Eds. 1997. Special issue on Blood Substitutes. Artif. Cells, Blood Substitutes & Immobilization Biotechnol. **25:** 1–241.
37. CHANG, T. M. S. 1997. Red Blood Cell Substitutes: Principles, Methods, Products and Clinical Trials. Karger Landes Systems. Georgetown, TX, 133 pp.
38. CHANG, T. M. S. 1993. Bioencapsulation in biotechnology. Biomat. Artifi. Cells & Immob. Biotechnol. **21:** 291–297.

Selected Aspects of the Microencapsulation of Mammalian Cells in HEMA-MMA[a]

MICHAEL V. SEFTON, JEONG R. HWANG, AND
JULIA E. BABENSEE

Department of Chemical Engineering and Applied Chemistry
University of Toronto
Toronto, Ontario, Canada M5S 3E5

We have used a submerged jet to microencapsulate various mammalian cells in a hydroxyethyl methacrylate-methyl methacrylate copolymer (HEMA-MMA) in order to isolate the cells from the immune system and permit their transplantation.[1,2] Pancreatic islets,[3] potentially for the treatment of insulin-dependent diabetes, dopamine-producing PC12 cells,[4] potentially for Parkinson's disease, or the liver cell line (HepG2, 5) have been among those that have been encapsulated within ~800 μm diameter capsules using the initial version of the submerged jet.[6] A second process has subsequently been developed to produce capsules as small as 300 μm in diameter.[7]

In the earlier submerged jet process, a cell suspension and polymer solution were pumped to a coaxial needle assembly and droplets of cell suspension surrounded by polymer solution were sheared off the needle tip by repeatedly withdrawing the needle from hexadecane. The two phase droplet then fell through the hexadecane to "refine" the core-and-shell morphology and into a gently stirred precipitation bath consisting of phosphate-buffered saline (PBS). A surfactant was used to lower the hexadecane-PBS interfacial tension to facilitate droplet penetration into the PBS. The polymer precipitated in the PBS to form a solid capsule. Droplet penetration through the hexadecane-PBS interface appeared to be the rate-limiting step to capsule production: 30 capsules/minute was the maximum production rate for a single needle assembly process. Another major concern with this process was the eccentricity of the capsules that were produced.[8] In the absence of a viscosity enhancer such as Ficoll 400 in the cell suspension, many of the capsules were seriously eccentric: adding Ficoll 400 at 20% (w/v) led to a reduction in eccentricity. Eccentricity is compensated for by increasing the polymer-to-cell ratio so that even at the thinnest part of the wall, there is adequate polymer present for the mechanical durability that is needed to withstand normal handling. Better centered capsules could have thinner and perhaps more permeable walls.

A modified version of the initial encapsulation process has been devised[7] in order to produce smaller (<600 μm diameter) capsules. The oscillating co-extrusion nozzle and stationary hexadecane interface was replaced with a stationary nozzle inserted in a rapidly flowing, co-axial hexadecane or other hydrophobic fluid stream. The shearing of the liquid cell suspension/polymer solution droplets was achieved

[a] We acknowledge the financial support of the Natural Science and Engineering Research Council and the Medical Research Council of Canada.

by the drag force of the hexadecane stream which also allowed for more precise control of the capsule sizes between 300 and 600 μm in diameter.

Since the initial work with alginate,[9] various methods have been used with varying degree of success in terms of the subsequent survival of the cells, the degree of cell proliferation in the confined space of the microcapsule, and the molecular weight cut-off[10] of the capsule membrane. There is a need to combine high capsule permeability to facilitate nutrient exchange with a well-defined molecular weight cutoff of ~100,000 to ensure adequate immunoisolation. The capsule permeability may be altered[6] by changing the structure of the capsule membrane, which can also be affected by the composition of the membrane-forming polymer solution. Here, the effect of HEMA-MMA concentration on the permeability of the capsule membrane was examined. Also the effect of poly(vinyl pyrrolidone), PVP, as a water-soluble, pore-forming additive, was investigated. PVP has been used as the pore-forming additive in membranes for ultrafiltration.[11,12]

Microencapsulation provides a physical barrier between encapsulated cells and the host immune system which alters the microenvironment of the cells; knowledge of its effects is necessary for the effective implementation of this technology. Conventional light and scanning electron microscopy techniques provide much of the required information, although sample preparation and examination are time consuming.[13] As an alternative, visualization of fluorescently stained cells by confocal microscopy allows the simultaneous examination of live and dead cells, distinguishable by different color staining, within a HEMA-MMA microcapsule. The time required to cut sections for conventional microscopy techniques is eliminated.

EXPERIMENTAL

Materials

HEMA-MMA (75 mole% HEMA) was synthesized,[14] and used as capsule-forming polymer. Triethylene glycol (TEG, MW 150, Aldrich) or poly(ethylene glycol) (PEG, MW 200) was used as the solvent; TEG facilitated the introduction of poly(vinyl pyrrolidone), PVP (MW 10000, Aldrich), as a pore-forming agent to the polymer solution.

Cells

HepG2 cells (ATCC) were routinely maintained in αMEM, supplemented with 100 U/mL penicillin, 100 mg/mL streptomycin and 10% fetal bovine serum (FBS: Sigma Chemicals, St. Louis, MO) on 25 cm^2 tissue culture flasks (Corning Glass Works, Corning, NY). The encapsulated cells were maintained in the same medium. In experiments where the protein concentration in tissue culture medium was to be determined, encapsulated cells were maintained with a hormonally defined medium (HDM[5]).

Preparation of Microcapsules

For small diameter capsules, HEMA-MMA microcapsules were prepared by the submerged jet technique described elsewhere.[7] HEMA-MMA solution was coextruded with core solution through a triple-barreled extrusion nozzle, with the core solution supplied to the center barrel. Polymer droplets were sheared off by the rapid flow of hexadecane (Aldrich) at 150 mL/min unless specified otherwise; this resulted in microcapsules ~450 μm in diameter. The nascent capsules passed through the hexadecane phase and into nonsolvent coagulant, forming solidified capsules. The coagulation bath consisted of a solution of Pluronic® L101 nonionic surfactant (100 ppm, BASF Chemicals) dissolved in PBS. The oscillating needle assembly was used to prepare larger diameter capsules.[6]

The medium for suspending cells contained either 20% w/v Ficoll® 400 ("regular capsules": Ficoll® 400 from Sigma) or 50% v/v Matrigel® ("Matrigel® capsules": Matrigel® from Collaborative Research, Bedford MA). Empty capsules without cells were made with 20% w/v Ficoll. Hexadecane (melting point: 19°C) was used for regular capsules and dodecane (melting point: −5°C) for Matrigel® capsules (both fluids from Sigma). During the extrusion of Matrigel®, the cell suspension and dodecane was kept at 3°C (by inserting the cell and dodecane tubing in a cold water bath) to prevent the gelation of Matrigel® in the needle assembly.

Standard capsules were made with 10% w/v polymer solutions in PEG 200. The concentration of HEMA-MMA in TEG was varied from 8 to 11% (w/v). The effect of PVP on capsule properties was determined by adding different amounts of PVP ranging from 0.1 to 0.3 of PVP/HEMA-MMA weight ratios to 10% (w/v) HEMA-MMA/TEG solution; *i.e.*, the total polymer concentration (PVP + HEMA/MMA) was 10 to 13% (w/v).

Determination of Microcapsule Permeability

The capsule permeability was determined at the individual capsule level by the method reported earlier.[19] Horseradish peroxidase (HRP, MW 40 kD, 1100 units/ mg, Sigma) was used as a model protein. HRP was loaded into the capsules by incubation in a 5 mg/mL HRP solution over a three day period (days 4 to 7); the loading was determined indirectly by mass balance knowing the amount released and the amount left in each capsule at the end of the release period. For the release, 7-days old capsules, one/well of a 96 well plate, were incubated with 300 μL of PBS release medium (phosphate-buffered saline, pH 7.4) at room temperature. The amount of HRP released was quantified by enzyme-chromogenic substrate assay using 3,3′,5,5′-tetramethylbenzidine (TMB) as the substrate for HRP.

Protein Secretion

The capsules were washed 3 times with PBS (5 minutes each) and once with HDM. The capsules were then incubated with a fixed volume of HDM and aliquots were removed at time = 0 and time = 18 h (for regular capsules) or 24 h (for Matrigel® capsules). The samples were frozen at −20° C until further analysis. The net accumulation of proteins between the indicated times were used to obtain an average secretion rate in ng/24 h/200 capsules. The details of the ELISA for α_1-acid glycoprotein (AG) are given elsewhere.[5]

Confocal Microscopy

The stains used to distinguish live and dead cells were the key components of the Molecular Probes (Eugene, OR) Live/Dead® Viability/Cytotoxicity Kit. Live cells were determined by the presence of intracellular esterase activity generating fluorescence upon the enzymatic hydrolysis of calcein-AM to calcein. Calcein-AM, the acetoxymethyl ester of calcein, is cell permeable and virtually non-fluorescent. Calcein is a fluorescent poly-anionic molecule that is well retained within live cells, much better than other commonly used stains, such as fluorescein diacetate. Dead cells were distinguished by the staining of nucleic acids with the nucleic acid stain, ethidium homodimer, which is excluded from live cells. In this way, live cells fluoresced green while dead cells fluoresced red.

Intact, unfixed (large) capsules were washed with Ca^{2+}/Mg^{2+}-free PBS to remove residual medium esterase activity, stained simultaneously with calcein-AM and ethidium homodimer at optimal concentrations of 10 μg/ml and 50 μg/ml, respectively, for 30 minutes, and washed with PBS. It was found that it was not possible to detect fluorescently stained cells within intact microcapsules by epifluorescent (UV source–halogen lamp) or confocal microscopy. This was presumably due to the scattering of light by the polymer membrane possibly compounded by the presence of ethidium homodimer taken up in the polymer wall. For this reason, the interior of cut-open capsules was examined.

The instrument used was a Confocal Laser Scanning Microscope (Ontario Laser Light Research Centre, OLLRC, University of Toronto, Toronto, Ontario, Canada), comprised of a Nikon Optiphot epifluorescent microscope, with a Bio Rad MRC600 detection system, interfacing with a Bio Rad data acquisition and analysis system. An argon-krypton laser (Ion Laser Technology Inc., Salt Lake City, UT, USA) supplied excitation wavelengths of 488 nm and 568 nm, thus exciting calcein and ethidium homodimer, respectively. The filter system used was that which is typically used for examination of double stained, FITC and Texas Red, samples.

RESULTS

Capsule Permeability to HRP

HEMA-MMA capsules were made with solutions of 8 to 11% polymer in TEG; the solution viscosity was within the processable range and the strength of the resulting capsule was sufficient to withstand the process. HEMA-MMA solutions of 6 or 7% (w/v) were not usable owing to the mechanical weakness of the resulting capsules.

Release of HRP from microcapsules was faster when a lower concentration of HEMA-MMA was used to prepare the capsules. For example, 9% (w/v) capsule membranes showed a more rapid increase in fractional HRP release compared to 10% (w/v) capsule membranes, suggesting a much higher permeability of the former capsules. The permeability coefficient (P_m) of the capsule membrane was estimated from the fractional release data.[21] The fractional release data of 8% (w/v) HEMA-MMA concentration could not be used owing to the failure to have sufficient points in the initial release period. Significant difference in P_m (FIG. 1) was found between 9% (w/v) HEMA-MMA capsule membranes (mean $= 26 \pm 6.4 \times 10^{-9}$ cm^2/sec) and 10% (w/v) HEMA-MMA capsule membranes (mean $= 0.4 \pm 0.5 \times 10^{-9}$ cm^2/sec).

The low molecular weight PVP used here was found to be quite soluble: as high as 0.3 PVP:HEMA-MMA ratio (w/w) could be added to a 10% (w/v) HEMA-MMA/TEG solution. HRP release from the resulting HEMA-MMA/PVP capsules (seven days after encapsulation) increased with only limited capsule-to-capsule variation. The corresponding estimated P_m of capsule membrane increased from 0.4 ($\pm$0.5) to 11 ($\pm$4.4) $\times 10^{-9}$ cm^2/sec as the PVP content increased from 0 to 0.3

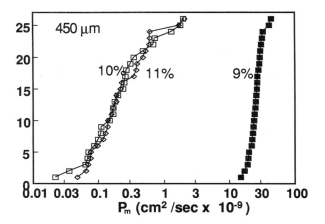

FIGURE 1. Distribution in the permeability coefficient of capsule membranes prepared with different HEMA-MMA concentrations. Mean permeability coefficients of capsules prepared with HEMA-MMA concentration of 9% (■), 10% (□), and 11% (◇) are 26 (±6.4), 0.39 (±0.51), and 0.37 (±0.48) × 10^{-9} cm²/sec, respectively. (± S.D.)

PVP:HEMA-MMA ratio (FIG. 2). This improvement in P_m presumably resulted from the significant difference in the "pore" structure of the capsule membranes.

Confocal Microscopy

Cell aggregates were found in the interior of fluorescently stained capsules (FIG. 3). The polymer capsule was visible in the red channel but not in the green channel because the polymer absorbed ethidium homodimer. The merging of the images of capsules from both red and green channels allowed for the imaging of both signals simultaneously. Live cells were of an oval/spherical shape and were completely fluorescent as viewed in the green channel. The signal from intensely fluorescent green cells spilled over into the red channel, presumably because of overlap of the calcein emission spectrum and the band pass of the red filter. Thus, in merged images, live cells were characterized by both solid green or yellow fluorescence. The signal from the nuclei of dead cells was detected in the red channel only. It was not possible to eliminate the green fluorescence from dead cells, although, a different staining pattern was observed: splotches of fluorescence as opposed to the solid fluorescence of live cells.

It was possible to observe an aggregate of cells by focusing through it and thus generating images at various planes. However, no signal in either the red or green channels, was detectable from an aggregate interior. Two possible reasons may be i) the inability of light to get in or out of an aggregate and ii) inadequate staining of the interior of an aggregate. An increase in the percent transmission of the emitted laser light from 1% to 10% to excite the sample did not allow the clear distinction of interior cells. An increase in the dye staining incubation time from 30 minutes to 45 or 60 minutes did not change the situation either.

Confocal microscopy clearly demonstrated the beneficial effect of adding Matri-

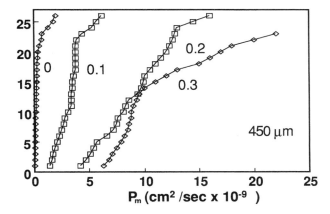

FIGURE 2. Distribution in the permeability coefficient of capsule membranes prepared with different contents of PVP. Mean permeability coefficients of capsules prepared with PVP:HEMA-MMA (wt/wt) ratio of 0 ($\Diamond$), 0.1 ($\blacksquare$), 0.2 ($\Box$), and 0.3 ($\blacklozenge$) are 0.39 ($\pm$0.51), 3.4 ($\pm$1.2), 9.4 ($\pm$3.1), and 11.3($\pm$4.4) $\times 10^{-9}$ cm^2/sec, respectively.

gel to HepG2 cell capsules. In the absence of Matrigel, viable cells were found in a large aggregate one week after encapsulation (FIG. 3a), but by two weeks, nuclei of dead cells were observed (FIG. 3b). However, in the presence of Matrigel (FIG. 3c), most of the HepG2 cells were viable at two weeks, presumably because of the presence of the attachment matrix in the otherwise nonadherent environment of the polymer capsule by itself. Within capsules containing Matrigel, cellular aggregates were more numerous, smaller and more uniformly distributed within the capsule core than capsules without Matrigel. This arrangement within Matrigel capsules may have contributed to their enhanced viability through more effective nutrient delivery and metabolic waste removal.

Protein Secretion

As a protein-release example,[5] human hepatoma, HepG2 cells, were used as a model for hepatocytes. Four plasma proteins which span the molecular weight range of interest (α_1-acid glycoprotein (AG; Mw 42 kD), α_1-antitrypsin (AT; Mw 52 kD), haptoglobin (Hap; Mw 98 kD) and fibrinogen (Fbg; Mw 340 kD)), were released into the surrounding medium by HepG2 cells from an aliquot of ~100 Matrigel containing capsules. Significantly more protein was released at day 7 as compared to day 3. There was no further increase in the amount secreted at day 14, except for AT. The higher amount of protein secreted is consistent with the increase in the number of cells per capsule. The amount of fibrinogen released, relative to α_1-acid glycoprotein, was lower for encapsulated cells as compared to control unencapsulated cells within Matrigel® in tissue culture, consistent with a sieving effect of the polymer membrane on the higher molecular weight protein, Fbg, relative to the smaller AG. HepG2 cells within small diameter capsules (~400 μm) also showed significantly lower Fbg:AG secretion rate ratio when compared to unencapsulated cells.[7] A comparison of large (~750 μm) and small (~400 μm) microcapsules is

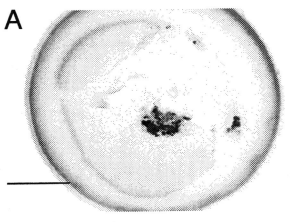

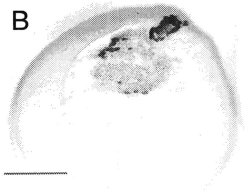

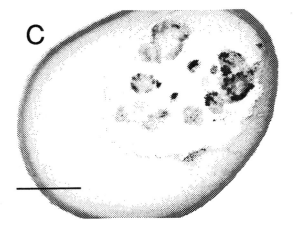

FIGURE 3. Merged (grey scale) images of confocal micrographs of HEMA-MMA microcapsules containing HepG2 cells in the absence of Matrigel, 1 week (**A**) and 2 weeks (**B**) after encapsulation and with Matrigel (**C**) 2 weeks after encapsulation. Dead cells and polymer (red in original image) are grey and live cells (green in original image) are black. Scale bar is 250 μm.

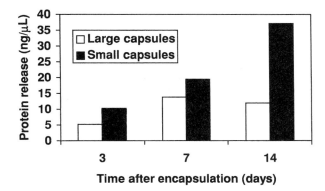

FIGURE 4. Comparison of acid glycoprotein release by small (~400 μm) and large (~750 μm) HEMA-MMA microcapsules containing HepG2 cells (initial encapsulation density: 5 × 10^6 cells/mL) in Matrigel. Large diameter capsules prepared by withdrawing nozzle assembly from stagnant hexadecade[5]; small diameter capsules prepared by pumping dodecane past a stationary nozzle. Capsules compared on the basis of equal intracapsule space: 11.3 μL/100 large capsules, 2.83 μL/200 small capsules.

shown in FIGURE 4. At all time points after encapsulation, and especially 14 days after encapsulation, there was more acid glycoprotein secreted by small microcapsules than by large ones when compared on the basis of equivalent core volume. This was attributed to the better use of internal volume and less degree of central necrosis in the case of smaller capsules.

DISCUSSION

Viable mammalian cells were encapsulated by an interfacial precipitation process in which liquid droplets from a submerged co-extrusion nozzle were sheared by a flowing fluid stream. Uniform HEMA-MMA microcapsules of controlled diameter were routinely produced. Human hepatoma (HepG2) cells retained an active metabolism inside capsules *in vitro*. Equally importantly, the encapsulated HepG2 cells were able to retain their functional state, as determined by the secretion of α_1-acid glycoprotein, among other proteins.

Encapsulation Process

In the submerged nozzle–liquid jet shearing scheme, the shearing frequency and microcapsule size were controlled by the flowing fluid velocity (*i.e.*, drag force exerted on the stationary droplet at the nozzle tip). The drag force was sufficient to produce HEMA-MMA capsules of ~400 μm diameter, as opposed to the previously utilized shearing scheme (the co-extrusion nozzle oscillating through an air-hexadecane interface) which gave ~750 μm diameter capsules. Although droplets of ~500 μm have been previously obtained using a co-axial airstream,[1] the higher viscosity of the hydrophobic fluid allowed us to use a lower velocity, or shear rate, at the nozzle tip. Velocity fluctuations are expected to be reduced accordingly, enabling us to obtain more uniformity among the capsules. More improvements in the present encapsulation scheme, however, will be needed at this stage. A thorough investigation of the various process parameters, such as fluid flow rates, solution densities/viscosities and apparatus design has been initiated to increase the fraction of acceptable capsules. The heterogeneity in the capsule permeability evident in FIGURES 1 and 2 has now been reduced by a needle design that is always centered and less sensitive to operator variability.

The morphological features of the present capsule membranes (not shown) were reported earlier[6]: a heterogeneous structure composed of dense 'skin' and macroporous 'trabecular' layers, similar to asymmetric phase-inversion membranes.[15,16] The thinner microcapsule membrane ($\sim$50 μm for smaller capsules as opposed to $\sim$100 μm in larger diameter), in addition to a reduction in capsule diameter has resulted in capsules of higher permeability coefficient.

Mechanism of Membrane Formation

The formation of a capsule was dependent on the polymer concentration which affected the viscosity of the capsule-forming solution. HEMA-MMA can be dissolved in TEG up to only 20% w/v. This indicates that the boundary of one-phase solution and gelation region for skin formation in the ternary phase diagram[17] is at a relatively low polymer concentration. Thus by losing a small amount of solvent at the interface, the solution even with a low concentration of polymer crosses the gelation boundary, to enter the gelation region. Polymer-polymer interaction is considerably favored in such solution crossing this boundary, increasing polymer saturation at the interface. The supersaturation of polymer at the interface presumably expedites rapid polymer aggregation before liquid-liquid demixing takes place.[18]

The formation of macrovoids in the capsule membrane can be described by the combination of the two demixing modes taking place at the internal and external surfaces of the capsule. Macrovoids are formed, according to Smolders,[19] from the growth of nuclei of solvent-rich (polymer-lean) phase after the instantaneous precipitation of polymer solution in a non-solvent. Freshly formed nuclei of solvent-rich phase grow by diffusion of solvent with the solution composition in front of fresh nuclei remaining stable. A higher content of solvent remaining in the polymer solution during demixing, therefore, can expedite the formation and growth of macrovoids. An experimental observation of demixing rates[20] shows that the diffusion of nonsolvent through the internal surface of a capsule takes place very slowly. This leads to a relatively high ratio of solvent to nonsolvent in much of the membrane, and this is a favorable condition for the formation of macrovoids in the external part of the capsule. That is, nuclei of the solvent rich phase formed immediately after instantaneous demixing (the start of precipitation) in the external part of the capsule grow until sufficient nonsolvent has diffused in to stop growth of the macrovoids by solidifying polymer rich phase.

The phase diagram[21] showed that the addition of PVP increased the nonsolvent tolerance of HEMA-MMA/TEG solution since the phase separation line was shifted towards the coagulant side. A strong interaction of hydrophilic PVP with HEMA-MMA hydrogel presumably expanded the homogeneous region on the phase diagram so that HEMA-MMA becomes swollen with PVP solution. Additional pores are then formed when PVP is leached out from the solidified polymer matrix.[12] Whether PVP (of this molecular weight) speeds up demixing,[22] as happens in other systems at higher molecular weights is unknown.

Protein Release

The small diameter HEMA-MMA capsules are expected to offer several advantages over the previously employed ~750 μm diameter capsules. The reduction of capsule diameter is expected to result in better utilization of the core volume. Because HEMA-MMA does not support cell attachment, cells grow within cellular aggregates of sizes considerably less then the core volume (*i.e.*, presumably due to growth-limiting factors implicit to three dimensional aggregate culture.[23] For example, CHO fibroblasts in large HEMA-MMA capsules proliferated within aggregates until an aggregate size of 50–150 μm was reached; there was a large void volume left in the capsule core (typical diameter >400 μm) giving rise to a low overall cell density.[8] Although this limitation was partly resolved by using an attachment matrix in the capsule core, there was still much empty space even after 1 month. This strategy is not useful for non-proliferating cells such as pancreatic islets; our previous experience indicated the presence of a large void volume for rat pancreatic islets in a significant fraction of large HEMA-MMA microcapsules.[3]

SUMMARY

Microencapsulation of live mammalian cells is one means of creating hybrid artificial organs, like an artificial pancreas or an artificial liver. In addition to creating and developing the methodologies for enclosing cells within the appropriate semipermeable and biocompatible membranes, novel techniques are needed to assess the various features of the resulting capsules. The small size of a capsule or its heterogeneity can lead to additional complexities that go beyond the problem of examining cell behavior in the presence of biomaterials. These problems are illustrated here by comparison of protein release by microencapsulated HepG2 cells within large and small HEMA-MMA (hydroxyethyl methacrylate–methyl methacrylate) capsules, by assessment of the effect of processing conditions on HEMA-MMA microcapsule permeability to horseradish peroxidase at the individual capsule level, and by a confocal microscopy technique for assessing intracapsule cell viability.

REFERENCES

1. SEFTON, M. V. & W. T. K. STEVENSON. 1993. Microencapsulation of live animal cells using polyacrylates. Adv. Poly. Sci. **107:** 145–198.
2. BABENSEE, J. E. & M. V. SEFTON. 199X. Protein Delivery by Microencapsulated Cells, in Protein Delivery: The Next Generation. K. Park, Ed. ACS Symposium Series. In press.
3. SEFTON, M. V. & L. KHARLIP. 1994. Insulin release from rat pancreatic islets microencapsulated in a HEMA-MMA polyacrylate. Pancreatic Islet Transplantation, Volume III: Immunoisolation of Pancreatic Islets. R. P. Lanza & W. L. Chick, Eds.: 107–117. R. G. Landes Company. Austin, TX.
4. ROBERTS, T., U. DE BONI & M. V. SEFTON. 1996. Dopamine secretion by PC12 cells microencapsulated in a hydroxyethyl methacrylate-methyl methacrylate copolymer. Biomaterials **17:** 267–275.
5. ULUDAG, H. & M. V. SEFTON. 1993. Microencapsulated human hepatoma cells: In vitro growth and protein release. J. Biomed. Mater. Res. **27:** 1213–1224.
6. CROOKS, C. A., J. A. DOUGLAS, R. L. BROUGHTON & M. V. SEFTON. 1990. Microencapsulation of mammalian cells in a HEMA-MMA copolymer: Effects on capsule morphology and permeability. J. Biomed. Mater. Res. **24:** 1241–1262.

7. ULUDAG, H., V. HORVATH, J. P. BLACK & M. V. SEFTON. 1994. Viability and protein secretion from human hepatoma (HepG2) cells encapsulated in 400 μm polyacrylate microcapsules by submerged nozzle-liquid jet extrusion. Biotechnol. Bioeng. **44:** 1199–1204.

8. ULUDAG, H. & M. V. SEFTON. 1993. Metabolic activity and proliferation of CHO cells in hydroxyethyl-methacrylate (HEMA-MMA) microcapsules. Cell Transplant. **2:** 175–182.

9. SUN, A. M. & F. LIM. 1980. Microencapsulated islets as bioartificial endocrine pancreas. Science **210:** 908.

10. KING, G. A., A. J. DAUGULIS, P. FAULKNER & M. F. A. GOOSEN. 1987. Alginate-polylysine microcapsules of controlled molecular weight cut-off for mammalian cell culture engineering. Biotechnol. Prog. **3:** 231.

11. TWEDDLE, T. A., O. KUTOWY, W. L. THAYER & S. SOURIRAJAN. 1983. Polysulfone ultrafiltration membranes. Ind. Eng. Chem. Progress Des. Develop. **22:** 320.

12. LAFRENIERE, L. Y., F. D. F. TALBOT, T. MATSUURA & S. SOURIRAJAN. Effect of polyvinyl pyrrolidone additive on the performance of polyethersulfone ultrafiltration membranes. Ind. Eng. Chem. Res. **26:** 2385.

13. BABENSEE, J. E., U. DE BONI & M. V. SEFTON. 1992. Morphological assessment of hepatoma cells (HepG2) microencapsulated in a HEMA-MMA copolymer with and without Matrigel. J. Biomed. Mater. Res. **26:** 1401.

14. STEVENSON, W. T. K., R. A. EVANGELISTA, M. E. SUGAMORI & M. V. SEFTON. 1987. Preparation and characterization of thermoplastic polymers from hydroxyalkyl methacrylates. J. Appl. Polym. Sci. **34:** 65.

15. ZEMAN, L. & L. DENAULT. 1992. Characterization of microfiltration membranes by image analysis of electron micrograph. Part I. Method development. J. Membrane Sci. **71:** 221.

16. ZEMAN, L. 1992. Characterization of microfiltration membranes by image analysis of electron micrographs. Part II. Functional and morphological parameters. J. Membrane Sci. **71:** 233.

17. WIJMANS, J. G., J. KANT, M. H. MULDER & C. A. SMOLDERS. 1985. Phase separation phenomena in solutions of polysulfone in mixtures of a solvent and a nonsolvent: Relationship with membrane formation. Polymer **26:** 1539.

18. REUVERS, A. J., F. W. ALTENA & C. A. SMOLDERS. 1986. Demixing and gelation behavior of ternary cellulose acetate solutions. J. Polym. Sci. Polym. Phys. **24:** 793.

19. SMOLDERS, C. A., A. J. REUVERS, R. M. BOOM & I. M. WIENK. 1992. Microstructures in phase-inversion membranes. Part 1. Formation of macrovoid. J. Membrane Sci. **73:** 259.

20. HWANG, J. R. & M. V. SEFTON. Effect of microcapsule diameter on the permeability of individual HEMA-MMA microcapsules. J. Controlled Release. In press.

21. HWANG, J. R. & M. V. SEFTON. 1995. The effects of polymer concentration and a pore forming agent (PVP) on HEMA-MMA microcapsule structure and permeability. J. Memb. Sci. **108:** 257–268.

22. BOOM, R. M., T. VAN DEN BOOMGAARD & C. A. SMOLDERS. 1994. Mass transfer and thermodynamics during immersion precipitation for a two-polymer system. Evaluation with the system PES-PVP-NMP-water. J. Membrane Sci. **90:** 231.

23. SUTHERLAND, R. M. 1988. Cell and environment interactions in tumor microregions: The multicell spheroid model. Science **240:** 177–184.

Microencapsulation of Cells

Medical Applications

ANTHONY M. SUN[a]

Department of Physiology
Faculty of Medicine
University of Toronto
1 King's College Circle
Toronto, Ontario, Canada, M5S 1A8

The concept of artificial cells was first demonstrated by Chang in 1964.[1] Since then a number of potential medical applications of artificial cells have been developed, including red blood cell substitutes, detoxification artificial liver, artificial kidney and immunosorbent and drug delivery systems. Most of these cells were prepared by encapsulating charcoal, enzymes, and biological substances. The encapsulation of living cells represents another important aspect of the artificial cell concept. It was proposed that immobilized encapsulated cells would be useful as transplanted tissue without the danger of immune rejection. The immobilized cells would act in the host as they had in the donor provided the surrounding membrane was impermeable to higher molecular weight antibodies but permeable to oxygen, glucose, other substances and/or internally generated hormones. Thus, the encapsulated cells would respond to external substrate concentrations (*e.g.*, blood glucose), and the required hormone (*e.g.*, insulin) would be secreted into the systemic circulation.

Another application of this concept is the encapsulation of cells which secrete substances with specific biological and medical applications, for example the production of monoclonal antibodies from hybridoma cells. Monoclonal antibodies secreted by encapsulated cells remain trapped inside the microcapsules and accumulate to a greater concentration than in the absence of encapsulation. To recover the antibodies, the microcapsules are separated from the culture medium and ruptured to release the antibodies. In the absence of encapsulation, the antibodies must be isolated from a large volume of culture medium.

A very exciting application of the microencapsulation concept is encapsulation of genetically modified cells which represents a novel approach to somatic gene therapy. Despite rapid progress in this field over the past years, three major obstacles are impeding the rapid transition between scientific research and medical treatment. Because somatic gene therapy requires the implantation of explanted cells, the first obstacle is associated with the same problems faced in any organ transplantation, which is to minimize or eliminate immunorejection after introduction of the genetically modified cells. The general protocol that has been devised to circumvent the problem of immunorejection includes reintroduction of the genetically modified cells after *in vitro* manipulation into the original donor. The other two obstacles impeding rapid progress in this field are associated with the inability to achieve efficient gene transfer and persistent gene expression in appropriate somatic cells.[2,3] In order to overcome the obstacles facing gene therapy, an alternate strategy was proposed that would allow nonsyngeneic recipients to receive the same engineered

[a] Tel: (416) 978-8781; Fax: (416) 978-4940; E-mail: Anthony.Sun@Utoronto.Ca

cell line under immunologically isolated conditions. This approach would not only eliminate the problem of immunorejection, but also provide a sustained delivery system of the recombinant products after transplantation.

It is clear that transplantation of mammalian cells or genetically engineered cells encapsulated in protective, biocompatible, and semipermeable membranes has great clinical potential for a wide range of diseases requiring enzyme or endocrine replacement therapy.

THE ALGINATE-POLYLYSINE-ALGINATE (APA) MICROCAPSULE

The original microencapsulation procedure was developed by Lim and Sun in 1980,[4] and since that time the technology has undergone a great number of critical modifications and improvements. In its present form the membrane is composed of polylysine sandwiched between two alginate layers.[5] The high degree of biocompatibility of the APA biocapsules was demonstrated in numerous *in vivo* transplantation experiments in which microencapsulated pancreatic islets remained functional for as long as 26 months.[6,7]

Capsule construction has improved considerably over the past years. It has been demonstrated that the capsule size is an important factor in the kinetics of insulin release by encapsulated pancreatic islets and in the easy access to nutrients and oxygen. Glucose tolerance in diabetic mice improved significantly after the mice received rat islets enclosed in capsules measuring 0.3 mm in diameter. By contrast, mice treated with islets enclosed in 0.8 mm capsules consistently experienced impaired glucose tolerance. The smaller capsules allow for: 1) increased cell viability, as encapsulated cells have easier access to oxygen and nutrients; 2) faster cell response to glucose fluctuations, since the dead space in the capsules is reduced; 3) significant reduction in the volume of capsules needed for transplants; and 4) less susceptibility to cell overgrowth on capsular surfaces, as the smaller capsules have greater mobility.

The development of the electrostatic droplet generator[8] resulted in considerably smaller capsules (0.25–0.35 mm in diameter) with improved sphericity, surface smoothness and, most importantly, capsule strength. When transplanted, the smaller capsules cause much less contact irritation, which in turn leads to a considerably smaller probability of cell overgrowth on capsular surfaces. *In vitro*, pancreatic islets encapsulated in the new capsules showed a response to glucose challenge which was comparable to that of free unencapsulated islets. The development of the droplet generator represents perhaps the single most important improvement in the microencapsulation procedure since its conception.

The chemical composition of the alginate has been considered by some investigators as crucial in attaining a high degree of biocompatibility of their microcapsules. The fibrosis of implanted microcapsules experienced by several groups was attributed to the mannuronic acid residues acting as cytokine inducers[9-12] while another study claimed that the final coating with a high mannuronic acid content alginate would actually reduce the amount of fibrosis around the microcapsules.[13] In our experience, the purity of the alginate—pyrogen and mitogen free—is much more important for the biocompatibility of the capsules than the alginate composition. However, the presence of both mannuronic and guluronic acids is very important for the construction of the capsule. The proper bonding between the COO^- groups of the two acids and the NH_2^+ of the polylysine is of a crucial importance for the strength of the resulting membrane and elimination of either mannuronic or guluronic acid would result in considerably weaker capsules.

The importance of the purity of the alginate was later confirmed by other investigators. Zimmerman et al.[14] have produced a method of preparing mitogen-free alginates. This work has incorporated the development of a mixed lymphocyte response assay to test the purity of the alginates and, as already suggested, has demonstrated that it is the purity and not the chemical composition of the alginate that affects the biocompatibility of the capsules. The nature of the contaminants was not determined in this study, but the authors commented that they could be oligomers of mannuronic and guluronic acids. Detailed descriptions of purification protocols such as that described by Zimmerman et al.[14] are essential if comparisons of encapsulated transplant experiments are to be made, and if the encouraging results of some groups are to be repeated by others who are not having the same degree of success. In summary, the construction of perfect capsules in terms of their size, sphericity, strength, surface smoothness, biocompatibility and purity of the component substances is of the uppermost importance for the proper physiological function and survival of the encapsulated graft.

MICROENCAPSULATION OF PARATHYROID CELLS AS A BIOARTIFICIAL PARATHYROID

Parathyroid transplantation has long been investigated in a hope of preventing long-term hypocalcemia in patients undergoing parathyroid operations secondary to parathyroid adenoma or hyperplasia. Severe hypocalcemia remains an unsolved therapeutic problem except when treated by autotransplantation. Again, the main obstacle to tissue transplantation is immunological rejection. Encouraged by success-ful transplants of encapsulated pancreatic islets, we studied the effects of trans-planted microencapsulated rat parathyroid cells on serum calcium and parathyroid hormone-midmolecule (PTH-M) levels in aparathyroid rats.[15]

Parathyroid cells were isolated from healthy rats and encapsulated in APA membranes. In vitro studies[16] demonstrated that both free and microencapsulated cells incubated with calcium-containing medium secrete parathyroid hormone (PTH). Microencapsulated cells were maintained in culture for five days, during which time they retained their Ca^{++}-dependent parathyroid hormone secretion.

In in vivo studies[15] rat parathyroid cells encapsulated in APA membranes were transplanted intraperitoneally into rats on which total parathyroidectomies had been performed. By three days post-transplantation, serum calcium and PTH-M concentrations had increased to near normal levels in the recipient animals and remained at a high level until the 12th week. Similar results were observed in a separate group of parathyroidectomized rats three days after free parathyroid cells were implanted, but within four weeks serum calcium and PTH-M concentrations had decreased almost to pretransplant values. No therapeutic effects were observed in rats injected with empty capsules or in the control group, which received no capsules or cells.

These results confirm the usefulness of semipermeable capsules in long-term hormone delivery systems and demonstrate that parathyroid cells encapsulated in a biocompatible membrane can serve effectively as a bioartificial parathyroid in the treatment of aparathyroid rats. Microencapsulation of parathyroid cells obviates the need for immunosuppressive therapy and pretreatment of the cells prior to implantation. The results reported here underline the need for investigations of possible future clinical uses of encapsulated parathyroid cells in the treatment of parathyroid hormone deficiency. A preliminary human experimentation protocol using human fetal tissue has been initiated in China and Taiwan.

MICROENCAPSULATION OF HEPATOCYTES

Current therapy for fulminant hepatic failure (FHF) is inadequate, with survival in the range of 10 to 20%. Liver transplantation has been performed in patients with FHF, with a success rate of 50%. However, liver transplantation is a formidable procedure, given the problem of rejection and the limited availability of donor livers, and it is associated with major, often lethal complications. Transplantation of hepatocytes is potentially a simpler, less hazardous treatment for FHF and permits the storage of hepatocytes for future use. However, the problem of immunological rejection must be solved before the technique can be applied clinically.

During the past years we investigated the use of encapsulated hepatocytes as a bioartificial organ in the treatment of FHF. In initial studies,[17,18] viable rat hepatocytes were encapsulated in alginate-polylysine-alginate membranes. The study demonstrated the short-term viability and functional characteristics of the encapsulated hepatocytes. Encapsulated rat hepatocytes were shown to survive and function for more than one week *in vitro* and up to one month *in vivo* in both normal rats and rats with galactosamine-induced FHF. In addition, encapsulated hepatocytes were found to synthesize urea. The results indicate that this system not only provides normal liver functions but also prevents immunological rejection by the host.

In our later study,[19] free hepatocytes harvested from normal rat livers by portal vein collagenase perfusion were encapsulated in APA membranes and transplanted into rats with galactosamine-induced FHF. The control group of animals received empty capsules. Intraperitoneal implantation resulted in marked improvements in the survival rate of the FHF rats. This improved rate at seven and fourteen days was statistically significant. Following the transplantation of encapsulated hepatocytes, the liver began to regenerate. By 21 days post-transplantation, this regeneration had progressed to the point where the viability of the transplanted hepatocytes was no longer critical to the survival of the rats. After encapsulation, hepatocytes remained viable for up to 30 days *in vitro*. The cultured encapsulated hepatocytes retained the capacity to synthetize albumin for up to three weeks. The results of this study strongly suggest that allografts of encapsulated hepatocytes can replace the functions of a liver damaged by toxins, drugs and acute disease, allowing the liver to fully recover. In sustaining the proper function of encapsulated hepatocytes, it is important to: 1) maintain the proper thickness and porosity of the membranes; 2) supply nutrients to the hepatocytes; 3) allow diffusion of metabolites and synthetic products; and 4) prevent an attack on the implants by the host immune system.

In a further study[20] we investigated the long-term viability of encapsulated hepatocytes *in vitro*. Viable hepatocytes were isolated from rats and encapsulated in biocompatible APA membranes. Urea formation, prothrombin and cholinesterase activity, the incorporation of tritiated leucine into intracellular proteins, and the immunolocation of synthetized albumin were monitored in culture. Despite a decrease in some of these activities, the cultured hepatocytes continued to function throughout the five week observation period maintaining cholinesterase activity and producing and excreting urea prothrombin into the medium. In addition, encapsulated hepatocytes were shown to synthetize albumin for up to five weeks. Scanning and transmission electron microscopy showed the cells to be embedded within the alginate matrix and to retain a globular shape. The results also confirmed that the semipermeability nature of the capsule membrane persisted throughout the five weeks.

The microencapsulation of hepatocytes has also been studied extensively by Chang *et al.*[21-23] They demonstrated that intraperitoneally implanted microencapsulated hepatocytes increased the survival time of galactosamine-induced fulminant hepatic failure in rats. Microencapsulated rat hepatocytes, unlike free hepatocytes, were not rejected after intraperitoneal injection into mice. In further experiments, the authors showed that microencapsulated hepatocytes transplanted intraperitoneally into Gunn rats effectively lowered bilirubin levels for more than three months.

MICROENCAPSULATION OF RECOMBINANT CELLS

Transkaryotic somatic gene therapy holds great promise in the treatment of a variety of endocrine, metabolic, and genetic diseases where morbidity results from a defect in the required gene. Despite rapid progress in this field over the past years, major obstacles associated with the use of autologous tissues as well as with the inability to achieve efficient gene transfers and persistent gene expression in appropriate somatic cells[2,3,24,25] are impeding the rapid transition between scientific research and medical treatment. In order to overcome these obstacles facing gene therapy, we propose an alternative strategy in somatic gene therapy that would allow nonsyngeneic recipients to receive the same engineered cell line under immunologically isolated conditions. This would involve expanding clones of transduced cell lines showing stable integration and sustained expression of the gene and encapsulating them with an APA membrane. This approach would not only eliminate the problem of immunorejection, but also provide a sustained delivery system of the recombinant products after transplantation. As a model, mouse fibroblasts transformed with the human growth hormone gene (Tlk⁻GH) were encapsulated with APA membrane. Long-term in $vitro$ studies showed that the encapsulation of the cells was physiologically compatible with growth and survival of the cells. Furthermore, there was a unique pattern of secretion of the human protein by the encapsulated cells: there was a phase of steady increase in the secretion of the human growth hormone by each cell, followed by a plateau phase. The most convincing evidence of the feasibility of this strategy was provided by the in $vivo$ study: BALB-C mice transplanted with encapsulated Ltk⁻GH cells had detectable serum levels of human growth hormone (hGH) for the duration of the study (115 days). Moreover, encapsulated cells recovered from a recipient one year after the transplantation continued to secrete high levels of hGH in culture.

The results of the in $vitro$ study clearly demonstrated that encapsulation of genetically modified mouse L-cells within the APA membrane system can provide an environment that is compatible with the maintenance of cell growth and expression of the gene product for an extended period of time. The finding that each cell within the capsule produced increasing levels of the recombinant protein before reaching a plateau phase demonstrates that the encapsulation of stably transfected cell lines can provide sustained delivery of the recombinant protein.

The success of this strategy to provide an effective long-term delivery system of the desired gene product was clearly demonstrated by the animal transplantation study. It was shown that over the course of the experiment of almost four months, animals transplanted with the microencapsulated cells had significantly higher levels of the human protein in the serum than their counterparts transplanted with unencapsulated cells. These results give a clear and convincing evidence of the ability of the microencapsulation strategy to provide a nutritionally supportive environment for the survival of the transduced cells. Furthermore, the development of the appropriate APA membrane for the purpose of the implantation clearly indicates that it can provide free passage of the recombinant products while maintaining the imunoisolating properties of the membrane.

We have demonstrated that encapsulation of genetically modified fibroblasts may represent a useful delivery system for recombinant proteins *in vivo*. One major advantage of this system is the ease with which the amount of protein to be delivered systematically can be controlled. These levels can be easily manipulated by number of capsules used for transplantation, as both cell growth and secretion of the gene product remain constant once the cells reach confluence within the capsules. This type of delivery system may be useful in the treatment of a number of diseases where sustained delivery of the missing protein is required, as a variety of cell lines transduced with the appropriated genes can be easily propagated and encapsulated for implantation into the affected individuals. Because genes for adenosine deaminase,[26] alpha-1-antitrypsine,[27] purine nucleoside phosphorylase,[28] and factor IX[29] have all been expressed successfully in cultured fibroblasts, and as more human disease-related genes are being cloned, this new approach to somatic gene therapy may provide a potential alternative to the treatment of metabolic and endocrine diseases.

An exciting example is the construction of genetically engineered β cells to be used for the treatment of diabetes mellitus. These may include cell lines of β-cell origin (*e.g.*, derived from insulinomas), or other types of cells which have been transfected with the insulin gene. The engineered cells must be capable of insulin synthesis, processing, storage and secretion. In addition, the insulin secretion should be regulated in the sense of closely mimicking the glucose-stimulated insulin secretion of the β cells of pancreatic islets.

TRANSPLANTATION OF MICROENCAPSULATED CHROMAFFIN TISSUE IN AN ANIMAL MODEL OF PARKINSON'S DISEASE

Transplantation of chromaffin tissue has been proposed as a possible treatment for Parkinson's disease. In our studies we investigated the effect of transplanting microencapsulated dopamine-producing bovine chromaffin tissue in a rat model of Parkinson's disease.

The adrenal modullae from slaughterhouse calves were dissociated and the cells encapsulated in APA microcapsules. In *in vivo* studies, the 6-hydroxydopamine hemiparkinsonian rat model was used to study the effects of striatal transplantation of bovine chromaffin cells. Following transplantation of 5,000 microencapsulated chromaffin cells, the recipients were challenged with apomorphine. The transplantation resulted in a marked reduction in rotational behavior in the recipient rats for up to 16 weeks. Thus, the results indicate that intrastritial transplantation of encapsulated chromaffin tissue leads to functional recovery in hemiparkinsonian rats. Consequently, such transplantation may represent a possible treatment for Parkinson's disease.

TRANSPLANTATION OF MICROENCAPSULATED PORCINE PANCREATIC ISLETS INTO SPONTANEOUSLY DIABETIC MONKEYS

For a number of years we studied transplantation of microencapsulated islets of Langerhans as novel treatment for diabetes mellitus. Recently, based on the results of our earlier experimentation we have conducted a pre-clinical study in which encapsulated porcine pancreatic islets were transplanted into naturally diabetic monkeys. All the diabetic animals displayed clinical features of type I diabetes mellitus including polyuria, polydypsia, polyphagia, weight loss and fatigue, persistent fasting hyperglycemia, persistent glycosuria and the need for daily injections of insulin. The pancreatic islets of a high degree of purity were isolated from large sows in excess of 200kg bodyweight, microencapsulated in APA membranes and implanted intraperitoneally into nine spontaneously diabetic cynomologus monkeys. Following one or two transplants of 3×10^4 to 7×10^4 islets per recipient, seven of the monkeys became insulin independent for periods ranging from 120 to 804 days with fasting blood glucose levels in the normoglycemic range. Glucose clearance rates in the transplant recipients were significantly higher than those before the graft administration and the insulin secretion during glucose tolerance tests was significantly higher compared to pretransplant tests. Porcine C-peptide was detected in all transplant recipients throughout their period of normoglycemia while none was found prior to the graft administration. Hemoglobin A_{1C} levels dropped significantly within two posttransplantation months. While ketones were detected in the urine of all recipients before the graft administration, all experimental animals became ketone-free two weeks post-transplantation. Capsules recovered from two recipients three months after restoration of normoglycemia were found physically intact with enclosed islets clearly visible. No clumping of the capsules was observed. In an *in vitro* static glucose challenge, the secretion of insulin in response to glucose stimulation of the recovered islets was found to be similar to freshly isolated islets. The capsules were free of cellular overgrowth. Examination of internal organs of two of the animals involved in our transplantation studies for the duration of two years revealed no untoward effect of the extended presence of the microcapsules.

Two of the nine recipients never became insulin independent, although their insulin requirement was significantly reduced to less than a half for a considerable period of time, 66 and 153 days for the two animals, respectively. Since these transplants were performed with porcine islets of a lesser degree of purity we can speculate that the contaminating exocrine cells may have caused damage to the encapsulated islet cells.

The long-term survival of the encapsulated xenograft which we previously demonstrated in rodents was reconfirmed in this preclinical study in primates. We have shown in a large animal model the ability of the encapsulated graft to achieve physiological glucose-insulin kinetics. Of equal importance is our finding that the until-now "elusive" porcine islets can be isolated with relative ease while retaining their physiological competence and that the immunoisolated porcine xenografts can effectively reverse diabetes in long-term experiments in primates. Ours is the first report on long-term discordant xenograft function resulting in a physiological glycemic control without recourse to immunosuppression in a large animal model. The results of this study warrant a clinical trial in human diabetics.

CONCLUSION

Our studies on microencapsulation and transplantation of pancreatic islets clearly show that this is the most promising approach to the problem of diabetes. Results of the preclinical study in spontaneously diabetic non-human primates prove unequivocally that the two major obstacles for future clinical studies, *i.e.*, the development of an adequate source of islets as well as the solution to the immunorejection problem, have been successfully overcome. The results of these studies will make the clinical application of our concept of islet transplantation possible in the near future. Similarly, the microencapsulation technology can be brought in the near future to clinical use in the treatment of other hormone deficiencies and potentially also in transkaryotic somatic gene therapy.

REFERENCES

1. CHANG, T. M. S. 1964. Semipermeable microcapsules. Science **146:** 524.
2. PALMER, T., G. ROSMAN, W. OSBORNE & R. MILLER. 1991. Genetically modified skin fibroblasts persist long after transplantation but gradually inactivate introduced genes. Proc. Natl. Acad. Sci. USA **88:** 1330–1334.
3. KANTOFF, K. W., A. P. GILLIO, J. R. MCLACHLIN et al. 1981. Expression of human adenosine in nonhuman primates after retrovirus-mediated gene transfer. J. Exp. Med. **166:** 219–234.
4. LIM, F. & A. M. SUN. 1980. Microencapsulated islets as bioartificial endocrine pancreas. Science **210:** 908.
5. SUN, A. M., G. M. O'SHEA & M. F. A. GOOSEN. 1983. Injectable, biocompatible islet microcapsules as a bioartificial pancreas. Prog. Artif. Organs **769:** 1983.
6. SUN, A. M., G. M. O'SHEA & H. GHARAPETIAN. 1985. Artificial cells containing islets as bioartificial pancreas. Prog. Artif. Organs **769:**
7. O'SHEA, G. M. & A. M. SUN. 1986. Encapsulation of rat islets of Langerhans prolongs xenograft survival in diabetic mice. J. Am. Diabetes Assoc. **35:** 943.
8. HOMMEL, M. & A. M. SUN. Droplet generation. Canadian patent 458605; 1984.
9. WEBER, C., S. ZABINSKI, T. KOSCHITZKY et al. 1990. The role of CD$^+$ helper T cells in the destruction of microencapsulated islet xenografts in NOD mice. Transplantation **49:** 396–404.
10. RICKER, A., S. STOCKBERGER & P. HALBAN. 1988. Hyperimmune response in microencapsulated xenogeneic tissue in non-obese mice. In The immunology of Diabetes Mellitus. M. Javorski, Ed.: 93–200. Elsevier, Amsterdam.
11. COLE, D. R., X. WATERFALL & J. D. BAYRD. 1989. Site modification of inflammatory response in alginate-polylysine-alginate microcapsules in BB/Edinburg rats. Diabetic Med. **6**(Suppl. 1): A41.
12. SOON-SHIONG, P., E. FELDMAN & R. NELSON. 1992. Successful reversal of spontaneous diabetes in dogs by intraperitoneal transplants of microencapsulated islets. Transplantation **54:** 769–774.
13. CLAYTON, H. A., N. J. M. LONDON, P. S. COLLOBY, P. R. F. BELL & P. E. L. JAMES. 1991. The effect of capsule composition on the biocompatibility of alginate-poly-L-lysine capsules. J. Microcapsulation **8:** 221–223.
14. ZIMMERMAN, U., G. KLOCK, K. FEDERLIN, H. HANNIG, M. KOWALSKI, R. G. BRETZEL, A. HORCHER & H. ENTEMANN. 1992. Production of mitogen contamination free alginate with variable ratios of mannuronic acid to guluronic acid by free flow electrophoresis. Electrophoresis **13:** 269–274.
15. FU, X. W. & A. M. SUN. 1989. Microencapsulated parathyroid cells as a bioartificial parathyroid: In vivo studies. Transplantation **47:** 432.
16. DARQUI, S. & A. M. SUN. 1987. Microencapsulation of parathyroid cells as a bioartificial parathyroid. Trans. Am. Soc. Artif. Intern. Organs **33:** 356.
17. SUN, A. M., Z. CAI, Z. SHI et al. 1986. Microencapsulated hepatocytes as a bioartificial liver. Trans Am. Soc. Artif. Intern. Organs **32:** 39.
18. SUN, A. M., Z. CAI, Z. SHI, F. MA & G. M. O'SHEA. 1987. Microencapsulated hepatocytes: In vitro and in vivo study. Biomater. Artif. Cells Org. **15:** 483.
19. CAI, Z., Z. SHI, G. M. O'SHEA & A. M. SUN. 1988. Microencapsulated hepatocytes for bioartificial liver support. Artif. Organs **19:** 388.
20. CAI, Z., Z. SHI, M. SHERMAN & A. M. SUN. 1989. Development and evaluation of a system of microencapsulation of primary cell hepatocytes. Hepatology **10:** 855.
21. WONG, H. & T. M. S. CHANG. 1986. Bioartificial liver: Implanted artificial cells microencapsulated living hepatocytes increases survival of liver failure rats. Int. J. Artif. Organs **9:** 355.
22. WONG, H., & T. M. S. CHANG. 1988. The viability and regeneration of artificial cell

microencapsulated rat hepatocytes xenograft transplants in mice. Biomater. Artif. Cells Artif. Organs **16:** 731.

23. BRUNI, S. & T. M. S. CHANG. 1989. Hepatocytes immobilized by microencapsulation in artificial cells: Effects of hyperbilirubinemia in Gunn rats. Biomater. Artif. Cells & Arif. Organs **17:** 403.

24. STEAD, R., W. KWOK, W. W. STORB & A. D. MILLER. 1988. Canine model of gene therapy: Inefficient gene expression in dogs reconstituted with autologous marrow infected retroviral vectors. Blood **71:** 742–747.

25. SANGOS, G. & F. H. RUDDLE. 1981. Mechanisms and applications of DNA-mediated gene transfer in mammalian cells—A review. Gene **14:** 1–10.

26. FLOWERS, M. E. D., M. A. R. STOCKSCHLAEDER, F. G. SCHUENING et al. 1990. Long-term transplantation of canine keratinocytes made resistant to G418 through retrovirus-medated gene transfer. Proc. Natl. Acad. Sci. USA **87:** 2349–2353.

27. GARVER, R. I., Jr., A. CHYTIL & S. KARLSSON. 1988. Production of glycosylated physiologically "normal" human alpha 1-antitrypsin by mouse fibroblasts modified by insertion of a human alpha antitrypsin cDNA using a retrovial vector. Proc. Natl. Acad. Sci. USA **84:** 1050–1054.

28. OSBORNE, W. R. A. & A. D. MILLER. 1988. Design of vectors for efficient expression of human purin nucleoside phosphorylase in skin fibroblasts from enzyme-deficient humans. Proc. Natl. Acad. Sci. USA **85:** 6851–6855.

29. ST. LOUIS, D. & I. M. VERMA. 1988. An alternative approach to somatic gene therapy. Proc. Natl. Acad. Sci. USA **85:** 3150–3154.

Models of Organ Regeneration Processes Induced by Templates

IOANNIS V. YANNAS

Fibers and Polymers Laboratory
Departments of Mechanical Engineering, and
Materials Science and Engineering
Massachussetts Institute of Technology
77 Massachussetts Avenue
Cambridge, Massachusetts 02139-4307

Regeneration templates are analogs of the extracellular matrix (ECM) which have been shown to induce at least partial organ regeneration in animals or humans who have lost significant organ mass owing to trauma or disease. The identification of an ECM analog as a regeneration template requires succesful performance both in qualitative and quantitative assays of the presumptive regenerate. Convincing evidence that regeneration has, in fact, occurred must be based on observation of definitive recovery of both structure and function in an anatomically well-defined defect. Furthermore, there must be evidence that the mass of the regenerated organ which forms in the absence of the template (spontaneous regeneration) is negligibly small relative to that which is induced in its presence.

The adult mammal generally does not regenerate organs that may have lost mass from disease or trauma. Loss of organ mass due to trauma is typically accompanied by contraction of the lesion and synthesis of scar tissue. Although most of our understanding of the spontaneous response to organ loss is derived from studies of skin wounds, there is evidence that contraction and scar synthesis are the obligatory results of wound healing in several other organ sites in the adult mammal. Several procedures have been developed since 1950 to assist humans who have suffered organ failure due to disease or trauma. Among these transplantation, autografting and implantation of "permanent" engineering prostheses are used most widely. Substantial research effort has also been expended in an attempt to synthesize organs *in vitro*. The subject of this review, organ regeneration, represents a fifth approach: *in vivo* synthesis of organs.

I will first summarize the evidence for regeneration of skin (in animals and humans), peripheral nerves (animals) and the knee meniscus (animals). The experimental parameters which must be adjusted to approriate levels in order for a definitive test of regeneration to be made will be reviewed next, followed by extensive modeling of the complex sequence of processes (mechanism) which ultimately lead to regeneration. It is expected that the empirical rules outlined in these sections will assist other workers who wish to experiment in this developing field. Finally, the structures of two regeneration templates will be briefly compared.

THE EVIDENCE FOR INDUCED REGENERATION IN THE ADULT MAMMAL

The adult mammalian dermis does not regenerate spontaneously.[1-3] Studies conducted since 1970 have shown that a porous graft copolymer of type I collagen and chondroitin 6-sulfate, a glycosaminoglycan (collagen-GAG copolymer), induces regeneration of the dermis in large areas of full-thickness skin loss in the guinea pig.[4–11] This finding has been extended to humans.[12–14] Regeneration of the dermis was demonstrated on the basis of conventional histological and ultrastructural studies, the use of small-angle laser light scattering studies from histological tissue, as well as on the basis of functional studies. The new integument was structurally and functionally competent but was totally lacking in hair follicles and other skin adnexa.

Early studies with this ECM analog emphasized keratinocyte seeding of the analog prior to grafting to achieve simultaneous regeneration of an epidermis as well as a dermis. It has since been recognized that, although seeding of the ECM analog with a minimal density of autologous, uncultured keratinocytes speeds up epidermal regeneration, cell seeding is not required either for regeneration of the epidermis nor for regeneration of the dermis. The combined evidence has served to identify a cell-free macromolecular network with highly specific structure, which has unprecedented morphogenetic activity.

Only one of several collagen-GAG matrices studied as described above was capable of preventing scar tissue formation and promoting dermal regeneration. The active ECM analog was characterized by a collagen/GAG ratio of 98/2 w/w, average pore diameter between 20 and 120 μm, and sufficiently high cross-link density to resist degradation by collagenases over about 10 days following grafting (average molecular weight between cross-links in the template, 12 kD). Several other very closely related ECM analogs showed either significantly reduced activity or no activity at all.[10] ECM analogs which showed high activity in promoting dermal regeneration also delayed significantly the onset of wound contraction.[10] The available evidence compels the conclusion that the activity of this insoluble network inside the wound bed depends critically on maintenance of a highly specific three-dimensional structure over a period of time between about 5 and 15 days. The active network has been referred to as dermis regeneration template (DRT). The observed activity of DRT, consisting in drastic modification of the outcome of the wound healing process, has not been duplicated so far by application on the wound bed of solutions of one or more growth factors or by application of suspensions of keratinocytes or fibroblasts.

A different ECM analog, also possessing a highly specific network structure, has induced regeneration of a partially functional sciatic nerve across a transected gap of 15 mm in the rat sciatic nerve.[15–18] In this animal model the nerve stumps at either side of the gap are inserted in a silicone tube (tubulation); in the absence of a tube, regeneration is decidedly absent and neuroma formation is invariably reported. It has been shown that spontaneous regeneration through the tube occurs reproducibly at a gap length of 5 mm whereas regeneration across a 15 mm gap is not observed.[19,20] The ECM analog which has been shown to possess the greatest activity so far, inducing regeneration across a 15 mm gap which was bridged by a tube that contained the ECM analog, is referred to as "nerve regeneration template" (NRT). It has an average pore diameter of 5 μm, an average molecular weight between crosslinks of 30–40 kD, a preferred orientation of pore channel axes in the direction of the nerve axis, and a 98/2 w/w ratio of type I collagen to GAG. The significant differences between the network structure of DRT and NRT are tabulated below (TABLE 1).

A third ECM analog has been reported capable of inducing regeneration of the canine meniscus following 80% transection.[21,22] Although the ECM used in these studies has been stated by the authors to be similar to that described earlier[10] its detailed structure was not reported.

TABLE 1. Structural Properties of Two Regeneration Templates

Design Parameter of ECM Analog	Dermis Regeneration Template	Nerve Regeneration Template
Degradation half-life *in vivo* (weeks)	1.5	6–8
Average pore diameter (μm)	20–120	5
Pore channel orientation	random	axial

In summary, evidence is accumulating that, under appropriate conditions, the adult mammal can be induced to regrow certain organs which are not regenerated spontaneously. The therapeutic avenues which are suggested by such evidence are novel and dramatic. However, many basic unanswered questions remain. Most pressing are questions on the detailed cell-biological mechanism by which active ECM analogs modify so spectacularly one or more of the processes involved in conventional wound healing.

DEFINITIVE EXPERIMENTAL IDENTIFICATION OF A REGENERATION TEMPLATE

Relative Value of Experimental Study of Organ Synthesis in Vitro *vs.* in Vivo

In vitro studies have traditionally been considered to be much more reproducible than *in vivo* studies. This widespread notion is based on the well-known fact that the error of a typical measurement *in vitro* is often an order of magnitude smaller than is the error in an equivalent measurement *in vivo*, e.g., the mass of a protein synthesized in a cell culture vs. the mass of tissue synthesized in a wound. In spite of a decided advantage in precision, conclusions reached by use of *in vitro* studies are typically burdened by an often-crippling systematic error when they are extrapolated to *in vivo* conditions. The reason, of course, is the far greater complexity of the organ relative to that of the cell and the attending necessity to decompose hypothetically a process at the scale of the organ to a number of processes at the scale of the cell in order to make study of the former more tractable. The systematic error originates in the series of assumptions made in order to bring about the desired simplification. One of the most common assumptions made is that the process at the organ scale is simply the sum of several cell processes each of which can be conveniently studied *in vitro*. This assumption disregards the extensive coupling effects which involve cells with different phenotypes in highly cooperative processes, e.g., the inflammatory process which follows any invasive surgical procedure. The presence of extensive coupling of cell function at the organ scale cancels the predictive value of an *in vitro* assay in which coupling is neglected. Another source of serious systematic error in the use of *in vitro* results to predict *in vivo* behavior arises from the almost universal failure to incorporate an active extracellular matrix *in vitro*.

Studies with experimental animals, on the other hand, suffer from the difficulty of isolating the desired synthetic process occurring at a specific anatomic site from the rest of the organ or even organism. Inability to isolate the experimental volume from its environment introduces uncontrolled variability which reduces greatly the value of conclusions reached. Because of the great value of *in vivo* data in predicting many clinical situations investigators have made a conscious effort to design experiments in which the experimental site is, for many practical purposes, conceptually, at least, isolated both from the organism and from the residual organ. Some of these efforts have been successful, as described below.

The Anatomically Well-defined Experimental Volume

The study of organ synthesis *in vivo* is potentially beset by lack of reproducibility in conditions from one wound to another in the same animal or from a wound in one animal to that in another. The problem of wound-to-wound variability was dramatically minimized, practically eliminated, in the pioneering experiments of Billingham and Medawar[1,2] who developed the concept of the anatomically constant wound. In their rodent models skin was routinely excised down to the *panniculus carnosus*, a layer of muscle which lies under the dermis. Such a wound consists of tissue substrate, including the exudate that flows into it, which is nearly identical from site to site in the plane (the third dimension is neglected in this example). The precise choice of dimensions of an anatomically constant wound varies with the goal of the investigator. In experiments in which the synthesis of peripheral nerve in rats has been studied, an anatomically constant wound has consisted in a gap, 10 or 15 mm long, along the axis of the nerve fiber. The experimental ECM, in the form of a rod-like matrix, has been placed inside a cylindrical prosthesis and the entire device has been grafted as a bridge for this gap in such a way that the nerve stumps are placed inside the tube and in full contact with the ECM analog.

Problems associated with isolation of a process occurring inside the experimental volume from the rest of the organism, and to some extent from the residual organ, can be approached effectively by taking advantage of the special anatomical features of the site. In a study of a synthetic process which is designed to replace lost organ mass the experimental volume is conveniently a gap of standardized geometry, selected to approximate the extent of organ loss in the clinical setting and to most effectively separate it from its living environment. Isolation of the experimental volume can be effected by bounding it with anatomically distinct tissues which belong to a neighboring organ, by an implanted device or by the atmosphere. Examples are: a gap in articular cartilage which is bounded by the bony end plate on one side and by synovial fluid on the other as a clinical model of a joint which has been compromised by osteoarthritis; a "full-thickness" skin lesion, bounded by muscle on the proximal side and by the atmosphere on the distal side, representing the massively burned patient; a gap in a peripheral nerve which is bounded tangentially by a silicone tube as a model of extensive trauma by laceration that typically leads to paralysis. Boundaries that are anatomically distinct from the organ under study provide a morphological and functional basis for separation of the acute or chronic synthetic events occurring inside the experimental volume from any chronic remodeling events which may occur outside it.

Since the experimental volume is typically continuous with the residual organ the question arises on the possibility of distinguishing newly synthesized tissue from mature tissue. A solution to this problem can, in principle, be based on the use of morphological techniques of sufficiently high resolution to distinguish between new and mature tissues of the same organ. The resolution requirements are obviously maximized, and the desired distinction becomes correspondingly more difficult, when the regenerate is mature and when it closely replicates physiological tissues adjacent to it.

An additional experimental problem is identification of flows of cells, by migration, or macromolecular regulators, by diffusion, into the experimental volume from the residual organ itself rather than from one of the neighboring organs. A model of the organ skin as a two-dimensional surface (a "membrane" in solid mechanics) leads to the prediction that a large enough gap on it is exposed to flows of cells and regulators primarily from the organ underneath (muscle) or the atmosphere over it; conversely, flows originating within the same organ (representing the third dimension) should be negligible by comparison. An approach to this problem which further isolated the experimental volume from the residual organ was approached in a study of skin regeneration induced by DRT by using the template in the form of an "island" graft. The "island" was located in the center of the full-thickness wound, sufficiently distant from the edges of the wound to eliminate the possibility of cell migration from tissues at the wound edges to the graft in the center of the wound for at least the first 14 days following generation of the wound and prompt grafting. A different approach, used in the study of peripheral nerve regeneration, consisted in modeling the injured nerve trunk as a one-dimensional rod (fiber) with a gap separating the two nerve stumps. The gap was ensheathed in an impermeable, cylindrical prosthesis made of silicone and filled with experimental ECM analogs which were in direct contact with the nerve stumps. In this design the experimental volume, simply equal to the volume of the cylinder bridging the gap, was isolated from the flow of cells and regulators originating anywhere outside the organ under study while being exposed only to flows originating in the residual organ itself.

The Experimental Volume as a Bioreactor for Study of Organ Synthesis

The process of *in vivo* synthesis is modeled as if it were taking place inside a bioreactor which is surrounded by the animal environment.[24,25] A wound in any of the organs is typically supplied with a continuous flow of exudate from the residual organ as well as from neighboring organs. Conditions inside the animal are subject to relatively strict homeostatic control, even when the experimental injury is of finite magnitude. This physiological environment accordingly becomes a thermal reservoir for the experimental volume.

The bioreactor feed consists of two components. The flow of exudate from surrounding tissues into the experimental volume starts seconds after formation of the wound bed by excision and constitutes the endogenous feed. Exudate consists of cells, cytokines and other diffusible components. Exudate typically does not contain ECM components; matrix components which are required for the synthesis are supplied exogenously in the form of an ECM analog. In the absence of a template the exudate is transformed into connective tissue which eventually becomes epithelialized and is referred to as scar or fibrotic tissue (repaired tissue). An organ consisting mostly of repaired tissue does not function physiologically. The template is therefore required to block the normal repair process in the experimental volume and to induce instead synthesis of a functional organ mass.

Spontaneous vs. Induced Regeneration

Mammals typically possess a very small but finite potential for spontaneous regeneration of most of their organs. For example, a cylindrical defect measuring less than about 1 cm in diameter in the long bone of many mammals is spontaneously refilled with apparently physiologic bone; a gap less than about 5 mm in the rat sciatic nerve is spontaneously synthesized as a relatively competent regenerate.

Organ mass which has been synthesized using the techniques described in this chapter must, therefore, be corrected for physiological organ mass which can be synthesized spontaneously at the same anatomically constant wound bed. This correction for "background" regeneration can be determined simply as the amount of organ mass synthesized in the absence of exogenous feed. Organ synthesis which has resulted from use of an exogenous feed is referred to as induced regeneration. It is clear that the net effect of the exogenous feed cannot be quantitatively appreciated until the data have been corrected for the contribution of background regeneration.

Apparent Necessity for a Regeneration Template Which Is Structured as an ECM Analog

The wound exudate typically contains substantial numbers of cells, such as blood cells and platelets, as well as considerable amounts of several cytokines, such as transforming growth factor β (TGF-β) and platelet derived growth factor (PDGF). The early exudate does not supply the experimental volume with components of ECM. While cells can migrate and cytokines can diffuse, the ECM is an insoluble and nondiffusible network that can do neither. ECM is eventually synthesized in the wound bed by the cells which have migrated to it; however, during the first 3–5 days of the wound healing process ECM components, such as collagen, are not being synthesized.[26] On the other hand, classic studies of organ development have shown without doubt that the early presence of specific ECM components is necessary for formation of physiological organs.[27,28]

The evidence presented in a preceding section strongly supports the conclusion that a specific ECM analog (template) suffices to induce regeneration. Evidence has also been cited above that the early exudate is free of ECM components and that specific components of the ECM are known to be necessary for development. In view of the inevitable close similarity between development and regeneration (both processes have the same end point though not the same mechanism) it is highly likely that, like development, regeneration also requires the presence of active ECM components.

Template Identification

In the model discussed here, the long-term experimental goal briefly consists in identifying a highly specific ECM analog which, when brought in contact with the exudate inside the experimental volume, blocks synthesis of scar and induces instead synthesis of a volume of physiological organ approximately equal to the experimental volume.

The conclusive evidence that an ECM analog possesses biological specificity is a performance assay in which the analog is tested directly for its ability to synthesize the desired organ. However, predictive assays can be used to speed up the screening process as well as to gain further insight into the mechanism of the regeneration process. It is necessary to establish a tentative correlation between the predictive assay and the performance assay. Such a correlation becomes firm when use of the predictive assay leads to identification of the ECM analog which exhibits maximal regenerative activity. For example, the degradation rate of an ECM analog can be determined by an *in vitro* assay which exposes it to a degradative enzyme under standardized conditions; the *in vitro* degradation rate is then correlated with *in vivo* degradation data determined by implanting the analog at the desired site in the animal model. Another assay is based on the ability of certain ECM analogs to inhibit contraction; in this case, the predictive assay is carried on *in vivo*, specifically at the wound bed where the desired synthesis will take place. On the basis of screening studies involving either predictive or performance assays it has been established that the structure of a template must satisfy certain requirements. The most important among these are the chemical composition, the average pore diameter and the degradation rate. Interestingly, the structures of templates which induce regeneration of skin and peripheral nerve are significantly different (TABLE 1).

RECENT ADVANCES IN THE MECHANISTIC UNDERSTANDING OF SKIN REGENERATION

In the search for understanding of the mechanism of regeneration induced by templates it has been important to identify a process associated with wound healing which could be considered to be a precursor of regeneration. Evidence has been presented that, of a large number of ECM analogs with similar structure, the analog which induces dermal regeneration most effectively (referred to above as dermis regeneration template) is the one which is capable of inhibiting the onset of wound contraction most effectively. On this basis it has been hypothesized above that there is a mutually exclusive relation between wound contraction and regeneration.

A test of this hypothesis was made in an amphibian species by a study of the extent of spontaneous regeneration under conditions of variable extent of wound contraction. The hypothesis would be supported if, other factors remaining constant, the extent of regeneration decreased as contraction became more dominant. This inverse relation is observed during the development of the North American bullfrog (*Rana catesbeiana*). Accordingly, certain characteristics of skin wound healing in *Rana catesbeiana* were studied grossly and histologically at various stages of development. The contraction kinetics of excisional, full-thickness skin wounds were monitored for 50 days in animals from four larval developmental stages (tadpoles) and from adults (frogs). Two sets of data were extracted from this study: the steady state value, *i.e.*, the percentage of original wound area which remained after contraction had ceased (a time-independent measurement) and the rate at which the steady state value was achieved (a kinetic measurement). The percentage of original wound area which remained after contraction had ceased (steady state value) in the four larval groups decreased steadily from 59.2 ± 6.8% for the least developed larvae to 9.9 ± 2.3% for the most developed ones; in adults it was less than 10%. This result was consistent with the conclusion that the job of wound closure was effected increasingly by wound contraction (and to a decreasing extent by regeneration) with increasing stage of development. Measurements of rate of wound closure showed that wounds in adults contracted at a much lower rate than for larvae; rates in adults were about 20% of rates in larvae. Histological observations at steady state showed that the morphological features characterizing the intact dermis and epidermis outside the wound bed in the larvae were also observed in qualitatively similar detail inside the wound bed. In contrast, in adults, the subepidermal connective tissue inside the wound bed was distinctly different from the physiological dermis outside and was classified as amphibian scar. We concluded that, during larval development, wound contraction increasingly displaced skin regeneration as a mechanism for wound closure.[23]

The results of this study supported the hypothesis that, at least in this amphibian species, wound contraction and regeneration appear to be mutually exclusive mechanisms of wound closure. Additional studies with mammals are, however, necessary before the hypothesis of mutual exclusivity between contraction and regeneration can be accepted in the context discussed here. However, studies of wound healing with mammalian fetuses are experimentally quite complicated.

MODELS OF THE MECHANISM OF REGENERATION

Overview of Models Which Simulate the Process of Regeneration

The evidence for regeneration described above requires the regeneration template to interact with components of the exudate (cells and cytokines) inside the experimental volume in such a way as to modify drastically the kinetics and mechanism of the spontaneous healing process which normally converts exudate to scar tissue. The processes by which such modification takes place will be described below as a sequence of model steps which constitute a hypothetical mechanism for the observed regeneration.[10,24,25] Each of these models is supported by one or more sets of data which will be briefly referred to. In summary, the desired mechanism requires the template surface to be adequately close and accessible to cells migrating from the exudate; migrating cells which have approached close enough require the template surface to be populated with the appropriate type and density of binding sites for certain cells and cytokines; such interaction must be allowed to proceed over the necessary time period; finally, when the interaction has successfully modified the kinetics and mechanism of wound healing away from repair, it is required that the template remove itself even as new tissue is being synthesized adjacent to the surface of the template.[10,24,25]

Proximity of Cells and Cytokines to Template Surface

Following implantation of the porous template into the wound bed there is need for transfer of cells and cytokines present in the exudate to the surface of the template. The exudate is pulled inside the capillaries (pore channels) of the template by surface tension, as described by:

$$P = 2\gamma/r \tag{1}$$

where r is the radius of the pore channel in a template undergoing wetting by exudate with an air-liquid surface tension of γ in dynes/cm. According to Eq. 1 the suction pressure P increases, and wetting is promoted, as the pore radius decreases. For example, water with an air-liquid surface tension of $\gamma = 72$ dyn/cm is pulled inside a pore radius of 100 μm with a suction pressure of almost one-hundredth of one atmosphere; the pressure increases almost to one full atmosphere when the pore radius decreases to 1 μm. Following flow of exudate inside the pore channels of a template with average pore diameter of 100 μm, cells and cytokines are within a distance of less than 50 μm from the template surface. This distance can be covered within no more than a few minutes by these components of the exudate.

Critical Cell Path Length; Maximum Dimension of Template

Cells from the solid-like tissue surrounding the experimental volume into the template require adequate nutrition during the entire time of residence in it. The complexity of nutritional requirements of the cell is simplified by defining a critical nutrient which is required for normal cell function; such a nutrient is assumed to be metabolized by the cell at a rate R mole/cm^3/s. The nutrient is pictured being transported from the solid-like tissue, where the concentration of nutrient is assumed to be a constant C_0 due to the presence of vascular supply, over a distance L through the exudate until it reaches the cell. In the early days following implantation of the template there is as yet no angiogenesis and the nutrient is, therefore, transported exclusively by diffusion, which is characterized by a diffusivity D cm^2/s. Dimensional analysis readily yields the cell lifeline number:

$$S = RL^2/DC_0 \qquad\qquad (2)$$

which can be used to compare the relative magnitude of the rate of nutrient consumption by the cell nutrient (numerator) and the rate of supply of nutrient to the cell by diffusion (denominator). If the rate of consumption of the critical nutrient exceeds greatly the rate of supply, $S \gg 1$; the cell must soon die. At steady state the rate of consumption of nutrient by the cell just equals the rate of transport by diffusion over the distance L. Under conditions of steady state, $S = O(1)$; at that point, the value of L becomes the critical cell path length, L_c, the longest distance away from the wound bed boundary along which the cell can migrate without requiring nutrient in excess of that supplied by diffusion. Alternatively, L_c is defined as the distance of migration beyond which cells require the presence of a vascular supply. For many cell nutrients of low molecular weight L_c is of order 100 μm. Use of S provides, therefore, an estimate of the maximum template dimension which can support cells.

Upper and Lower Bound of Template Pore Diameter

Having successfully migrated onto the template surface a host cell is visualized interacting with binding sites on the surface. The surface density of binding sites can be expressed as Φ_b, equal by definition to the number of sites N_b per unit surface of template. Another way of expressing Φ_b (more usefully expressed in terms of quantities measurable by optical microscopy) is in terms of the volume density of binding sites ρ_b (number of sites per unit volume porous template) and the specific surface of the template expressed in units of mm^2/cm^3:

$$\Phi_b = N_b/A = \rho_b/\sigma \qquad\qquad (3a)$$

Assuming that each cell is bound to (an *a priori* unknown number of) χ binding sites, there will be N_b/χ bound cells per unit surface; the volume density of cells will be $\rho_c = \rho_b/\chi$ and the surface density of cells will be:

$$\Phi_c = \Phi_b/\chi = N_b/\chi A = \rho_b/\chi\sigma = \rho_c/\sigma \qquad\qquad (3b)$$

Observations of myofibroblast density inside templates with pore diameter of about 10 μm have yielded typical values of the volume density, ρ_c, of order 10^7 myofibroblasts per cm^3 porous template. For a template of average pore diameter

10 μm the specific surface σ is calculated to be approximately 8×10^4 mm^2/cm^3 template; therefore, 1 cm^3 porous template is characterized by a cell surface density of $\Phi_c = \rho_c/\sigma = 10^7/8 \times 10^4 = 125$ cells/mm^2. For a template of identical composition but average pore diameter as large as 300 μm, Φ_c is the same as above; however, the specific surface is calculated to be only about 3×10^3 mm^2/cm^3 template. In this case, the volume density of cells is, accordingly, only $\rho_c = \Phi_c \cdot \sigma = 125 \times 3 \times 10^3 = 3.75 \times 10^5$ per cm^3 porous template. We conclude that the template which has the smaller average pore diameter (10 μm) has a volume density of myofibroblasts which is about 27 times lower than with the template which has the larger pore diameter (300 μm). These considerations suggest a maximum pore diameter requirement for the template, simply to ensure a specific surface which is large enough to bind an appropriately large number of cells.

Additional reflection makes it obvious that cells originating in the wound bed cannot migrate inside the template and eventually reach binding sites on its surface unless the template has an average pore diameter large enough to allow for this. There is, therefore, a requirement for a minimum pore diameter for the template, about equal to the characteristic diameter of the cells (of order 5 μm). Thus, the pore diameter of the regeneration template is limited both by an upper and a lower bound. This conclusion is in agreement with the experimental evidence which shows that ECM analogs, identical in chemical composition but differing only in average pore diameter, show maximum activity (inhibition of onset of wound contraction, consistent with regeneration rather than scar formation) when the average pore diameter lies between 20 and 120 mm.[10] Further evidence has shown that, when other structural parameters of the template remain constant, loss of the 20–120 μm porous structure of the template by simple evaporation at room temperature (a process which yields an ECM analog with average pore diameter of less than 1 μm) leads to synthesis of a scar capsule at the surface of the grafted analog, evidence of a barrier to cell migration inside an implant.[29]

Template Residence Time

A template must be in place long enough to induce the appropriate synthetic processes to take place, but it must disappear in timely fashion so as not to interfere with these same processes which it induces. The time period necessary to induce synthesis will be taken to be of the same order as that required to complete the wound healing process at that anatomical site. (In general, the rate of wound healing is quite different in tissues such as, for example, the dermis and the sciatic nerve.) Since the template is an insoluble (and, therefore, nondiffusible) three-dimensional network, it follows that cells which are bound on it become immobilized and their migration is, accordingly, arrested. Not only cells are prevented from migrating to locations which are appropriate for synthesis of a new organ but, in addition, the laying down of newly synthesized ECM by the cells in the space of the wound bed is probably blocked physically by the presence of the template. These considerations suggest strongly that the persisting insolubility of the template will increasingly interfere with the synthesis of the new organ at that site. The template is, accordingly, required to become diffusible (by degradation to small molecular fragments) and thereby remove itself from the wound bed in order not to interfere with cellular processes which lead to the emerging organ.

The simplest model which can accommodate these two requirements is one which requires synchronization of the two processes: organ synthesis and template degradation.[6,10] This model leads directly to the hypothesis of isomorphous tissue replacement:

$$t_d/t_s = O(1) \qquad (4)$$

In Eq. **4** t_d denotes a characteristic time constant for degradation of the template at the tissue site where a new organ is synthesized with a time constant of t_s. The degradation rate can be estimated by histological observation of the decrease in mass of template fragments at various times.[11,30] A closer estimate of t_d has been obtained by measuring the kinetics of disintegration of the macromolecular network using rubber elasticity theory.[4] An alternate procedure consists of monitoring the kinetics of mass disappearance of a radioactively labeled template. A rough estimate of t_s can be obtained by observing the timescale of synthesis of new tissue during healing (in the absence of a template) at the anatomical site.[31] Using the latter approach it has been estimated that t_s for the regenerating dermis is of order 3 weeks[31] and of order 6 weeks for the regenerating peripheral nerve.[16] These estimates allow adjustment of t_d for the template, by adjustment of the cross-link density and GAG content, to levels which are approximately equal to the value of t_s, as the latter is dictated by the nature of the anatomical site.

The isomorphous tissue replacement hypothesis has received some experimental support from observations that when the ratio in Eq. **4** was adjusted to values much smaller than one (by implanting a rapidly degradaing ECM analog, for which $t_d \ll t_s$) the wound healing process resulted in contraction and synthesis of scar, as would have been the case if the template was missing. It was also observed that when the ratio in Eq. **4** was much larger than 1 (by implanting an ECM analog which degraded very slowly, so that $t_d \ll t_s$) the ECM analog was surrounded by a capsule of scar tissue.[31] Even though this limited evidence cannot be used to test the hypothesis of Eq. **4** conclusively, it is, at the least, compatible with a template half-life which has both lower and an upper bounds. Direct experimental support for this conclusion is afforded by experimental evidence based on studies of inhibition of wound contraction by several ECM analogs with defined structure. These studies have shown that, of several ECM analogs studied, the dermal regeneration template was the analog which degraded at a rate corresponding to a half-life of about 1.5 to 2 weeks; ECM analogs which degraded at much slower or much faster rates were not active.[10]

The simplest template structure which can participate in this disappearing act with minimum harm to the host is one in which the template undergoes degradation by enzymes of the wound bed to non-toxic low-molecular weight fragments that diffuse rapidly away from the site of organ synthesis.[31]

Chemical Composition of Template

Interactions which are developmentally significant are known to involve cells, growth factors and ECM components. The latter include the collagens, elastin, several proteoglycans as well as cell adhesion molecules such as fibronectin and laminin. Since development and induced regeneration have a common endpoint we will assume that the required cell-matrix binding events in each case are similar, though not identical; if so, the identity of matrix components in each case must also be similar. This presumptive similarity between developmental and regenerative mechanisms has been previously referred to briefly in terms of the hypothetical rule: regeneration recapitulates ontogeny;[9] however, we emphasize the lack of detailed evidence for such an identity. In the dermis, as well as in the connective tissue of peripheral nerves, type I collagen is present in greatest abundance whereas the most prominent glycosaminoglycans in the dermis are dermatan sulfate and chondroitin 6-sulfate (dermis); in peripheral nerves, type I collagen and sulfated proteoglycans have also been prominently observed.[32]

Although quite richly endowed with undifferentiated cells and growth factors the early exudate of a spontaneously healing skin wound is free of ECM components and is, therefore, lacking in components which are known to be required for development. As pointed out above, this lack of ECM components is hypothetically associated with the absence of synthetic processes which lead to a physiological organ.

These hypothetical considerations are consistent with the choice of Type I collagen and at least one of the proteoglycans or glycosaminoglycans (GAGs) as basic structural components of regeneration templates. Although several efforts have been made to replace the use of ECM analogs in templates with synthetic polymers there is, at this time, no firm evidence that synthetic polymers can induce regeneration of the dermis or of a peripheral nerve in lesions where the physiological structures are not regenerated spontaneously.

There is considerable experimental evidence linking the biological activity of the dermis regeneration template to its detailed structural features (TABLE 1). Two ECM analogs, one of which was prepared with a GAG while the other was prepared with the corresponding proteoglycan, showed the same actitvity in an *in vivo* assay (inhibition of onset of wound contraction) which predicts dermal regeneration.[33] This result suggested that the dermal regeneration template can be constructed using a GAG, rather than the corresponding proteoglycan, without loss of activity. The necessity for a covalently cross-linked network of collagen and the sulfated GAG derived from the observation that these two macromolecules form an ionic complex spontaneously at acidic pH; however, the complex is dissociated at neutral pH, i.e., under conditions which prevail following implantation.[34] To preserve the chemical composition of the ECM analog *in vivo* over the period suggested by the residence time considerations discussed above it was, therefore, necessary to introduce a certain density of covalent bonds between collagen chains and GAG molecules, *i.e.*, to form a collagen-GAG graft copolymer.[34] There is evidence that an increase in the fraction of GAG in the copolymer increases the resistance of the macromolecular network to degradation by mammalian collagenases.[4] Such resistance also increases with the density of collagen-collagen cross-links and collagen-GAG cross-links.[29,35] A review of the effect of each of these structural features of the dermis regeneration template on inhibition of the onset of wound contraction can be made based on the published evidence.[10,33] This review suggests that the chemical composition and the detailed pore structure of the dermal regeneration template contribute about equally to its activity. A similar study of the relation between structure and activity for the nerve regeneration template has not been made.[10,24,25]

REFERENCES

1. BILLINGHAM, R. E. & P. B. MEDAWAR. 1951. The technique of free skin grafting in mammals. J. Exp. Biol. **28**: 385–394.
2. BILLINGHAM, R. E. & P. B. MEDAWAR. 1955. Contracture and intussusceptive growth in the healing of extensive wounds in mammalian skin. J. Anat. **89**: 114–123.
3. PEACOCK, E. E., JR. & W. VAN WINKLE, JR. 1976. Wound repair, second edition. W. B. Saunders. Philadelphia.
4. YANNAS, I. V., J. F. BURKE, C. HUANG & P. L. GORDON. 1975. Suppression of in vivo

degradability and of immunogenicity by reaction with glycoaminoglycans. Polymer Repr. Am. Chem. Soc. **16:** 209–214.

5. YANNAS, I. V., J. F. BURKE, P. L. GORDON & C. HUANG. 1977. Multilayer membrane useful as synthetic skin. US Patent 4,060,081.

6. YANNAS, I. V., J. F. BURKE, M. UMBREIT & P. STASIKELIS. 1979. Progress in design of an artificial skin. Fed. Proc. **38:** 988.

7. YANNAS, I. V., J. F. BURKE, M. WARPEHOSKI, P. STASIKELIS, E. M. SKRABUT, D. ORGILL & D. J. GIARD. 1981. Prompt, long-term functional replacement of skin. Trans. Am. Soc. Artif. Intern. Organs **27:** 19–22.

8. YANNAS, I. V., J. F. BURKE, D. P. ORGILL & E. M. SKRABUT. 1982. Wound tissue can utilize a polymeric template to synthesize a functional extension of skin. Science **215:** 174–176.

9. YANNAS, I. V., D. P. ORGILL, E. M. SKRABUT & J. F. BURKE. 1984. Skin regeneration with a bioreplaceable polymeric template. *In* American Chemical Symposium Series, No. 256. C. G. Gebelein, Ed.: 191–197.

10. YANNAS, I. V., E. LEE, D. P. ORGILL, E. M. SKRABUT & G. F. MURPHY. 1989. Synthesis and characterization of a model extracellular matrix that induces partial regeneration of adult mammalian skin. Proc. Natl. Acad. Sci. USA **86:** 933–937.

11. MURPHY, G. F., D. P. ORGILL & I. V. YANNAS. 1990. Partial dermal regeneration is induced by biodegradable collagen-glycosaminoglycan grafts. Lab. Invest. **63:** 305–313.

12. BURKE, J. F., I. V. YANNAS, W. C. QUINBY, JR., C. C. BONDOC & W. K. JUNG. 1981. Successful use of a physiologically acceptable artificial skin in the treatment of extensive skin injury. Ann. Surg. **194:** 413–428.

13. HEIMBACH, D., A. LUTERMAN, J. BURKE, A. CRAM, D. HERNDON, J. HUNT, M. JORDAN, W. MCMANUS, L. SOLEM, G. WARDEN & B. ZAWACKI. 1988. A multi-center randomized clinical trial. Artificial dermis for major burns. Ann. Surg. **208:** 313–320.

14. STERN, R., M. MCPHERSON & M. T. LONGAKER. 1990. Histologic study of artificial skin used in the treatment of full-thickness thermal injury. J. Burn Care Rehabil. **11:** 7–13.

15. YANNAS, I. V., D. P. ORGILL, J. SILVER, T. V. NORREGAARD, N. T. ZERVAS & W. C. SCHOENE. 1987. Regeneration of sciatic nerve across 15-mm gap by use of a polymeric template. *In* Advances in Biomedical Polymers. C. G. Gebelein, Ed.: 1–9. Plenum. New York.

16. CHANG, A. S., I. V. YANNAS, S. PERUTZ, H. LOREE, R. R. SETHI, C. KRARUP, T. V. NORREGAARD, N. T. ZERVAS & J. SILVER. 1990. Electrophysiological study of recovery of peripheral nerves regenerated by a collagen-glycosaminoglycan copolymer matrix. *In* Progress in Biomedical Polymers. C. G. Gebelein, Ed.: 107–120. Plenum. New York.

17. CHANG, A. S. & I. V. YANNAS. 1992. Peripheral nerve regeneration. *In* Neuroscience Year (Supplement 2 to the Encyclopedia of Neuroscience). B. Smith & G. Adelman, Eds.: 125–126. Birkhäuser. Boston, MA.

18. LANDSTROM, A. & I. V. YANNAS. 1996. Peripheral nerve regeneration. *In* Encyclopedia of Neuroscience. B. Smith & G. Adelman, Eds. Birkhäuser, Boston, MA. In press.

19. LUNDBORG, G., L. B. DAHLIN, N. DANIELSEN, R. H. GELBERMAN, F. M. LONGO, H. C. POWELL & S. VARON. 1982. Nerve regeneration in silicone chambers: Influence of gap length and of distal stump components. Exp. Neurol. **76:** 361–375.

20. LUNDBORG, G. 1987. Nerve regeneration and repair: A review. Acta Orthop. Scand. **58:** 145–169.

21. STONE, K. R., W. G. RODKEY, R. J. WEBBER, L. MCKINNEY & J. R. STEADMAN. 1990. Collagen-based prostheses for meniscal regeneration. Clin. Orthop. **252:** 129–135.

22. STONE, K. R., R. J. WEBBER, W. G. RODKEY & J. R. STEADMAN. 1989. Prosthetic meniscal replacement: In vitro studies of meniscal regeneration using copolymeric collagen prostheses. Arthroscopy **5:** 152.

23. YANNAS, I. V., J. COLT & Y. C. WAI. 1996. Wound contraction and scar synthesis during development of the amphibian *Rana catesbeiana*. Wound Rep. Regen. **4:** 31–41.

24. YANNAS, I. V. 1995. Regeneration templates. *In* The Biomedical Engineering Handbook. J. D. Bronzino, Ed.: 1619–1635. CRC Press. Boca Raton, FL.

25. YANNAS, I. V. 1996. In vivo synthesis of tissues and organs. *In* Textbook of Tissue

Engineering. R. P. Lanza, R. S. Langer & W. L. Chick, Eds. R. G. Landes/Academic Press. New York.

26. McPherson, J. M. & K. A. Piez. 1988. *In* The Molecular and Cellular Biology of Wound Repair. R. A. F. Clark & P. M. Henson, Eds.: 471–496. Plenum. New York.
27. Hay, E. D., Ed. 1981. Cell biology of extracellular matrix. Plenum. New York.
28. Loomis, W. F. 1986. Developmental Biology. Macmillan. New York.
29. Yannas, I. V. 1981. Use of artificial skin in wound management. *In* The Surgical Wound. P. Dineen, Ed.: 171–190. Lea and Febiger. Philadelphia, PA.
30. Yannas, I. V., J. F. Burke, C. Huang & P. L. Gordon. 1975. Correlation of *in vivo* collagen degradation rate with *in vitro* measurements. J. Biomed. Mater. Res. **9:** 623–628.
31. Yannas, I. V. & J. F. Burke. 1980. Design of an artificial skin. Part. I. Design principles. J. Biomed. Mater. Res. **14:** 65–68.
32. Rutka, J. T., G. Apodaca, R. Stern & M. Rosenblum. 1988. The extracellular matrix of the central and peripheral nervous systems: structure and function. J. Neurosurg. **69:** 155–170.
33. Shafritz, T. A., L. C. Rosenberg & I. V. Yannas. 1994. Specific effects of glycosamino-glycans in an analog of extracellular matrix that delays wound contraction and induces regeneration. Wound Rep. Reg. **2:** 270–276.
34. Yannas, I. V., J. F. Burke, P. L. Gordon, C. Huang & R. H. Rubenstein. 1980. Design of an artificial skin. Part II. Control of chemical composition. J. Biomed. Mater. Res. **14:** 107–131.
35. Yannas, I. V. 1988. Regeneration of skin and nerves by use of collagen templates. *In* Collagen: Biotechnology, vol. III. M. Nimni, Ed.: 87–115. CRC Press. Boca Raton, FL.

Neonatal Porcine Islets as a Possible Source of Tissue for Humans and Microencapsulation Improves the Metabolic Response of Islet Graft Posttransplantation

GREGORY S. KORBUTT,[a] ZILIANG AO,[a]
MIKE FLASHNER,[b] AND RAY V. RAJOTTE[a,c]

[a]Surgical-Medical Research Institute
University of Alberta
Edmonton, Alberta, Canada, T6G 2N8

[b]Metabolex, Inc.
Hayward, California 94545

CLINICAL ISLET TRANSPLANTATION

Current methods for treating insulin-dependent (Type 1) diabetes mellitus do not prevent transient episodes of hyperglycemia.[1] Recurrent hyperglycemia has been suggested to cause chronic lesions which can culminate in renal failure, blindness, heart disease, neuropathy, or atherosclerosis.[2] Recently the Diabetes Control and Complications Trial demonstrated that long-term intensive insulin treatment was associated with a reduced risk of developing diabetes-related complications.[3] This intensive therapy, however, can result in harmful side effects due to recurrent hypoglycemia, and the extraordinary effort required in self-monitoring and in providing ongoing management for these patients may exceed the capabilities of many individuals and their health care providers. An attractive alternative is to transplant insulin-producing tissue, which can offer a more physiological approach for precise restoration of glucose homeostasis, thereby reversing the metabolic and neurovascular complications of diabetes. Compared to vascularized pancreatic grafts, transplantation of isolated islets offers a number of advantages. For example, donor islet tissue can be tested and/or pretreated before implantation, thus allowing the possibility of using grafts with defined metabolic or immunological characteristics.

Since 1974, 236 adult human islet allografts have been performed in European and North American centers.[4] A detailed analysis of 75 type 1 diabetics (C-peptide negative) transplanted with adult islet allografts from 1990 to 1993 showed a 1 year patient survival of 95% and a graft survival (defined by basal C-peptide >1 ng/ml) of only 28%.[5] Eight of these patients were insulin independent for >1 year, of which two were from our program in Edmonton.[6,7] Insulin independence in these

[c]Author to whom correspondence should be addressed: Dr. Ray V. Rajotte, Director, Surgical-Medical Research Institute, 1074 Dentistry/Pharmacy Building, University of Alberta, Edmonton, Alberta, Canada, T6G 2N8; Tel: (403) 492-3386; Fax: (403) 492-1627; E-mail: rrajotte@gpu.srv.ualberta.ca

individuals was attributed to the implantation of a sufficient β cell mass, which was often achieved by combining freshly isolated islets with cryopreserved tissue from multiple donors.[6-8] Irrespective of the relatively low success of human islet transplantation, the results do demonstrate that this form of therapy is capable of correcting hyperglycemia in man—thus supporting the concept that islet transplantation can achieve the fundamental aim of restoring carbohydrate metabolism.

PORCINE ISLETS AS A SOURCE OF DONOR TISSUE

If islet transplantation is to become a widespread treatment for type I diabetics, solutions must be found for increasing the availability of insulin-producing tissue and to over come the need for continuous immunosuppression. In an attempt to overcome this 'islet supply' problem, insulin-producing tissue from abundant and accessible sources are being considered for clinical transplantation. These include: 1) porcine[9-13] and bovine[14] islets, 2) fish-brockman bodies,[15] 3) genetically engineered insulin-secreting cell lines,[16-18] and 4) *in vitro* production of human fetal[19] or adult[20] β cells. The use of fetal porcine islet cells for treating Type 1 diabetics was examined by Groth and associates in Sweden.[10] Although there was no evidence to indicate engraftment of the fetal cells, all patients tolerated the procedure well and no adverse side effects were recorded.[10] Despite this failure, porcine islets still represent the most likely practical solution to the 'islet supply' problem, since pigs are inexpensive, readily available, ethically acceptable, and they exhibit morphological and physiological characteristics comparable to man. Porcine insulin is also structurally similar to human insulin and has been used safely for treating Type I diabetics for decades, and pigs can be raised under gnotobiotic (microbe-free) conditions if necessary.

Unfortunately, despite many reports on the isolation of adult porcine islets, factors such as age, breed, and quality of organs adversely affect the final yield,[21,22] and once isolated adult porcine islets are fragile and difficult to maintain in tissue culture.[13,23,24] In contrast, tissue culture of collagenase digested fetal porcine pancreas produces viable islet-like cell clusters,[9,11] which have the ability to cure diabetic nude mice within 2 months posttransplantation.[9] A general finding, however, in rat,[25-28] porcine,[9] and human[29] fetal pancreatic β cells is that they exhibit a poor insulin secretory response to glucose, and the onset and maturation of glucose-induced insulin secretion is more evident in the postnatal period.[25-28] We therefore developed a simple, standardized procedure for isolating large numbers of neonatal porcine islets with a reproducible and defined cellular composition.[30]

Neonatal porcine islets were prepared from 1 to 3 day old piglets by collagenase digestion and tissue culture at 37°C for nine days. After the period of tissue culture, the average number of neonatal porcine islet equivalents recovered per pancreas was 48,000 (range = 28,210–90,966). As opposed to adult pancreatic islets which are known to consist of approximately 80–90 percent endocrine cells, the neonatal porcine islets were shown to consist primarily of fully differentiated endocrine (35%) and endocrine precursor cells (57%). *In vitro* viability assessment of the cultured islets demonstrated that in the presence of 20 mM glucose, the islets were capable of releasing 7-fold more insulin than at 2.8 mM glucose, and when exposed to 20 mM glucose in combination with 10 mM theophylline, the stimulation index increased to 30-fold as compared to basal release. When 2000 neonatal islets were transplanted into alloxan diabetic nude mice (n = 10), 100 percent of the recipients became normoglycemic within 6–8 weeks posttransplantation and remained euglycemic until the graft-bearing kidney was removed at 100 days follow-up, after which all recipients returned to a hyperglycemic state. Examination of the grafts derived from normalized mice revealed that they were largely composed of insulin-positive cells, and their cellular insulin content was 5- to 20-fold higher than at the day of transplantation.

Although neonatal porcine islet grafts are unable to correct diabetes immediately after transplantation, they eventually develop the capacity to establish and maintain normoglycemia long-term in nude mice.[30] This delay in achieving euglycemia is most likely related to the fact that neonatal porcine islets are not fully developed and are composed of only 25% β cells and thus, the resulting grafts contain relatively few β cells at the time of implantation (i.e., 6×10^5 β cells/2000 neonatal porcine islets). This seems more plausible than the possibility that neonatal porcine β cells exhibit an immature or poor glucose sensitivity and/or insulin secretory capacity prior to transplantation. Many studies have shown that the fetal β cell has a poor insulin response to glucose, which is rapidly converted to a more adult pattern after birth.[25-28] In our experiments, 9-day cultured neonatal porcine β cells were capable of secreting considerable amounts of insulin in response to an in vitro glucose challenge. These secretory rates are significantly higher than those observed for fetal pig islet cells,[9,11] suggesting that in the pig, neonatal β cells are more responsive to glucose than fetal β cells. It is therefore plausible that the latent period for correcting diabetes is not related to the functional capacity of neonatal porcine islets but rather to an inadequate mass of implanted β cells. For example, following transplantation, neonatal porcine islet grafts are likely subsequently supplemented by the growth and/or differentiation of new β cells so that a critical mass is obtained, which ultimately results in normoglycemia. It is also possible that key growth factors originating from the transplanted tissue itself, as well as perhaps from the hyperglycemic recipient, promotes an increase in β cell mass in vivo.

Since our data has demonstrated that neonatal porcine islets have an inherent ability for growth both in vitro and in vivo,[30] one approach to more rapidly correct diabetes is to enhance the growth and proliferation of new β cells in vitro prior to transplantation so that the islets contain a majority of endocrine cells. Furthermore, the ability to differentiate islet endocrine tissue in vitro would not only facilitate neonatal porcine islet transplantation as a therapy, it could ultimately provide a better understanding of islet growth, so that new therapies can be potentially developed for treating diabetes. Nonetheless, our results demonstrate that the neonatal porcine pancreas can be used for the isolation of a large number of functionally viable islet cells and due to their ready availability and inherent capacity to proliferate and differentiate, they constitute an attractive source of insulin-producing tissue for studies of islet cell neogenesis or as a source of xenogeneic islet cells for clinical transplantation.

Before neonatal porcine islets can be considered for application in man, several key immunological problems need to be solved. For instance, xenotransplantation between discordant species (e.g., pig-to-man) has been hindered by the occurrence of hyperacute rejection (HAR), a process believed to be initiated when naturally occurring xenoreactive antibodies in the recipients sera bind to antigens present on the surface of endothelial (and other) cells within the xenograft. Antibody binding in turn activates complement, which rapidly destroys the transplanted organ or tissue.[31-35] All of these effects are the result of endothelial cell activation and lysis by the combined action of recipient antibodies and complement.[34,35] The most important target for these antibodies has been identified as the carbohydrate Galα(1–3)Galβ1,4GlcNAc.[36-41] This epitope is present in high concentrations on all porcine endothelial cells[41,42] and has recently been detected on fetal porcine islet cells.[43,44] Rapid *in situ* destruction of an islet graft has been described in a rabbit-to-primate model,[45] and when fetal porcine islet cells were transplanted into Type I diabetics, there was no immediate evidence to indicate graft function.[10] Therefore before porcine pancreatic islets can be considered a potential source of islets for transplantation into diabetic recipients the issue of whether these grafts will be susceptible to damage by natural antibody mediated hyperacute rejection needs to be elucidated. In a recent study, we performed Western Blots to determine if membrane proteins present on neonatal porcine islets are recognized by xenoreactive antibodies present in human sera.[46] Immunoblots of freshly isolated neonatal porcine islets with human AB sera detected the presence of 14 antigens (MW 24–164 kD) and 4 antigens (MW 101–150 kD) to which antiserum against human IgM and IgG bound, respectively. The most prominent antigens with IgM reactivity had MWs of 36 and 65 kD, whereas for IgG, the most intensely-reactive antigen had a MW of 120 kD. When membrane fractions of porcine aortic endothelial cells and LLC-PK1 cells (a porcine renal tubular epithelial cell line) were analyzed, predominant antigens were shown to have MWs comparable to those observed for neonatal porcine islets. After culturing the islets for 5 days, the total number of xenoreactive antigens binding IgM decreased to 11 and for IgG, to 3. Furthermore, the prominent antigens at 36 and 65 kD with IgM reactivity present in freshly isolated islets exhibited a decreased intensity of binding following the culture period.

Incubation of 5 day cultured neonatal porcine islets for 18 h in the presence of heat-inactivated human AB serum containing rabbit complement resulted in a 55% loss of cellular insulin mass ($p < 0.0001$) and a 45% reduction in recoverable DNA content ($p < 0.0001$) when compared to control islets incubated in the same pool of human serum without rabbit complement. Electron micrographs of islets incubated in human serum with complement demonstrated numerous degranulated or necrotic β cells. In contrast, control islets incubated in human sera without complement were composed of ultrastructurally intact cells with the presence of well-granulated β cells. The functional viability of the different neonatal porcine islet cell suspensions was tested by comparing the percentages of cellular insulin that was released at low (2.8 mM), high (20 mM) and high glucose plus 10 mM theophylline. Control islets incubated in human serum in the absence of complement, released 4.9-fold more insulin at 20 mM glucose than at 2.8 mM glucose, and when exposed to 20 mM glucose in combination with 10 mM theophylline, the stimulation index increased to approximately 30-fold as compared to basal release. When neonatal porcine islets were examined for their secretory activity after an 18 h incubation with human serum and rabbit complement, they released significantly higher levels ($p < 0.001$) of insulin in response to 2.8 mM glucose and lower amounts ($p < 0.001$) when challenged with 20 mM glucose plus theophylline than that observed in control preparations. Therefore, the calculated stimulation indices after incubation with either 20 mM glucose or 20 mM glucose plus 10 mM theophylline were significantly lower when the islets were treated with human serum containing rabbit complement.

Since human natural antibodies of both IgG and IgM subtypes are capable of binding to antigens present on neonatal porcine islets and that exposure to human AB serum and complement significantly reduces islet cell survival and viability, neonatal porcine islet grafts will likely be subjected to antibody-mediated destruction if implanted in man. If this is the case, identification of the pertinent antigens and clarification of the mechanisms behind this form of rejection may lead to the development of effective strategies for preventing acute xenorejection of porcine neonatal islet cell grafts. Furthermore, since this form of rejection involves the binding of xeno-reactive antibodies to islet cells and the subsequent activation of complement one potential approach to prevent this reaction is to place the islet grafts in an immunoisolation barrier in order to block the binding of the hosts antibodies.

MICROENCAPSULATION OF PANCREATIC ISLETS

Compared with whole organ transplantation, grafting of isolated islets offers more alternatives for developing strategies to prevent tissue rejection. For example, prevention of experimental islet rejection has been accomplished by placing islets in immunoisolation devices constructed of semipermeable membranes separating donor tissue from the recipients immune system. These devices consist of synthetic membranes which allow diffusion of low molecular weight substances (*i.e.*, glucose, insulin) yet exclude cellular contacts between donor and host cells as well as passage of large molecular weight molecules (*i.e.*, immunoglobulins). Islets have been immunoisolated by placing them in: biohybrid chambers anastomosed to the vascular system[47]; diffusion chambers or hollow fibers[48]; and microcapsules.[49] Biohybrid chambers as well as diffusion chambers are however limited in their long-term use, since islet survival may be compromised by a reduced availability of nutrients caused by extensive fibrosis around the device. One appealing approach is microencapsulation, where individual islets are surrounded by a biocompatible membrane that functions as a barrier to the host's immune system.

The viability of microencapsulated islets following transplantation, in animal models devoid of immunologic factors, has been poorly characterized. This basic information is essential as it provides insight into the long-term metabolic function of microencapsulated islet grafts. We have therefore recently conducted a study in which we compared the function of defined quantities of alginate microencapsulated and non-encapsulated canine islet grafts when transplanted into diabetic athymic nude mice. Briefly, canine islets were isolated from mongrel dogs using collagenase perfusion, automated dissociation, and Ficoll purification, as previously described.[50] Isolated islets were cultured overnight at 22°C then microencapsulated with highly purified alginate using an electrostatic generator that produces uniform capsules of 200–350 μm in diameter. After an additional overnight culture period, defined numbers of encapsulated (intraperitoneally) and non-encapsulated (intraperitoneally and beneath the kidney capsule) were transplanted into alloxan-induced diabetic nude mice.

Transplantation of 1000 unencapsulated islets under the kidney capsule of diabetic nude mice was unable to correct hyperglycemia in all recipients, whereas, 75% of the animals implanted with 2000 unencapsulated islets (renal subcapsule) achieved euglycemia. These data therefore demonstrate that 2000 canine islets is the minimal mass required to obtain normoglycemia in nude mice when the grafts are transplanted beneath the kidney capsule. On the other hand, when 4000 unencapsulated islets were placed intraperitoneally only 1 of 8 recipients achieved euglycemia. Intraperitoneal transplantation of grafts consisting of 500 or 1000 encapsulated islets was shown to consistently correct diabetes in 70% and 100% of the animals, respectively—indicating that a significantly lower mass is needed when the islets are encapsulated and transplanted intraperitoneally. In addition, recovery of the capsules at 100 days posttransplantation showed structurally intact islets with no signs of fibrosis on the microcapsule.

These data clearly demonstrate that alginate microencapsulation improves the long-term metabolic function of canine islets grafts and indicates that the intraperitoneum is a suitable site for the implantation of encapsulated islets. Furthermore, since recipients of microencapsulated islet grafts exhibited similar responses during an oral glucose tolerance test to those of age-matched normal controls, these results also show that an encapsulated islet graft placed intraperitoneally not only corrects basal hyperglycemia but can produce normal glucose tolerance.

The use of isolated islet preparations as grafts also offers the advantage that donor tissue can be stored prior to transplantation. This creates the possibility of combining isolates from multiple donors, after adequate quality control. Clinical islet transplantation however, requires conditions for preserving islet grafts with a minimal loss in viable beta cells. Since extracellular matrices have been reported to enhance islet cell survival *in vitro*,[51] we recently compared the recovery and functional viability of alginate microencapsulated canine islets during long-term tissue culture. In these experiments, canine islets were isolated and microencapsulated as described above, then a paired study was conducted to compare the recovery and functional viability of encapsulated and non-encapsulated islets during three weeks of tissue culture at 22°C.

After one, two, and three weeks in tissue culture, islet recovery (*i.e.*, islet equivalents) for the non-encapsulated group was 63, 56, and 24 percent, compared to 92, 89, and 71 percent for encapsulated islets ($p < 0.05$ at all time points). During a static incubation assay at 2.8 mM glucose and 20 mM glucose plus 50 μm IBMX, similar amounts of insulin were secreted from encapsulated and nonencapsulated islets when measured at all three time points. Compared to basal release at 2.8 mM glucose, the increase of stimulated insulin release at 20 mM glucose plus IBMX by nonencapsulated islets was 19- (1 week), 10- (2 weeks), and 9- (3 weeks) fold higher—while the stimulation indexes from encapsulated islets were 21-, 12-, and 10-fold higher than basal release, respectively. Following 3 weeks of culture, 2000 islets transplanted intraperitoneally (encapsulated) achieved euglycemia in 100% of the animals for >100 days, whereas when 2000 non-encapsulated grafts were placed beneath the renal capsule only 33% of the recipients maintained normoglycemia for over 100 days posttransplantation.

This comparative study on recovery and function of canine pancreatic islets following 1 to 3 weeks culture clearly demonstrates that microencapsulation with highly purified alginate can be successfully used for storage of islet grafts for prolonged periods without a significant loss of islet cell mass. Microencapsulation achieves this protective effect likely by preventing islet deterioration during culture and ultimately enhances their survival during long-term tissue culture.

Clinical islet transplantation has been facilitated by low temperature banking which is a procedure Rajotte developed a number of years ago.[52] To determine if microencapsulated canine islets survive cryopreservation, we assessed the recovery and *in vivo* function of microencapsulated canine islets following the freeze-thaw process. Canine islets were isolated and encapsulated as described above. A defined number of encapsulated and non-encapsulated islets were cryopreserved in multiple glass freezer tubes using step-wise addition of the cryoprotectant dimethyl sulfoxide (DMSO), nucleation at -7.4°C, and slow cooling at 0.25°C/min to -40°C before plunging and storage in liquid nitrogen.[52] After storage, islets are thawed rapidly (200°C/min), and the DMSO removed from the intracellular compartment by using a 0.75 M sucrose dilution.[52] Islets were then cultured for 24 hours (22°C) before being assessed for recovery and *in vivo* function after transplantation into alloxan-induced diabetic nude mice.

Following cryopreservation and overnight culture the mean recovery of encapsulated islets was 88% as compared to 76% for unencapsulated islets ($p < 0.05$). Transplantation of 1000 or 2000 cryopreserved encapsulated islets into the peritoneal cavity corrected diabetes in 100% of the recipients for >100 days posttransplantation. In contrast, implantation of 2000 cryopreserved non-encapsulated islets under the kidney capsule achieved euglycemia in only 33% of the animals at 100 days posttransplantation. These data therefore prove that alginate microencapsulated islets can be successfully cryopreserved and when thawed they continue to exhibit the metabolic potential to correct diabetes long-term in nude mice.

CONCLUSION

Twenty-five years ago, diabetes was successfully corrected in rats by intra-portal transplantation of isogeneic islets. Today, islet transplantation has become clinically applicable, resulting in insulin-independence long-term in some Type 1 diabetics. The clinical potential of islet transplantation will however only be fully realized by its ability to correct glucose homeostasis at an early stage of the disease and to prevent the development of chronic complications associated with diabetes. The avoidance of chronic immunosuppression is definitely the ideal scenario for islet transplantation and studies in animal models suggest that microencapsulation may help accomplish this goal. Nonetheless, even if islet transplantation becomes the treatment of choice for diabetes, the supply of cadaveric human pancreata will become a major limiting step. Based upon our recent findings, we hypothesize that neonatal porcine islets are likely to provide the first abundant, practical source of insulin-producing tissue which will allow the widespread application of islet transplantation to treat Type 1 diabetics. Even though the transfer of such approaches to a clinical setting is far from being perfect, the establishment of concise, well controlled step-by-step protocols in both basic and clinical research can potentially facilitate their application in man.

REFERENCES

1. NATHAN, D. M. 1992. The rationale for glucose control in diabetes mellitus. Endocrinol. Metab. Clin. N.A. **21:** 221–235.
2. NATHAN, D. M. 1993. Long-term complication of diabetes mellitus. N. Engl. J. Med. **328:** 1676–1685.
3. AMERICAN DIABETES ASSOCIATION. 1993. Position Statement, Implications of the Diabetes Control and Complications Trial. Diabetes **42:** 1555–1558.
4. INTERNATIONAL ISLET TRANSPLANT REGISTRY. 1995. Newsletter No. 6, vol. 5.
5. HERING, B. J., C. C. BROWATZKI, A. SCHULTZ, R. G. BRETZEL & K. FEDERLIN. 1993. Clinical islet transplantation—registry report, accomplishments in the past and future research needs. Cell Transplant. **2:** 269–282.
6. WARNOCK, G. L., N. M. KNETEMAN, E. RYAN, R. E. SEELIS, A. RABINOVITCH & R. V. RAJOTTE. 1991. Normoglycemia after transplantation of freshly isolated and cryopreserved pancreatic islets in type 1 (insulin dependent) diabetes mellitus. Diabetologia **34:** 55–58.
7. WARNOCK, G. L., N. M. KNETEMAN, E. RYAN, A. RABINOVITCH & R. V. RAJOTTE. 1992. Long term follow up after transplantation of insulin-producing pancreatic islets into patients with type 1 diabetes mellitus. Diabetologia **35:** 89–95.
8. SCHARP, D. W., P. E. LACY, J. V. SANTIAGO, C. S. McCULLOUGH, L. G. WEIDE, L. FALGUI et al. 1990. Insulin independence after islet transplantation in type 1 diabetic patients. Diabetes **39:** 515–518.
9. KORSGREN, O., L. JANSSON, D. EIZIRIK & A. ANDERSSON. 1991. Functional and morphological differentiation of fetal porcine islet-like clusters after transplantation into nude mice. Diabetologia **34:** 379–386.
10. GROTH, C. G., O. KORSGREN, A. TIBELL, J. TOLLEMAR, E. MOLLER, J. BOLINDER, J.

OSTMAN F. R. REINHOLD, C. HELLERSTROM & A. ANDERSSON. 1994. Transplantation of porcine fetal pancreas to diabetic patients. Lancet **344:** 1402–1404.

11. LUI, X., K. F. FEDERLIN, R. G. BRETZEL, B. J. HERING & M. D. BRENDAL. 1991. Persistent reversal of diabetes by transplantation of fetal pig proislets into nude mice. Diabetes **40:** 858–866.

12. DAVALLI, A. M., Y. OGAWA, L. SCALIA, Y-J. WU, J. HOLLISTER, S. BONNER-WEIR & G. C. WEIR. 1995. Function, mass and replication of porcine and rat islets transplanted into diabetic nude mice. Diabetes **44:** 104–111.

13. RICORDI, C., C. SOCCI, C. DAVALLI, C. STAUDACHER, P. BARO, A. VERTOVA, I. SASSI, F. GAVAZZI, G. POZZA & V. DICARLO. 1989. Isolation of the elusive pig islet. Surgery **107:** 688–694.

14. MARCHETTI, P., R. GIANNARELLI, S. COSIMI, P. MASIELLO, A. COPPELLI, P. VIACAVA & R. NAVALESI. 1995. Massive isolation, morphological and functional characterization, and xenotransplantation of bovine pancreatic islets. Diabetes **44:** 375–381.

15. WRIGHT, J. R., S. POLVI & H. MACLEAN. 1992. Experimental transplantation with principal islets of teleost fish (Brockman Bodies). Long-term function of tilapia islet tissue in diabetic nude mice. Diabetes **41:** 1528–1532.

16. FERBER, S., H. BELTRANDELRIO, J. H. JOHNSON, R. J. NOEL, L. E. CASSIDY, S. CLARK, T. C. BECKER, S. D. HUGHES & C. B. NEWGARD. 1994. GLUT-2 gene transfer into insulinoma cells confers both low and high affinity glucose-stimulated insulin release. J. Biol. Chem. **269:** 11523–11529.

17. KNAACK, D., D. M. FIORE, M. SURANA, M. LEISER, M. LAURANCE, D. FUSCO-DEMANE, O. D. HEGRE, N. FLEISCHER & S. EFRAT. 1994. Clonal insulinoma cell line that stable maintains correct glucose responsiveness. Diabetes **43:** 1413–1417.

18. EFRAT, S., D. FUSCO-DEMANE, H. LEMBERG, O. EMRAN & X. WANG. 1995. Conditional transformation of a pancreatic beta-cell line derived from transgenic mice expressing a tetracycline-regulated oncogene. Proc. Natl. Acad. Sci. USA **92:** 3576–3580.

19. KOVER, K. & W. V. MOORE. 1989. Development of a method for isolation of islets from human fetal pancreas. Diabetes **38:** 917–924.

20. HAYEK, A., G. M. BEATTIE, V. CIRULLI, A. D. LOPEZ, C. RICORDI & J. S. RUBIN. 1995. Growth factor/matrix-induced proliferation of human adult b-cells. Diabetes **44:** 1458–1460.

21. SOCCI, C., C. RICORDI, A. M. DAVALLI, C. STAUDACHER, P. BARO, A. VERTOVA, M. FRESCHI, F. GAVAZZI, S. BRAGHI, G. POZZA & V. DICARLO. 1989. Selection of donors significantly improves pig islet isolation yield. Horm. Metab. Res. **25**(Suppl. 1): 32–35.

22. KIRCHHOF, N., B. J. HERING, V. GEISS, K. FEDERLIN & R. G. BRETZEL. 1994. Evidence for breed-dependent differences in porcine islets of Langerhans. Transplant. Proc. **26:** 616–617.

23. VAN DEIJNEN, J. H. M., C. E. HULSTAERT, G. H. J. WOLTERS & R. VAN SCHILFGAARDE. 1992. Significance of the peri-insulinar extracellular matrix for islet isolation from the pancreas of the rat, dog, pig. Diab. Nutr. Metab. **5**(Suppl. 1): 151–154.

24. MARCHETTI, P., E. H. FINKE, C. SWANSON, A. GERASIMIDI-VAZEOU, D. W. SCHARP, R. NAVALESI & P. E. LACY. 1992. The potential of porcine islet xenotransplantation in the therapy of diabetes. Diab. Nutr. Metab. **5**(Suppl. 1): 151–154.

25. ASPLUND, K., S. WESTMAN & C. HELLERSTRÖM. 1969. Glucose stimulation of insulin secretion from the isolated pancreas of foetal and new born rats. Diabetologia **5:** 260–262.

26. ASPLUND, G. 1973. Dynamics of insulin release from the foetal and neonatal rat pancreas. Europ. J. Clin. Invest. **3:** 338–344.

27. RHOTEN, W. B. 1980. Insulin secretory dynamics during development of rat pancreas. Am. J. Physiol. **239:** E57–E63.

28. HOLE, R. L., M. C. M. PIAN-SMITH & G. W. G. SHARP. 1988. Development of the biphasic response to glucose in fetal and neonatal rat pancreas. Am. J. Physiol. **254:** E167–E174.

29. TUCH, B. E., A. JONES & J. R. TURTLE. 1985. Maturation of the response of human fetal pancreatic explants. Diabetologia **28:** 28–31.

30. KORBUTT, G. S., J. F. ELLIOTT, Z. AO, D. K. SMITH, G. L. WARNOCK & R. V. RAJOTTE.

1996. Large scale isolation, growth, and function of porcine neonatal islet cells. J. Clin. Invest. **97:** 2119–2129.

31. PLATT, J. L., G. M. VERCELLOTTI, A. P. DALMASSO, A. J. MATAS, R. M. BOLMAN, J. S. NAJARIAN & F. H. BACH. 1990. Transplantation of discordant xenografts: A review of progress. Immunol. Today **11:** 450.

32. AUCHINCLOSS, H. JR. 1988. Xenogeneic transplantation. A Review. Transplantation **46:** 1.

33. PLATT, J. L. & F. H. BACH. 1991. The barrier to xenotransplantation. Transplantation **52:** 937.

34. BALDWIN, W. M., III, S. K. PRUIT, R. B. BRAUER, M. R. DAHA & F. SANFLIPPO. 1995. Complement in organ transplantation—Contributions to inflammation, injury and rejection. Transplantation **59:** 797–808.

35. SCHILLING, A., W. LAND, E. PRATSCHKE, K. PIELSTICKER & W. BRENDEL. 1976. Dominant role of complement in the hyperacute xenograft rejection reaction. Surgery, Gynecol. & Obst. **142:** 29–32.

36. PLATT, J. L., R. J. FISCHEL, A. J. MATAS, S. A. REIF, R. M. BOLMAN & F. H. BACH. 1991. Immunopathology of hyperacute xenograft rejection in a swine-to-primate model. Transplantation **52:** 214–220.

37. GALILI, U. 1993. Interaction of the natural anti-Gal antibody with alfa-galactosyl epitopes: A major obstacle for xenotransplantation in human. Immunol. Today **14:** 480.

38. SANDRIN, M. S., H. A. VAUGHAN, P. L. DABOWSKI & I. F. MCKENZIE. 1993. Anti-pig IgM antibodies in human serum react predominantly with Galα(1-3)Gal epitopes. Proc. Natl. Acad. Sci. USA **90:** 11391–11395.

39. COOPER, D. K., A. H. GOOD, E. KOREN, R. ORIOL, A. J. MALCOLM, R. M. IPPOLITO, F. A. NEETHLING, Y. YE, E. ROMANO & N. ZUHDI. 1993. Identification of α-galactosyl and other carbohydrate epitopes that are bound by human antipig antibodies: Relevance to discordant xenografting in man. Transplant. Immunol. **1:** 198–205.

40. VAUGHAN, H. A., B. E. LOVELAND & M. SANDRIN. 1994. GALα(1,3)GAL is the major xenoepitope expressed on pig endothelial cells recognized by naturally occurring cytotoxic human antibodies. Transplantation **58:** 879–882.

41. ORIOL, R., Y. YE, E. KOREN & D. K. COOPER. 1993. Carbohydrate antigens of pig tissues reacting with human natural antibodies as potential targets for hyperacute vascular rejection in pig-to-man organ xenotransplantation. Transplantation **56:** 1433–1442.

42. SANDRIN, M. S. 1994. Distribution of the major xenoantigen ((galα1,3)gal) for pig-to-human xenografts. Transplant. Immunol. **112:** 293.

43. MCKENZIE, I. F., M. KOULMANDA, T. E. MANDEL, P-X. XING & M. S. SANDRIN. 1995. Pig-to-human xenotransplantation: The expression of Galα(1-3)Gal epitopes on pig islet cells. Xenotransplantation **2:** 1–7.

44. RYDBERG, L., C. G. GROTH, E. MOLLER, A. TIBELL & B. E. SAMUELSSON. 1995. Is the Galα(1,3)Gal epitope a major target for human xenoantibodies on pig fetal islet cells? Xenotransplantation **2:** 148–153.

45. HAMELMANN, W., D. W. GRAY, T. D. CAIRNS, T. OZASA, D. J. FERGUSON, A. CAHILL, K. I. WELSH & P. J. MORRIS. 1994. Immediate destruction of xenogeneic islets in a primate model. Transplantation **58:** 1109–1114.

46. KORBUTT, G. S., L. J. ASPESLET, R. V. RAJOTTE, G. L. WARNOCK, Z. AO, J. EZEKOWITZ, A. J. MALCOM, A. KOSHAL & R. W. YATSCOFF. 1996. Natural human antibody-mediated destruction of porcine neonatal islet cell grafts. Xenotransplantation **3:** 207–216.

47. MONACO, A. P., T. MAKI, H. OZATO, M. CARRETA, S. J. SULLIVAN, K. M. BORLAND, M. D. MAHONEY, W. L. CHICK, T. E. MULLER, J. WOLFRUM & B. SOLOMON. 1991. Transplantation of islet allografts and xenografts in totally pancreatectomized diabetic dogs using the hybrid artificial pancreas. Am. Surg. **214:** 339–362.

48. LACY, P. E., O. D. HEGRE, A. GERASIMIDI-VAZEOU, F. T. GENTILE & K. E. DIONNE. 1991. Maintenance of normoglycemia in diabetic mice by subcutaneous xenografts of encapsulated islets. Science **254:** 1782–1874.

49. SUN, Y., X. MA, D. ZHOU, I. VACEK & A. M. SUN. 1996. Normalization of diabetes in spontaneously diabetic cynomologus monkeys by xenografts of microencapsulated porcine islets without immunosuppression. J. Clin. Invest. **98:** 1417–1422.

50. Ao, Z., K. Matayoshi, J. R. T. Lakey, R. V. Rajotte & G. L. Warnock. 1993. Survival and function of purified islets in the omental pouch site of outbred dogs. Transplantation **56:** 524–529.
51. Brendal, M. D., S. S. Kong, R. Alejandro & D. H. Mintz. 1994. Improved functional survival of human islets of Langerhans in three-dimensional matrix culture. Cell Transplant. **3:** 427–435.
52. Rajotte, R. V., G. L. Warnock, L. C. Bruch & A. W. Procyshn. 1983. Transplantation of cryopreserved and fresh rat islets and canine pancreatic fragments: Comparison of cryopreservation protocols. Cryopreservation **20:** 169–184.

Alginate-based Microcapsules for Immunoprotected Islet Transplantation[a]

ULRIKE SIEBERS,[b] ANDREA HORCHER,
REINHARD G. BRETZEL, KONRAD FEDERLIN, AND
TOBIAS ZEKORN

Medizinische Klinik III und Poliklinik
Justus-Liebig-Universität
Rodthohl 6
D-35385 Giessen, Germany

Insulin-dependent diabetes mellitus is still a disease of major concern in health care. Although metabolic control can be achieved by insulin treatment, even the intensified therapy regimen is not able to prevent all secondary complications as has been shown in the DCCT study. Moreover, tight metabolic control which is essential to improve the long-term prognosis of the disease is accompanied by a higher risk for severe hypoglycemic events.[1] Therefore, an ideal diabetes treatment would provide insulin delivery by a closed loop system. Replacement of the insulin producing cell by islet transplantation is an attractive therapeutic approach and successful clinical islet transplantations have already documented this.[2,3] But, islet transplantation necessitates a permanent immunosuppressive drug therapy with the risk of side effects. Thus, at the moment only patients with advanced secondary complications, most of them in need of a kidney transplant for endstage renal failure, have been considered for islet cell transplantation. Transplantation of encapsulated islets could potentially circumvent this problem and offer an attractive alternative perhaps even for a xenogeneic approach.

Microencapsulation of islets for transplantation was introduced by Lim and Sun in 1980[4] using alginate-polylysine capsules. In principle, this technique is still used by most of the researchers although some modifications, for example concerning the concentrations of the different solutions, have been introduced.[5,6] We have developed an alginate-based microcapsule by complexing the alginate with barium instead of calcium.[7] The affinity of barium to alginate is higher than that of calcium, so that an additional complexation with a polyamino acid like poly-l-lysin is not necessary to provide biostability.[7] Other encapsulation materials, for example agarose, have been tested by only a few groups.[8]

Characteristics of Alginate

Alginate, the encapsulation material most commonly used, is a collective name for a variety of substances that share their origin from seaweeds and their general

---

[a] This work was supported by a grant from the Bundesminister für Forschung und Technologie, Bonn, Germany (FKZ 0702480A).
[b] Address correspondence to Dr. Siebers at Institut für Humangenetik, Universität Münster, Vesaliusweg 12-14, D-48149 Münster, Germany; Tel: 49-251-8355412; Fax: 49-251-8356995.

composition of 1–4 linked β-D-mannuronic acid and alpha-L-guluronic acid. The M and G subunits may occur as homopolymeric regions (M-blocks or G-blocks) or show an alternating structure (MG-blocks). The overall M:G ratio and the distribution of the different blocks throughout the individual alginate seem to influence not only the biomechanical properties of the gel but also its immunogenicity *in vitro* and *in vivo*. Otterlei *et al.*[9] showed that poly-M-blocks were potent stimulators of TNF-alpha release by human monocytes *in vitro* whereas poly-G-blocks did not increase production of TNF-alpha, IL-1 or IL-6. Nevertheless, isolated poly-M-blocks were much more efficient than high-M alginates (by approximately a factor of 10). The same group[10] postulated an involvement of the LPS receptor CD 14 in this process. Data from our own work suggest that high-M alginates do not necessarily induce a higher stimulation of IL-1 release of human mononuclear cells than high-G alginates (unpublished data).

Biocompatibility of Alginate

The impact of the M : G ratio for biocompatibility of the capsules is controversial. Soon-Shiong *et al.*[11] observed a cellular overgrowth of 90% of the capsules when high-M alginate was used whereas alginate capsules of low M content were largely free of overgrowth. In contrast, Clayton *et al.*[12] reported the weakest reaction in high-M alginates. This contradiction might be due to different animal models and different implantation sites but moreover the influence of other features of alginates (*e.g.*, molecular size, viscosity, charges, impurities) have to be taken into account. Zimmermann *et al.*[13] analyzed raw alginate by free flow electrophoresis and showed that commercial alginates contained at least 10–20 fractions with different electrophoretic mobility which induced lymphocyte proliferation *in vitro*. After purification lymphocyte proliferation *in vitro* was reduced to background levels and the inflammatory response *in vivo* was attenuated.[14]

Microencapsulated Transplantation

Successful transplantation of microencapsulated islets has been demonstrated by several groups in different animal models including rodent models of chemically induced diabetes[15,16] and autoimmune models of diabetes like the BB-rat[17] and the NOD mouse.[18] There are also reports on graft failure especially in the autoimmune recipients[19] and in xenotransplantation.[20] Moreover, the results must be cautiously interpreted since normalized blood glucose values do not necessarily prove graft function, especially in fasting animals. Chicheportiche *et al.*[21] clearly demonstrated that after transplantation of microencapsulated porcine islets into streptozotocin diabetic rats normoglycemia was sustained although no porcine insulin could be detected by HPLC. Fritschy *et al.*[22] showed that in rats transplanted with microencapsulated allogeneic islets non-fasting blood glucose levels were normalized but insulin response in the glucose tolerance test was severely impaired.

In the analysis of the possible mechanisms of graft failure after microencapsulated transplantation, unspecific inflammatory processes towards the material and the procedure have to be considered as well as specific immunological interactions between the grafted tissue and the immune system of the host via the semipermeable membrane.

TABLE 1. Initial and Long-Term (>100 days) Graft Function after Intraperitoneal Transplantation of 3500 Microencapsulated Islets in STZ Diabetic Lewis Rats for Syngeneic vs. Allogeneic (Wistar) vs. Immunomodulated Allogeneic Islets

	Primary Graft Function	Long-term Graft Function
Syngeneic mc islets	6/7	6/7
Allogeneic mc islets	9/12	2/12
Immunomodulated allo mc islets	10/10	7/10

Data are given as number of functioning grafts/total number of transplanted animals. Graft function was assumed if non-fasting blood glucose was below 11 mmol/L.

EXPERIMENTAL RESULTS AND DISCUSSION

Transplantation Experiments

Transplantation of islets encapsulated in barium alginate beads into streptozo-tocin diabetic rat recipients resulted in normoglycemia in the non-fasting animal. Rat islets were isolated by ductal distension and collagenase digestion followed by a purification on a BSA gradient. Islets were cultured overnight under standard conditions prior to encapsulation. For encapsulation islets were suspended in a 2% w/v suspension of purified alginate (kindly provided by Prof. U. Zimmermann, Lehrstuhl für Biotechnologie, Universität Würzburg, Germany) and droplets were formed by a spraying technique using a homemade nozzle with a surrounding air stream.[7] Hydrogel formation was achieved by complexing the alginate with a 20 mMol solution of bariumchloride. Afterwards, the islets were washed three times with buffered sodiumchloride and cultured for 12 hours before transplantation. In the case of immunomodulated islets, a low-temperature culture of 14 days at 22 Celsius was performed prior to encapsulation; 3500 microencapsulated islets were transplanted into the peritoneal cavity of streptozotozin-diabetic Lewis rats. Trans-plantation was performed in three categories: syngeneic (Lewis-to Lewis), allogeneic (Wistar-to-Lewis), allogeneic with immunomodulation (Wistar-to-Lewis, low-tem-perature culture). Graft function was assumed if the non-fasting, random blood glucose level was below 11 mMol. Transplantation of non-encapsulated syngeneic islets unexpectedly revealed the need for a higher number of islets for the correction of diabetes in the intraperitoneal site[16] indicating a protective effect of the matrix. After syngeneic microencapsulated transplantation 6 out of 7 animals showed an initial normalization of the blood glucose values and all of the primary functioning grafts remained so until the end of the experiment at day 105. In contrast, allogeneic transplantation (Wistar-to-Lewis) resulted in an initial graft function of about 75% with a decline over time leading to a percentage of approximately 20% of functioning grafts after 105 days. However, when allogeneic islets were pretreated with immu-noaltering low temperature culture prior to encapsulation, a long-term function of 70% was achieved which was not significantly different from the syngeneic controls (TABLE 1). These results indicate that an interaction between the grafted tissue and the host takes place despite the barrier of the capsule impeding direct cell to cell contact.[23] Histologically, capsules that were retrieved after graft failure showed an increased overgrowth by fibroblasts and inflammatory cells.

Tissue Reaction towards Encapsulated Islets beneath the Kidney Capsule

Transplantation of a subtherapeutic dose of encapsulated islets beneath the kidney capsulse of non-diabetic Lewis rats resulted in an increasing reaction from syngeneic to allogeneic and xenogeneic grafts (Figs. 1–3). The inflammatory response towards the capsule containing allogeneic or xenogeneic cells may be due to allo- or xenoantigens that are released out of the alginate gel. Unexpectedly, encapsulated syngeneic islets also caused a minor reaction whereas empty microcapsules produced from the same alginate preparation did not show any cellular overgrowth on the light microscopical level. Interestingly, this reaction could not be observed after transplantation of non-encapsulated islets beneath the kidney capsule in the syngeneic model. Explanations for this observation are still highly speculative. We hypothesize that some islet products, perhaps even insulin itself, may act as growth factors. Moreover, after transplantation of non-vascularized tissue a certain percentage of the cells presumably are prone to cell death due to hypoxia and/or malnutrition. In case of encapsulated grafts, the host effector mechanisms to eliminate cell debris, especially the phagocytes, are not able to reach the necrotic cells and therefore the frustrane reaction might result in an increased fibrous tissue

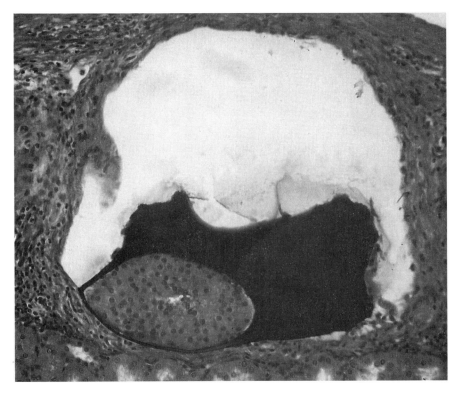

FIGURE 1. *Syngeneic* microencapsulated islets beneath the kidney capsule of Lewis rat 21 days after transplantation. H.-E. staining (magnification × 200).

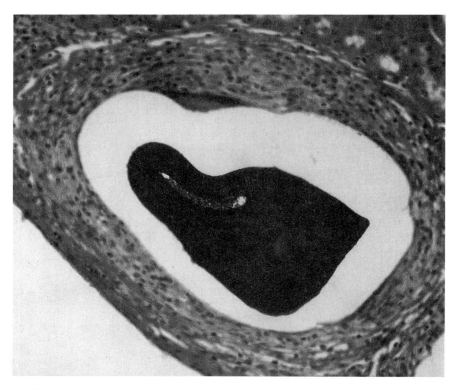

FIGURE 2. *Allogeneic* (Wistar) microencapsulated islets beneath the kidney capsule of Lewis rat 21 days after transplantation. H.-E. staining (magnification × 200).

formation. These findings underline that not only specific immunological interactions but as well non-specific mechanisms are involved in fibrogenicity.

Cellular Reaction towards Encapsulated Islets in Vitro (MLIC)

In vitro, a cellular immune response against encapsulated islets occurred during the mixed lymphocyte islet culture (MLIC), probably due to antigen release. After coculture of mouse splenocytes with rat islets the proliferation was significantly reduced in case of encapsulated islets compared with naked islets, but in comparison to empty microcapsules there was still an induction of a cellular reaction by the encapsulated graft.[24] The data for alginate polylysine and barium alginate capsules did not differ in this respect. Weber *et al.*[25] demonstrated an induction of IgG and IgM antibody production after encapsulated xenotransplantation. Empty capsules themselves did not initiate a humoral response. Thus, recognition occurs on a humoral level as well.

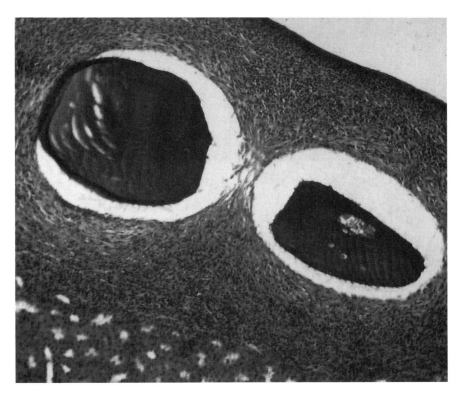

FIGURE 3. *Xenogeneic* (porcine) microencapsulated islets beneath the kidney capsule of Lewis rat 21 days after transplantation. H.-E. staining (magnification × 100).

Summary and Outlook

In conclusion, our own data, as well as studies by other groups, suggest that encapsulation of tissue in alginate-based microcapsules as they are currently used does not provide a strict immunoisolation. Encapsulation creates rather a sort of immunoprivileged transplantation site preventing direct cell to cell contact. Activation of the host's immune system by specific and unspecific factors that are released by the encapsulated graft via the semipermeable membrane seem to play a crucial role as a trigger of the cellular and humoral response. This might result in a vicious circle for example of macrophage activation by islet products leading to further islet damage presumably via cytokine release and other substances which are known to be toxic to islet cells such as nitric oxide or free radicals. In order to avoid these deleterious effects, modifications of the molecular cut off of the capsule and/or modulation of the grafted tissue prior to encapsulation are necessary. From the immunological point of view, the factors initiating and triggering the reaction should be identified in order to provide a rationale for the technical development. Further progress in encapsulation technology is an indispensable prerequisite to improve transplantation outcome. This will hopefully lead to successful transplantation without the need for long-term immunosuppression.

SUMMARY

Islet transplantation is a promising therapeutic approach for the treatment of insulin-dependent diabetes mellitus. Nevertheless, its broader clinical use is hampered by the shortage of human organ donors as well as the need for a permanent immunosuppressive drug therapy in order to avoid rejection. Microencapsulation shall help to overcome this problem by creating an immunoprotected transplantation site. Biocompatibility of the encapsulation material and the possible immuno-interaction of the grafted tissue and the host immune system need to be examined very carefully. In transplantation experiments, we could show that the long-term function of the graft is dependent on the species of the islet donor, indicating that there has to be a recognition of the encapsulated islet despite the encapsulation membrane. This could be confirmed by *in vitro* data in the mixed lymphocyte islet culture (MLIC). Moreover, morphological studies of the tissue reaction towards encapsulated syngeneic vs. allogeneic vs. xenogeneic encapsulated islets reveal that the greater the difference between donor and recipient species the greater the amount of fibrous tissue formation. Thus, for the outcome of transplantation experiments, not only the material-related biocompatibility but as well the reaction towards the whole device (consisting of the capsule plus the encapsulated tissue) are crucial. Therefore, immunoprotection does not only comprise the protection of the grafted tissue from the host immune effector mechanisms but as well the inhibition of the recognition of the graft by the host immune system.

ACKNOWLEDGMENTS

The authors thank Claudia Fett, Gabriele Gruber and Uta Röhm for excellent technical assistance. Moreover, we thank Dr. G. Klöck and Prof. U. Zimmermann (Institut für Biotechnologie, Universität Würzburg, Germany) for supplying us with purified alginates.

REFERENCES

1. DCCT RESEARCH GROUP. 1993. The effect of intensive treatment of diabetes on the development and progression of long-term complications in insulin-dependent diabetes mellitus. New Engl. J. Med. **329:** 977–986.
2. SCHARP, D. W., P. E. LACY, J. V. SANTIAGO, C. S. MCCULLOUGH, L. G. WEIDE, L. FALQUI, P. MARCHETTI, R. L. GINGERICH, A. S. JAFFE, P. E. CRYER *et al.* 1990. Insulin independence after islet transplantation into type I diabetic patient. Diabetes **39:** 515–518.
3. CARROLL, P. B., C. RICCORDI, H. R. RILO, P. FONTES, R. KHAN, A. G. TZAKIS, R. SHAPIRO, J. J. FUNG & T. E. STARZL. 1992. Intrahepatic human islet transplantation at the university of Pittsburgh: Results in 25 consecutive cases. Transplant. Proc. **24:** 3038–3039.
4. LIM, F. & A. M. SUN. 1980. Microencapsulated islets as bioartificial endocrine pancreas. Science **210:** 908–910.
5. CALAFIORE, R., N. KOH, F. CIVANTOS, F. L. SHIENVOLD, S. D. NEEDELL & R. ALEJANDRO.

1986. Xenotransplantation of microencapsulated canine islets in diabetic mice. Trans. Ass. Am. Phys. **99:** 29–33.

6. FRITSCHY, W. M., G. H. J. WOLTERS & R. VAN SCHILFGAARDE. 1991. Effect of alginate polylysine alginate microencapsulation on in vitro insulin release from rat pancreatic islets. Diabetes **40:** 37–43.

7. ZEKORN, T., A. HORCHER, U. SIEBERS, G. KLÖCK, U. ZIMMERMANN, K. FEDERLIN & R. G. BRETZEL. 1992. Barium-cross-linked alginate beads: A simple one-step-method for successful immuno isolated transplantation of islets of Langerhans. Acta Diabetologica **29:** 99–106.

8. IWATA, H., H. AMEMIYA, T. MATSUDA, H. TAKANO, R. HAYASHI & T. AKUTSU. 1992. Agarose for a bioartificial pancreas. J. Biomed. Mater. Res. **26:** 967–977.

9. OTTERLEI, M., A. SUNDAN, G. SKJAK-BRAEK, L. RYAN, O. SMIDSROD & T. ESPEVIK. 1993. Similar mechanisms of action of defined polysaccharides and lipopolysaccharides: Characterization of binding and tumor necrosis factor alpha induction. Infect. Immunity **61/5:** 1917–1925.

10. ESPEVIK, T., M. OTTERLEI, G. SKJAK-BRAEK, L. RYAN, S. D. WRIGHT & A. SUNDAN. 1993. The involvement of CD 14 in stimulation of cytokine production by uronic acid polymers. Eur. J. Immunol. **23:** 255–261.

11. SOON-SHIONG, P., M. OTTERLEI, G. SKJAK-BRAEK, O. SMIDSROD, R. HEINTZ, R. P. LANZA & T. ESPEVIK. 1991. An immunologic basis for the fibrotic reaction to implanted microcapsules. Transplant. Proc. **23:** 758–759.

12. CLAYTON, H. A., N. J. M. LONDON, P. S. COLLOBY, P. R. F. BELL & R. F. L. JAMES. 1991. The effect of capsule composition on the biocompatibility of alginate-poly-l-lysine capsules. J. Microencapsulation **8:** 221–233.

13. ZIMMERMANN, U., G. KLÖCK, K. FEDERLIN, K. HANNIG, M. KOWALSKI, R. G. BRETZEL, A. HORCHER, H. ENTENMANN, U. SIEBERS & T. ZEKORN. 1992. Production of mitogen-contamination free alginates with variable ratios of mannuronic acid to guluronic acid by free flow electrophoresis. Electrophoresis **13:** 269–274.

14. ZEKORN, T., G. KLÖCK, A. HORCHER, U. SIEBERS, M. WÖHRLE, M. KOWALSKI, M. W. ARNOLD, K. FEDERLIN, R. G. BRETZEL & U. ZIMMERMANN. 1992. Lymphoid activation by different crude alginates and the effect of purification. Transplant. Proc. **24:** 2952–2953.

15. AR'RAJAB, A., S. BENGMARK & B. AHREN. 1991. Insulin secretion in streptozotocin-diabetic rats transplanted with immunoisolated islets. Transplantation **51:** 570–574.

16. SIEBERS, U., A. HORCHER, R. G. BRETZEL, G. KLÖCK, U. ZIMMERMANN, K. FEDERLIN & T. ZEKORN. 1993. Transplantation of free and microencapsulated islets in rats: Evidence for the requirement of an increased islet mass for transplantation into the peritoneal site. Int. J. Art. Org. **16:** 35–38.

17. FAN, M. Y., Z. P. LUM, X. W. FU, L. LEVESQUE, I. T. TAI & A. M. SUN. 1991. Reversal of diabetes in BB rats by transplantation of encapsulated pancreatic islets. Diabetes **39:** 519–522.

18. LUM, Z. P., I. T. TAI, M. KRESTOW, J. NORTON, I. VACEK & A. M. SUN. 1991. Prolonged reversal of diabetic state in NOD mice by xenografts of microencapsulated rat islets. Diabetes **40:** 1511–1516.

19. COLE, D. R., M. WATERFALL, M. MCINTYRE & J. D. BAIRD. 1992. Microencapsulated islet grafts in the BB/E rat: A possible role for cytokines in graft failure. Diabetologia **35:** 231–237.

20. DARQUY, S., D. CHICHEPORTICHE, F. CAPRON, C. BOITARD & G. REACH. 1990. Comparative study of microencapsulated rat islets implanted in different diabetic models in mice. *In* Methods in Islet Transplantation Research. K. Federlin, R. G. Bretzel & B. J. Hering, Eds.: 209–213. G. Thieme Verlag.

21. CHICHEPORTICHE, D., S. DARQUY, J. LEPEINTRE, F. CAPRON, P. A. HALBAN & G. REACH. 1990. High-performance liquid chromatography analysis of circulating insulins distinguishes between endogenous insulin production (a potential pitfall with streptozotocin diabetic rats) and islet xenograft function. Diabetologia **33:** 457–461.

22. FRITSCHY, W. M., J. H. STRUBBE, G. H. J. WOLTERS & R. VAN SCHILFGAARDE. 1991.

Glucose tolerance and plasma insulin response to intravenous glucose infusion and test meal in rats with microencapsulated islet allografts. Diabetologia **34:** 542–547.

23.   HORCHER, A., U. SIEBERS, R. G. BRETZEL, K. FEDERLIN & T. ZEKORN. 1995. Transplantation of microencapsulated islets in rats: Influence of low temperature culture before or after the encapsulation procedure on the graft function. Transplant. Proc. **27:** 3232–3233.

24.   ZEKORN, T. D. C., U. ENDL, A. HORCHER, U. SIEBERS, R. G. BRETZEL & K. FEDERLIN. 1995. Evidence for an antigen-release induced cellular response against alginate-polylysine encapsulated islets. Xenotransplantation **2:** 116–119.

25.   WEBER, C., V. D'AGATI, L. WARD, M. COSTANZO, R. RAJOTTE & K. REEMTSMA. 1993. Humoral reaction to microencapsulated rat, canine and porcine islet xenografts in spontaneously diabetic NOD mice. Transplant. Proc. **25:** 462–463.

Alginate/Polyaminoacidic Coherent Microcapsules for Pancreatic Islet Graft Immunoisolation in Diabetic Recipients

RICCARDO CALAFIORE,[a] GIUSEPPE BASTA,[a]
GIOVANNI LUCA,[a] CARLO BOSELLI,[b]
ANDREA BUFALARI,[b] GIAN MARIO GIUSTOZZI,[b]
LUIGI MOGGI,[b] AND PAOLO BRUNETTI[a]

[a]Departments of Internal Medicine and Endocrine
and Metabolic Sciences
University of Perugia
Via E. Dal Pozzo
06126 Perugia, Italy

[b]Istituto di Clinica Chirurgica
Policlinico Monteluce
06100 Perugia, Italy

BACKGROUND

Pancreatic islet cell transplantation could result in restoration of normoglycemia, thereby allowing for withdrawal of exogenous insulin treatment, in patients with insulin-dependent diabetes mellitus (IDDM). However, the invariable requirement for general pharmacological immunosuppression, in order to prevent islet graft-directed immune destruction, strictly limits progress of this approach into clinical trials. Moreover, owing to immunosuppression-related restrictions, only patients with IDDM, who also require transplant of another major organ (*e.g.*, liver, kidney) are usually enrolled in combined liver- or kidney-islet graft trials. Unfortunately this procedure, if ethically correct, invariably cuts off the majority of IDDM-patients, who while not requiring solid organ transplantation, could potentially benefit from this strategy. Finally, the restricted availability of cadaveric human donor pancreata represents, an additional, significant limiting factor.

ISLET GRAFT IMMUNOISOLATION

A potential approach that may circumvent continuous requirement for pharmacological immunosuppression,[1] also offering the opportunity to employ nonhuman tissue (*i.e.*, porcine) as a resource for donor islets, could be islet graft immunoisolation within permselective and biocompatible artificial membranes.[12] These physical barriers, while securing normal biochemical exchange, would interdict access to humoral as well as cellular mediators of the host's immune system.

[a] Tel: +39-75-578-3682; Fax: +39-75-585-2067; E-mail: islet©unipg.it
[b] Tel: +39-75-572-2097; Fax: +39-75-578-3258.

Two different immunoisolatory membrane types have been so far described: 1) macro-devices; 2) microcapsules. The former, that may be variously configured (*i.e.*, planar, laminar, tubular *etc.*), and are implantable into either extra- or intra-vascular sites, in spite of preliminary and even recent encouraging reports,[3] have, so far, missed their ambitious goal towards human applicability, possibly owing to technical problems, depending upon either their excessive size, or tissue-loading restrictions.

On the contrary, microcapsules generally formulated with alginic acid (AG) derivatives, eventually but not necessarily, complexed with polyaminoacids (PA), have gained, over time, evidence of function, mainly in rodents, but also in a limited number of higher mammals, and very preliminarily, in patients with IDDM. The historical recipe, that has represented the cornerstone technology for islet microencapsulation over the past 15 years, consisted of generating islet cell containing AG microdroplets. These were mechanically extruded into a bath comprised of an oppositely charged cation, thereby turning into 600–800 μm hydrogel microspheres, and were finally overlayered with an aminoacidic polycation solution.[4] These AG/PA microcapsules, whose preparative method has been subsequently modified in other laboratories,[5] performed very satisfactorily in rodent animal models of either spontaneous (NOD mice, BB rats) or streptozotocin (STZ)-induced diabetes, where hyperglycemia was fully and consistently reversed over very long periods of time, upon allo- or xenogeneic encapsulated islet transplantation, in our as well as other laboratories.[6,7] Biocompatibility of these membranes was assessed by intraperitoneal graft of empty AG/PA microcapsules in experimental animal models, which was not usually associated with any inflammatory cell infiltration. Generally, success rate of this experimental system depended upon employment of both, highly purified, endotoxin-free biopolymers, and correct microencapsulation procedure, yielding a final molecular weight cut-off (MWCO) that would approximately range from 50 to 70 kD.

Attempts to scale up the microencapsulation system to diabetic higher mammals, and ultimately patients, unfolded, however, a series of technical problems. For instance, unlike successful results accomplished elsewhere,[8] our own experience with intraperitoneal graft of microencapsulated either allogeneic canine, or xenogeneic porcine islets into dogs with spontaneous or artificially-induced diabetes, was consistent with only partial, but never full remission of hyperglycemia. To explain the gap between rodent and canine graft trial results, we speculated that the "encapsulated islet mass/peritoneal surface ratio," while eventually suitable for small size animals, probably was inadequate for large mammals. Each dog, in fact, received an intraperitoneal graft of approximately 80 ml of islet-containing microcapsules, carrying an islet mass which would putatively result in significant metabolic effects. We consistently observed, regardless of whether our dogs, that never took immunosuppressive agents, received grafts of allo-/xenogeneic or autologous islet-containing microspheres, a more or less intense inflammatory infiltrate surrounding the implanted capsules. Of course, the microcapsular fibrotic overgrowth clearly impaired trans-membrane gas/nutrient fluxes.

However, in successful trials of microencapsulated islet transplantation, conducted elsewhere in either dogs, or one patient with IDDM,[9] where normoglycemia apparently was achieved and sustained for long, though ultimately finite, periods of time, the recipients undertook an immunosuppressive course of Cyclosporin. In our opinion, the addition of this drug disturbed the interpretation about whether the transient graft-induced remission of hyperglycemia and subsequent withdrawal of exogenous insulin, solely depended on the capsular barrier's immunoisolatory properties, or rather required a pharmacological extra-protection. Moreover, it still is unclear whether the large volume of islet-containing microcapsules, grafted in the

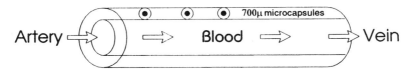

FIGURE 1. Schematic representation of microencapsulated islet containing co-axial vascular prosthesis.

above-mentioned patient,[9] could have triggered a mechanically related inflammatory response. On this purpose, the not necessarily immunologic nature of the peritoneal reactivity was well documented by our own experiments where fibrotic cell overgrowth of encapsulated canine islet autografts was observed over long periods of transplant. Now, it is acknowledged that very recent reports seem to indicate that large AG, PA-uncovered microcapsules, measuring an average 800–1000 μm in equatorial diameter, were able to protect bovine or porcine islet xenografts, and restore long-term normoglycemia in diabetic mice.[10] It also is true, however, that these results were achieved only in a mouse diabetic animal model, whose weakness in terms of immune competence is well known, and not in higher mammals, where low-dose immunosuppression was apparently necessary to obtain an even temporary remission of hyperglycemia.

In an attempt to explore alternative, potentially suitable graft sites for our islet-containing microcapsules, we employed a special vascular coaxial prosthesis, directly anastomosed to blood vessels (FIG. 1). We speculated that such a vascular implant site would significantly improve nutrient and insulin kinetics, thus permitting access to smaller encapsulated islet volumes, as compared with those required by the peritoneal cavity. This assumption was proven to be correct, looking at preliminary results achieved by our vascular implant trials of microencapsulated allo- or xenogeneic islets into nonimmunosuppressed insulin-dependent dogs and patients. In the former, full remission of hyperglycemia and subsequent exogenous insulin withdrawal were accomplished in 2 out of 6 animals, receiving porcine or human encapsulated islet xenografts, with the rest of the dogs showing substantial decline in daily exogenous insulin consumption, within near normal mean blood glucose (MBG) levels.[11] In pilot human clinical studies, we provided evidence of function of encapsulated human islets, embodied within a double chamber vascular prosthesis, which had been grafted as arterial by-passes or A-V shunts, in 2/4 patients with insulin-dependent diabetes. In these responders, C-peptide (CPR) levels significantly rose, as compared to pre-transplant baseline values, and in one case, peaked after 20 days, when the patient was able to discontinue exogenous insulin supplementation, for 1 week (pt. 1). Insulin requirements dropped down by 50–75% of the beginning values, within near normal MBG values (both responder pt. 1 and pt. 2).[12]

DEVELOPMENT OF COHERENT MICROCAPSULES

In light of both our significant experience accumulated with transplant in diabetic high mammals, and the at least theoretical benefits which would derive from reducing the encapsulated islet graft volume, we have undertaken the difficult task of developing a new prototype of coherent microcapsules (CM). The rationale was to generate novel micromembranes that while retaining biocompatibility and immu-

FIGURE 2. Coherent vs. conventional-size microcapsules.

noselective properties, already validated in conventional AG/PA microcapsules, would be able to envelop each individual islet very tightly, so as to eliminate any redundant, idle, dead space between islet and capsule's membrane, a major pitfall of conventional-size microspheres[13] (FIG. 2). Although based on the already-established AG/PA formulation, the originality of our method derived from the completely different and innovative fabricative principle.

Fabricative Procedure

Briefly, following a novel procedure, the isolated islet suspension was thoroughly mixed within a two-phase aqueous emulsification process with poly-ethylene glycol, AG and ficoll. The islet containing emulsion microdroplets underwent immediate gelling upon reaction on calcium chloride, thus becoming solid microspheres, which were then sequentially coated with poly-L-ornithine (PLO) and AG at appropriate molar ratios, so as to avoid any coat wrinkling (FIG. 3).

Morphology of CM and Islet Viability

Light microscopy examination of either empty or islet-containing CM thin sections, upon fixation and staining with Hematoxylin-Eosin (H&E) (FIG. 4), was associated with both full morphologic integrity of multilayered membrane, and virtual elimination of any space between membrane and islet. The enveloped either rat, or canine, or porcine or human islets fully retained their viability at the end of the preparative process as well as after time of *in vitro* culture maintenance. These findings were also confirmed by either scanning or transmission electron microscopy[14] (FIG. 5) and finally laser confocal microscopy examination.

In Vitro *Function of Rat Islets Enveloped in CM*

Batches of rat islets in CM were statically and sequentially incubated for 2-hour time periods, with glucose at different concentrations, showing retention of functional competence by physiologic insulin secretory kinetics in response to glucose stimulation (FIG. 6).

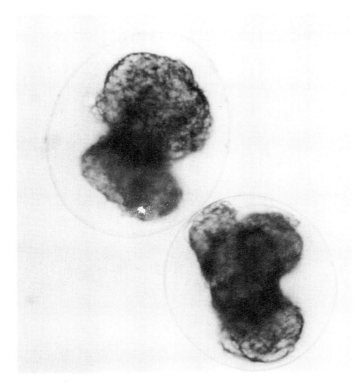

FIGURE 3. Photomicrograph of freshly prepared rat-islet-containing CM under light microscopy.

In Vitro *Immunobarrier Competence of CM*

Either free or encapsulated Wistar/Furth (W/F) rat islets were co-cultured with alloreactive Lewis (Lw) rat splenocytes. Lw splenocyte proliferation occurred with free control, but not encapsulated W/F rat islets, thus confirming immunoprotection from cell-mediated immune aggression. Moreover, either free or encapsulated W/F rat islets were exposed to islet cell antibody (ICA+) positive human sera (>60 JDF U); using a second fluorescein-conjugated (FITC) polyclonal antibody as a revealing system, a classic immunofluorescence pattern was shown by free but not encapsulated islets, thus confirming CM impermeability to Ig.[15]

Biocompatibility

Implant of empty CM beneath the kidney capsule of normal CD-1 mice was associated with complete absence of any inflammatory cell reaction at 30 days of graft, thus proving full acceptance of CM biomaterials.

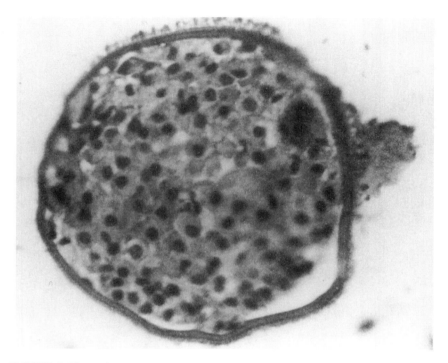

FIGURE 4. Photomicrograph of rat-islet-containing coherent microcapsules (Hematoxylin-Eosin, 40×).

In Vivo *Immunobarrier Competence*

Graft of W/F rat-islet-containing CM beneath the renal sub-capsular space of normal CD-1 mice was associated with full retention of the enveloped islet cell viability and no inflammatory cell overgrowth of the membranes, at 30 days of transplant, upon kidney retrieval and histological examination after H&E staining.

Diabetes Correction and Higher Mammal Viability Studies

Rodents

So far of 5 CD-1 mice with STZ-induced diabetes, receiving intraperitoneal graft of W/F rat-islet-containing CM, all recipients showed normalization of blood glucose for at least 1 month, throughout 90 (2/5) and 140 (1/5) days of transplant. Graft explantation by peritoneal lavage from the animals undergoing recurrence of hyperglycemia, after the initial remission, showed CM that contained no more viable islets but were not surrounded by any inflammatory cell reaction either.

So far of 5 Lw rats with STZ-induced diabetes, transplanted with allogeneic W/F rat islets in CM either intraperitoneally (n = 3), or beneath the renal sub-

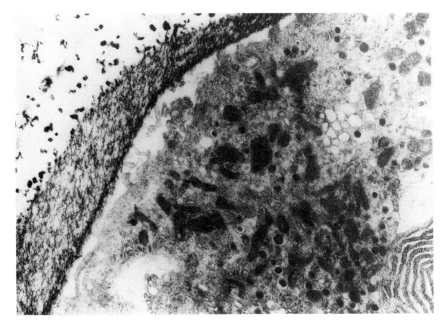

FIGURE 5. Transmission electron photomicrograph of rat-islet-containing coherent microcapsules (× 4600).

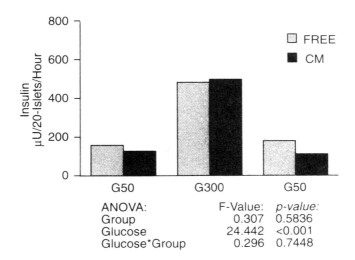

FIGURE 6. *In vitro* insulin secretory patterns of rat-islet-containing coherent microcapsules. coherent microcapsules.

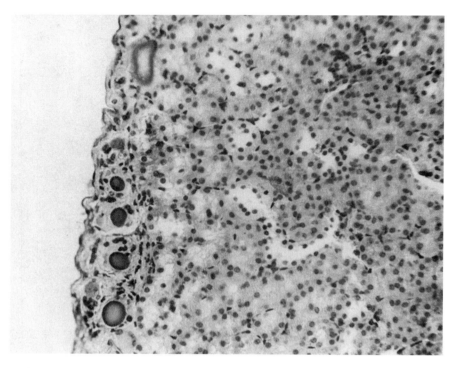

FIGURE 7. Histological section of empty CM in the renal sub-capsular space after 30 days of graft in normal CD-1 mice.

capsular space (n = 2), all showed full normalization of blood glucose which was sustained for at least 30 days in all recipients, and went on for over 80 days in 2/5 recipients. No signs of inflammatory cell reaction were observed upon graft retrieval, with the renal eventually performing better than the peritoneal grafts.

Higher Mammals

Since CM offer the unique opportunity to implant immunoisolated islets within an extremely thin volume, a major advantage associated with this microcapsule type consists of permitting access to graft sites which were previously interdicted to conventional-size microcapsules. These, as above emphasized, were usually implanted in the peritoneal cavity, since, due to their final graft size (120–180 ml in a human recipient) they would not fit any other site. On the contrary, a putative corrective dose of >85% pure, human islets, if enveloped within CM, would occupy only 5–7 ml, thereby becoming eligible for alternative graft sites, including parenchymatous organs.

For this purpose we have begun to explore implantation of allogeneic porcine islets in CM into multiple sites including liver, spleen and omentum of normal pigs.

Initial data seem to demonstrate that CM fully prevent allograft rejection and do not provoke any significant inflammatory cell overgrowth of the capsules. Consequences of these preliminary data on an eventual extension of these technologies into larger cohorts of higher mammals, man included, are implicit.

CONCLUSION

We have established a new prototype of minimal volume AG/PA microcapsules which retain immunoisolatory, biocompatibility and functional properties that seem to match those of conventional-size microcapsules. Since CM tightly envelop each islet, any redundant space between membrane and islet is virtually eliminated. Consequently, these microcapsules occupy an extremely thin space, thus addressing a major problem associated with conventional-size microspheres. Upon demonstration of *in vitro* and *in vivo* CMs' immunoisolatory capacity, retention of enveloped islet viability, and full biocompatibility, we have initiated transplant of either nondiscordant xenogeneic, or allogeneic rat-islet-containing CM into diabetic mice and rats, respectively. Full remission of hyperglycemia was accomplished in 100% of the recipients for at least 1 month, and sustained in some of them for extraordinary long periods of time, throughout 140 days of post-transplant follow-up. Since islet-containing CM final graft volume would not exceed a few ml, in a large mammal, alternative and multiple implant sites might be considered for graft with these new membranes. This opportunity could potentially help resolution of technical problems, associated with conventional-size microcapsules, by permitting access to multiple sites which might better suit requirements for both engraftment capability and metabolic function of the implanted islets.

REFERENCES

1. WARNOCK, G. L., N. M. KNETEMAN, E. A. RYAN, A. RABINOVITCH & R. V. RAJOTTE. 1992. Long-term follow-up after transplantation of insulin producing pancreatic islets into patient with type I diabetes mellitus. Diabetologia **35:** 89–95.
2. COLTON, C. K. 1995. Implantable biohybrid artificial organs. Cell Transplantation **4(4):** 415–436.
3. MAKI, T., I. OTSU, J. J. O'NEIL, K. DUNLEAVY, C. J. P. MULLON, B. A. SOLOMON & A. P. MONACO. 1996. Treatment of diabetes by xenogeneic islets without immunosuppression: Use of a vascularized bioartificial pancreas. Diabetes **45(3):** 342–347
4. LIM, F. & A. M. SUN. 1980. Microencapsulated islets as bioartificial endocrine pancreas. Science **210:** 908–910.
5. CALAFIORE, R., G. BASTA, A. FALORNI, F. CALCINARO, M. PIETROPAOLO & P. BRUNETTI. 1992. A method for the large-scale production of microencapsulated islets: In vitro and in vivo results. Diab. Nutr. Metab. **5:** 23–29.
6. FAN, M. Y., Z. P. LUM, X. W. FU, L. LEVESQUE, I. T. TAI & A. M. SUN. 1990. Reversal of diabetes in BB rats by transplantation of encapsulated pancreatic islets. Diabetes **39:** 519–522.
7. LUM, Z. P., I. T. TAI, M. KRESTOW, J. NORTON, I. VACEKL & A. M. SUN. 1991. Prolonged reversal of diabetic state in NOD mice by xenografts of microencapsulated rat islets. Diabetes **40:** 1511–1516.
8. SOON-SHIONG, P., E. FELDMAN, R. NELSON, J. KOMTEDEBBE, O. SMIDSROD, G. SKJAK-BRAEK, T. ESPEVIK, R. HENITZ & M. LEE. 1992. Successful reversal of spontaneous diabetes in dogs by intraperitoneal microencapsulated islets. Transplantation **54:** 769–774.
9. SOON-SHIONG, P., R. HEINTZ, N. MERIDETH, Q. X. YAO, Z. YAO, T. ZHENG, M. MURPHY,

M. K. MOLONEY, M. SCHMEHL, M. HARRIS, R. MENDEZ, R. MENDEZ & P. A. SANFORD. 1994. Insulin-independence in a type I diabetic patient after encapsulated islet transplantation. Lancet **343:** 950–951.

10. LANZA, R. P., W. M. KUHTREIBER, D. ECKER, J. E. STARUK & W. L. CHICK. 1995. Xenotransplantation of porcine and bovine islets without immunosuppression using uncoated alginate microspheres. Transplantation **59:** 1378–1384.

11. BRUNETTI, P., G. BASTA, A. FALORNI, F. CALCINARO, M. PIETROPAOLO & R. CALAFIORE. 1991. Immunoprotection of pancreatic islet grafts within artificial microcapsules. Int. J. Artif. Organs **14:** 789–791.

12. CALAFIORE, R., G. BASTA, A. FALORNI, G. BROTZU, D. ALFANI, R. CORTESINI & P. BRUNETTI. 1991. Vascular graft of microencapsulated human pancreatic islets in nonimmunosuppressed diabetic recipients: Preliminary results. Diab. Nutr. Metab. **4:** 45–48.

13. BASTA, G., L. OSTICIOLI, M. E. ROSSODIVITA, P. SARCHIELLI, C. TORTOIOLI, P. BRUNETTI & R. CALAFIORE. 1995. Method for fabrication of coherent microcapsules: A new, potential immunoisolatory barrier for pancreatic islet transplantation. Diab. Nutr. Metab. **8:** 105–112.

14. BASTA, G., M. E. ROSSODIVITA, L. OSTICIOLI, G. LUCA, P. BRUNETTI & R. CALAFIORE. 1996. Ultrastructural examination of pancreatic islet containing alginate/polyaminoacidic coherent microcapsules. J. Submicrosc. Cytol. Pathol. **28(2):** 209–213.

15. CALAFIORE, R., G. BASTA, P. SARCHIELLI, G. LUCA, C. TORTOIOLI & P. BRUNETTI. 1996. A rapid qualitative method to assess in vitro immunobarrier competence of pancreatic islet containing alginate/polyaminoacidic microcapsules. Acta Diabetologica **33:** 150–153.

Immunoisolation Strategies for the Transplantation of Pancreatic Islets

ROBERT P. LANZA[a] AND WILLIAM L. CHICK

BioHybrid Technologies Inc.
910 Boston Turnpike
Shrewsbury, Massachusetts 01545

Diabetes mellitus is a leading cause of morbidity and premature mortality in the world. For seventy-five years—since the discovery of insulin—there has been no major new therapy for the disease. There is hope that the transplantation of islets of Langerhans will not only eliminate the need for daily insulin injections, but will prove effective in preventing or retarding the development of complications associated with diabetes. In fact, restoration of normal glucose metabolism has already been achieved in diabetic patients by the transplantation of isolated human islets.[1] Unfortunately, the requirement for immunosuppressive drugs exposes these patients to a wide variety of problems, sometimes causing serious complications such as cancer, infection, renal failure and/or osteoporosis. Ultimately, however, the goal of islet transplantation is to treat patients without immunosuppression. Encapsulation of islets in immunoisolation devices offers a distinct advantage in this respect. Unlike solid organs, islets can be readily isolated from the immune system of the host by a selectively permeable membrane without interfering with their physiological function. Low molecular weight substances such as nutrients, oxygen, and insulin are exchanged across the membrane while immunocytes, antibodies and other immune rejection effector mechanisms are excluded.[2] These systems may also modulate the bidirectional diffusion of antigens, cytokines and other smaller immunological moieties based on the characteristics of the selectively permeable membrane and matrix support.

Immunoisolation has the potential not only to allow allogeneic transplantation without immunosuppression, but also to allow the use of animal cells and tissues that would otherwise be nearly impossible to engraft. In the form of a vascular implant (FIG. 1A), the islets can be distributed in a chamber surrounding the membrane, and the device implanted as a shunt in the vascular system.[3-5] Alternatively, the islets can be encapsulated within diffusion chambers (tubular and planar configurations) (FIG. 1B)[6-9] or spherical micro- or macrocapsules (FIG. 1C)[8,9] and placed intraperitoneally,[6-9] subcutaneously[10,11] or in other sites.[12] Results in diabetic animals indicate that these systems can function for periods of several months to more than a year.[13,14] Furthermore, results in spontaneously diabetic animals indicate that both conventional transplant rejection and autoimmune beta cell destruction can be blocked. However, these data also suggest that because of limitations in functional islet longevity, periodic replenishment of islets will be required in patients. In some designs this may pose significant difficulties. Use of biodegradable materials may well help to solve this potential problem by allowing absorption and excretion of implants when the islet cells which they contain become functionally inactive.

[a] Address for correspondence: Robert P. Lanza, M.D., Director, Transplantation Biology, BioHybrid Technologies Inc., 910 Boston Turnpike, Shrewsbury, Massachusetts 01545; Tel: (508) 842-4460; Fax: (508) 842-7535; E-mail: rtla@aol.com

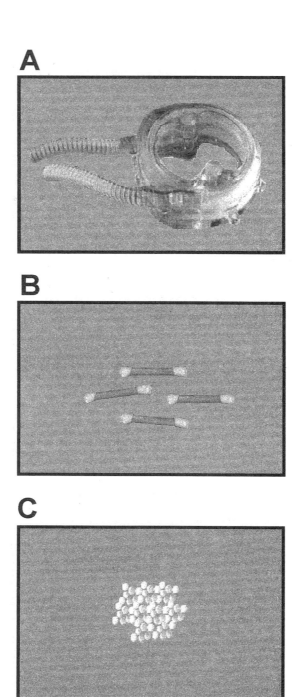

FIGURE 1. Immunoisolation strategies. In the form of a vascular implant (**A**), islets can be distributed in a chamber surrounding a permselective membrane, and the device implanted as a shunt in the vascular system. Alternatively, islets can be immunoisolated within diffusion chambers (tubular or planar configurations) (**B**) or spherical micro- or macrocapsules (**C**) and placed in extravascular sites.

VASCULAR DEVICES

The modern era of biohybrid device development began approximately 2 decades ago with the introduction of islet-containing perfusion devices implanted as AV shunts. The original perfusion devices utilized bundles of capillary fibers seeded on their outside surfaces with isolated islet cells.[15] However, the use of these small diameter fibers as vascular implants was limited to short-term studies because of problems with clotting.[16–18] A device which utilized a coiled tubular membrane with an inner diameter of 5–6 mm was subsequently found to have improved biocompatibility with respect to blood clotting.[19,20] The function of this perfused artificial pancreas was evaluated in diabetic pancreatectomized dogs by implanting devices seeded with canine islet allografts (FIG. 2A).[3] In 2 animals, the devices were removed a year after implantation. In both cases, the exogenous insulin required to control blood glucose concentrations increased by more than 20 U/day after device removal. Data from the implantation of devices containing xenogeneic islets were limited but did indicate that discordant xenografts were also feasible.[19,20] One dog which received devices containing bovine islets demonstrated excellent control of glucose levels for almost 2 months without exogenous insulin. The results using porcine islets showed substantially decreased insulin requirement for up to >9 months.

However, a number of issues remain which appear to limit the therapeutic potential of this approach. Perhaps most importantly, data suggested that the size and geometry of perfusion devices imposed a limitation on the amount of islet tissue that could be transplanted into a patient using a single unit. At present, 2 devices would be required to treat a patient with an insulin requirement of approximately 30–40 U/day. Attempts to lengthen the tubular membrane, thereby increasing insulin secretion, failed because of clotting. In addition, the glycemic control provided by the perfusion device design clearly was not optimal. Nevertheless, much was learned from these studies. They represent an important step toward developing simpler, more viable strategies for transplanting islets using immunoisolation.

EXTRAVASCULAR CHAMBERS

Numerous types of extravascular chambers have also been evaluated.[1,21] The key advantage of these devices, of course, is that they do not require major vascular surgery—particularly in diabetic patients who often have significant vascular disease. Diffusion-based chambers are typically tubular or planar designs; although many geometries have been studied, the most significant progress has been achieved with cylindrical polyacrylonitrile-polyvinyl chloride (PAN-PVC) membrane chambers having a smooth outer skin.[6,22,23] Porcine, bovine, and canine islets transplanted i.p. within these chambers restored normoglycemia in spontaneously diabetic BB and STZ rats for periods of several months to >year.[14,23] While these membranes solved many of the early problems associated with diffusion chambers (e.g., fibrosis, abscess formation, adhesions), studies in large animals closer to man will be required before clinical trials can be contemplated. Experiments in totally pancreatectomized, severely diabetic dogs have in fact already been performed in our laboratory.[6] They indicated that canine islet implants can provide long-term correction of hyperglycemia without the use of immunosuppressive drugs. Insulin independence was achieved for >10 weeks in dogs with preimplantation insulin requirements of 30–40 U/day (FIG. 2B).

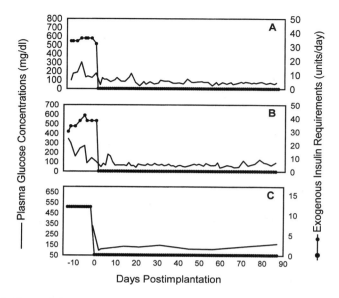

FIGURE 2. Successful treatment of diabetes in dogs using different immunoisolation strategies. Exogenous insulin requirements (●) and blood glucose concentrations (—) before and after implantation of (**A**) a vascular device, (**B**) tubular diffusion chambers, and (**C**) microspheres containing canine islets.

Despite these encouraging results, a number of technical and safety issues critical to the wide scale clinical success of these devices must be addressed. These include long-term biocompatibility, membrane breakage, and suitability for retrieval. Experiments have demonstrated the feasibility of long-term immunoisolation of islets by artificial [PAN-PVC] membranes and the long-term biocompatibility of the membrane versus the graft and versus the recipient.[14,22] These data indicate that islet implants can provide correction of hyperglycemia in dogs and rodents for up to >year without the use of immunosuppressive drugs. Histological examination of the chambers revealed that they were biocompatible. However, most of the implants ultimately failed because of membrane breakage. By 6–8 months postimplantation most of the chambers in dogs had broken. The membranes used in these studies were relatively fragile and susceptible to breakage. An increase in the membrane wall thickness may minimize this problem. Because of limitations imposed by islet longevity, membrane chambers will also eventually require localization and removal. It is unclear whether the devices could be removed by laparoscopy. Surgical excision might be necessary if the chambers were to become fibroencapsulated. Open surgery, of course, carries risk of infection and would involve a more extensive procedure.

MICROCAPSULES

Over the past decade, several methods for microencapsulating islets have been investigated. Microcapsules offer a number of distinct advantages over the use of other encapsulation devices, including 1) greater surface to volume ratio, 2) ease of implantation, and, if necessary, 3) retrievability by lavage and aspiration. Most of the procedures for fabricating microspheres involve extruding a mixture of cells and sodium alginate using a droplet generation device into a $CaCl_2$ solution. The negatively charged gelled droplets can then be coated with positively charged agents such as poly-L-lysine (PLL) to form a permselective membrane.

Small Animal Models

Microencapsulation has been successfully used to reverse diabetes in rodents using islet allografts and concordant (rodent-to-rodent) islet xenografts without immunosuppression.[24–27] Although prolongation of survival of discordant islets has also been achieved with the alginate-PLL technique, these studies have been performed in mice, and have usually required adjunctive treatment with immunosuppressive agents.[28,29] Recently, prolongation of discordant xenograft survival in diabetic mice has been achieved in our laboratory without immunosuppression using alginate microspheres without the synthetic PLL membrane.[30] Uncoated alginate spheres containing porcine and bovine islets routinely reversed hyperglycemia after i.p. injection into diabetic mice. The ability of uncoated microspheres to achieve marked prolongation of discordant xenograft survival is surprising, as the destruction of the grafts might have been expected to occur based on the presence of circulating preformed natural antibodies in the recipients. Our data suggest that complement would also have had access to the encapsulated islet grafts. An explanation for the immunoprotective effect of the alginate spheres also needs to accommodate the fact that cytokines, nitric oxide and other toxic moieties are small enough to diffuse readily into the gel matrix, yet did not induce dysfunction or destruction of the islet graft.

Preliminary experiments suggest that uncoated alginate spheres containing porcine and bovine islets can also reverse hyperglycemia in diabetic rats for extended periods of time (>25 weeks).[31] However, these results have required the use of larger spheres and/or adjunctive treatment with immunosuppressive agents. Of course, the goal of encapsulated islet transplantation is to eliminate the need for immunosuppression altogether. Toward that end, we have developed a new type of encapsulation technology that allows transplantation of islets across a wide species barrier without immunosuppression. These selectively permeable "microreactors" are fabricated from biodegradable polymers which are slowly absorbed and excreted from the body. The microreactors can simply be injected under the skin, or placed i.p. or in other extravascular sites using a needle and syringe. Moreover, the rate of degradation of the microreactors can be adjusted to correspond to the functional longevity of the encapsulated islets. We have successfully tested these microreactors using discordant islet xenografts in several animal models (FIGS. 3 and 4). In one set of experiments, porcine islets were immobilized in reactors and implanted into the peritoneum of NOD mice, and diabetic rats and rabbits. Diabetes was reversed in the animals for periods of several weeks to months without any immunosuppression (FIGS. 1 and 2).

Large Animal Model

Experiments in spontaneously diabetic dogs have also been performed in our laboratory using canine islets encapsulated inside uncoated alginate microspheres.

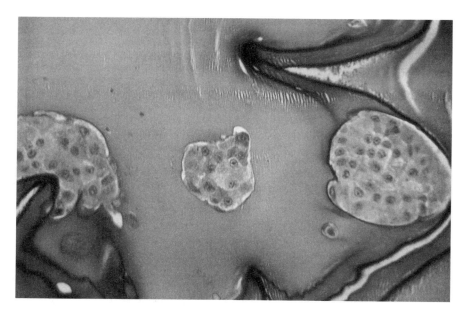

FIGURE 3. Encapsulated porcine islets retrieved from the peritoneal cavity of a rat 20 weeks after xenotransplantation. No immunosuppression was used in this study.

Although low-dose CsA was also administered, by 3 weeks postimplantation the levels of the drug were below detectable limits by HPLC. Intraperitoneal implantation of the microspheres completely supplanted exogenous insulin therapy in the dogs for 60 to >175 days (FIG. 2C). Patrick Soon-Shiong et al.[32] have also reported successful long-term implantations of microencapsulated allografts in larger animals. They treated spontaneous diabetes in dogs that were administered CsA. However, these microspheres were PLL-coated. The implants maintained euglycemia for 63 to 172 days, comparable to the results obtained in our laboratory without the use of a synthetic PLL membrane.

More recently, we have tested our new type of microreactors in dogs using discordant islet tissue. Bovine islets were implanted i.p. in either uncoated alginate spheres or in the new type of selectively permeable microreactors for periods of several weeks. No islets survived in the uncoated alginate spheres, even with the use of triple immunosuppressive therapy (CsA, immuran, and prednisone). However, when the islets were immobilized within the new selectively permeable microreactors, viable tissue was observed both with and without immunosuppression. Immunohistochemical staining of selectively permeable microreactors recovered from these dogs revealed well-granulated α, β, and δ cells consistent with functionally active hormone synthesis and secretion. To test further the secretory function of the islets, the explanted microreactors were incubated in media containing either basal or stimulatory concentrations of glucose. The islets responded with an approximately 4–6-fold average increase above basal insulin secretion. These results, together with data generated using porcine islets transplanted into NOD mice and diabetic rats and rabbits, indicate that long-term survival of discordant islet xeno-

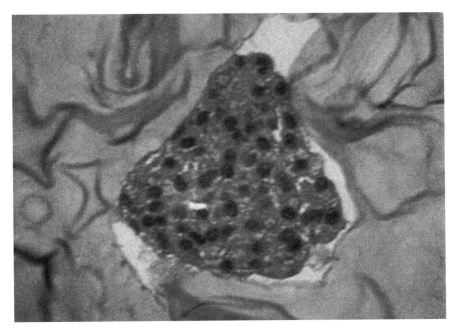

FIGURE 4. Encapsulated porcine islet retrieved from the peritoneal cavity of a spontaneously diabetic NOD mouse one month after xenotransplantation. No immunosuppression was used in this study.

grafts can be achieved in both rodents and dogs without immunosuppressive drugs using microreactors fabricated from biodegradable materials. It will be important to obtain FDA approval to bring this new approach to xenotransplantation to clinical reality.

SUMMARY

The currently limited supply of human pancreatic glands, and the fact that multiple glands may be required to isolate sufficient numbers of islets to treat a single patient, indicate that techniques must be further developed and refined for xenografting of isolated islets from animal sources to diabetic patients. An increasing body of evidence using immunoisolation techniques strongly suggests that this will be achieved during the next few years. Several different types of systems employing selectively permeable membranes and matrix supports for cells have been successfully tested in animals, including devices anastomosed to the vascular system as arteriovenous (AV) shunts, tubular membrane chambers, and spherical micro- and macrocapsules. Results in diabetic animals indicate that these systems can function for periods of several months to >year without the use of any immunosuppression. Our data suggest that this approach has the potential not only to allow the transplantation of islets across wide species barriers, but that it can be achieved using injectable microreactors fabricated from biodegradable polymers. The use of these various immunoisolation systems to transplant islets and other cells and tissues offers the opportunity to revolutionize current therapy for many human diseases.

REFERENCES

1. BRETZEL, R. G., B. J. HERING, A. O. SCHULTZ, C. GEIER & K. FEDERLIN. 1996. International Islet Transplant Registry report. In 1996/97 Yearbook of Cell and Tissue Transplantation. R. P. Lanza & W. L. Chick, Eds.: 153–160. Kluwer Academic Press. Dordrecht.
2. LANZA, R. P., J. L. HAYES & W. L. CHICK. 1996. Encapsulated cell technology. Nature Biotechnol. 14: 1107–1111.
3. SULLIVAN, S. J., T. MAKI, K. M. BORLAND, M. D. MAHONEY, B. A. SOLOMON, T. E. MULLER, A. P. MONACO & W. L. CHICK. 1991. Biohybrid artificial pancreas: Longterm implantation studies in diabetic, pancreatectomized dogs. Science 252: 718–721.
4. LANZA, R. P., S. J. SULLIVAN, A. P. MONACO & W. L. CHICK. 1992. The hybrid artificial pancreas: Diffusion and vascular devices. In Pancreatic Islet Cell Transplantation. C. Ricordi, Ed.: 223–237. R. G. Landes. Austin, TX.
5. MONACO, A. P., T. MAKI, H. OZATO, M. CARRETTA, S. J. SULLIVAN, K. M. BORLAND, M. D. MAHONEY, W. L. CHICK, T. E. MULLER, J. WOLFRUM & B. SOLOMON. 1991. Transplantation of islet allografts and xenografts in totally pancreatectomized diabetic dogs using the hybrid artificial pancreas. Ann. Surg. 214: 339–362.
6. LANZA, R. P., K. M. BORLAND, P. LODGE, M. CARRETTA, S. J. SULLIVAN, T. E. MULLER, B. A. SOLOMON, T. MAKI, A. P. MONACO & W. L. CHICK. 1992. Treatment of severely diabetic, pancreatectomized dogs using a diffusion-based hybrid pancreas. Diabetes 41: 886–889.
7. RACE, J. M., M. LEGRELLE, J. P. BETHOUX, P. H. CUGNENC & J. J. ALTMAN. 1994. Macroencapsulation in small animals. In Pancreatic Islet Transplantation: Volume III, Immunoisolation of Pancreatic Islets. R. P. Lanza & W. L. Chick, Eds.: 133–138. R. G. Landes. Austin, TX.
8. LIM, F. & A. M. SUN. 1980. Microencapsulated islets as bioartificial endocrine pancreas. Science 210: 908.
9. GOOSEN, M. F. A. 1994. Fundamentals of microencapsulation. In Pancreatic Islet Transplantation: Volume III, Immunoisolation of Pancreatic Islets. R. P. Lanza & W. L. Chick, Eds.: 21–43. R. G. Landes. Austin, TX.
10. LACY, P. E., O. D. HEGRE, A. GERASIMIDI-VAZEOU, et al. 1991. Maintenance of normoglycemia in diabetic mice by subcutaneous xenografts of encapsulated islets. Science 254: 1282.
11. VALENTE, U., M. FERRO, C. CAMPISI, et al. 1980. Allogeneic pancreatic islet transplantation by means of artificial membrane chambers in 13 diabetic recipients. Transplant. Proc. 12: 223.
12. ICARD, P., F. PENFORNIS, C. GOTHEIL, et al. 1990. Tissue reaction to implanted bioartificial pancreas in pigs. Transplant. Proc. 22: 724.
13. LANZA, R. P., S. J. SULLIVAN & W. H. CHICK. 1992. Islet transplantation with immunoisolation. Diabetes 41: 1503–1510.
14. LANZA, R. P., A. M. BEYER, J. E. STARUK & W. L. CHICK. 1993. Biohybrid artificial pancreas: Longterm function of discordant islet xenografts in streptozotocin diabetic rats. Transplantation 56: 1067.
15. CHICK, W. L., A. A. LIKE & V. LAURIS. 1975. Beta cell culture on synthetic capillaries: An artificial endocrine pancreas. Science 187: 847–849.
16. TZE, W. J., F. C. WONG & I. M. CHEN. 1976. Implantable artificial endocrine pancreas unit used to restore normoglycemia in the diabetic rat. Nature 264: 466–467.
17. WHITTEMORE, A. D., W. L. CHICK, P. M. GALLETTI, et al. 1977. Effects of the hybrid artificial pancreas in diabetic rats. Trans. Am. Soc. Artif. Intern. Organs 13: 336–340.
18. SUN, A. M., W. PARISIUS, G. M. HEALY, et al. 1977. The use in diabetic rats and monkeys

of artificial capillary units containing cultured islets of Langerhans. Diabetes **26:** 1136–1139.

19. LANZA, R. P., B. A. SOLOMON, A. P. MONACO & W. L. CHICK. 1994. Devices implanted as AV shunts. R. P. Lanza & W. L. Chick, Eds.: 154–168. Pancreatic Islet Transplantation: Volume III, Immunoisolation of Pancreatic Islets. R. G. Landes. Austin, TX.

20. MAKI, T., I. OTSU, J. J. O'NEILL, *et al.* 1996. Treatment of diabetes by xenogeneic islets without immunosuppression. Diabetes **45:** 342–347.

21. COLTON, C. K. 1995. Implantable biohybrid artificial organs. Cell Transplant. **4:** 415–436.

22. LANZA, R. P., D. H. BUTLER, K. M. BORLAND, *et al.* Xenotransplantation of canine, bovine, and porcine islets in diabetic rats without immunosuppression. Proc. Natl. Acad. Sci. USA **88:** 11100–11104.

23. LANZA, R. P., K. M. BORLAND, J. E. STARUK, *et al.* 1992. Transplantation of encapsulated canine islets into spontaneously diabetic BB/Wor rats without immunosuppression. Endocrinology **131:** 637–642.

24. LIM, F. & A. M. SUN. 1980. Microencapsulated islets as bioartificial endocrine pancreas. Science **210:** 908–910.

25. O'SHEA, G. M., M. F. A. GOOSEN & A. M. SUN. 1984. Prolonged survival of transplanted islets of Langerhans encapsulated in a biocompatible membrane. Biochim. Biophys. Acta **804:** 133–136.

26. FAN, M. Y., Z. P. LUM, X. W. FU, *et al.* 1990. Reversal of diabetes in BB rats by transplantation of encapsulated pancreatic islets. Diabetes **39:** 519–522.

27. LUM, Z. P., I. T. TAI, M. KRESTAW, *et al.* 1991. Prolonged reversal of the diabetic state in NOD mice by xenografts of microencapsulated rat islets. Diabetes **40:** 1511–1516.

28. CALAFIORE, R., D. JANJIC, N. KOH & R. ALEJANDRO. 1987. Transplantation of microencapsulated canine islets into NOD mice: Prolongation of survival with superoxide dismutase and catalase. Clin. Res. **35:** 499A.

29. RICKER, A., V. BHATIA, S. BONNER-WEIR & G. EISENBARTH. 1987. Microencapsulated xenogeneic islet grafts in the NOD mouse. Dexamethasone and inflammatory response. Cold Spring Harbor Symposium. October, 1987. p. 53A.

30. LANZA, R. P., W. M. KÜHTREIBER, D. ECKER, *et al.* 1995. Xenotransplantation of porcine and bovine islets without immunosuppression using uncoated alginate microspheres. Transplantation **59:** 1377–1384.

31. LANZA, R. P., D. ECKER, W. M. KÜHTREIBER, *et al.* 1995. A simple method for transplanting discordant islets into rats using alginate gel spheres. Transplantation **59:** 1486–1487.

32. SOON-SHIONG, P., E. FELDMAN, R. NELSON, *et al.* 1993. Long-term reversal of diabetes by the injection of immunoprotected islets. Proc. Natl. Acad. Sci. USA **90:** 5843–5847.

Immunoisolation of Adult Porcine Islets for the Treatment of Diabetes Mellitus

The Use of Photopolymerizable Polyethylene Glycol in the Conformal Coating of Mass-isolated Porcine Islets

RONALD S. HILL,[a,c] GREG M. CRUISE,[b]
STEVE R. HAGER,[a] FRANCIS V. LAMBERTI,[a]
XIAOJIE YU,[a] CARRIE L. GARUFIS,[a] YAO YU,[a]
KAREN E. MUNDWILER,[a] JOHN F. COLE,[a]
JEFFERY A. HUBBELL,[b] ORION D. HEGRE,[a]
AND DAVID W. SCHARP[a]

[a]Neocrin Company
Irvine, California 92718
[b]California Institute of Technology
1200 East California Boulevard
Pasadena, California 91125

Results from the Diabetes Control and Complications Trial (DCCT) demonstrate the benefit of tight glucose control on reducing the vascular complications associated with Type I diabetes.[1] Results from islet allo-transplantation clinical studies clearly demonstrate the ability to achieve the desired level of tight glucose control in the absence of exogenous insulin therapy and without the major risk of such intensive insulin therapy—life threatening episodes of hypoglycemia.[2-4] However, allo-transplantation requires immunosuppression—an unacceptable risk to the newly diagnosed Type I patient with diabetes. Even with the advent of improved and safer immunosuppressive agents, islet allo-transplantation will not have widespread application owing to the shortage of human pancreata.[5]

The goal of the immunoisolation approach is to permit the efficacious transplantation of immunologically disparate islets in the absence of chronic immunosuppression.[6] By encapsulating the insulin producing cells behind a permselective barrier, the cellular and humoral arms of the immune system are prevented from attacking and rejecting the transplant. Because of the shortage of human (allogeneic) islets, alternative sourcing (xenogeneic) is required. Thus the immunoprotective barrier is designed to protect against the immune mediators of xenogeneic rejection (FIG. 1).

ISLET SOURCING

Following extensive animal testing, Neocrin Company has selected a porcine breed in which mass islet isolation can be accomplished from young donors. Classic

[c] Address correspondence to: Ronald S. Hill, Ph.D., Director of Preclinical Studies and Islet Production, Neocrin Company, 31 Technology Drive, Suite 100, Irvine, CA 92718; Tel: (714) 727-1942; Fax: (714) 727-1718; e-mail: rshill@neocrin.com

FIGURE 1. Therapeutic effect of encapsulated islets—the concept of immunoisolation for the protection of physiologically responsive primary porcine islet cells. The preclinical results indicate that PEG encapsulated islets, when transplanted by injection into the peritoneum, achieve *in vivo* functionality similar to islet cells in the native pancreas, absorbing nutrients, monitoring blood glucose levels, and secreting appropriate levels of insulin. The studies also indicate that PEG encapsulation allows these cells to function normally while avoiding the need for chronic immunosuppression.

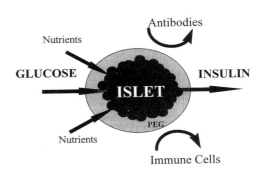

islet isolation methods[7] have been adapted for the efficient procurement of islets from such "market weight" pigs at yields and purities that now make widespread clinical application of islet xenotransplantation (in combination with immunoisolation) a feasible consideration.

A Safe Product: Bioburden and Control

Disease control and surveillance within the donor source herd is essential for such a clinical product. As a first step, the establishment and maintenance of a "closed," Specific Pathogen Free (SPF) herd is required.[8] In addition, the transmission of zoonoses (diseases of one species capable of infecting another) is a safety concern with xenotransplantation. Known porcine zoonotic agents (bacterial, fungal, viral) have been identified and risk management protocols have been implemented. These involve stringent monitoring of the animals at various levels of product production and include the following.

Herd

Serological testing of the breeding stock is in place, monitoring for specific pathogen exposure. Two-site segregated early weaning production techniques are used to reduce the risk of disease transmission.[9] A quarterly slaughter check is conducted on the breeding herd. An example of results obtained from the herd monitoring is shown in TABLE 1. Animals are maintained on a controlled, defined diet.

Individual Donor Animals

Donors are vaccinated against certain agents (swine influenza virus, encephalomyocarditis, Leptospira) and titers monitored. Animals are monitored for passive immunity against certain other agents. Each group of donors is processed in an

TABLE 1. Quarterly Donor Breeding Herd Monitoring

Date	SPF Status	No. Pigs	Vesicular Stomatitis Virus	Bovine Viral Diarrhea Virus	Porcine Reproductive Respiratory Syndrome Virus	Toxoplasmosis	Trichinellosis
7/10/95	Passed	32	0	—	—	0	0
10/9/95	Passed	32	0	0	0	0	0
1/8/96	Passed	36	0	—	—	0	0
4/8/96	Passed	34	0	0	0	0	0
7/8/96	Passed	36	0	0	0	0	0

Notes: The number of pigs sampled provides at the 95% confidence level that one or more positive animals would be detected having a condition at 10% prevalence.

"all-in/all-out" manner.[10] Prior to pancreas processing, donors are quarantined for a minimum of four weeks at Neocrin's SPF Swine Unit. Individual donors are tested serologically for vesicular stomatitis, toxoplasmosis and trichinellosis. At the time of excision of the pancreas, clinical and pathological examinations of the donor are conducted. An example of the results obtained from the individual donor monitoring is shown in TABLE 2. Pancreata from animals that fail to pass the above monitoring are not used for islet isolation.

Islets

Following excision of the pancreas and its preparation for digestion, transport and preservation solutions are monitored for sterility. In-process monitoring for bioburden continues and the final islet product is again screened for endotoxin and mycoplasma as well as bacterial and fungal contamination. In addition, implementation of viral screening of the final islet product (by co-culture and by PCR) is in progress. An example of the results obtained from the processed islet monitoring is shown in TABLE 3. Our data show that any contamination found early in the process is substantially reduced or eliminated by subsequent processing steps. These data were generated prior to the institution of GMP (Good Manufacturing Practice) requirements which would eliminate any lots demonstrating contamination.

TABLE 2. Donor Pig Monitoring during Quarantine: Database Summary Since Full Implementation of Plan on 7/3/95 with Animals Born in February 1995

Pathology Examination[a] n = 826		Vesicular Stomatitis Serology (SVN/CF) n = 754		Toxoplasmosis Serology (MAT) n = 754		Trichinellosis Serology (ELISA) n = 766	
Positive	%	Positive	%	Positive	%	Positive	%
6	0.73	0	0	0	0	0	0

[a] The pathology examination is done immediately after pancreas excision. Pathology detected included lung discoloration with or without fibrin (3), enlarged visceral nodes draining lesioned organs (3), and a tumor (1). These donors would be rejected.

TABLE 3. Microbiological Monitoring of Pancreatic Tissue Processing: 4,927 In-process Samples

Sample Type	No. Samples Tested	No. Samples Positive	% Positive Samples
Pancreas	495	70	14.1
Islets Post-Purification	1495	55	3.7
Islets Pre-Culture	1389	20	1.4
Islets Post-culture	1548	38	2.5

In addition to the above, assessment of unknown potential porcine zoonotic agents (*i.e.*, retrovirus) continues by the Company and by regulatory authorities.[11,12] The possibility exists of recombinant events leading to unique pathogens. The Company views this as remote and of low risk. In addition, preliminary data indicate that permselective membranes, with transport properties similar to those of the Neocrin product, are viral retentive, further reducing the risk of a "clinically relevant" recombinant event. In our view, the far-reaching benefits to the health of the diabetic population far outweigh the risk.

An Efficacious Product: Viability, Purity and Potency and in Vivo Function

TABLE 4 provides an example of the post processing viability, purity and potency of porcine islets produced at Neocrin. At production levels currently attainable, adequate numbers of high quality porcine islets can be produced to take the Company through Phase III clinical trials. Process development steps are currently underway that will allow scale-up to commercial levels.

With this experience, we have been able to establish stringent release criteria for porcine islet preparations: sterile, mycoplasma free, negative endotoxin, viability of >80%, purity of >80% and an acceptable potency level (1.5× stimulation of insulin secretion with high glucose; 5× stimulation with high glucose and IBMX).

TABLE 4. Isolated Porcine Islet Product

	Viability[a]	Purity[b]	Stimulation Index[c]
Analysis Period I[d]	92.0 ± 0.3	94.0 ± 0.3	10.5 ± 0.3
Analysis Period II[e]	97.0 ± 0.1	96.0 ± 0.2	20.3 ± 4.6

[a] Fluorescein diacetate-ethidium bromide viability stain at 24 hr post-isolation (N > 750).
[b] Dithizone positive tissue/total tissue counts × 100 (N > 750).
[c] Ratio of 30 min insulin release at 16.7 mM glucose + 1mM IBMX/30 minute insulin release at 3 mM glucose (N > 50).
[d] Jan–Dec 1995 for viability and purity; Jan-April 1996 for stimulation index.
[e] Jan–Dec 1996 for viability and purity; May-August 1996 for stimulation index.
All values mean ± SEM.

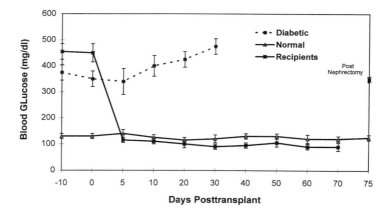

FIGURE 2. Porcine islet function in athymic diabetic mice: Streptozotocin-induced diabetes in the athymic mouse results in persistent hyperglycemia (*dashed line*) and significant mortality within the first month post-induction. Normal control animals run nonfasting blood glucose values of around 120 mg/dl (*triangles*). Following transplantation of free porcine islets beneath the kidney capsule (*stars*), diabetic animals return to normoglycemia and remain normoglycemic until graft removal.

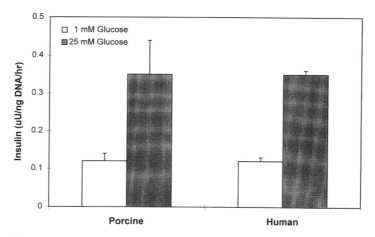

FIGURE 3. Insulin secretion: comparison *in vitro* of porcine and human islets. Collagenase-isolated human and porcine islets were tested in static incubation (modified RPMI with 1% bovine serum albumin at 37°C in 5% CO_2/air) for insulin release in response to glucose stimulation. On a cellular basis, similar amounts of insulin were released under stimulatory conditions suggesting near-equivalency of the two types of islets.

Using the athymic diabetic mouse model, porcine islets can be clearly demonstrated to function *in vivo*. FIGURE 2 shows the data from animals that were transplanted with porcine islets at the kidney subcapsular site. As has been observed previously, a prompt return of recipient blood glucose levels to donor islet-driven normoglycemic values (in this case ~90 mg/dl—normal porcine blood glucose) is observed. Upon removal of the transplanted islets, recipients return to the pretransplant diabetic state.

The equivalency of porcine islets with human islets with regard to insulin secretion are shown in FIGURE 3. Batches of islets were incubated in static culture for 30 minute periods under high and low glucose conditions. The insulin released was then determined by radioimmunoassay and values expressed on a per ng DNA per hour basis. These data suggest that dosages required to treat patients with porcine islets will be similar to those using human islets.

IMMUNOISOLATION BY ENCAPSULATION

Cellular as well as humoral immunity appears to be involved in the rejection of xenogeneic grafts.[13] Immunoisolation by encapsulation attempts to protect the

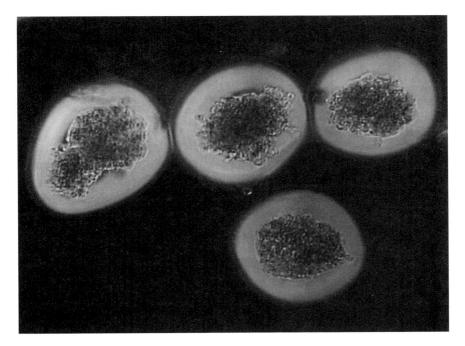

FIGURE 4. Four porcine islets (mean diameter ~ 100 μm) are shown with their PEG coatings. The interfacial polymerization results in an opaque layer of cross-linked PEG extending from the islet surface out about 30 μm terminating in a more translucent zone of about 10 μm. Coating thickness can be varied by controlling the PEG composition and the conditions of polymerization. Phase contrast microscopy, 400×.

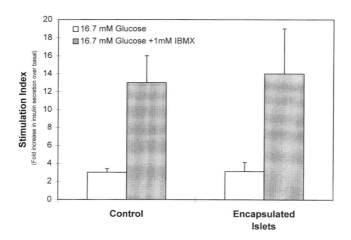

FIGURE 5. Insulin secretory responsiveness: comparison *in vitro* of control and encapsulated islets. Free porcine islets and PEG encapsulated islets were tested in static incubation (modified RPMI with 1% bovine serum albumin at 37°C in 5% CO_2/air) for insulin release in response to glucose stimulation and glucose + IBMX stimulation. These data were compared to insulin release under basal conditions (2.8 mM glucose) and a stimulation index calculated from the ratio of the stimulated value/the basal value. Insulin release was equivalent from encapsulated islets compared to free islets indicating that the presence of the coating did not significantly interfere with the production and release of the islet cell product.

donor tissue from damage using permselective membranes. These membranes are constructed with "functional" pores that prevent the ingress of the immune mediators while still permitting the ingress and egress of nutrients, metabolites and, in the case of islets, insulin. A variety of materials have been investigated; a variety of geometries have been tested.[14,15]

Neocrin's approach utilizes photopolymerizable polyethylene glycol diacrylate (PEG-DA) to form conformal coatings around individual islets.[16] This approach optimizes the loading density (one islet/capsule = 100%) thus minimizing the "size" or volume of the transplant while reducing diffusion distances thus permitting more efficient transport of nutrients, oxygen and insulin across relatively "tight" (higher molecular weight exclusionary) membrane structures.[17]

Photopolymerizable PEG-DA

The backbone starting compounds, polyethylene glycol, are Generally Regarded As Safe (GRAS). Their chemistry is defined and PEG is available in a variety of molecular weights (chain lengths). Neocrin's method for acrylation of the PEG results in a highly purified product with a high degree of acrylation and little if any biologically relevant by-products. Current production levels are adequate through Phase III clinical trials.

Conformal Coating Process

Neocrin's proprietary encapsulation process[18] involves the interfacial polymerization of the PEG-DA molecules at the surface of the islet resulting in a conformal

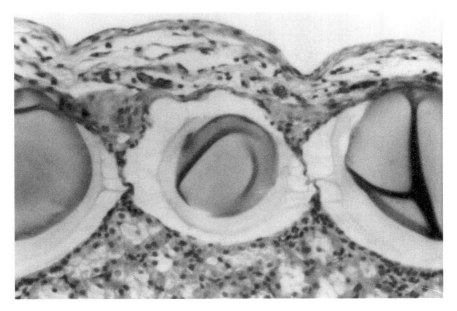

FIGURE 6. Three PEG coated substrate beads (mean diameter ~ 100 μm) are shown at the rat kidney subcapsular site, two weeks following implantation. The relatively clear zone between the host tissue and the opaque bead is where the PEG coat was; artifactual changes due to dehydration during histologic processing have altered the morphology to some extent. The recipient's reaction to the cross-linked polymer is minimal. Hematoxylin and eosin, 400×.

membrane. The membrane structure extends out from and covers the entire islet surface, for a controllable distance: 10–100 μm (FIG. 4). The PEG-DA monomers are cross-linked by free radicals generated when a photoinitiator (Eosin Y) on the islet surface is activated by laser light. The permselective properties of the generated conformal membrane are determined by a number of factors including the concentration and molecular weight of the PEG-DA monomer. Nominal molecular weight cutoffs of less than 30 kD can be attained.[19] Control of the encapsulation process maintains a high viability of cells by limiting radical generation to that needed to achieve optimal polymerization. The process is done under sterile conditions and is easily scaleable. Postencapsulation cell viabilities for 200 consecutive runs averaged 94 ± 1.0%.

In FIGURE 5, insulin release from encapsulated islets is compared to insulin release from unencapsulated islets. Static incubations were carried out, *in vitro*, for 30 minutes under basal and various stimulatory conditions. The ratio of insulin release under stimulatory conditions to release under basal conditions was expressed as a Stimulation Index. Encapsulated islets released insulin in response to glucose and other secretagogues in a manner similar to unencapsulated islets.

Biocompatibility of PEG Membranes

PEG coatings can be generated on any surface to which the photoinitiator can be attached. Relatively inert substrate microspheres (100–200 μm diameter) have

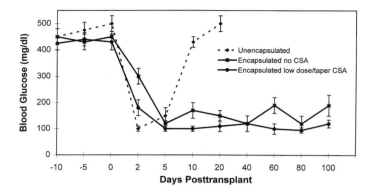

FIGURE 7. Reversal of diabetes with encapsulated islets: PEG conformal-coated porcine islets transplanted to outbred rats. Xenotransplantation of unencapsulated porcine islets to diabetic outbred rats resulted in a temporary reversal of hyperglycemia, followed by a rapid return to the diabetic state within 5–10 days (*dashed line*). Cyclosporine (CSA) treatment of such hosts did not alter the course of islet rejection (data not shown). In contrast, PEG encapsulated islets implanted to similar diabetic outbred rats produced a near-normoglycemic state out to 100 days posttransplantation (*stars*). Low dose/tapered CSA treatment of such recipients resulted in a more stable reversal of the diabetes (*circles*).

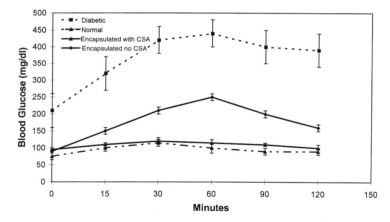

FIGURE 8. Oral glucose tolerance test: outbred rat recipients reversed of hyperglycemia following encapsulated porcine islet transplantation. Outbred diabetic rats were reversed of their hyperglycemia by transplantation of encapsulated porcine islets. Oral glucose tolerance testing revealed a normal response on the part of CSA treated recipients (*triangles-solid line*) when compared to non-diabetic controls (*triangles-dashed line*) and a near-normal response in non-immunosuppressed recipients (*diamonds-solid line*); greatly improved over diabetic controls (*square-dashed line*).

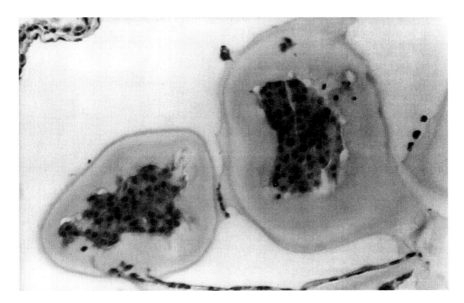

FIGURE 9. Two PEG coated islets are shown, recovered following >100 days posttransplantation at the intraperitoneal site of an outbred rat. Host reaction is minimal consisting of at most a single layer of peritoneal macrophages. Healthy viable islet tissue is present. Hematoxylin and eosin, 400×.

been used to examine the inherent biocompatibility of the cross-linked PEG polymer. FIGURE 6 shows the histological appearance of such a coated bead and its PEG coat after two weeks at the kidney subcapsular site in a normal rat. Very little host reaction is observed. In most cases it is restricted to a single layer of non-activated macrophages. No fibrosis is apparent and inflammation is minimal indicating that PEG crosslinked polymer, when manufactured and crosslinked under optimal conditions, is highly biocompatible.

XENOGENEIC IMMUNOPROTECTION

Intraperitoneal transplantation of unencapsulated porcine islets to streptozotocin diabetic outbred rats was followed by a temporary amelioration of hyperglycemia with a return to the diabetic state within 7–10 days (FIG. 7). Thus hyperacute rejection (measured in minutes to hours), as observed in whole organ transplantation, does not occur with porcine islets in this host.

Preliminary studies involving the intraperitoneal transplantation of PEG-encapsulated porcine islets demonstrate long-term reversal of hyperglycemia in a significant number of recipients. The addition of temporary (30 days) tapering low dose cyclosporine treatment (10, 5, 2.5, 1.25 mg/kg) of the recipients increased the number of successful reversals of the diabetic state (FIG. 7). Oral glucose tolerance tests (2 g/kg) on these reversed animals demonstrated near normal responses (FIG. 8).

Histological examination of recovered transplant tissue has confirmed the presence of viable encapsulated porcine islet tissue at greater than 100 days post-transplantation in this xenogeneic model (FIG. 9).

Studies in the rodent model continue, directed at optimizing the permselective nature of the PEG conformal membrane (polymer chain-length, polymer concentration, polymerization conditions) for xenogeneic transplantation.

SUMMARY

Functional porcine islets, free of known pathogens, can serve as a source of insulin producing cells for the treatment of experimentally induced insulin dependent Diabetes Mellitus.

Porcine islets can be conformally coated (microencapsulated) with a covalently linked, stable permselective membrane while maintaining islet viability and function.

The PEG conformal coating is immunoprotective in a discordant xenograft animal model (porcine islets to rat).

REFERENCES

1. THE DIABETES CONTROL AND COMPLICATIONS RESEARCH GROUP. 1993. The effect of intensive insulin treatment of diabetes on the development and progression of long-term complications in insulin dependent diabetes mellitus. N. Engl. J. Med. **329:** 977–986.
2. International Islet Transplant Registry, Newsletter No. 6, Vol 5, 1995.
3. SCHARP, D. W., P. E., LACY, J. V. SANTIAGO, C. S. McCULLOUGH, L. G. WEIDE, L. FALGUI, et al. 1990. Insulin independence after islet transplantation in type 1 diabetic patients. Diabetes **39:** 515–518.
4. WARNOCK, G. L., N. M. KNETEMAN, E. RYAN, A. RABINOVITCH & R. V. RAJOTTE. 1992. Long term follow up after transplantation of insulin-producing pancreatic islets into patients with type 1 diabetes mellitus. Diabetologia **35:** 89–95.
5. United Network for Organ Sharing 1996 Annual Report: The U.S. scientific registry of transplant recipients and the organ procurement and transplantation network. ISBN 1-886651-13-2; ISSN 1076-8874.
6. SCHARP, D. W., N. S. MASON & R. E. SPARKS. 1984. Islet immunoisolation: The use of hybrid artificial organs to prevent islet tissue rejection. World J. Surg. **8:** 221–229.
7. SCHARP, D. W., J. LONG, M. FELFMEIER, et al. 1985. Automated methods of mass islet isolation. In Methods of Diabetes Research, Vol. 1, Part C. J. Larner & S. L. Pohl, Eds.: 225–236. Wiley. New York.
8. NATIONAL SPF SWINE ACCREDITING AGENCY, INC. 1995. Rules and regulations. Conrad, IA 50621.
9. Segregated Early Weaning. National Hog Farmer Blueprint Series for Top Managers: Volume 39, No. 10, Fall 1994.
10. LINDQVIST, J. O. 1974. Animal health and environment in the production of fattening pigs. Acta Vet. Scand. (Suppl.) **51:** 1–78.
11. MURPHY, F. A. 1996. The public health risk of animal organ and tissue transplantation into humans. Science **273:** 746–747.
12. MATTHEWS, P. J. & G. W. BERAN. 1996. Assessment of public health aspects of porcine xenotransplantation. In Advances in Swine in Biomedical Research. Tumbleson & Schook, Eds.: 163–169. Plenum Press. New York.
13. AUCHINCLOSS, H. 1988. Xenogeneic Transplantation. A Review. Transplantation **46:** 1.
14. COLTON, C. 1995. Implantable biohybrid artificial organs. Cell Trans. **4:** 415–436.
15. LANZA, R. P. & W. L. CHICK, Eds. 1994. Pancreatic Islet Transplantation, Volume III: Immunoisolation of Pancreatic Islets. R. G. Landes Co. Austin, TX.

16. SAWHNEY, A. S., C. P. PATHAK & J. A. HUBBELL. Modification of islet of Langerhans surfaces with immunoprotective Poly(ethylene glycol) coatings via interfacial photopolymerization. Biotech. Bioeng. **44:** 383–386.
17. AVGOUSTINIATOS, E. & C. COLTON. 1996. Design consideration in immunoisolation. *In* Textbook of Tissue Engineering. R. G. Landes Co. Austin TX.
18. HUBBELL, J. A., C. P. PATHAK, A. S. SAWHNEY, N. P. DESAI & S. F. A. HOSSAINY. Gels for encapsulation of biological materials. US Patent No. 5,529,914.
19. CRUISE, G. M. 1997. Interfacially Polymerized Poly(ethylene glycol) Diacrylate Membranes upon Islets of Langerhans for Use as a Bioartificial Pancreas. Ph.D. Dissertation, University of Texas at Austin.

Application of AN69® Hydrogel to Islet Encapsulation

Evaluation in Streptozotocin-induced Diabetic Rat Model[a]

PH. PREVOST, S. FLORI, C. COLLIER, E. MUSCAT,[b]
AND E. ROLLAND

Bioartificial Organs Department
HOSPAL R&D International
13, Avenue de Lattre de Tassigny
69881 Meyzieu cedex, France

The idea of using encapsulation for living cells, creating a bioartificial organ, was born in 1964.[1] Since this date, many polymers have been used with more or less success: the slow development of their usage in applications such as diabetes or hepatic failure could have two main reasons. Firstly, the complex mechanisms of the immune system render the concept of immunoisolation by a permselective membrane less obvious. Secondly, no material seems to fit perfectly with the concept of biocompatibility defined as "the ability to perform with an appropriate host response, in a specific application."[2]

Because the polymer AN69® (polyacrylonitrile-sodium methallylsulfonate) is a reference in biocompatibility in the field of hemodialysis, several teams have used it for encapsulating hepatocytes[3-5] or islets.[6-8] HOSPAL has started a program of bioartificial organs development using the AN 69®: BIORGAN, EUREKA which receved a label in June 1993. Diabetes is a pertinent and rigorous model to evaluate the properties of this material. The following study is the first description of AN 69® hydrogel–encapsulated islet isograft in streptozotocin-induced (STZ) diabetic rats. The aim of this work is to evaluate the biocompatibility of the AN 69® hydrogel by comparing the efficacy of free versus encapsulated islets transplanted to mitigate diabetes, as performed for alginate.[9]

MATERIALS AND METHODS

Animals

Male Lewis rats (Iffa-Credo, l'Arbresle France), weighing 220–260 g were rendered diabetic at day 0 (D0) by intravenous injection of STZ 65 mg/kg: Sigma, St. Louis, MO, USA). Rats are fed and watered *ad libitum*. Blood glucose and diuresis were monitored for 1 week to ensure the onset of diabetes: fasting blood glucose (measured by tail bleedings using the glucose oxydase method: Accu check

[a] BIORGAN is an EUREKA project. This work was supported by the French Ministère de l'Enseignement Supérieur et de la Recherche.
[b] Author to whom correspondence should be addressed.

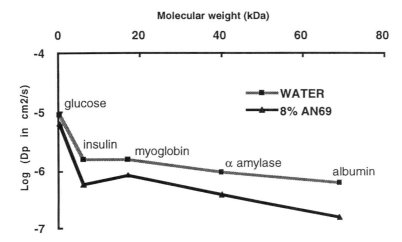

FIGURE 1. *In vitro* evaluation of an 8% AN 69® hollow fiber permeability.

Glucose, Boehringer Mannheim, Germany) exceeded 350 mg/dl for two consecutive determinations and diuresis exceeded 100 ml per 24 H on D5.

Islet Isolation

Pancreatic islets were isolated from adult male Lewis rats (220–270 g) by a standard collagenase digestion and purified on Ficoll (Sigma) discontinuous density gradient. The mean yield is 990 islets per pancreas and the viability, assessed by red neutral dye, is over 94%. Islets were cultured overnight in RPMI 1640 medium supplemented with 10% fetal calf serum (FCS) at 37°C in a humidified atmosphere at 5% CO_2 in air.

Encapsulation

HOSPAL has developed an AN 69® hydrogel process for islet encapsulation. Hollow fibers are manufactured by a wet/wet process using the phase inversion principle based on solvent/non-solvent/polymer ternary diagram. The solvent is dimethylsulfoxide (Sigma), the non-solvent is a saline solution (NaCl 9 g/l, Sigma), and the polymer is AN 69®, a polyacrylonitrile-sodium methallylsulfonate copolymer (HOSPAL, Meyzieu, France).

The resulting hollow fibers have an 80% water content, an insulin diffusion coefficient of $5.2 \ 10^{-7}$ cm²/s, a stress at breaking of 0.32 N/mm² and a molecular weight cut-off about 80,000 Da (FIG. 1). Their dimensions are 120 cm long, 1065 μm internal diameter and 140 μm wall thickness.

The hollow fibers were filled with islets suspended in agarose (0.15% w/v, Sigma) at the final concentration of 10,000 islets per ml and closed with surgical clips (Merlin Medical, Bron, France).

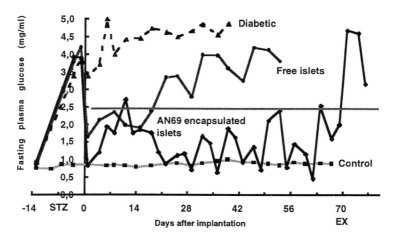

FIGURE 2. Mean body weight in Lewis rats. STZ = streptozotocin injection (D-7); EX = explantation (D70); n = 6 except for group 3 (n = 4 during 3 weeks, then n = 3).

Experimental Design

Recipient rats are anesthesized using Zoletil (20 mg/kg, Reading, Carros, France) followed by Halothane (Belamont, Paris France). 6000 free islets (group 2; n = 6) or 9000 encapsulated islets (group 3; n = 4) are introduced into the peritoneal cavity through a midline incision. The wound is closed in two layers. Group 1 (n = 6) and group 4 (n = 6) represent respectively normal control and diabetic control rats. Weight and fasting glycemia are evaluated twice a week. The encapsulated islets grafts were removed respectively at D54, D61, D63 and D70 (n = 3). After the explantation at D70, one rat died. Animals of group 2 (n = 6) and 3 (n = 2) are sacrificed respectively 54 and 77 days after transplantation. Animals of the group 2 (n = 5) were sacrificed 54 days after STZ injection.

Implants and pancreas are retrieved from peritoneal cavity, fixed in formaldehyde and stained with Masson trichrome and hematoxylin-eosin safron (HES) respectively.

RESULTS

Body weight, fasting glucose plasma and diuresis evolution are shown in FIGURES 2, 3 and 4. In group 3, after 3 weeks, one rat who had improved returned to the diabetic state: the implant removed at 4 weeks appears to be contaminated.

Fasting Plasma Glucose Level

If normoglycemia is defined as a fasting plasma glucose level inferior to 250 mg/dl, the free islets transplantation reverses the hyperglycemia immediately but for 3 weeks only. After 3 weeks, animals become hyperglycemic with glucose

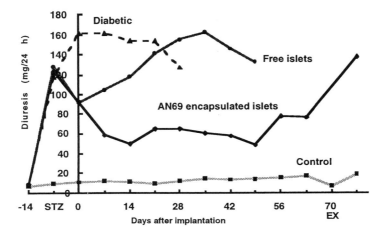

FIGURE 3. Mean fasting plasma glucose level in Lewis rat. STZ: streptozotocin injection (D-7); EX: explanation (D70); n = 6 except for group 3 (n = 4 during 3 weeks, then n = 3).

concentrations rising from 240 ± 20 to 420 ± 4 mg/dl. At the opposite, AN69® encapsulated islets recipients remain at normoglycemia for at least 70 days. The mean glycemia from D1 to D70 is 122 ± 1 mg/dl, compared to 88 ± 6 mg/dl (group 1), 266 ± 2 mg/dl (group 2), and 443 ± 10 mg/dl (group 4). After the explantation (D70), hyperglycemia of the two surviving rats returns to the diabetic level.

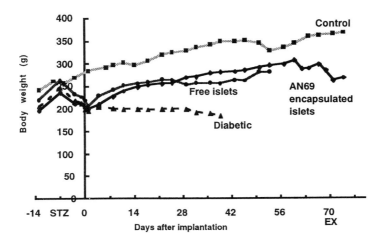

FIGURE 4. Mean diuresis in Lewis rats. STZ: streptozotocin injection (D-7); EX: explantation (D70); n = 6 except for group 3 (n = 4 during 3 weeks, then n = 3).

Diuresis

Daily diuresis evolution confirms previous results. The mean diuresis from D1 to D70 is 13 ± 1 ml/24 H (group 1), 123 ± 1 ml/24 H (group 2), 78 ± 1 ml/24 H (group 3) and 161 ± 1 ml/24 H (group 4).

Body Weight

During the period D1–D32, the daily mean gain in body weight is 1.7 g (group 1), 1.1 g (group 2), 2.1 g (group 3) and -0.4 g (group 4), and during the overall period (D1–D70), 1.2 g (group 1) and 0.5 g (group 3). Compared to control rat, the gain of body weight during the period D1–D32 is better (Student t-test, $p > 0.05$) for AN69® encapsulated islets transplanted rats: this could be due to compensation because of the dramatic body weight decrease after the STZ injection. For group 2, the body weight gain is 1.6 g/day for the period D0–D18. It decreases to 0.6 g per day for the period D18–D53, concomitantly with the return to hyperglycemia.

Morphological Studies

Morphological evaluation of recipient rat pancreata revealed that islets have almost completely disappeared. Some groups of endocrine cells survive (10–100 cells). During explantation, we observe that the area of the AN 69® implant remains intact. No tissue necrosis nor cellular inflammation was observed (except for the contaminated one). The AN 69® implant is covered with epiploon. The light micrographs show a connective tissue composed of several layers of fibroblasts (data not shown).

DISCUSSION

This study shows that AN 69® encapsulated islets isograft is able to reverse diabetes for at least 70 days, assessed by 3 parameters: body weight, fasting plasma glucose, and diuresis.

Both the return to the diabetic state after explantation and pancreata micrographs demonstrate that these results are not due to pancreata regeneration. Although the clinical state and body weight are quite normal, neither glycemia nor diuresis completely returned to a normal level. The AN 69® biocompatibility, as evaluated by macroscopic observation, is satisfactory. The host reaction to the implant is reduced to a thin layer of fibroblasts.

In contrast, free islets isograft reverse diabetes for only 3 weeks. This could be due to an insufficient number of islets (6000 compared to 9000 encapsulated islets), low-quality islets, or the non-physiological situation of the islets.

The model we choose is rather severe, because islets are grafted into a hyperglycemic animal, which has been demonstrated to be very deleterious. This could explain the high number of islets necessary to reverse the diabetes.

SUMMARY

The polymer AN69 (polyacrylonitrile-sodium methallylsulfonate) is a reference in biocompatibility in the field of hemodialysis. Its use for the encapsulation of living cells has been already described, but this study is the first description of AN69® hydrogel–encapsulated islet isograft in streptozotocin (STZ) diabetic rats. The aim of this work is to evaluate the biocompatibility of the AN69® hydrogel by comparison of the efficacy of free versus encapsulated islets transplanted to balance diabetes. Pancreatic islets are isolated from adult male Lewis rats by a standard collagenase digestion and purified on Ficoll density gradients. The AN69® hollow fiber is obtained by coextrusion of an 8% AN69® collodion.

The hollow fiber is filled with islets suspended in agarose at the final concentration of 10,000 islets/ml, closed with surgical clips and implanted. The recipients are rendered diabetic by intravenous injection of STZ. The experimental design includes 4 groups of 8 rats: group 1: control, group 2: diabetic rats intraperitoneally implanted with 6000 free islets, group 3: diabetic rats intraperitonally implanted with 9000 encapsulated islets, group 4: diabetic control. Weight and fasting glycemia are evaluated twice a week, diuresis once a week.

After free islet implantation, rat survival is improved with glycemia below 250 mg/dl during 22 days. Compared to group 2, the status of group 3 is better, with a glycemia below 250 mg/dl during at least 70 days. This tends to demonstrate the biocompatibility of AN69® and is the first step of the validation of the use of AN69® for living cell encapsulation.

REFERENCES

1. CHANG, T. M. S. 1964. Semi-permeable microcapsules. Science **146:** 524–525.
2. WILLIAMS, D. F. 1990. Biocompatibility: Performance in the surgical reconstruction of man. Interdisciplinary Sci. Rev. **15**(1): 20–33.
3. ROGER, V. *et al.* 1995. A good model of experimental acute hepatic failure: 95% Hepactectomy treatment by transplantation of hepatocytes. Submitted.
4. BALLADUR, P. *et al.* 1995. Transplantation of allogenic hepatocytes without immunosuppression: Long term survival. Surgery **117**(2): 189–194.
5. HONIGER, J. *et al.* Permeability and biocompatibility of a new hydrogel used for encapsulation of hepatocytes. Submitted.
6. KESSLER, L. *et al.* 1992. Diffusion properties of an artificial membrane used for Langerhans islets encapsulation: An *in vitro* test. Biomaterials **13**(1): 44–49.
7. KESSLER, L. *et al.* 1991. *In vitro* and *in vivo* studies of the properties of an artificial membrane for pancreatic islet encapsulation. Horm. Metab. Res. **23:** 312–317.
8. HONIGER, J. *et al.* 1994. Preliminary report on cell encapsulation in a hydrogel made of a biocompatible material, AN 69®, for the development of a bioartificial pancreas. Int. J. Artif. Organs **17**(1): 46–52.
9. CLAYTON, H. *et al.* 1992. The transplantation of encapsulated islets of Langerhans into the peritoneal cavity of the Biobreeding rat. Transplantation **54**(3): 558–559.

Treatment of Severe Liver Failure with a Bioartificial Liver[a]

STEVE C. CHEN,[b] CLAUDY MULLON,[c]
ELAINE KAHAKU,[b] FRED WATANABE,[b]
WINSTON HEWITT,[b] SUSUMU EGUCHI,[b]
YVETTE MIDDLETON,[b] NIKOLAOS ARKADOPOULOS,[b]
JACEK ROZGA,[b] BARRY SOLOMON,[c] AND
ACHILLES A. DEMETRIOU,[b,d]

[b]The Liver Support Unit, Department of Surgery
Cedars-Sinai Medical Center
UCLA School of Medicine
Los Angeles, California 90048

[c]Grace Biomedical, Inc.
Lexington, Massachusetts 02173

Patients with severe acute liver failure represent a major challenge despite advances in critical care.[7-9] Severe fulminant hepatic failure (FHF) has a high mortality (in some series approaching 90%) without OLT.[10] There is a need to stabilize these patients until an organ becomes available for transplant. In many instances, severe FHF patients deteriorate so rapidly owing to development of cerebral edema and intracranial hypertension, that they no longer qualify for OLT owing to irreversible brain damage. There is thus a need to develop a liver support system to maintain these patients alive and neurologically intact prior to OLT.

We have developed and extensively tested a porcine hepatocyte-based bioartificial liver (BAL).[3-5] Here we report our clinical experience with the BAL. This study demonstrated that the BAL system appears to have significant beneficial effects. The survival achieved by combining BAL treatment(s) as either a bridge to transplant or spontaneous recovery with standard supportive measures, in this group of FHF patients with significant neurologic dysfunction is the best reported in the literature.

METHODS

Patients

Twenty-eight patients underwent 54 BAL treatments; among them, were 27 adults (42.8 ± 2.9 years of age, 14 male and 13 female) and one child (10-year-old

[a] Grants in support of this research were received from Grace Biomedical Inc., W.R. Grace, Co. and The Cedars-Sinai Research Institute.

[d] Author to whom correspondence should be addressed: Achilles A. Demetriou, M.D., Ph. D., 8700 Beverly Boulevard, Suite 8215, Los Angeles, CA 90048; Tel: (310) 855-5884; Fax: (310) 967-0139.

TABLE 1. Patient Demographics, Etiologies, Encephalopathy Stage and Treatment Outcomes of Group I Fulminant Hepatic Failure (FHF) Patients and Group II Primary Non-Function (PNF) Patients

PT	Age	Sex	Etiology	Encephalopathy	BAL TX #	Bridge Time (Hr)	Outcome
Group I: FHF Patients							
1.	35	F	HCV	II	1	32	OLT, Recovered
2.	10	M	Indeterminate	IV	1	34.5	OLT, Recovered
3.	18	F	Acetaminophen	IV	3	58	OLT × 2, Recovered
4.	34	M	Indeterminate	III/IV	1	20	OLT, Recovered
5.	24	M	Indeterminate	IV	2	58	OLT, Recovered
6.	50	F	Acetaminophen	IV	2	30	OLT, Recovered
7.	49	M	HBV	IV	2	31	OLT × 2, Recovered
8.	31	F	Indeterminate	IV	1	33.5	OLT, Recovered
9.	52	F	Indeterminate	IV	3	60	OLT, Recovered
10.	34	F	Ischemic Liver	IV	1	19	OLT, Recovered
11.	51	M	Indeterminate	IV	2	42	OLT × 2, Recovered
12.	47	F	Acetaminophen	III/IV	2	No OLT	Recovered
13.	18	F	Acetaminophen	IV	2	20	OLT × 2, Recovered
14.	56	F	HBV	IV	3	71	OLT, Recovered
15.	26	F	Indeterminate	III/IV	1	31	OLT × 2, Recovered
Group II: PNF Patients							
1.	58	M	Indeterminate	IV	1	36	OLT, Recovered
2.	61	F	HAV, HBV	IV	3	21	OLT, Recovered
3.	26	F	Autoimmune	IV	1	8 Days	OLT, Recovered

boy). All procedures were conducted in full compliance with the ethical standards of the institutional committee for the protection of human subjects, in accordance with the Declaration of Helsinki. Patients belonged to one of three groups. Patient demographics, disease etiology, hepatic encephalopathy stage (Trey, Davidson Classification) and outcome are summarized in TABLES 1 and 2. Group I (n = 15) patients had no previous history of chronic liver disease, fulfilled all diagnostic criteria of FHF, and were candidates for OLT. On admission, patients were listed

TABLE 2. Patient Demographics, Etiologies, Encephalopathy Stage and Treatment Outcomes of Group III "Acute-on-Chronic" Patients

PT	Age	Sex	Etiology	Encephalopathy	BAL TX #	Outcome
1.	33	M	ETOH	III/IV	1	OLT, Recovered
2.	45	M	ETOH, HBV, HCV	IV	2	Death, 14 Days
3.	46	M	ETOH, HBV	IV	1	Death, 1 Day
4.	64	M	ETOH	IV	1	Death, 7 Days
5.	52	F	Autoimmune	IV	4	Death, 10 Days
6.	58	M	HBV	IV	2	Death, 4 Days
7.	55	M	PBC	III/IV	2	OLT × 2, Recovered
8.	39	F	HCV	IV	3	Death, 9 Days
9.	70	M	HCC	III/IV	1	Death, 4 Days
10.	57	M	ETOH	IV	5	Death, 20 Days

on a national transplant waiting list with the highest priority status (UNOS Status 1). Fourteen FHF patients were in deep stage IV hepatic encephalopathy (coma) and one was in stage II. Group II (n = 3) patients had undergone OLT and in the immediate postoperative period developed primary graft non-function with rapid deterioration and development of stage IV encephalopathy. All three patients were listed for urgent (UNOS status 1) re-transplantation. Group III patients (n = 10) experienced acute exacerbation of chronic liver disease due to various etiologies. These "acute-on-chronic" patients were not candidates for transplantation at the time of BAL treatment, mostly because of sepsis and/or evidence of continued alcohol abuse. All patients were in stage III/IV encephalopathy.

We have established a multi-disciplinary Liver Support Unit (LSU) to provide optimal, focused care to patients with severe acute liver failure. In addition to utilizing a computerized, on-line clinical data collection system (CareVue 9000 Clinical Information System, Hewlett-Packard, Andover, MA), we have developed and standardized diagnostic and therapeutic protocols to allow meaningful, accurate data collection and analysis. Immediately upon admission, patients were evaluated and treated with standard supportive measures to correct electrolyte, metabolic, respiratory, coagulation and hemodynamic abnormalities. Hemodynamically stable patients were evaluated with head computerized tomography (CT). Intracranial pressure monitors were placed at the bedside by a neurosurgeon in patients with evidence of brainstem dysfunction (decerebrate features) and/or cerebral edema on CT.

BAL treatment was instituted in all patients who did not respond to standard therapeutic measures including hyperventilation, mannitol and lactulose administration, metabolic and hemodynamic support. Each BAL treatment lasted 6 hours preceded by an hour period of plasma separation to ensure the patients' ability to tolerate the extracorporeal circuit. No plasma exchange was carried out. All patients continued to receive standard measures throughout their hospital course. Vital signs, urinary output, arterial blood gases and central hemodynamic parameters were monitored continuously. Neurologic monitoring and assessment (clinical examination, CLOCS, Glasgow Coma Score (GCS), ICP, CPP) were carried out at hourly intervals.[11] Liver function tests, coagulation tests, complete blood cell count and electrolyte, ammonia, lactate, amino acid, creatinine and blood urea nitrogen (BUN) levels were determined at the start, mid-point and end of each BAL treatment and then serially during the post-BAL period until either the patients were transplanted or underwent another BAL treatment. Sodium citrate was used as an anticoagulant to prevent thrombosis in the system. Plasma ionized calcium levels were monitored closely and hypocalcemia was prevented by continuous infusion of calcium chloride. "Bridge Time" was the interval (hours) between beginning of the first BAL treatment to transplantation.

Bioartificial Liver (BAL)

The design of the current BAL system evolved from laboratory and pilot clinical experiments carried out by our group.[3–6,12,13] The system has been standardized and in the last 21 patients of the series reported here, we used a BAL circuit (HepatAssist™ 2000, FIG. 1) built by Grace Biomedical Inc. (Lexington, MA); it consists of a high-flow plasma re-circulation loop through a reservoir (Harmac Inc., Buffalo, NY), a column loaded with 300 g of cellulose-coated activated charcoal (Adsorba 300C, Gambro, Hechingen, Germany), an oxygenator (Capiox 308, Terumo, Japan), a water bath (Temp Marq, Marquest, CO) and a hollow-fiber module

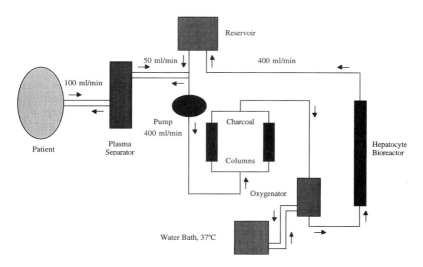

FIGURE 1. Schematic representation of the Bioartificial Liver (BAL) support system.

(Microgon Inc., Laguna Hills, CA) seeded with 5×10^9 viable porcine hepatocytes on microcarriers (Cytodex 3, Pharmacia, Sweden).[14] The bioreactor has porous fibers (0.2 μm) with total internal surface area ~6,000 cm², external surface area ~7,000 cm², wall thickness of 62 μm and extra-fiber volume ~200 ml. Blood is removed from a patient through a large-bore double-lumen catheter placed in the right superficial femoral vein at a rate of 90–100 ml/min and is separated into plasma and blood cells by a plasma separator (Spectra, COBE, Lakewood, CO). The plasma is directed to the BAL at a rate of ~50 ml/min where it is recirculated at 400 ml/min.

Hepatocyte Preparation

Methods of hepatocyte isolation, enrichment, attachment to microcarriers, cryo-preservation and storage have been described elsewhere.[3-5,15] Freshly isolated hepatocytes were used initially and cryopreserved hepatocytes have been used to treat the last 13 patients. All future treatments will continue utilizing cryopreserved cells as the physiologic and clinical effects of the two types of cells appear to be identical. The initial viability of freshly isolated hepatocytes was consistently greater than 90% and that of cryopreserved cells greater than 70%. For each treatment, 5 billion viable cells were used. At the end of each treatment, a sample of microcarrier-anchored hepatocytes was taken from the bioreactor for direct light microscopic examination and assessment of viability.

Statistical Analysis

Statistical analyses were conducted using paired Student t-test to compare immediately pre- and post-treatment values. A p value < 0.05 was considered statistically significant. Data are expressed as means $\pm$ standard errors.

RESULTS

Plasma Separation and BAL Perfusion

Patients in all groups were treated with the BAL 1–5 times as shown in TABLES 1 and 2. With the exception of a patient who experienced an episode of transient hypotension requiring discontinuation of a treatment, patients remained hemodynamically stable during treatments, there were no technical problems during plasma separation and no adverse reactions due to the use of porcine hepatocytes were noted. Hepatocyte viability at the end of BAL treatments varied from 10–90%, suggesting a significant degree of variability of patient plasma toxicity.

BAL Treatment Outcome

The treatment end-point of the study is patient survival. Patients are followed for a minimum of six months post-treatment at our clinic. Patients are now 2 to 62 months post-treatment (24.0 ± 3.3 months). Secondary endpoints include overall clinical neurologic improvement, improved brainstem function as assessed by CLOCS, a decrease in ICP and an increase in CPP, following each treatment. The number of BAL treatment(s), bridge time to OLT and patient outcome data are summarized in TABLES 1 and 2.

In Group I, all FHF patients survived. Fourteen patients in this group were bridged to OLT for 38.6 ± 4.5 hours ranging from 19 to 71 hours. The remaining patient with FHF experienced a remarkable and steady improvement following two BAL treatments. She was removed from the urgent transplant waiting list after five days and fully recovered without undergoing a liver transplant. Four patients were initially transplanted with an ABO incompatible liver and later required retransplantation with an ABO compatible organ. No unusual patterns of rejection were noted. One patient required retransplantation owing to organ-size discrepancy. In Group II, all patients were bridged to retransplantation and survived. These patients were bridged from 21 hours to 8 days. For Group III "acute-on-chronic" patients, the treatment end-points were less clear since patients were not OLT candidates on admission. Although these patients demonstrated transient beneficial effects from BAL treatment(s) (TABLES 3 and 4), they eventually succumbed to sepsis and multiple organ failure due to progressive deterioration of liver function and no possibility to undergo liver transplantation. However, two patients did recover from the acute event and later underwent successful transplantation after meeting the appropriate selection criteria. Thus, mortality only occurred in the non-transplant candidate group, resulting in an overall survival of 71% for all three groups of patients and 100% for the FHF and PNF groups.

Neurologic and Hemodynamic Effects of the BAL

In Group I, we observed significant neurologic improvement. Patients with brain edema and intracranial hypertension, experienced a dramatic reversal of the decerebrate state: posturing, rigidity, anisocoria and sluggish pupil reactivity were lessened by the end of the treatment(s); in addition, patient responsiveness to external stimuli increased. Brainstem function improvement was quantified using the CLOCS (TABLE 4).[11] One patient who recovered without OLT, demonstrated remarkable neurologic improvement as she woke up from hepatic coma and began

TABLE 3. Effect of Bioartificial Liver (BAL) Treatment on Metabolic Parameters and Liver Function Tests in Group III "Acute-on-Chronic" Patients

	Pre-BAL	Post-BAL	p
Glucose (mg/dl)	144 ± 10	174 ± 12	0.003
Lactate (mmol/l)	6.3 ± 1.0	5.4 ± 0.7	0.7
pH	7.46 ± 0.01	7.44 ± 0.01	0.3
Ammonia (mmol/l)	165.8 ± 28.1	115.9 ± 14.4	0.03
Albumin (g/dl)	2.9 ± 0.1	2.6 ± 0.1	0.00001
AST (U/l)	668 ± 416	728 ± 455	0.2
ALT (U/l)	259 ± 118	233 ± 119	0.2
Alk. Phos. (U/l)	114 ± 10	122 ± 25	0.7
Total Bilirubin (mg/dl)	26.0 ± 3.0	21.9 ± 2.5	0.00002
Direct Bilirubin (mg/dl)	13.4 ± 2.0	11.1 ± 1.6	0.002
Indirect Bilirubin (mg/dl)	11.5 ± 2.1	10.1 ± 1.8	0.001
PT (sec)	21.6 ± 1.1	21.6 ± 0.7	0.9
Fibrinogen (mg/dl)	151.8 ± 18.9	126.4 ± 15.1	0.002

to respond to verbal commands during the second BAL treatment. BAL treatment resulted in reduction in ICP from 17.2 ± 2.0 to 9.8 ± 1.3 mmHg ($p = 0.0008$). This was accompanied by an increase in CPP from 65.9 ± 3.3 to 74.3 ± 2.5 mmHg ($p = 0.01$). The beneficial effects in ICP, CPP and CLOCS were more dramatic in patients who had abnormal ICP values (ICP: 21.6 ± 2.1 to 8.7 ± 2.6 mmHg, $p = 0.004$; CPP: 67.7 ± 4.2 to 79.7 ± 4.1 mmHg, $p = 0.008$; CLOCS: 19.2 ± 1.2 to 27.1 ± 1.4, $p = 0.00001$). In Groups II and III, similar trends were observed (TABLE 4). However, statistically significant improvement was shown only in brainstem function (CLOCS: 21.0 ± 3.6 to 26.4 ± 3.6, $p = 0.02$) in Group III. In all three groups, patients remained hemodynamically stable (TABLE 5).

Effect of the BAL on Serum Liver Function Tests

BAL effects on serum liver function tests are summarized in TABLES 3 and 6. Serum ammonia levels were lowered in Groups I and III. There was also a decrease

TABLE 4. Effect of Bioartificial Liver (BAL) Treatment on Intracranial Pressure (ICP), Cerebral Perfusion Pressure (CPP), Glasgow Coma Score (GCS) and Comprehensive Level of Consciousness Score (CLOCS)

	Pre-BAL	Post-BAL	p
Group I: FHF Patients			
ICP (mmHg)	17.2 ± 2.0	9.8 ± 1.3	0.0008
CPP (mmHg)	65.9 ± 3.3	74.3 ± 2.5	0.01
GCS	7.1 ± 0.5	7.3 ± 0.5	0.5
CLOCS	24.4 ± 1.7	31.0 ± 1.4	0.00001
Group II: PNF Patients			
GCS	5.0 ± 1.1	7.0 ± 1.4	0.2
CLOCS	29.7 ± 7.4	31.7 ± 7.9	0.5
Group III: "Acute-on-Chronic" Patients			
ICP (mmHg)	11.7 ± 0.8	12.5 ± 1.8	0.6
CPP (mmHg)	80.2 ± 5.2	90.5 ± 9.3	0.2
GCS	7.3 ± 0.5	7.6 ± 0.5	0.4
CLOCS	27.7 ± 2.1	32.0 ± 1.3	0.02

TABLE 5. Effect of Bioartificial Liver (BAL) Treatment on Hemodynamics

	Pre-BAL	Post-BAL	p
Group I: FHF Patients			
Heart Rate (/min)	100 ± 4	99 ± 3	0.8
MAP (mm/Hg)	87 ± 2	83 ± 2	0.1
CVP (mm/Hg)	8 ± 1	8 ± 1	0.8
PCW (mm/Hg)	13 ± 2	10 ± 1	0.3
SVRI (dyne/sec/cm^5/m^2)	1405 ± 128	1699 ± 197	0.3
CI (L/min/m^2)	4.6 ± 0.4	3.7 ± 0.2	0.06
Group II: PNF Patients			
Heart Rate (/min)	102 ± 5	91 ± 3	0.1
MAP (mm/Hg)	79 ± 3	88 ± 6	0.2
CVP (mm/Hg)	14 ± 2	15 ± 3	0.9
PCW (mm/Hg)	11 ± 2	10 ± 1	0.6
SVRI (dyne/sec/cm^5/m^2)	1329 ± 257	1780 ± 409	0.09
CI (L/min/m^2)	6.5 ± 2.5	6.4 ± 2.6	0.7
Group III: "Acute-on-Chronic" Patients			
Heart Rate (/min)	101 ± 3	100 ± 3	0.8
MAP (mm/Hg)	80 ± 3	82 ± 4	0.3
CVP (mm/Hg)	13 ± 1	14 ± 1	0.4
PCW (mm/Hg)	15 ± 1	15 ± 1	0.6
SVRI (dyne/sec/cm^5/m^2)	987 ± 478	1019 ± 113	0.7
CI (L/min/m^2)	5.8 ± 0.4	5.4 ± 0.3	0.1

in transaminase activities and bilirubin levels in all groups. No significant effects were observed in plasma clotting factor activity (data not shown) and prothrombin time (PT).

Effect of the BAL on Plasma Amino Acid Profile and Encephalopathic Index

Plasma amino acid levels were measured at the start and the end of each treatment. The ratio of branched chain amino acids (BCAA: leucine, isoleucine and valine) to aromatic amino acids (AAA: phenylalanine and tyrosine) felt to be an index of the degree of encephalopathy was calculated.[16,17] There was a significant ($p < 0.01$) increase in the BCAA/AAA ratio from 0.75 ± 0.07 to 0.98 ± 0.07. The increase was due to a decrease in aromatic amino acid levels.

DISCUSSION

Severe acute liver failure, whether occurring in the setting of FHF and PNF or superimposed on chronic liver disease, is associated with high mortality.[7-10] Despite improved critical care, many of these patients succumb to brainstem herniation with rapid neurologic deterioration because of failure to arrest the progression of cerebral edema. Urgent liver transplantation has become the only clinically effective treatment for patients with FHF. Similarly, patients with PNF need urgent retransplantation. In patients with acute exacerbation of chronic disease, the goal is to allow them to recover from the acute process and then electively undergo OLT if they fulfill appropriate selection criteria. The problem remains organ shortage.[18] Thus, there is a need for a liver support system to provide a "bridge" to OLT.

TABLE 6. Effect of Bioartificial Liver (BAL) Treatment on Metabolic Parameters and Liver Function Tests in Group I FHF Patients and Group II PNF Patients

	Pre-BAL	Post-BAL	p
Group I: FHF Patients			
Glucose (mg/dl)	128 ± 9	177 ± 12	0.0007
Lactate (mmol/l)	5.8 ± 1.3	5.3 ± 1.3	0.1
pH	7.53 ± 0.02	7.47 ± 0.02	0.05
Ammonia (mmol/l)	163 ± 10	132 ± 9	0.006
Albumin (g/dl)	3.3 ± 0.1	2.6 ± 0.1	0.00004
AST (U/l)	1374 ± 381	880 ± 204	0.01
ALT (U/l)	1282 ± 281	792 ± 190	0.0007
Alk. Phos. (U/l)	125 ± 13	92 ± 10	0.000002
Total Bilirubin (mg/dl)	18.6 ± 2.3	15.2 ± 1.9	0.00002
Direct Bilirubin (mg/dl)	8.9 ± 1.3	6.9 ± 1.0	0.00001
Indirect Bilirubin (mg/dl)	9.7 ± 1.2	8.3 ± 1.1	0.002
PT (sec)	21.8 ± 1.3	22.3 ± 0.9	0.7
Fibrinogen (mg/dl)	162 ± 10	115 ± 8	0.000004
Group II: PNF Patients			
Glucose (mg/dl)	117 ± 26	144 ± 24	0.06
Lactate (mmol/l)	13.1 ± 2.9	13.2 ± 2.2	0.9
pH	7.46 ± 0.1	7.40 ± 0.06	0.2
Ammonia (mmol/l)	81.0 ± 8.7	91.0 ± 13.3	0.3
Albumin (g/dl)	3.7 ± 0.3	2.7 ± 0.1	0.01
AST (U/l)	5661 ± 2613	2821 ± 1291	0.1
ALT (U/l)	2139 ± 704	1633 ± 544	0.05
Alk. Phos. (U/l)	108 ± 15	83 ± 9	0.03
Total Bilirubin (mg/dl)	19.1 ± 2.2	14.7 ± 1.7	0.009
Direct Bilirubin (mg/dl)	3.8 ± 1.3	3.1 ± 0.8	0.2
Indirect Bilirubin (mg/dl)	18.1 ± 2.3	13.9 ± 1.3	0.05
PT (sec)	21.6 ± 1.8	23.0 ± 2.1	0.5
Fibrinogen (mg/dl)	166.7 ± 29.6	120.7 ± 21.0	0.06

Investigators have attempted to provide temporary liver support with various techniques: cross-circulation,[19,20] whole liver perfusion,[21,22] hemadsorption,[20,23-25] hemodialysis,[26,27] plasma exchange,[28] total body wash-out,[29] use of microsomal enzymes bound to artificial carriers,[30] and other procedures.[31-35] However, none of these strategies succeeded in gaining wide clinical use. An effective artificial liver support device should provide all essential liver functions which are either impaired or lost in severe liver failure including detoxification, biotransformation, and biosynthesis. Because of incomplete understanding of the pathophysiology of liver failure, hepatic encephalopathy and cerebral edema, most investigators believe that such task could only be achieved by utilizing biologically active components.

Recently, there has been renewed interest in the use of *ex vivo* whole liver perfusion to treat patients with severe liver failure.[36,37] Human livers rejected for transplantation have been used for *ex vivo* perfusion with promising results.[36] However, this strategy remains impractical owing to shortage of organs and inability to procure an organ on short notice to treat FHF patients. Certainly, it would appear that a liver demonstrating such a significant level of metabolic support in *ex vivo* perfusions should be transplanted. Others explored the possibility of treating FHF patients with *ex vivo* perfusions using porcine livers. Unfortunately, these procedures are technically cumbersome and although promising, in a recent report, only 1 out of 4 patients with acute liver failure was successfully bridged to OLT. [37]

We have completed a clinical study to examine primarily the safety of the BAL. We have arrived at a standardized system-design, cell-processing and cryopreservation methods. Use of cryopreserved cells makes the system practical as it allows distribution of cells from a central facility to many user sites. Our clinical outcome data appear promising and thus justify continuing to study this approach to treating patients with acute liver failure. The survival data in the FHF/PNF group which had significant neurologic dysfunction (with one exception, patients were in deep stage IV coma with a Glasgow coma scale score of 7 or less), are the best reported in the literature with any combination of therapeutic modalities including transplantation.

The reason for the 100% survival in the FHF/PNF group appears to be the arrest and/or reversal of cerebral edema with neurologic improvement. All patients were able to fully recover neurologically. Statistically significant changes were seen in various plasma biochemical parameters (glucose increase, transaminases, alkaline phosphatase and bilirubin reduction), but the significance of these findings is not clear. Reduction in liver enzyme levels was seen after a treatment with the BAL; there was a return to baseline several hours post-treatment with another reduction following a subsequent treatment. A similar pattern was observed with the post-treatment hyperglycemia, with blood glucose levels returning to baseline between BAL treatments. Of interest is the observed reduction in plasma ammonia and the levels of aromatic amino acids in view of their proposed roles in the pathogenesis of hepatic encephalopathy.[16,17] The observed reduction in fibrinogen levels is felt to be due to binding to the plasma separation tubing.

In summary, we have developed a novel extracorporeal liver support system based on high-flow plasma perfusion through a charcoal column, a membrane oxygenator, water heater and a hollow-fiber bioreactor with viable porcine hepatocyte aggregates anchored by collagen-coated microcarriers. A multi-center, randomized, prospective study including a control group receiving standard management is the next phase of our clinical studies.

SUMMARY

Orthotopic liver transplantation (OLT) is the definitive therapy for severe liver failure.[1] However, many patients die before an organ becomes available, mostly from cerebral edema.[2] To provide temporary liver support, we developed a bioartificial liver (BAL) based on porcine hepatocytes and a charcoal column.[3-6] Fifty-four consecutive BAL treatments were carried out in three groups of patients: Group I (n = 15) patients presented with FHF were listed for emergent OLT, Group II (n = 3) patients with primary non-function (PNF) of their liver grafts required urgent re-transplantation and Group III (n = 10) patients with acute exacerbation of chronic liver disease were not candidates for OLT. Patients were managed in a critical care unit receiving maximal standard support. Each BAL treatment was conducted for 6 hours. In Group I, all patients showed significant neurologic improvement, intracranial pressure (ICP) decreased and cerebral perfusion pressure (CPP) increased; other significant improvements, included lowered plasma ammonia and liver enzymes and increased glucose. One patient recovered spontaneously without OLT, all other patients were "bridged" to OLT, and recovered. Group II: PNF patients showed similar benefits. Group III: Chronic liver patients demonstrated transient beneficial effects after BAL treatment(s), however, most (n = 8) eventually succumbed to sepsis and multiple organ failure as they were not candidates for OLT; two patients, recovered, later were successfully transplanted and survived. Our clinical experience demonstrates that the BAL can serve as a bridge to OLT in patients with acute liver failure.

REFERENCES

1. SHEIL, A. G. R., G. W. McCAUGHAN, H. ISAI, *et al.* 1991. Acute and subacute fulminant hepatic failure: The role of liver transplantation. Med. J. Australia **154**: 724–728.
2. O'GRADY, J. G., A. E. S. GIMSON, C. J. O'BRIEN, *et al.* 1988. Controlled trials of charcoal hemoperfusion and prognostic factors in fulminant hepatic failure. Gastroenterology **94**: 1186–1192.
3. NEUZIL, D. F., J. ROZGA, A. D. MOSCIONI, *et al.* 1993. Use of a novel bioartificial liver in a patient with acute liver insufficiency. Surgery **113**: 340–343.
4. ROZGA, J., M. D. HOLZMAN, M.-S. RO, *et al.* 1993. Hybrid bioartificial liver support treatment of animals with severe ischemic liver failure. Ann. Surg. **217**: 502–511.
5. ROZGA J., F. WILLIAMS, M.-S. RO, *et al.* 1993. Development of a bioartificial liver: Properties and function of a hollow-fiber module inoculated with liver cells. Hepatology **17**: 258–265.
6. DEMETRIOU, A. A., J. ROZGA, L. PODESTA, *et al.* 1995. Early clinical experience with a bioartificial liver. Scand. J. Gastroenterol. **30**(Suppl 208): 111–117.
7. TREY, C. & C. DAVIDSON. 1970. The management of fulminant hepatic failure. Prog. Liver Dis. **3**: 282–298.
8. O'GRADY, J., S. W. SCHALM & R. WILLIAMS. 1993. Acute liver failure: Redefining the syndromes. Lancet **342**: 273–275.
9. BERNUAU, J. & J. P. BENHAMOU. 1993. Classifying acute liver failure. Lancet **342**: 252.
10. PAPPAS, S. C. 1988. Fulminant hepatic failure and need for artificial liver support. Mayo Clin. Proc. **63**: 198–200.
11. STANCZAK, D. E., J. G. WHITE III, W. D. GOUVIEW, *et al.* 1984. Assessment of level of consciousness following severe neurological insult. J. Neurosurg. **60**: 955–960.
12. DEMETRIOU, A. A. Ed. 1994. Support of the acutely failing liver. Medical Intelligent Unit, R. G. Landes Co. Austin, TX.
13. ROZGA, J., E. LePAGE, A. D. MOSCIONI, *et al.* 1994. Clinical use of a bioartificial liver to treat fulminant hepatic failure. Ann. Surg. **219**: 538–546.
14. KONG, L. B., S. CHEN, A. A. DEMETRIOU & J. ROZGA. 1995. Matrix-induced liver cell aggregates (MILCA) for bioartificial liver use. Int. J. Artif. Organs **18**: 43–49.
15. MORSIANI, E., J. ROZGA, H. C. SCOTT, *et al.* 1995. Automated liver cell processing facilitates large scale isolation and purification of porcine hepatocytes. ASAIO J. **41**: 155–161.
16. RECORD, C. O., B. BUXTON, R. A. CHASE, *et al.* 1976. Plasma and brain amino acids in fulminant hepatic failure and their relationship to hepatic encephalopathy. Eur. J. Clin. Invest. **6**: 387–394.
17. JAMES, J. H., B. JEPPSON, U. ZIPARO & J. E. FISCHER. 1979. Hyperammonemia, plasma amino acid imbalance and blood brain amino acid transport: A unified theory of portal hepatic encephalopathy. Lancet **ii**: 772–775.
18. LEE, W. 1994. Acute liver failure. N. Engl. J. Med. **329**(25): 1862–1872.
19. BURNELL, J. M., C. RUNGE, F. C. SAUNDERS, E. D. THOMAS & W. VOLWILER. 1973. Acute hepatic failure treated by cross circulation. Arch. Intern. Med. **132**: 493–498.
20. BIHARI, D., R. D. HUGHES, A. E. S. GIMSON, *et al.* 1983. Effects of serial resin hemoperfusion in fulminant hepatic failure. Int. J. Artif. Organs **6**: 299–302.
21. PARBHOO, S. P., I. M. JAMES, A. AJDUKIEWICZ, *et al.* 1971. Extracorporeal pig liver perfusion in treatment of hepatic coma due to fulminant hepatitis. Lancet **ii**: 659–665.
22. ABOUNA, G. M., J. S. COOK, L. M. A. FISHER, *et al.* 1972. Treatment of acute hepatic coma by ex vivo baboon and human liver perfusion. Surgery **71**: 537–546.
23. GIMSON, A. E. S., P. J. MELLON, S. BRAUDE, *et al.* 1982. Earlier charcoal haemoperfusion in fulminant hepatic failure. Lancet **ii**: 68–83.
24. SMITH, J. W., S. MATSUBARA, T. HORIUCHI, *et al.* 1982. Sorption-filtration therapy for

chronic liver disease in vivo testing and clinical correlation. Trans. Am. Soc. Artif. Intern. Organs **28:** 215–219.

25. O'GRADY, J. G., A. E. S. GIMSON, C. J. O'BRIEN, *et al.* 1988. Controlled trials of charcoal hemoperfusion and prognostic factors in fulminant hepatic failure. Gastroenterology **94:** 1186–1192.

26. SILK, D. B. A., P. N. TREWBY, R. A. CHASE, *et al.* 1977. Treatment of fulminant hepatic failure by polyacrylonitrile-membrane haemodialysis. Lancet **ii:** 1–3.

27. DENIS, J., P. OPOLON, V. NUSINOVICI, *et al.* 1978. Treatment of encephalopathy during fulminant hepatic failure by hemodialysis with high permeability membrane. Gut **19:** 787–793.

28. REDEKER, A. G. & H. S. YAMAHIRO. 1973. Controlled trial of exchange transfusion therapy in fulminant hepatitis. Lancet **ii:** 3–6.

29. COOPER, G. N., K. E. KARLSON, G. H. A. CLOWES, *et al.* 1977. Total body washout and exchange. A valuable tool in acute hepatic coma and Reye's syndrome. Am. J. Surg. **133:** 522–530.

30. DENTI, E. & M. P. LUBOZ. 1974. Preparation and properties of gel-entrapped liver cell microsomes. *In* Artificial Liver Support. R. Williams and I. M. Murray Lyon, Eds.: 148–152. Pitman Medical.

31. USAMI, M., H. OHYANAGI, S. NISHIMATSU, *et al.* 1989. Therapeutic plasmapheresis for liver failure after hepatectomy. Trans. Am. Soc. Artif. Intern. Organs. **35:** 564–567.

32. OLUMIDE, F., A. ELIASHIV, N. KRALIOS, *et al.* 1977. Hepatic support with hepatocyte suspensions in a permeable membrane dialyzer. Surgery **82:** 599–606.

33. YANAGI, K., K. OOKAWA, M. SHUICHI, *et al.* 1989. Performance of a new hybrid artificial liver support system using hepatocytes entrapped within a hydrogel. Trans. Am. Soc. Artif Intern. Organs **35:** 570–572.

34. MATSUMURA, K. N., G. R. GUEVARA, H. HUSTION, *et al.* 1987. Hybrid bioartificial liver in hepatic failure: Preliminary clinical report. Surgery **101:** 99–103.

35. SAITO, S., K. SAKAGAMI & K. ORITA. 1987. A new hybrid artificial liver using a combination of hepatocytes and biomatrix. Trans. Am. Soc. Artif. Intern. Organs **33:** 459–462.

36. FOX, I. J., A. N. LANGNAS, C. F. OZAKI, *et al.* 1993. Successful application of extracorporeal liver perfusion for the treatment of fulminant hepatic failure: A technology whose time has come. Am. J. Gastroenterol. **88:** 1876–1881.

Molecular Regulation of Liver Regeneration[a]

BETSY T. KREN,[b] JANEEN H. TREMBLEY,[c,e]
GUANGSHENG FAN,[b] AND CLIFFORD J. STEER[b,d,f]

[b]Department of Medicine
[c]Department of Genetics and Cell Biology
[d]Department of Cell Biology and Neuroanatomy
University of Minnesota Medical School
Minneapolis, Minnesota 55455

The liver constitutes one of the few, normally quiescent tissues in the adult animal that has the capacity to regenerate in response to cell loss through physical, infectious or hepatotoxic injury. The most popular experimental model to study hepatic regeneration was reported by Higgins and Anderson in 1931 in which they described the surgical removal of two-thirds of the liver in rats.[1] In the remaining lobes, the majority of hepatic cells rapidly reenter the growth cycle and begin to replicate. The "regeneration" of the liver after 70% partial hepatectomy (PH) is a precise, highly regulated process which appears to be controlled by many of the same factors responsible for the liver's fetal development. Restoration of liver mass is governed by functional rather than anatomical factors, occurs by compensatory hyperplasia of the remnant tissue and, therefore, does not represent true regeneration. In the paradigm of "hepatic regeneration" after PH, liver function recovers quickly following the restoration of histologically normal tissue. The liver appears to have an optimal functional mass and as the remnant tissue grows, its shape is largely determined by external pressure. Reorganization of lobular architecture is a dynamic process involving both dissolution and deposition of extracellular matrix.[2]

The kinetics of cell replication displayed by hepatocytes after PH are well described and, in general, represent a fairly synchronized process.[3–6] The exact timing of DNA synthesis after PH varies with the age of the animal and can be modified by hormones and dietary manipulations. For younger adult rats, the basal rate of DNA synthesis is unchanged in the first 12 hours (prereplicative phase) after which there is a wave of DNA synthesis in hepatocytes which peaks at about 24 hours and then gradually declines. Hepatocytes located in the periportal area

[a] This work was supported in part by grants from the Minnesota Medical Foundation and National Institutes of Health (RO1 DK44649) to C.J.S. and a grant-in-aid from the Graduate School, University of Minnesota to J.H.T.

[e] Present address: St. Jude Children's Research Hospital, Department of Tumor Cell Biology, 332 North Lauderdale, P.O. Box 318, Memphis, TN 38101. Tel: (901) 495-2156; Fax: (901) 495-2381; E-mail: janeen.trembley@stjude.org

[f] Corresponding author: Clifford J. Steer, M.D., Department of Medicine, Box 36 UMHC, University of Minnesota Medical School, 420 Delaware Street, S.E., Minneapolis, MN 55455. Tel: (612) 624-6648; Fax: (612) 625-5620; E-mail: steer001@maroon.tc.umn.edu

replicate earlier than those located towards the central veins and DNA synthesis in nonparenchymal, Ito and bile ductular cells is usually delayed by about 24 hours. Typically, mitosis occurs 6 to 8 hours following DNA replication.[7] Both DNA synthesis and mitosis exhibit the same pattern of distribution within the remnant lobe. One to several rounds of DNA synthesis takes place, each successive round exhibiting less synchrony until the original liver mass is restored. Liver growth then ceases and the hepatocytes resume a quiescent state. In regeneration after PH, restoration of liver mass results from the capacity of adult hepatocytes to divide and does not appear to involve stem cell replication. In a young adult rat, as many as 95% of the hepatocytes undergo at least a single cycle of replication to restore the original size of the liver. The basic steps which occur during liver regeneration from certain toxic injuries are similar to those after PH.[5] The major differences relate to the triggering events, expression of the immediate-early genes and the involvement of a population of undifferentiated liver progenitor cells which persist in the adult liver.

METABOLIC CHANGES

Numerous metabolic changes take place during the prereplicative phase of liver regeneration. They include increases in intracellular pH, cAMP levels, Na^+/K^+ ATPase activity, pools of ornithine and lysine, RNA and mRNA levels as well as ornithine decarboxylase activity and polyamine synthesis.[5] In fact, it has been postulated that increased Na^+ fluxes into hepatocytes are necessary to initiate their replication. A number of serum factors have been implicated as responsible for these early changes in the regenerating liver, including insulin, glucagon, norepinephrine, vasopressin, epidermal growth factor, as well as other hepatocyte growth inducers.[3,8] To date, no mediator has been identified which is solely responsible for triggering hepatocytes to enter the cell cycle. During the early phase, all hepatic cells are primed to undergo transition from a G_0 resting state to a G_1 replicative state.[4,5,9] It is well established that this G_0/G_1 transition occurs simultaneously in all hepatic cells beginning almost immediately after PH, perhaps triggered by factors already present in the blood or liver. Although the total amount of cytoplasmic mRNA increases significantly during the first 12 hours after PH, the actual rate of synthesis is increased only for the first several hours.

HEPATIC GROWTH FACTORS

The stimulus for regeneration is influenced by numerous factors including nutrient excess and/or metabolic overload. However, the initiation of hepatocyte replication is critically dependent on the interaction of growth factors with their cell surface receptors. Regeneration represents a complex scheme of stimulatory and inhibitory effects on cell growth. Most growth regulators can be described as either complete mitogens or comitogens.[3] Complete mitogens are substances which are by themselves able to stimulate hepatocyte replication in chemically defined media and in the absence of serum. Examples include epidermal growth factor, transforming growth factor α, heparin binding growth factors, keratinocyte growth factor and hepatocyte growth factor. Comitogens are substances which affect hepatocyte growth in an indirect manner and are best characterized as growth triggers. Basically they enhance the growth effects of the complete mitogens but by themselves are

TABLE 1. Hepatic Growth Regulators

Hormones and Nutrients
Adrenal cortical hormones
Catecholamines
Estrogens and androgens
Insulin and glucagon
Nutrients
Parathyroid hormone, calcium and vitamin D
Prolactin
Prostaglandins
Thyroid hormones
Vasopressin
Polypeptide Growth Factors
Augmenter of liver regeneration
Epidermal growth factor
Growth hormone and insulin-like growth factors
Heparin-binding growth factors
Hepatic stimulatory substance
Hepatocyte growth factor
Hepatopoietins
Keratinocyte growth factor
Transforming growth factor α
Tumor necrosis factor α
Miscellaneous hepatotrophic factors
Growth Inhibitory Factors
Hepatocyte proliferation inhibitor
Interleukin 1β
Transforming growth factor β
Other growth inhibitors

SOURCE: Modified from Bucher & Strain.[8]

nonmitogenic. Examples include the estrogens and androgens, vasopressin and the angiotensins, insulin, glucagon and norepinephrine. The three major growth inhibitors which have been identified include transforming growth factor-β (TGF-β), interleukin 1β and hepatocyte proliferation inhibitor.[3,8] According to Bucher and Strain, hepatic growth regulators can be grouped into several broad categories (TABLE 1).[8] The hormones and nutrients represent the relatively low-molecular weight factors. Polypeptide growth factors include the larger molecular weight subtances which are derived either from serum and/or liver. The inhibitory factors are few in number and appear to be higher molecular weight proteins.

Hormones and Nutrients

Adrenal cortical hormones have been reported to induce hepatic enlargement due mainly to their hypertrophic effects. Although PH results in elevated plasma levels of certain cortical hormones, the increase may simply be due to a reduced capacity of the liver remnant to process the molecules. Their effects on growth vary considerably and no definitive conclusion can be made regarding their role in liver regeneration.

Catecholamines appear to be effective modulators of hepatocyte growth. The work of several investigators has suggested a role for adrenergic hormones in the regulation of liver regeneration. Blockade of α_1-adrenergic receptor by prazolsin or surgical hepatic denervation significantly depresses the 24 hour peak of DNA synthesis after PH.[10] Hepatocytes isolated from regenerating liver are very sensitive to norepinephrine during the prereplicative phase of the cell cycle. Its increase after PH is thought to be a potential source of stimulation of the α_1-adrenergic receptor and subsequent activation of protein kinase C and mobilization of calcium from intracellular stores by phosphatidylinositol diphosphate (PIP_2). Interestingly, norepinephrine has been shown to suppress the growth-inhibiting effects of TGF-β. Vasopressin and the angiotensins also act through receptors which enhance PIP_2 turnover and may play a role in liver regeneration. In fact, vasopressin may be involved in the mediation of effects by the sympathetic nervous system on the regenerating liver.

Nutrients are critical effectors of cell growth and availability is clearly essential for maximal regenerative activity.[11] An early prereplicative event found in the liver remnant following PH is an increased pool of free amino acids. The accumulation results primarily from enhanced translocation of amino acids across the plasma membrane. It has been reported that system A amino acid transporters are increased in the regenerating liver 2 to 24 hours post-PH.[12] System A appears to perform a unique role in the secondary active transport of neutral amino acids to meet the metabolic demands of the regenerating liver. Moreover, it has been demonstrated that hepatocytes pass through a priming stage before they replicate[13] and that nutrients, particularly, protein are important for this process. Rats denied protein for several days underwent a burst of hepatic DNA synthesis and mitosis when refed amino acids in contrast to normally fed or starved animals. The livers of protein-deprived rats exhibited significantly increased mRNA levels for several of the proto-oncogenes as well as p53. It was suggested that hepatocytes pass through a priming stage prior to proliferation and that replicative competence without DNA synthesis can be induced in normal liver by changes in nutritional state. Interestingly, the inducible cellular proliferative response was preserved by controlling calorie intake despite reduced expression of certain proto-oncogenes.[14]

It is well established that insulin and glucagon act as comitogens in optimizing DNA synthesis and liver regeneration. Likewise, parathyroid hormone, calcium and vitamin D also appear to be important factors in the regulation of liver regeneration.[8] The step-by-step control of progression of replicating hepatocytes through the cell cycle is dependent on calcium ions. Hepatic regeneration is greatly reduced in parathyroidectomized animals due to their inability to respond to the thyroid-dependent hypocalcemia caused by partial hepatectomy. It is thought that vitamin D3 plays a essential role in regulating a set of replication-linked genes, c-myc, c-myb, and histone H4, which are critical for rapid cell proliferation. In vitamin D depletion, hypocalcemia retards DNA synthesis and liver mass recovery. Normocalcemia contributes to DNA synthesis, but fails to sustain mitosis and compensatory liver growth to a level comparable to that found after repletion of D3 and/or 1,25 dihydroxyvitamin D3, the major biologically active metabolite of vitamin D3.[15]

Prolactin administration increases thymidine kinase and ornithine decarboxylase activity in liver. However, little information is available to implicate it as a key regulator of hepatic regeneration. Prostaglandins may play a role in the regulation of liver regeneration. It has been reported that an early prostaglandin- or thromboxane-mediated process in stimulated hepatocytes is involved in their subsequent entry into mitosis. The process appears to be separate from the early events leading to DNA synthesis. Thyroid hormones appear to elicit a hyperplastic response in the liver. However, much of their stimulatory action may be indirect and reflect extensive metabolic changes thoughout the body.

Polypeptide Growth Factors

Epidermal growth factor (EGF) is a potent mitogen for numerous cell types including those derived from liver. It is the most frequently used polypeptide to induce hepatocyte DNA synthesis in culture. Although insulin is not essential for EGF-stimulated mitogenesis, it is required for the full magnitude of the response. Interestingly, only low-affinity EGF receptors are expressed in isolated hepatocytes. It has been suggested that they are the true mitogenic-response receptors in contrast to the high affinity receptors which function to prevent EGF from interacting with the low-affinity receptors. The role of EGF in liver regeneration is unresolved. A decline in the number of EGF receptors and their related tyrosine kinase activity occurs within 8 hours post-PH. No significant changes in EGF plasma concentrations have been reported during the regenerative process. Relatively large amounts of EGF are produced in mouse salivary glands and their removal is associated with a significant delay in peak DNA synthesis after PH.[16] Similarly, removal of Brunner's glands and administration of EGF antiserum both significantly reduced liver regeneration in rats. Treatment of sialoadenectomized mice with EGF restored the normal pattern of DNA synthesis in the regenerating liver.

Transforming growth factor α (TGF-α) is also a potent mitogen for hepatocytes in primary culture. It is synthesized as a 160 amino acid precursor which is anchored in the plasma membrane and cleaved to a 50 amino acid processed molecule.[5] It shares 35% amino acid sequence homology with EGF and binds to the EGF receptor. TGF-α is developmentally regulated in the liver and produced by replicating hepatocytes *in vivo* and *in vitro*. The concentration of the protein in hepatic tissue is low in adult rats, but increases significantly after PH. TGF-α mRNA levels begin to increase 4 hours after PH and peak at 18 to 24 hours, paralleling the kinetics of DNA synthesis in the regenerating liver.[17] Although the mechanisms involved in its induction are unknown, TGF-α appears to represent an important autocrine regulator of hepatocyte growth. Like EGF, its mitogenic effect is also suppressed by TGF-β.

The synthesis of insulin-like growth factors (IGF) 1 and 2, originally known as the somatomedins, is thought to be regulated by interaction of growth hormone with its hepatic receptors.[8] There is evidence to suggest that IGFs may play a role in regulation of liver growth as autocrine factors. For example, it has been demonstrated that IGF-1 receptors are expressed in regenerating rat liver and not in hepatocytes from normal adult rat and human livers. One of the most abundant liver-specific early genes in regenerating liver encodes the rat homolog of the low-molecular weight IGF-binding protein.[18] It was suggested that IGF-1 and its binding protein interact with hepatocytes through IGF-1 and/or novel receptors. Growth hormone does appear to enhance and accelerate hepatic regeneration particularly if administered prior to surgical resection.

Heparin-binding growth factors (HBGF), also termed fibroblast growth factors, are mitogenic for a wide variety of cell types including hepatocytes. They require heparin for their activity and are inactive in its absence. HBGF-1, or acidic fibroblast growth factor (aFGF), is potentially an important factor in liver regeneration. After PH, a significant increase in HBGF-1 transcripts was observed at 24 hours.[19,20] Expression occurred in both hepatocytes and nonparenchymal cells and persisted for 7 days after PH. HBGF-1 was stimulatory to rat hepatocytes in culture and more refractory to the inhibitory effects of TGF-β than was EGF. It was suggested that this growth factor is an early autocrine stimulus that drives hepatocyte DNA synthesis prior to or concurrent with the EGF/TGF-α stimulus.[19] Expression of a 25 kD form of HBGF-2 (basic FGF) has been shown to increase in regenerating liver.[8]

Hepatic stimulatory substance (HSS) was first described in 1974. It was originally derived from cytosolic extracts of normal weanling and regenerating rat livers. Since then it has been demonstrated in many other species. Of the mitogens discussed, it is unique because it is liver specific. No activity has been demonstrated on other cell types. The peptide has recently been purified to homogeneity and exhibits an apparent molecular mass of 7.5 kD.[21] It has been shown to induce rapid influx of sodium and calcium and increases in protein phosphorylation. It appears to activate genes at the G_1/S cell cycle transition and thus may regulate a cell's commitment to DNA synthesis. HSS has limited growth-promoting effects on normal hepatocytes in primary culture. However, in the presence of EGF it produces dramatic increases in DNA synthesis in cultured hepatocytes from regenerating liver. It significantly augments regenerative growth and is a potent mitogen for several hepatoma cell lines. Although its role in the regulation of liver regeneration is undefined, it is a unique liver-specific mitogen which functions as a true autocrine factor.

There has been a growing interest in defining the putative role of hepatocyte growth factor (HGF) in liver regeneration. It was originally identified as hepatopoietin A in a chromatographic fraction of serum from hepatectomized rats. It is the most potent mitogen for mature hepatocytes and was initially purified from rat platelets in 1986.[22,23] It is synthesized as a 728 amino acid precursor which is cleaved into a disulfide-linked heterodimer composed of a 69 kD α-subunit and a 34 kD β-subunit. The HGF receptor was identified as the product of the c-*met* proto-oncogene, which encodes a 190 kD glycosylated transmembrane protein containing a tyrosine kinase domain on the β subunit. The receptor is expressed by many different tissues and cell lines. In the liver the growth factor is produced only by nonparenchymal cells and not hepatocytes, and its mRNA and protein levels increase markedly after PH. HGF and its two mRNA transcripts are most abundant in lipocytes, with smaller amounts present in Kupffer and endothelial cells. HGF increases rapidly in the blood after PH. The increase 2 to 4 hours post-PH occurs well before peak DNA synthesis and coincides with the observed increase in plasma norepinephrine levels. The rapid rise of HGF in plasma following PH, however, is probably not due to *de novo* synthesis, but rather to decreased removal of the molecule by the compromised liver.[24] It has been suggested that the combination of HGF as mitogen and norepinephrine as comitogen serves to provide the signal which initiates the first round of DNA synthesis during liver regeneration. Although HGF is a heparin-binding growth factor, heparin diminishes its mitogenic activity as does TGF-β.

HGF has been shown to be a remarkable pleiotropic factor. It is not only a potent hepatocyte mitogen, but also stimulates the growth of epithelial cells from a number of tissues. In transformed cells, HGF acts as a motogen to induce migration and spreading. In fact, "scatter factor" which induces epithelial and endothelial cell migration has recently been shown to be HGF. Additionally, HGF acts as a morphogen and induces epithelial tubule formation. Taken together, the growth factor has a remarkable ability to restore liver mass, promote cell migration during the architectural remodeling and influence differentiation—all factors inherent in the process of liver regeneration. The precise relationship between HGF and liver regeneration remains to be established. Although many questions are still unanswered, it remains a remarkably exciting growth factor which appears to be important in numerous facets of hepatocyte repair and replication.

Hepatopoietin B is a 500 dalton molecule which has also been isolated from the serum of hepatectomized rats.[3] It is considered a complete hepatocyte mitogen and, interestingly, appears to be a glycolipid. It also interacts synergistically with both HGF and EGF. Little other information is available concerning its role in liver regeneration.

Tumor necrosis factor α (TNF-α) appears to act as a paracrine factor to promote liver regeneration after PH.[25] Pre-treatment with antibodies to the cytokine has been shown to significantly inhibit increases in serum IL-6 concentrations which normally follow PH. It also blunted [³H]thymidine incorporation into DNA at 24 hours post-PH and suppressed the expression of proliferation-specific antigens by both parenchymal and nonparenchymal cells through 72 hours post-PH. Other reports have identified additional substances with potential hepatotrophic effects. For example, an unusual quality of two powerful immunosuppressive agents, FK 506 and cyclosporine, is augmentation of the regenerative response after PH.[26] It has been suggested that this effect is independent of immunological pathways and probably involves an as yet undefined second messenger system. Recently, this mechanism has been elucidated and appears to involve the binding of a new growth factor, augmenter of liver regeneration (ALR), found in hepatocyte cytosol to these immunosuppresive molecules.[27]

Growth Inhibitory Factors

Numerous unanswered questions exist regarding the role of growth-inhibitory factors in liver regeneration. TGF-β is the paradigm multifunctional cytokine whose actions are dependent on numerous factors including cell type, state of differentiation and growth conditions.[28,29] In general, TGF-β is growth-stimulatory for cells of mesenchymal origin and growth-inhibitory for cells of epithelial origin. TGF-β is known to exist in at least five different isoforms which are 60 to 80% identical in amino acid sequence. Three of the isoforms (TGF-β1, TGF-β2, and TGF-β3) are present in mammalian liver. TGF-β1 is a potent inhibitor of DNA synthesis for rat, mouse and human hepatocytes in culture.[5] The inhibitory effect appears to occur just prior to the G_1/S transition.[30] Although the exact mechanisms are unknown, TGF-β1 has been shown to inhibit cyclin E-dependent kinase activity,[31] and has been linked to suppression of retinoblastoma protein phosphorylation.[32] It is synthesized and secreted in a latent high molecular weight form which is devoid of biological activity. The active molecule is a homodimeric 25 kD polypeptide. The liver plays a major role in regulating circulating levels of TGF-β1. The molecule is cleared rapidly by the liver with a half-life of 2.2 minutes in rats. It elicits a potent inhibitory effect on hepatocyte replication as well as liver-derived epithelial cells. The inhibitory action does not appear to result from direct competition with known mitogens. It is involved in the regulation of fetal hepatic growth and appears to play a key role in the control of liver regeneration. The timing of the elevations of TGF-β1, TGF-β2 and TGF-β3 mRNAs in the regenerating liver varies.[33] Following PH, only the increase in steady-state mRNA levels for TGF-β1 are sustained beyond 4 hours, while those for TGF-β2 and -β3 peak within 4 hours and then decline. Interestingly, following PH both the endothelial cells as well as hepatocytes express increased levels of TGF-β1 transcripts in contrast to the quiescent liver in which the mRNAs are restricted to nonparenchymal cells.[34] It has been reported that intravenously administered TGF-β1 at the time of surgery and 11 hours post-PH substantially reduced the number of hepatocytes engaged in DNA synthesis.[35] The inhibitory effect was transient, however, and administration of TGF-β1 regularly for 5 days failed to suppress recovery of liver mass. It is somewhat paradoxical that increased expression of TGF-β mRNA occurs during maximal hepatocyte proliferative activity.

Hepatocytes express type I and type II TGF-β receptors but do not express the betaglycan type III receptor. Following PH, there is a small decrease in the number of type II receptors and an appearance of a new population of higher affinity TGF-β1 receptors. In contrast, insulin-like growth factor-II/mannose 6-phosphate receptors are up-regulated during liver regeneration and may be responsible for the observed increase in uptake of the latent TGF-β1 phosphomannosyl glycoprotein complex.[36] Expression of the receptor coincided with the increase in TGF-β1 observed initially in periportal and then perivenous hepatocytes. The results are consistent with the observation that hepatocytes from regenerating livers are capable of activating latent TGF-β1 complexes *in vitro*, in contrast to normal hepatocytes.

Members of the TGF-β family of cytokines are not the only potential inhibitors of liver regeneration. It has been shown that interleukin 1β suppresses proliferation of adult rat hepatocytes in primary culture. Hepatocyte proliferation inhibitor is a 15 kD polypeptide which also inhibits hepatocyte proliferation in culture and is not inhibited by anti-TGF-β antibodies.[3] Activin, a member of the TGF-β family of proteins, acts as an inhibitor of DNA synthesis and like TGF-β increases in expression during liver regeneration.[5] Recently, it has been reported that nonparenchymal cells in culture from 24-hour regenerating livers release a 14 to 17 kD factor which acts as a potent inhibitor of the proliferative response by hepatocytes to EGF, HGF and TGF-α.[37] Thus, in contrast to the large number of hepatotrophic factors identifed, very few inhibitors of liver regeneration have been identified and characterized. Moreover, it is unlikely that a single inhibitory substance determines the extent to which a liver regenerates, just as no single factor appears to control the initiation of the regenerative process. Realistically, this complex paracrine, autocrine, hormonal and neurally regulated process is subject to growth inhibition resulting from an interplay of molecules, factors and pathways, including those typically associated with apoptosis, or programmed cell death.

PRIMARY RESPONSE GENES

As indicated above, one of the initial metabolic changes undergone by the liver in the early stages of regeneration post-PH is a rapid change in the rate of RNA synthesis and overall mRNA steady-state levels. In fact, more than 70 immediate-early genes induced in regenerating liver after PH have been identified, of which 41 are novel.[38,39] Genes rapidly induced in transition from the normally quiescent state of the liver to the growth phase are called immediate-early genes and include certain proto-oncogenes.[40,41] They appear to be transcribed in response to mitogenic stimuli and are independent of protein synthesis, in contrast to delayed-early genes.[42] Their response is of enormous complexity and appears to be necessary for subsequent cellular events. The complexity may, in fact, allow for the rapid cellular growth reponse observed after PH. Proto-oncogene expression in the regenerating rat liver provided some of the earliest examples of a regulated, cell cycle-dependent response to PH.[43] Although the exact role of proto-oncogenes in the regenerative process is unknown, there is sufficient evidence to suggest they are critical regulators of cell growth and proliferation. Steady-state mRNA levels of c-*fos* and c-*jun* increase almost immediately after PH, peak at 15 to 30 minutes and return to basal levels within 2 hours. c-*myc* increases more slowly, peaks at 2 to 4 hours and returns to near basal levels by 12 hours. Additional smaller peaks have been observed for c-*fos* at 8 hours and c-*myc* at 18 as well as 36 hours, but all are short-lived. Both of these nuclear proto-oncogenes are expressed abundantly in many types of proliferating cells and are induced early in the transition from G_0 to G_1. It has been shown that the c-*fos* protein complexes with that of c-*jun* to form the transcriptional activating factor AP-1. In contrast to the very early expression of c-*fos* and c-*myc*, the levels of the tumor suppressor gene p53 transcript increase between 8 and 16 hours and return to normal by the onset of the first wave of DNA synthesis. Expression of members in the *ras* gene family of proto-oncogenes begins during the prereplicative phase, peaks at cell division and slowly returns to normal by 72 to 96 hours. The increased expression of these proto-oncogenes appears to be highly regulated and specific, since the steady-state levels of c-*mos*, c-*abl* and c-*src* remain invariant during liver regeneration after PH. Certain variations in proto-oncogene expression may influence the nature of the proliferative response. In this regard, it is interesting that the hyperplastic response of the liver to the peroxisome proliferators nafenopin and cyproterone acetate occurs without detectable changes in transcript expression for either c-*fos* or c-*myc*.[44]

There are additional immediate-early genes which are rapidly induced in regenerating liver and, by definition, do not require new protein synthesis for increased expression. These include the gene encoding insulin-like growth factor binding protein, LRF-1 (liver regeneration factor 1) and RL/IF-1 (regenerating liver inhibitory factor 1).[18,45,46] LRF-1 codes for a leucine zipper protein which complexes with c-*jun* and functions as a transcription factor. RL/IF-1 binds to the NF-κB transcription factor in cytosol and inhibits its nuclear translocation. It inhibits DNA binding not only of NF-κB but also other transcription factors involved in cell replication. However, within minutes after PH, PHF (partial hepatectomy factor) is increased several thousand fold and is capable of binding to DNA NF-κB sites and inducing transcription of those particular genes.

CONTROL OF GENE EXPRESSION

Three characteristic temporal patterns of immediate-early, delayed-early as well as growth-related and liver-specific gene expression appear to characterize the regulation of liver regeneration[9] (FIG. 1). One pattern of induction has two peaks coincident with the first and second G_1 phases of the hepatic cell cycles, with the initial peak representing the immediate-early genes. A second pattern parallels the major growth period of the liver ending 60 to 72 hours post-PH, and includes the delayed-early and growth-regulated genes. The third pattern includes liver-specific genes which exhibit maximal expression after the growth period. The reentry of liver cells into a proliferative state results in the discrete appearance of transcripts for many different genes. Transcriptional and/or posttranscriptional processes control the steady-state expression of mRNAs, yet for many of the induced transcripts, substantial changes in transcriptional activity are not observed (TABLE 2). In fact, numerous genes expressed in the regenerating liver are probably controlled at the posttranscriptional level, including those modulated at the immediate-early phase of the cell cycle.[16,47-57] Posttranscriptional control of mRNA expression occurs primarily by nuclear processing of heterogeneous nuclear (hn) RNA, nucleocytoplasmic transport of mature mRNA and mRNA stability.

The regulation of mRNA stability is thought to play an important role in eukaryotic gene expression by modulating the abundance of the different transcripts. However, the notion is based almost entirely on results generated from tissue culture studies. In contrast, very few reports have addressed this important issue in an *in vivo* model of tissue growth. The remaining portion of this review will examine the results of using the unique model of regenerating liver to investigate mRNA stability and cyclin gene expression during the cell cycle of adult differentiated cells *in vivo*.

Time Post-PH (h)

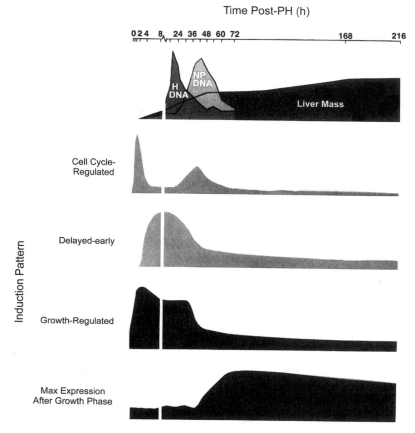

FIGURE 1. Representative patterns and temporal expression of regulated genes in regenerating rat liver post-PH. The patterns of DNA synthesis in hepatocytes (H) and nonparenchymal cells (NP) as well as restoration of liver mass through 216 hours after PH are indicated at the top. The induction patterns of the four classes of regulated genes are shown with the classification listed at left. (Modified from Haber *et al.*[9])

mRNA Stability

The half-lives of many mRNAs are modulated in response to exogenous stimuli, cell cycle phase, and state of differentiation. In fact, mRNA levels often correlate more closely with transcript stability than with transcriptional activity. It is well established that mRNAs exhibit varying half-lives in a given cell and the stability of a single mRNA can be temporally and spatially modulated.[58] In mammalian cells, mRNA half-lives can vary by orders of magnitude. Can one assume then that this posttranscriptional process plays a key regulatory role in expression of steady-state transcript levels following PH?

A subset of the genes listed in TABLE 2 as well as others have been studied to establish the role of mRNA stability in modulating their mRNA steady-state levels

TABLE 2. Genes Whose Steady-state Transcript Levels Are Modulated during Liver Regeneration but Exhibit No Change in Transcription Rate during Liver Regeneration

bcl-2	ornithine decarboxylase
bcl-x	glutathione S-transferases
bax	multidrug resistance
p53	P450IIB1
MDM-2	P450IIE1
H-ras	cholesterol 7α-hydroxylase
cyclin A	HMG-CoA reductase
cyclin B1	low density lipoprotein receptor
cyclin D1	asialoglycoprotein receptor
cyclin D3	procollagen $\alpha_1(I)$
cyclin E	procollagen $\alpha_1(III)$
CDK1	procollagen $\alpha_1(IV)$
connexin 32	fibronectin
connexin 26	laminin
HNF-1	TGF-β_1
HNF-4	growth arrest specific gene

SOURCE: From references 48–53, 55, 56.

in regenerating rodent liver.[16,48,53–57,59,60] The majority of the mRNAs exhibited modulations in steady-state mRNA levels at the same time points post-PH. Genes with transcriptional rate changes insufficient to account for the alterations in their steady-state levels post-PH as well as those with no transcriptional changes have been investigated. The *in vivo* chemical half-lives of the selected mRNA transcripts were determined by northern blot analyses of poly(A)$^+$-enriched RNA isolated after administration of the transcriptional inhibitors actinomycin D and α-amanitin. A summary of the results of the studies is presented in TABLE 3. The transcripts for TGF-β_1, procollagens $\alpha_1(I)$ and $\alpha_1(III)$, ornithine decarboxylase, cyclin B$_1$, p21, H-*ras*, multidrug resistance, *bcl*-x, *bax*, EGF receptor, *MDM*-2, and p53 exhibited increased stability post-PH corresponding to increased mRNA steady-state levels. Moreover, decreased stability of the cyclin B$_1$ and *bcl*-x transcripts occurred prior to the loss of the mRNA species. Intermediate increases in *bax* and ornithine decarboxylase mRNA half-lives paralleled increasing abundance of steady-state levels, while p53 transcript half-life at 24 hours was between that observed at 0 and 6 hours, demonstrating that continued loss of the transcript was associated with decreasing half-life. No changes in transcript stability for hemopexin, fibronectin, retinoblastoma or PFK-2/FBPase-2 were detected at times of altered steady-state transcript abundance. The immediate-early proto-oncogene c-*myc* exhibited a surprising threefold increase in mRNA half-life at 6 hours post-PH, in contrast to hemopexin whose transcriptional activation post-PH was also insufficient to account for the increased transcript steady-state levels observed. P450IIE1 and the hepatic gap junction proteins connexins 32 (β_1) and 26 (β_2) exhibited significant decreases in transcript abundance at 24 and 12 hours post-PH, respectively. The connexin transcripts half-lives were decreased significantly at 12 hours post-PH relative to pre-PH levels. Interestingly, the P450IIE1 transcript revealed an extremely prolonged half-life at both 0 and 24 hours following PH, suggesting that other posttranscriptional mechanisms are involved in its regulation, such as hnRNA processing and/or nucleocytoplasmic transport. However, certain *trans*-acting factors required for modulating the decay of P450IIE1 mRNA in liver may have been reduced by

TABLE 3. Transcript Half-lives of Genes Modulated during Liver Regeneration

Gene	mRNA half-life ($t_{1/2}$)		
	0 h $t_{1/2}$ (h)	Time Post-PH (h)	$t_{1/2}$ (h)
p53	1.2	6	2.3
		24	1.8
MDM-2	14 min	24	2.1
retinoblastoma	40 min	6	40 min
c-*myc*	9 min	6	31 min
H-*ras*	4.7	24	>12
bax	2.8	24	4.3
		40	>8
bcl-x_L	27 min	6	106 min
		12	26 min
cyclin B1		24	>12
		48	2.4
p21	30 min	3	4.5
procollagen α_1(I)	2.9	48	>12
procollagen α_1(III)	9.9	48	>12
fibronectin	2.5	48	2.5
TGF-β1	2.7	48	3.8
EGF receptor	2.8	4	3.6
connexin 32	10.9	12	3.8
connexin 26	6.1	12	3.7
multidrug resistance	2.2	24	>12
P450IIE1	>12	24	>12
ornithine decarboxylase	2.5	12	4.7
		24	>12
6-phosphofructo-2-kinase/fructose-2,6-bisphosphatase	2.5	2	2.5
hemopexin	>12	18	>12

SOURCE: From references 16, 48, 53–57, 59, 60.

the inhibition of transcription,[58] thus preventing transcript degradation from taking place. In conclusion, the data from several laboratories suggest that mRNA stability is a significant factor in the posttranscriptional modulation of transcript steady-state levels during liver regeneration.

It is important to understand the mechanisms by which transcript stability is modulated during liver regeneration following partial hepatectomy. The translational activity of a transcript is known to affect its stability as well as *trans*-acting protein factors. Early tissue culture studies revealed that some mRNA decay processes are coupled to translation. In fact, it has recently been shown that selective translational control of ribosomal protein mRNAs is an important regulatory mechanism during the course of liver development and regeneration.[61] It now appears that most mRNAs require their own translation to be degraded and the requirement for translation may occur at several points in the decay pathway. Translational inhibitors such as cycloheximide inhibit the decay of a variety of mRNAs containing AU-rich sequences. However, since cycloheximide blocks overall translation within a cell, the studies do not establish whether it is the translation of the specific mRNA or the synthesis of a labile protein that is required for more rapid degradation.

The effect of protein synthesis inhibitors on the disappearance of specific mRNAs and the stability of the transcript pre- and post-PH has been investigated.

Studies have indicated that transcript expression for the tumor suppressors, the hepatic connexins, H-*ras*, ornithine decarboxylase and cyclin B$_1$ was significantly affected by inhibition of protein synthesis.[48,53-55] Moderate transcriptional rate changes were observed only for the proto-oncogenes following cycloheximide administration.[47] Inhibition of protein synthesis post-PH induced some transcripts (H-*ras*, p53 and retinoblastoma), prevented the disappearance of others (cyclin B$_1$, p53, connexin 26, retinoblastoma), and had no effect on the temporal patterns of expression of a third subset (*MDM*-2, c-*fos*, c-*myc*, c-*jun*, *jun* B and *jun* D). Thus, translational activity or *trans*-acting labile protein factors may be a component of posttranscriptional stability regulation.

Further evidence supporting the role of *trans*-acting factors in modulating transcript stability during liver regeneration comes from the increased stability of the transcripts for p21 from 30 min to 6.5 hours[57] and for the EGF receptor from 3.6 to 11.2 hours[16] after inhibition of protein synthesis with cycloheximide. Moreover, up regulation at times post-PH coincident with increased transcript stability is observed for a novel homolog of the 70 kD c-*myc* coding region determinant binding protein whose binding increases the stability of the transcript.[62] Similar modulation of both *trans*-acting RNA binding proteins that stabilize the transferrin receptor mRNA was observed during periods of increased transcript abundance post-PH.[63] Interestingly, the novel c-*myc* coding region determinant-binding protein identified from quiescent as well as regenerating liver appears to be a 172 kD protein homologue of the previously identified 70 kD binding protein.[62] Moreover, the transferrin receptor mRNA binding protein predominantly induced during liver regeneration is the second form of the protein identified in rodent liver and is normally present in much lower abundance than the initially characterized cytosolic protein. These data suggest that during liver regeneration, modulation of *trans*-acting factors involved in regulating transcript stability is different from that observed in cultured cells, perhaps reflecting differences between *in vivo* and *in vitro* cellular metabolism. In addition, results from our laboratory indicate that increased translational activity of the mRNAs for connexin 32 and ornithine decarboxylase is observed at times post-PH concurrent with increased stability of the transcript. Thus, the translational activity of a transcript as well as *trans*-acting protein factors are involved in controlling the posttranscriptional stabilization of mRNAs *in vivo*, as has been reported previously for cells in culture.

Another mechanism for controlling transcript turnover rates *in vitro* is the rate of poly(A) tail shortening.[58] A regulatory role of the poly(A) tail in mRNA degradation has been suggested by the observation that removal of the poly(A) tail precedes mRNA degradation.[64-66] Moreover, the key AU-rich sequence that effectively destabilizes mRNAs has recently been identified and was shown to induce rapid deadenylation of transcripts.[67] Recent purification of a mammalian 3' to 5' exoribonuclease capable of degrading polysome-associated deadenylated mRNAs but not poly(A)-intact transcripts supports the role of the poly(A) tail in regulating transcript stability.[68] It is well known that cellular activation can lead to increased steady-state levels of mRNAs by mechanisms that decrease mRNA degradation. Thus, the role of poly(A) tail shortening in modulating the decay rates of the gap junction connexin 32 and ornithine decarboxylase mRNAs was investigated at 0 and 12 hours post-PH. These times reflect when their respective transcript stabilities are oppositely regulated.[48,55] The rate of poly(A) tail removal was increased for both transcripts coincident with decreased mRNA stability. These data imply that the rate of deadenylation of specific transcripts during hepatic regeneration following PH is another factor involved in modulating mRNA decay.

Change in transcript stability is only one posttranscriptional mechanism during liver regeneration responsible for the regulation of steady-state transcript levels. Increases in mRNA stability alone are insufficient to fully acount for the dramatic coincident increases in steady-state levels observed post-PH in many cases. Additionally, no alterations in stability for retinoblastoma, p450IIE1, fibronectin and other transcripts were detected following PH even though their respective steady-state levels were dramatically modulated, suggesting that other posttranscriptional mechanisms are involved. Numerous posttranscriptional nuclear processing events as well as the transport of the mature mRNA to the cytoplasm occur prior to degradation of the transcript in the cytoplasm. Many of these processing events appear to be highly regulated, including nucleocytoplasmic transport of the mature mRNA.[69] During liver regeneration following PH the efficiency of processing hnRNA into mature mRNA is increased coincident with increased steady-state cytoplasmic mRNA levels.[70] Moreover, following PH, modulation in the biosynthesis of the spliceosomal UsnRNAs involved in splicing the hnRNAs is observed.[71] Furthermore, one of the novel insulin-induced delayed-early genes identified in hepatocytes is a regulator of alternative pre-mRNA splicing[39] and fibronectin transcripts are alternatively spliced in quiescent versus regenerating liver.[72] These data suggest that alternative splicing or changes in processing rates may play an important posttranscriptional role in modulating steady-state transcript abundance. Furthermore, modulation of the stability of the hnRNA in the nucleus is known to occur in quiescent liver[73] suggesting an additional nuclear posttranscriptional mechanism involved in regulating transcript steady-state levels.

The role of methylation in transcriptional regulation of gene expression is well established, however, a number of recent studies suggest that DNA methylation might also influence the subsequent processing of certain RNAs.[74-76] It has been reported that methylation-deficient diets led to hypomethylation of genomic DNA encoding H-*ras* and c-*myc* and increased expression of their transcripts in rat liver, possibly by posttranscriptional events.[77] Southern blot analyses were performed to determine if a correlation existed between transcript stability and genomic methylation status of the respective allele during liver regeneration. Genomic DNA was digested using three restriction endonucleases, *Msp* I, *Hpa* II and *HinP*1 I, whose 4 nucleotide recognition sites contain CpG nucleotides and whose cleavage is dependent on the methylation state of the cytosine residue. Increased mRNA stability for c-*myc*, H-*ras*, ornithine decarboxylase, and p53 was associated with decreased methylation at some of the restriction endonuclease sites of their DNAs encoding the hnRNAs.[55] In contrast, the control genes asialoglycoprotein receptor and P450IIE1, which showed no alterations in mRNA stability, exhibited no changes in genomic methylation patterns. It is possible that the observed changes in methylation status resulted from formation of hemimethylated DNA during S phase. However, the altered methylation patterns of the c-*myc* and p53 genes at 6 hours as well as the ornithine decarboxylase studies at 12 hours post-PH do not support the hemimethylation premise. Furthermore, the lack of change in genomic methylation status for both asialoglycoprotein receptor and P450IIE1 at 24 hours following PH strongly suggests that the observed changes were not merely a result of DNA replication. Finally, it has been shown that *Hpa* II is unable to cleave hemimethylated DNA.[75] This association between increased transcript stability and decreased methylation status of the genomic DNA suggests another possible and intriguing posttranscriptional mechanism involved in controlling steady-state transcript levels. Whether it affects the nuclear processing of the hnRNA or is involved in altering the cytoplasmic degradation rate remains to be determined.

Cyclin Gene Expression

Much of the information available on cyclin expression in liver was obtained using the PH model of liver regeneration. Entrance into G_1 and the cell cycle is marked by a similar pattern of cyclin and cyclin-dependent kinase (CDK) gene and proto-oncogene induction and expression as observed in other model systems.[43,49,78] Many of the cyclins demonstrate dramatic patterns of cell cycle-related expression at the transcript level following PH in both rat and mouse. Cyclins D_1 and D_3 exhibit induced transcript abundances which fluctuate and peak coincident with the G_1 phase of the cell cycles following PH in rat, whereas cyclin D_2 is undetectable at all time points examined.[49,79] Cyclins C and E are also induced during liver regeneration; however less apparent cycling of their transcript levels is observed.[49,78] Cyclins C and D_3 represent the only cyclin genes with readily detectable transcript expression in quiescent rat liver. In normal liver transcripts for cyclins A, B_1 and B_2 are negligible, but following PH they exhibit patterns of transcript induction and abundance coincident with the $S/G_2/M$ phases of the cell cycle in the rat.[49,54,78,80]

CDKs also exhibit alterations in transcript expression post-PH. CDK1 transcripts in the rat mirror those of cyclin B_1 through 96 hours, whereas CDKs 4 and 5 exhibit no dramatic changes in transcript expression during the first 48 hours of rat liver regeneration.[49,79,81,82] Mouse liver regeneration has been less extensively studied than rat; however many of the cyclin genes demonstrate similar patterns of induction as those observed in rat with a predictable 12–18 hour delay.[49,79] Cyclin and CDK expression in athymic nude mice following PH is both diminished and delayed compared to normal mice, as is their capacity to regenerate their liver.[49,83] Although the cyclin genes exhibit dramatic transcript induction following PH in both mouse and rat, as shown in TABLE 2, there is no detectable change in transcription rate for cyclins A, B_1, C, D_1, D_3 and E during liver regeneration.[49,54] Similarly, CDK1 also exhibits invariant transcription activity during mouse liver regeneration.[49] Cyclin B_1 does, however, exhibit changes in mRNA stability during rat liver regeneration (TABLE 3),[54] yet these changes can not entirely explain the extent of transcript induction. Thus, the mechanisms involved in the cycling pattern of transcript expression for the various cyclin and CDK genes following PH remain unclear.

In contrast to oscillating transcript expression, most cyclin and CDK proteins do not exhibit significant changes following PH. Cyclin A protein levels are induced by PH, whereas cyclin B_1 protein is present in quiescent liver and fluctuates minimally during rat liver regeneration.[80,82,84] Cyclin D_1 protein is detectable in resting rat liver and varies less than twofold from baseline levels during regeneration, in contrast to its mRNA steady-state levels which increase by as much as 10-fold.[79,81] Interestingly, in mice post-PH, cyclin D_1 protein levels are induced by greater than 20-fold following PH as are its transcript levels.[79] It is somewhat surprising that the cyclin D_1 gene is differentially regulated in these two rodent models of liver regeneration following surgical resection. However, disparate regulation of cyclin D between mouse and human cells has been noted in other systems.[85] Cyclin D_1 protein is associated with its partner kinase CDK4 during liver regeneration in both rodent models.[79] Cyclin D_1 is also abundant in freshly isolated rat hepatocytes yet diminishes significantly by 6 hours in culture media lacking certain growth factors. In contrast to the *in vivo* stimulus of PH, cultured rat hepatocytes stimulated to proliferate using HGF resulted in a fivefold increase in cyclin D_1 mRNA and a 20-fold increase in protein product. Cyclin E protein is also present in resting rat liver and varies minimally in abundance during regeneration.[81]

In quiescent liver CDK2 protein is detected and its steady-state levels increase following PH.[81,84] CDK4 and CDK5 proteins are also present in resting mouse and rat liver, but minimal changes in abundance were observed during regeneration.[79] CDK1 protein is present at very low levels in quiescent liver, and is dramatically induced during regeneration in a pattern mirroring that of its mRNA.[79,82,84] During liver regeneration following PH, CDK1- and CDK2-associated histone H_1 kinase activities have been assayed and coincide with the predicted phases of the cell cycle. A single peak of CDK2-associated histone H_1 kinase activity is exhibited during S-phase of the first round of hepatocyte replication following PH. In contrast, CDK1-associated kinase activity has two peaks, one in S and one in M-phase.[78,81]

Overall, cyclin/CDK gene expression post-PH is governed primarily through posttranscriptional mechanisms and significant uncoupling of steady-state transcript and protein levels are observed. Thus, translational and/or posttranslational control of gene expression is also an important regulatory mechanism post-PH. Similar uncoupling of transcripts and protein steady-state levels have been noted for a number of other genes following PH in rat liver. The tumor suppressor genes, retinoblastoma and p53[86] as well as the apoptosis-associated genes *bcl-2*, *bax* and *bcl*-x$_L$[56] are examples of other gene groups exhibiting this type of regulation. It has been suggested by others observing a similar uncoupling of protein and transcript steady-state levels for *bcl-2 in vivo* in normal but not oncogenic tissue[87] that translational and/or posttranslational control of gene expression is also lost during the transformation process.

CONCLUDING REMARKS

Thus, in summary, the regenerating liver following PH provides a viable model to investigate the commonalities and differences in controlling gene expression at multiple levels in differentiated cells *in vivo* and *in vitro*. Genetic changes in transformed and immortalized cells allowing them to continue growth and replication in an artificial environment have resulted in altered expression for key cell cycle-regulatory genes. Aberrant regulation of cyclin genes has been noted in several cell lines, and these cells respond differently to certain chemicals.[88,89] Immortalization and transformation of cells is also known to alter their RNA metabolism and processing[90] and most tissue culture studies to date have utilized these types of cells. In addition, transfected plasmid encoded RNAs are not processed in a fashion similar to their endogenous counterparts.[91] Moreover, numerous observed differences exist between transcriptional and posttranscriptional control of transcripts and their protein products in *in vitro* cell culture systems and *in vivo* in the regenerating rodent liver. Taken together, these data indicate that verification of tissue culture study results *in vivo* becomes essential to understanding the "correct" factors, pathways and mechanisms involved in regulating gene expression in adult differentiated mammalian cells. It is through a coordinated approach using both *in vitro* and *in vivo* model systems that a comprehensive understanding of the factors, mechanisms and pathways involved in the posttranscriptional regulation of gene expression will emerge.

ACKNOWLEDGMENTS

We would like to thank all the individuals who made the cDNAs available for conducting our own studies and Dr. Peter Leeds, University of Wisconsin for communicating unpublished data on the c-*myc* CRD binding protein.

REFERENCES

1. HIGGINS, G. M. & R. M. ANDERSON. 1931. Experimental pathology of the liver. I. Restoration of the liver of the white rat following partial surgical removal. Arch. Pathol. **12:** 186–202.
2. MARTINEZ-HERNANDEZ, A. & P. S. AMENTA. 1995. The extracellular matrix in hepatic regeneration. FASEB J. **9:** 1401–1410.
3. MICHALOPOULOS, G. K. 1990. Liver regeneration: Molecular mechanisms of growth control. FASEB J. **4:** 176–187.
4. FAUSTO, N. & E. M. WEBBER. 1993. Control of liver growth. Crit. Rev. Euk. Gene Exp. **3:** 117–135.
5. FAUSTO, N. & E. M. WEBBER. 1994. Liver regeneration. *In* The Liver: Biology and Pathobiology, 3rd edition. I. M. Arias, J. L. Boyer, N. Fausto, W. B. Jacoby, D. Schachter & D. A. Shafritz, Eds.: 1059–1084. Raven Press. New York.
6. FAUSTO, N. 1996. Hepatic regeneration. *In* Hepatology: A Textbook of Liver Disease. 3rd edition. D. Zakim & T. D. Boyer, Eds.: 32–58. W. B. Saunders Co.. Philadelphia.
7. GRISHAM, J. W. 1962. A morphologic study of deoxyribonucleic acid synthesis and cell proliferation in regenerating rat liver; autoradiography with thymidine-H³. Cancer Res. **22:** 842–849.
8. BUCHER, N. L. R. & A. J. STRAIN. 1992. Regulatory mechanisms in hepatic regeneration. *In* Wright's Liver and Biliary Disease. Pathophysiology, Diagnosis and Management. G. H. Millward-Sadler, R. Wright & M. J. P. Arther, Eds.: 258–274. W. B. Saunders Co. London.
9. HABER, B. A., K. L. MOHN, R. H. DIAMOND & R. TAUB. 1993. Induction patterns of 70 genes during nine days after hepatectomy define the temporal course of liver regeneration. J. Clin. Invest. **91:** 1319–1326.
10. CRUISE, J. L., S. J. KNECHTLE, R. R. BOLLINGER, C. KUHN & G. MICHALOPOULOS. 1987. α_1-Adrenergic effects and liver regeneration. Hepatology **7:** 1189–1194.
11. DIEHL, A. M. 1991. Nutrition, hormones, metabolism and liver regeneration. Sem. Liver Dis. **11:** 315–320.
12. FOWLER, F. C., R. K. BANKS & M. E. MAILLIARD. 1992. Characterization of sodium-dependent amino acid transport activity during liver regeneration. Hepatology **16:** 1187–1194.
13. MEAD, J. E., L. BRAUN, D. A. MARTIN & N. FAUSTO. 1990. Induction of replicative competence ("priming") in normal liver. Cancer Res. **50:** 7023–7030.
14. HIMENO, Y., R. W. ENGELMAN & R. A. GOOD. 1992. Influence of calorie restriction on oncogene expression and DNA synthesis during liver regeneration. Proc. Natl. Acad. Sci. USA **89:** 5497–5501.
15. ÉTHIER, C., R. KESTEKIAN, C. BEAULIEU, C. DUBÉ, J. HAVRANKOVA & M. GASCON-BARRÉ. 1990. Vitamin D depletion retards the normal regeneration process after hepatectomy in the rat. Endocrinology **126:** 2947–2959.
16. NOGUCHI, S., Y. OHBA & T. OKA. 1992. The role of transcription and messenger RNA stability in the regulation of epidermal growth factor receptor gene expression in regenerating mouse liver. Hepatology **15:** 88–96.
17. STRÖMBLAD, S. & G. ANDERSSON. 1993. The coupling between transforming growth factor-α and the epidermal growth factor receptor during rat liver regeneration. Exp. Cell Res. **204:** 321–328.
18. MOHN, K. L., A. E. MELBY, D. S. TEWARI, T. M. LAZ & R. TAUB. 1991. The gene encoding rat insulinlike growth factor-binding protein 1 is rapidly and highly induced in regenerating liver. Mol. Cell. Biol. **11:** 1393–1401.
19. KAN, M., J. HUANG, P.-E. MANSSON, H. YASUMITSU, B. CARR & W. L. MCKEEHAN 1989. Heparin-binding growth factor type 1 (acidic fibroblast growth factor): A potential biphasic autocrine and paracrine regulator of hepatocyte regeneration. Proc. Natl. Acad. Sci. USA **86:** 7432–7436.
20. MARSDEN, E. R., Z. HU, K. FUJIO, H. NAKATSUKASA, S. S. THORGEIRSSON & R. P. EVARTS. 1992. Expression of acidic fibroblast growth factor in regenerating liver and during hepatic differentiation. Lab. Invest. **67:** 427–433.

21. LaBRECQUE, D. R., G. STEELE, S. FOGERTY, M. WILSON & J. BARTON. 1987. Purification and physical-chemical characterization of hepatic stimulator substance. Hepatology **7:** 100–106.

22. MICHALOPOULOS, G. K. & R. ZARNEGAR. 1992. Hepatocyte growth factor. Hepatology **15:** 149–155.

23. MATSUMOTO, K. & T. NAKAMURA. 1992. Hepatocyte growth factor: Molecular structure, roles in liver regeneration, and other biological functions. Crit. Rev. Oncogenesis **3:** 27–54.

24. APPASAMY, R., M. TANABE, N. MURASE, R. ZARNEGAR, R. VENKATARAMANAN, D. H. VAN THIEL & G. K. MICHALOPOULOS. 1993. Hepatocyte growth factor, blood clearance, organ uptake, and biliary excretion in normal and partially hepatectomized rats. Lab. Invest. **68:** 270–276.

25. AKERMAN, P., P. COTE, S. Q. YANG, C. McCLAIN, S. NELSON, G. J. BAGBY & A. M. DIEHL. 1992. Antibodies to tumor necrosis factor-α inhibit liver regeneration after partial hepatectomy. Am. J. Physiol. **263:** G579-G585.

26. FRANCAVILLA, A., T. E. STARZL, M. BARONE, Q.-H. ZENG, K. A. PORTER, A. ZEEVI, P. M. MARKUS, M. R. M. VAN DEN BRINK & S. TODO. 1991. Studies on mechanisms of augmentation of liver regeneration by cyclosporine and FK 506. Hepatology **14:** 140–143.

27. FRANCAVILLA, A., M. HAGIYA, K. A. PORTER, L. POLIMENO, I. IHARA & T. E. STARZL. 1994. Augmenter of liver regeneration: Its place in the universe of hepatic growth factors. Hepatology **20:** 747–757.

28. ROBERTS, A. B. & M. B. SPORN. 1990. The transforming growth factor-βs. *In* Handbook of Experimental Pharmacology. Peptide Growth Factors and Their Receptors. M. B. Sporn & A. B. Roberts, Eds.: 419–472. Springer-Verlag. Heidelberg.

29. STEER, C. J. 1992. The TGF-β receptor(s)–hepatic expression and functional properties. *In* Hepatic Endocytosis of Lipids and Proteins. E. Windler & H. Greten, Eds.: 92–114. W. Zuckschwerdt Verlag. München.

30. THORESEN, G. H., M. REFSNES & T. CHRISTOFFERSEN. 1992. Inhibition of hepatocyte DNA synthesis by transforming growth factor β_1 and cyclic AMP: Effect immediately before the G_1/S border. Cancer Res. **52:** 3598–3603.

31. KOFF, A., M. OHTSUKI, K. POLYAK, J. M. ROBERTS & J. MASSAGUÉ. 1993. Negative regulation of G1 in mammalian cells: Inhibition of cyclin E-dependent kinase by TGF-β. Science **260:** 536–539.

32. LAIHO, M., J. A. DeCAPRIO, J. W. LUDLOW, D. M. LIVINGSTON & J. MASSAGUÉ. 1990. Growth inhibition by TGF-β linked to suppression of retinoblastoma protein phosphorylation. Cell **62:** 175–185.

33. JAKOWLEW, S. B., J. E. MEAD, D. DANIELPOUR, J. WU, A. B. ROBERTS & N. FAUSTO. 1991. Transforming growth factor-β (TGF-β) isoforms in rat liver regeneration: Messenger RNA expression and activation of latent TGF-β. Cell Reg. **2:** 535–548.

34. BISSELL, D. M., S.-S. WANG, W. R. JARNAGIN & F. J. ROLL. 1995. Cell-specific expression of transforming growth factor-β in rat liver. Evidence for autocrine regulation of hepatocyte proliferation. J. Clin. Invest. **96:** 447–455.

35. RUSSELL, W. E., R. J. COFFEY JR., A. J. OUELLETTE & H. L. MOSES. 1988. Type β transforming growth factor reversibly inhibits the early proliferative response to partial hepatectomy in the rat. Proc. Natl. Acad. Sci. USA **85:** 5126–5130.

36. JIRTLE, R. L., B. I. CARR & C. D. SCOTT. 1991. Modulation of insulin-like growth factor-II/mannose 6-phosphate receptors and transforming growth factor-β1 during liver regeneration. J. Biol. Chem. **266:** 22444–22450.

37. WOODMAN, A. C., C. A. SELDEN & H. J. F. HODGSON. 1992. Partial purification and characterization of an inhibitor of hepatocyte proliferation derived from nonparenchymal cells after partial hepatectomy. J. Cell. Physiol. **151:** 405–414.

38. MOHN, K. L., T. M. LAZ, J.-C. HSU, A. E. MELBY, R. BRAVO & R. TAUB. 1991. The immediate-early growth response in regenerating liver and insulin-stimulated H-35 cells: Comparison with serum-stimulated 3T3 cells and identification of 41 novel immediate-early genes. Mol. Cell. Biol. **11:** 381–390.

39. DIAMOND, R. H., K. DU, V. M. LEE, K. L. MOHN, B. A. HABER, D. S. TEWARI & R. TAUB. 1993. Novel delayed-early and highly insulin-induced growth response genes. Identification of HRS, a potential regulator of alternative pre-mRNA splicing. J. Biol. Chem. **268:** 15185–15192.

40. HERSCHMAN, H. R. 1991. Primary response genes induced by growth factors and tumor promoters. Annu. Rev. Biochem. **60:** 281–319.

41. MCMAHON, S. B. & J. G. MONROE. 1992. Role of primary response genes in generating cellular responses to growth factors. FASEB J. **6:** 2707–2715.

42. LANAHAN, A., J. B. WILLIAMS, L. K. SANDERS & D. NATHANS. 1992. Growth factor-induced delayed early response genes. Mol. Cell Biol. **12:** 3919–3929.

43. THOMPSON, N. L., J. E. MEAD, L. BRAUN, M. GOYETTE, P. R. SHANK & N. FAUSTO. 1986. Sequential protooncogene expression during rat liver regeneration. Cancer Res. **46:** 3111–3117.

44. CONI, P., G. SIMBULA, A. C. DE PRATI, M. MENEGAZZI, H. SUZUKI, D. S. R. SARMA, D. G. M. LEDDA-COLUMBANO & A. COLUMBANO. 1993. Differences in the steady-state levels of c-*fos*, c-*jun* and c-*myc* messenger RNA during mitogen-induced liver growth and compensatory regeneration. Hepatology **17:** 1109–1116.

45. HSU, J.-C., T. LAZ, K. L. MOHN & R. TAUB. 1991. Identification of LRF-1, a leucine-zipper protein that is rapidly and highly induced in regenerating liver. Proc. Natl. Acad. Sci. USA **88:** 3511–3515.

46. TEWARI, M., P. DOBRZANSKI, K. L. MOHN, D. E. CRESSMAN, J.-C. HSU, R. BRAVO & R. TAUB. 1992. Rapid induction in regenerating liver of RL/IF-1 (an IκB that inhibits NF-κB, BelB-p50, and c-Rel-p50) and PHF, a novel κB site-binding complex. Mol. Cell. Biol. **12:** 2898–2908.

47. MORELLO, D., A. LAVENU & C. BABINET. 1990. Differential regulation and expression of *jun*, c-*fos* and c-*myc* proto-oncogenes during mouse liver regeneration and after inhibition of protein synthesis. Oncogene **5:** 1511–1519.

48. KREN, B. T., N. M. KUMAR, S-q. WANG, N. B. GILULA & C. J. STEER. 1993. Differential regulation of multiple gap junction transcripts and proteins during rat liver regeneration. J. Cell Biol. **123:** 707–718.

49. ALBRECHT, J. H., J. S. HOFFMAN, B. T. KREN & C. J. STEER. 1993. Cyclin and cyclin-dependent kinase 1 mRNA expression in models of regenerating liver and human liver diseases. Am. J. Physiol. **265:** G857–G864.

50. FLODBY, P., P. ANTONSON, C. BARLOW, A. BLANCK, I. PORSCH-HALLSTROM & K. G. XANTHOPOULOS. 1993. Differential patterns of expression of three C/EBP isoforms, HNF-1, and HNF-4 after partial hepatectomy in rats. Exp. Cell Res. **208:** 248–256.

51. LEE, S. J. & T. D. BOYER. 1993. The effect of hepatic regeneration on the expression of the glutathione S-transferases. Biochem. J. **293:** 137–142.

52. FERRERO, M., M. A. DESIDERIO, A. MARTINOTTI, C. MELANI, A. BERNELLI-ZAZZERA, M. P. COLOMBO & G. CAIRO. 1994. Expression of a growth arrest specific gene (gas-6) during liver regeneration: Molecular mechanisms and signalling pathways. J. Cell. Physiol. **158:** 263–269.

53. TREMBLEY, J. H., B. T. KREN & C. J. STEER. 1994. Posttranscriptional regulation of cyclin B messenger RNA expression in the regenerating rat liver. Cell Growth & Differ. **5:** 99–108.

54. KREN, B. T., A. L. TEEL & C. J. STEER. 1994. Transcriptional rate and steady-state changes of retinoblastoma mRNA in regenerating rat liver. Hepatology **19:** 1214–1222.

55. KREN, B. T., J. H. TREMBLEY & C. J. STEER. 1996. Alterations in mRNA stability during rat liver regeneration. Am. J. Physiol. **270:** G763–G777.

56. KREN, B. T., J. H. TREMBLEY, S. KRAJEWSKI, T. BEHRENS, J. C. REED & C. J. STEER. 1996. Modulation of the apoptosis-associated genes, *bcl-2*, *bcl-x* and *bax* during rat liver regeneration. Cell Growth & Differ. **7:** 1633–1642.

57. ALBRECHT, J. H., A. H. MYER & M. Y. HU. 1997. Regulation of cyclin-dependent kinase inhibitor p21$^{WAFI/Cip/Sdil}$ gene expression in hepatic regeneration. Hepatology **25:** 557–563.

58. ROSS, J. 1995. mRNA stability in mammalian cells. Microbiol. Rev. **59:** 423–450.

59. ROSA, J. L., A. TAULER, A. J. LANGE, S. J. PILKIS & R. BARTRONS. 1992. Transcriptional and posttranscriptional regulation of 6-phosphofructo-2-kinase/fructose-2,6-bisphosphatase during liver regeneration. Proc. Natl. Acad. Sci. USA **89:** 3746–3750.

60. ALBRECHT, J. H., U. MULLER-EBERHARD, B. T. KREN & C. J. STEER. 1994. Influence of transcriptional regulation and mRNA stability on hemopexin gene expression in regenerating liver. Arch. Biochem. Biophys. **314:** 229–233.

61. ALONI, R., D. PELEG & O. MEYUHAS. 1992. Selective translational control and nonspecific posttranscriptional regulation of ribosomal protein gene expression during development and regeneration of rat liver. Mol. Cell. Biol. **12:** 2203–2212.

62. LEEDS, P., B. T. KREN, J. M. BOYLAN, N. A. BETZ, C. J. STEER, P. A. GRUPPUSO & J. ROSS. 1997. Developmental regulation of CRD-BP, an RNA-binding protein that stabilizes c-*myc* mRNA *in vitro*. Oncogene **14:** 1279–1286.

63. CAIRO, G. & A. PIETRANGELO. 1994. Transferrin receptor gene expression during rat liver regeneration. Evidence for post-transcriptional regulation by iron regulatory factor$_B$, a second iron-responsive element-binding protein. J. Biol. Chem. **269:** 6405–6409.

64. SHYU, A.-B., J. G. BELASCO & M. E. GREENBERG. 1991. Two distinct destabilizing elements in the c-*fos* messenger trigger deadenylation as a first step in rapid mRNA decay. Genes & Dev. **5:** 221–234.

65. BREWER, G. & J. ROSS. 1988. Poly(A) shortening and degradation of the 3' A+U-rich sequences of human c-*myc* mRNA in a cell-free system. Mol. Cell Biol. **8:** 1697–1708.

66. SACHS A. & E. WAHLE. 1993. Poly(A) tail metabolism and function in eucaryotes. J. Biol. Chem. **268:** 22955–22958.

67. ZUBIAGA A. M., J. G. BELASCO & M. E. GREENBERG. 1995. The nonamer UUAUUUAUU is the key AU-rich sequence motif that mediates mRNA degradation. Mol. Cell Biol. **15:** 2219–2230.

68. CARUCCIO N. & J. ROSS. 1994. Purification of a human polyribosome-associated 3' to 5' exoribonuclease. J. Biol. Chem. **269:** 31814–31821.

69. JARMOLOWSKI, A., W. C. BOELENS, E. IZAURRALDE & I. W. MATTAJ. 1994. Nuclear export of different classes of RNA is mediated by specific factors. J. Cell Biol. **124:** 627–635.

70. BAKI, L. & M. N. ALEXIS. 1994. The efficiency of nuclear processing of the tyrosine aminotransferase mRNA transcript increases after partial hepatectomy. Eur. J. Biochem. **225:** 797–803.

71. RAY, R., C. K. PANDA, B. K. CHAKRABORTY, S. MUKHERJI, K. CHAUDHURY & J. ROYCHOUDHURY. 1994. Changes in UsnRNA biosynthesis during rat liver regeneration. Mol. Cell. Biochem. **141:** 71–77.

72. CAPUTI, M., C. A. MELO & F. E. BARALLE. 1995. Regulation of fibronectin expression in rat regenerating liver. Nucleic Acids Res. **23:** 238–243.

73. GOUMAZ, M. O., H. SCHWARTZ, J. H. OPPENHEIMER & C. N. MARIASH. 1994. Kinetic modeling of the response of precursor and mature rat hepatic mRNA-S14 to thyroid hormone. Am. J. Physiol. **266:** E1001–E1011.

74. NAMBU, S., K. INOUE & H. SASAKI. 1987. Site-specific hypomethylation of the c-*myc* oncogene in human hepatocellular carcinoma. J. Cancer Res. **78:** 695–704.

75. JOST, J.-P. 1993. Nuclear extracts of chicken embryos promote an active demethylation of DNA by excision repair of 5-methyldeoxycytidine. Proc. Natl. Acad. Sci. USA **91:** 4684–4688.

76. INGELBRECHT, I., H. VAN HOUDT, M. VAN MONTAGU & A. DEPICKER. 1994. Posttranscriptional silencing of reporter transgenes in tobacco correlates with DNA methylation. Proc. Natl. Acad. Sci. USA **91:** 10502–10506.

77. WAINFAN, E. & L. A. POIRIER. 1992. Methyl groups in carcinogenesis: Effects on DNA methylation and gene expression. Cancer Res. **52:** 2071s–2077s.

78. LU, X. P., K. S. KOCH, D. J. LEW, V. DULIC, J. PINES, S. I. REED, T. HUNTER & H. L. LEFFERT. 1992. Induction of cyclin mRNA and cyclin-associated histone H1 kinase during liver regeneration. J. Biol. Chem. **267:** 2841–2844.

79. ALBRECHT, J. H., M. Y. HU, & F. B. CERRA. 1995. Distinct patterns of cyclin D1 regulation in models of liver regeneration and human liver. Biochem. Biophys. Res. Commun. **209:** 648–655.

80. ZINDY, F., E. LAMAS, X. CHENIVESSE, J. SOBCZAK, J. WANG, D. FESQUET, B. HENGLEIN & C. BRECHOT. 1992. Cyclin A is required in S phase in normal epithelial cells. Biochem. Biophys. Res. Commun. **182:** 1144–1154.

81. LOYER, P., D. GLAISE, S. CARIOU, G. BAFFET, L. MEIJER & C. GUGUEN-GUILLOUZO. 1994. Expression and activation of cdks (1 and 2) and cyclins in the cell cycle progression during liver regeneration. J. Biol. Chem. **269:** 2491–2500.

82. TREMBLEY, J. H., J. O. EBBERT, B. T. KREN & C. J. STEER. 1996. Differential regulation of cylin B1 RNA and protein expression during hepatocyte growth *in vivo*. Cell Growth & Differ. **7:** 903–916.

83. ALBRECHT, J. H., J. S. HOFFMAN, B. T. KREN & C. J. STEER. 1994. Changes in cell cycle-associated gene expression in a model of impaired liver regeneration. FEBS Lett. **347:** 157–162.

84. CASTRO, A., M. JAUMOT, M. VERGES, N. AGELL & O. BACHS. 1994. Microsomal localization of cyclin A and cdk2 in proliferating rat liver cells. Biochem. Biophys. Res. Commun. **201:** 1072–1078.

85. BATES, S., D. PARRY, L. BONETTA, K. VOUSDEN, C. DICKSON & G. PETERS. 1994. Absence of cyclin D/cdk complexes in cells lacking functional retinoblastoma protein. Oncogene **9:** 1633–1640.

86. FAN, G., R. XU, M. W. WESSENDORF, X. MA, B. T. KREN & C. J. STEER. 1995. Expression of retinoblastoma and retinoblastoma-related proteins in regenerating rat liver and primary hepatocytes. Cell Growth & Differ. **6:** 1463–1476.

87. CHLEQ-DESCHAMPS, C. M., D. P. LEBRUN, P. HUIE, D. P. BESNIER, R. A. WARNKE, R. K. SIBLEY & M. L. CLEARY. 1993. Topographical dissociation of BCL-2 messenger RNA and protein expression in human lymphoid tissues. Blood **81:** 293–298.

88. GONG, J., B. ARDELT, F. TRAGANOS & Z. DARZYNKIEWICZ. 1994. Unscheduled expression of cyclin B1 and cyclin E in several leukemic and solid tumor cell lines. Cancer Res. **54:** 4285–4288.

89. GONG, J., F. TRAGANOS & Z. DARZYNKIEWICZ. 1995. Growth imbalance and altered expression of cyclins B1, A, E, and D3 in MOLT-4 cells synchronized in the cell cycle by inhibitors of DNA replication. Cell Growth & Differ. **6:** 1485–1493.

90. URLAUB, G., P. J. MITCHELL, C. J. CIUDAD & L. A. CHASIN. 1989. Nonsense mutations in the dihydrofolate reductase gene affect RNA processing. Mol. Cell. Biol. **9:** 2868–2880.

91. MALYANKAR, U. M., S. R. RITTLING, A. CONNOR & D. T. DENHARDT. 1994. The mitogen-regulated protein/proliferin transcript is degraded in primary mouse embryo fibroblast but not 3T3 nuclei: Altered RNA processing correlates with immortalization. Proc. Natl. Acad. Sci. USA **91:** 335–339.

In Vitro Organogenesis of Liver Tissue[a]

LINDA G. GRIFFITH,[b,e] BEN WU,[c] MICHAEL J. CIMA,[c]
MARK J. POWERS,[b,d] BEVERLY CHAIGNAUD,[d] AND
JOSEPH P. VACANTI[d]

[b]Department of Chemical Engineering
Center for Biomedical Engineering
Massachusetts Institute of Technology
Cambridge, Massachusetts 02139

[c]Department of Materials Science and Engineering
Massachusetts Institute of Technology
Cambridge, Massachusetts 02139

[d]Department of Surgery
Harvard Medical School and Children's Hospital
Boston, Massachusetts 02115

Orthotopic liver transplantation is currently the only clinically accepted therapy for most patients suffering from liver failure. It is relatively successful: the one year survival rate for patients receiving a liver transplant is 80–85%.[1] A severe shortage of donor organs exists, though, and has stimulated investigation into many alternative approaches for treating liver failure. Because the liver carries out so many vital functions, virtually all current efforts are cell-based tissue engineering approaches.

Hepatic failure arises from a heterogeneous and diverse assortment of liver diseases and liver insults, including viral infection, alcoholic cirrhosis, drug poisoning, cancer, and autoimmune destruction.[2] Some patients who now become candidates for a transplant could perhaps recover liver function if instead treated on a short-term (<1 week) basis with an extracorporeal liver assist device.[3] Indeed, the early clinical results discussed by Demetriou and coworkers in this volume suggest great promise for treating such patients in the near future. The predominant fraction of patients presenting with hepatic failure, however, will ultimately require liver replacement regardless of the success of extracorporeal assist devices. Strategies which complement liver transplantation must be developed if this entire patient population is to be successfully treated.

Cell transplantation, in which a small amount of donor tissue is dissociated into individual cells and transplanted as a cell suspension or in conjunction with a polymer support, is an attractive approach to liver replacement for several reasons. Based on studies in animals which have shown that transplanted cells can double 12 or more times,[4] only a small amount of donor tissue would likely be needed. This would greatly expand the donor pool: one liver could be used for many patients, living related donors could be used, and in some cases the patient's own cells may

[a] This work was supported by an NSF PYI award to L.G.G., the Whitaker Foundation, Therics, Inc., Advanced Tissue Sciences, and the Center for Biomedical Engineering at MIT.
[e] Author to whom correspondence should be addressed: Chemical Engineering, MIT 66-556, Cambridge, MA 02139; Tel: (617) 253-0013; Fax: (617) 258-8224; E-mail: griff@mit.edu

Perfusion Culture System

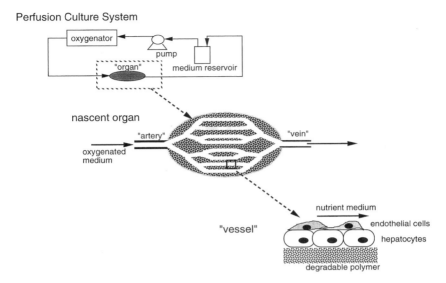

FIGURE 1. Schematic of an *in vitro* organogenesis approach. Cells are isolated from tissue and seeded in a biodegradable polymer scaffold which has branching internal channels (*center*). Isolated cells organize histotypically on the small scale of the channels. The cell-polymer construct is maintained *in vitro* in a perfusion circuit.

be suitable provided they are either freed from the diseased extracellular matrix or are transfected with a missing gene. Furthermore, cell transplantation can potentially be carried out in the early stages of the disease, and the patient's own liver can be left intact until the functional viability of the transplanted cells is demonstrated.

While some liver diseases, particularly genetic deficiencies, might be treated by injecting cell suspensions directly into the liver,[5] the most general approach involves transplantation of cells in conjunction with some type of support to an ectopic, non-diseased site. Several animal models have shown that such ectopic cell transplants can remain viable and carry out liver functions. An inherent problem in cell transplantation is the high metabolic demand of liver. In native liver tissue, each hepatocyte is in almost direct contact with blood; only a thin layer of endothelium intervenes.[6] Cells are transplanted without a vascular supply and thus the scale of an implant is limited to the diffusion distance of oxygen in hepatic tissue, about 0.1 mm.[7,8] The time scale for development of vascularity in the implant (even in the presence of angiogenic factors) is on the order of days, and the time scale for cell death due to oxygen deprivation is on the order of hours.

To address the issue of oxygen diffusion limitations, and thus scale up the mass of cells which can be implanted, we are focusing on developing a vascularized "mini-liver" *in vitro*. This mini-liver comprises an inlet "artery" which branches sequentially to smaller and smaller vessels feeding a liver "parenchyma," and an outlet "vein" which drains the tissue (FIG. 1). We envision that such a construct can be anastomosed in to the portal vein, just upstream of the blood supply of the native liver, and can be induced to grow at the expense of the native liver after it is in place. Our approach to constructing such a mini-liver *in vitro* is to seed a scaffold made from biodegradable polymers with the constituent cells of the tissue, and allow the organ to develop in a recirculating reactor system where oxygenated medium is pumped through the construct. During this *in vitro* culture phase, the cells must organize into appropriate structures while the scaffold degrades, so that upon implantation blood flows past endothelialized surfaces.

This approach hinges on the ability to create complex hierarchical scaffolds with features (*i.e.,* channels and walls, or "vessels" and "parenchymal space") controlled at the 100-micron size scale. To accomplish this, we are using one of a family of solid-free form fabrication (SFF) techniques. SFF techniques build complex 3-D objects as a series of very thin 2-D slices, using a CAD representation of the object to drive an additive fabrication process. Our approach, the Three Dimensional Printing process (3DP™ process), is the most versatile of these because it is adaptable to almost any material.[9] Devices with gradients in composition and locally controlled surface chemistry can be constructed

The 3DP™ process was originally developed for rapid prototyping of ceramic parts and is now being used for direct manufacture of ceramic, metal, and polymer parts. Devices are constructed by first spreading a powder in a thin (0.05–0.15 mm) layer on top of a piston. An ink-jet printhead then prints a liquid binder into the layer wherever the particles are to be bonded together to form the solid part of the object. Colloidal silica is a commonly-used binder in ceramic systems, and organic solvents such as chloroform are suitable for polymer systems. Each printed droplet is 50–80 microns in diameter and its position is controlled by the CAD program. After the first layer is printed, the piston is then dropped, and the whole process of spreading powder and printing is repeated. Very complex scaffolds can be created because the whole object is supported by the powder bed during the build process, thus allowing formation of channels and overhangs, and multiple printheads containing different solutions can be used to modify surface chemistry and composition locally. At the end, the scaffold is taken from the powder bed and the loose powder is removed.

We have adapted this technique from its original applications in ceramics and metals to fabrication of polymer devices. Our major focus has been construction of devices from biodegradable surgical polymers such as polylactide and polylactide-co-glycolide bonded with chloroform.[10] We can now control the size of walls or channels in such polymer devices to a scale of ~200 microns. As described below, this degree of resolution is perhaps sufficient for creating mini-liver scaffolds.

In this paper, we first describe our basic design principles for creating a vascularized mini-liver *in vitro*. These include: cell types, physico-chemical basis of creating organized cell structures on the necessary scale from mixtures of cells, and mass and momentum transport limitations. We then describe experiments directed at demonstrating the feasibility of this approach. Simple branching scaffolds were fabricated by the 3DP™ process and evaluated for their ability to support attachment and reorganization of mixed hepatocyte/endothelial cell cultures.

DESIGN PRINCIPLES

Our ultimate objective is to create a structure which includes both large blood vessels (for anastomosis into the portal vein) and liver parenchyma. Our initial focus is liver parenchyma.

The initial clinical objective is to augment or replace primary hepatic metabolic functions except for biliary secretion. It is unknown whether lack of a biliary

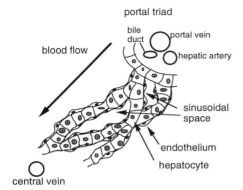

FIGURE 2. Basic structural arrangement of liver parenchyma (not to scale). Blood flows from the portal vein and hepatic artery (portal triad) to the central vein through sinusoidal spaces comprising plates of hepatocytes lined with endothelium.

drainage system will adversely affect the new tissue *in vivo*. The native liver is irreversibly damaged by cholestasis upon interruption of existing biliary drainage, but ectopically transplanted cells[11] and long-term 3-D tissue cultures of hepatocytes function in its absence, perhaps due to downregulation of secretion.

At a minimum, then, the synthesized tissue must comprise a mixture of hepatocytes, the major metabolically functional cells in the liver, and endothelial cells, which provide non-thrombogenic sinusoidal and vessel linings. The basic functional unit of the liver is the acinus (FIG. 2), and comprises plates of hepatocytes (lined on either side by endothelial cells) arranged so that blood flows through sinusoids from the portal triad (portal vein, hepatic artery, and bile duct) to the central vein. The scale of the acinus is ~1 mm. How should we arrange donor hepatocytes and endothelial cells to suitably reconstruct native tissue structure and function? Our working hypothesis is that mixtures of isolated cells can spontaneously form suitable tissue structures over a scale the size of an acinus if provided with an appropriate environment.

The concept of cell sorting as an important phenomenon in development dates back to classic experiments by Holtfreter, in which dissociated fragments of amphibian embryos were shown to adhere and develop *in vitro* in an analogous fashion to natural *in vivo* development. An elegant theoretical and experimental analysis by Steinberg presents compelling evidence that these sorting phenomena are biophysical in nature and arise from differential cell-cell adhesion forces; *i.e.,* sorting in mixed cell populations occurs much like phase separation occurs in mixtures of immiscible liquid molecules.[12] In reconstruction of a macroscopic piece of liver tissue, the polymer support can serve on the one hand as a template to locally facilitate the sorting process (on the scale of hundreds of microns) and on the other hand to provide an appropriate macroscopic arrangement of multiple acini (on the scale of tens of millimeters).

Cell-substrate adhesion forces, in addition to cell-cell adhesion forces, are expected to play a key role in formation of tissue structures from mixed cell populations in 3-D devices. Using substrata coated with systematically varied densities of extracellular matrix (ECM) proteins, we have demonstrated that the propensity of isolated hepatocytes to form multicellular aggregate structures depends on the cell-substrate adhesion strength,[13] with low values of adhesion strength favoring aggregate formation. Cell-substrate adhesion strength can be modulated in 3DP™

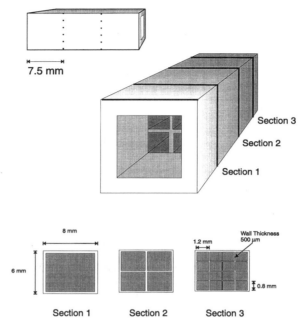

FIGURE 3. Structure of branching 3-D polymer scaffolds.

devices by coating the surfaces with specific densities of cell adhesion molecules during manufacture. Thus, the effects of systematic variations in cell-substrate adhesion strength on the formation of sinusoidal structures can be investigated. In this study, we use devices constructed from biodegradable polyesters which intrinsically allow formation of multicellular aggregates without an ECM coating.[14] Since the scale over which natural reorganization occurs is unknown, we designed a simple scaffold which incorporates three scales of channels (FIG. 3). In this preliminary design, the inlet channel has inner dimensions of 6.4×4.8 mm and branches ultimately to 16 channels of dimensions 0.8×1.2 mm, with 0.5 mm thick walls separating the channels.

Because cells are in direct contact with the perfusion medium during culture, a critical issue in scaffold design is the effects of fluid flow during perfusion. Fluid flow rates must be high enough to provide all cells down the length of the flow path with adequate nutrients, and yet not so high that cells are sheared off the surface during the early phase of culture. (Ultimately, the fluid flow rate will be determined by the available pressure drop in the circulatory system *in vivo*.)

We can estimate the flow rate needed for cell survival based on the cell mass and literature values for nutrient consumption rates. Under standard culture conditions, oxygen is the limiting nutrient, and we specify that the oxygen concentration should not drop more than 50% from the inlet to the outlet. The volumetric oxygen consumption rate, Q_{O_2}, is about $2\text{–}6 \times 10^{-5}$ mmol/cm^3 cell mass-s for metabolically active cells.[15] Native liver is about 50% by volume cells; the scaffold contains <5% by volume cells at the time it is set up *in vitro*. The flow rate, F, required to maintain the oxygen concentration at the desired level immediately after seeding is thus at most $F = 0.05V \dfrac{Q_{O_2}}{0.5C_{O_2,inlet}}$, for given value of inlet oxygen concentration $C_{O_2,inlet}$.

The concentration of oxygen in 5% CO_2/humidified air-saturated culture medium at 37°C is 0.16×10^{-3} mmol/ml and the scaffold void volume is 0.5 cm^3. The required flow rate to maintain the initial cell mass is thus 1 ml/min and would increase to 10 ml/min if the entire void volume of the scaffold achieves tissue-like density.

The fluid force acting to dislodge the cells can be calculated from the shear stress at the wall. The shear stress at the wall for fully developed laminar flow in a square channel is $\tau_w = \dfrac{8F_sQ_c\mu}{w^3}$, where F_s is a shape factor for non-circular conduits (0.89), μ is the fluid viscosity (0.7 cP), Q_c is the volumetric flow rate in the channel, and w is the channel width. In the smallest (highest stress) channels ($w = 0.8$ mm), at a flow rate of 2 ml/min, the wall shear stress is 0.02 Pa. Assuming the cell morphology is a hemispherical cap with radius r_p and height h, the distractive force acting on the cells can then be obtained from the relation $F_d = 2.15\pi(r_p^2 + h^2)\tau_w$. Typical values of r_p and h obtained for hepatocytes are 16.6 μm and 12.8 μm respectively; the sum of the squares varies by less than a factor of two for hepatocytes on low (0.01 μg/cm^2) and high (1 μg/cm^2) matrix densities and thus direct comparison of τ_w gives a fair comparison of detachment probabilities for the range of morphologies exhibited by hepatocytes on substrates of interest for use in the 3-D scaffold. For comparison, the mean shear stress required to detach hepatocytes cultured on a low surface density of ECM (0.01 μg/cm^2), where spreading is impaired, is 7 Pa and that for the high ECM, 105 Pa. The shear stresses encountered by cells attached to the walls in the channel in the perfusion setup are thus within an acceptable range, once cell attachment has occurred.

MATERIALS AND METHODS

Device Fabrication

PLLA (Mw = 132,000) and PLGA (65L:35G, M_w = 53,000) were provided in pellets (>2 mm) from Ethicon, Inc. (Somerville, NJ). Pellets were cooled in liquid nitrogen and cryogenically milled in an Ultra Centrifugal Mill (Glen Mills Inc., Clifton, NJ) with a continuous liquid nitrogen supply. The milled powder was dried under vacuum for 72 hr, then sieved and characterized. No change in Mw occurred as a result of the processing. Powder in the size range 45–75 mm was used in these experiments.

Devices were fabricated by printing chloroform into a mixed powder containing 25% PLLA and 75% PLGA. Devices were printed in 31 consecutive layers, each 200 μm thick. The relevant printing parameters include: print head speed = 60 cm/s, binder flow rate 20 μl/s (80 μm diameter droplets), and horizontal interline spacing = 200 μm (center-to-center). Devices were constructed in batches of 27 and the processing (printing) time for a batch was approximately 3 hr. The resulting devices consisted of an inlet channel with inner dimensions of 6.4 × 4.8 mm, branching ultimately to 16 channels of dimensions 0.8 × 1.2 mm, with 0.5 mm thick walls separating the channels. The length of each section was 0.75 cm. The total surface area contained in the device, based on the macroscopic channel dimensions, was 9.5 cm^2. Surface roughness (see Fig. 4) likely increased this by at least a factor of 2.

After construction, the entire powder bed (containing devices and unprinted powder) and its supporting plate were removed from the 3DP™ machine and placed in a nitrogen glove box for 48 hours to allow most residual solvent to evaporate under dry conditions. Further solvent removal was accomplished by vacuum drying (0.001 torr) for 72 hours. Loose (unprinted) powder was removed from the channels after drying was complete. The devices were sterilized with ethylene oxide and soaked in culture medium for 24 hours prior to seeding.

Device Characterization

Device microstructural morphology was investigated using scanning electron microscopy (SEM) on samples sputter-coated with gold. Surface molecular composition was assessed with X-ray photoelectron spectroscopy (XPS) using a Surface Science Instruments SSX100 spectrometer at the joint Harvard-MIT surface analytical facility. Monochromatic Al K$_\alpha$ (1486.6 eV) radiation was used to probe the core levels. An electron flood gun operating at 5.0 eV and a nickel grid placed several millimeters over the samples were used to compensate for charge. A survey scan was conducted to determine elemental composition and high resolution carbon-1s scans were performed to distinguish among the different carbon bonding environments. Surface Science Instruments software was used to fit the spectra using 100% Gaussian peaks. Peak areas were used to determine the relative amounts of each type of carbon bond.

Cell Isolation, Seeding, and Culture

Primary hepatocytes were isolated from adult Lewis rats with a modification of Seglen's two step collagenase perfusion procedure.[16,17] Viability following isodensity Percoll purification was 85–95%. Primary endothelial cells were isolated from bovine aortas using a scraping technique and expanded *in vitro* using a culture medium comprising DMEM supplemented with 10% fetal bovine serum.

Initial experiments for suitability of the matrices for culture were conducted by seeding 2.5 × 10^6 endothelial cells (~125,000 − 250,000 cells/cm^2) on the device and maintaining the devices in static cultures (in petri dishes) for up to 5 weeks. Mixed cell cultures were initiated by mixing 2.5 × 10^6 endothelial cells (from culture) and 2.7 × 10^6 hepatocytes (freshly isolated) in DMEM supplemented with 10% fetal bovine serum, and seeding devices in static culture. These devices were maintained in static culture or in a continuous perfusion culture.

For continuous perfusion culture, a sleeve of silastic tubing (Cole Parmer) was fitted over the device so that the channels ran lengthwise down the device; the tubing was easily attached to the perfusion circuit after seeding. The perfusion circuit comprised a recirculation reservoir from which medium was pumped (via a peristaltic pump) at a flow rate of 1.5 ml/min through an 8 ft. length of silastic tubing for oxygenation, through the device, and returned to the medium reservoir. A 45 min static attachment period was allowed before perfusion was started.

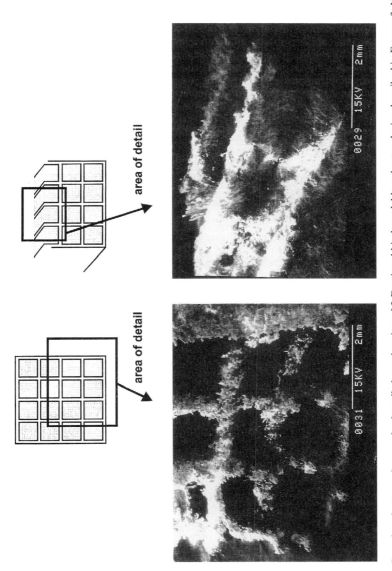

FIGURE 4. Scanning electron micrograph of small-channel region of 3-D printed biodegradable polyester device described in FIGURE 3. Note that the surface is textured owing to the mechanism of construction.

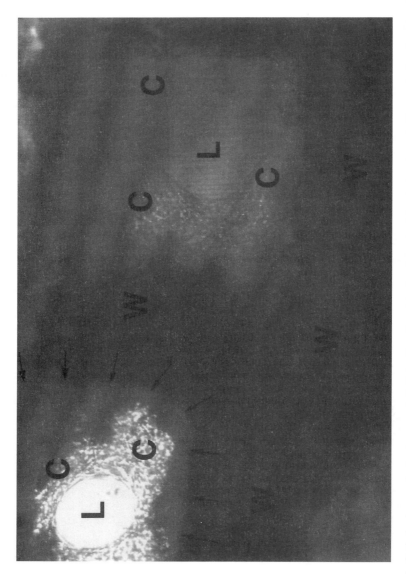

FIGURE 5. Optical micrograph of primary endothelial cells cultured in the channels of the device shown in FIGURE 4 after 5 weeks of culture. The walls of the device (W) appear as dark regions, and the cells (C) have lined the channels and extended toward the center, rounding the square channels (*e.g.*, demarcated by arrows) off and forming a central lumen (L). The channel diameter is on the order of 800 μm.

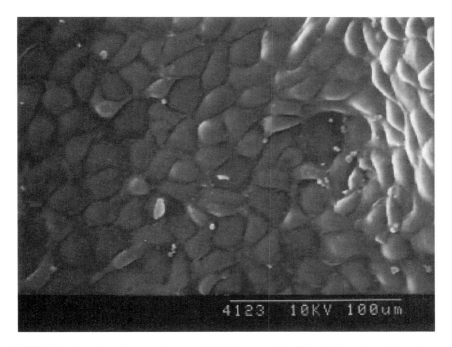

FIGURE 6. Scanning electron micrograph of primary endothelial cells after 4 weeks in culture. The cells were cultured as described in FIGURE 5.

Microscopy

Samples were prepared for scanning electron microscopy (SEM) by fixation, dehydration, and critical point drying. Samples were sputter-coated with gold and examined in a Hitachi SEM.

Endothelial cell viability was ascertained via uptake of acetylated low density lipoprotein (Ac-LDL) labeled with 1,1′-dioctadecyl-3,3,3′,3′-tetramethylindocarbo-cyanine perchlorate (DiI) (Biomedical Technologies, Inc.; Stoughton, MA). Cells were incubated for 4 hours in medium containing 10 μg/ml DiI-Ac-LDL at 37°C and were subsequently rinsed twice with medium. The fluorescent DiI label is not degraded by lysosomal enzymes and can be visualized by optical microscopy.

RESULTS AND DISCUSSION

The 3DP™ printing process enabled construction of devices with a branching internal architecture using degradable polyesters. The microscopic internal structure of the device comprised square channels with highly textured walls (FIG. 4). The wall texture results from the interplay of chloroform binder and polymer powder during the printing process. The channel wall is created by printing a line of sequential overlapping chloroform droplets. When a droplet of chloroform impinges on

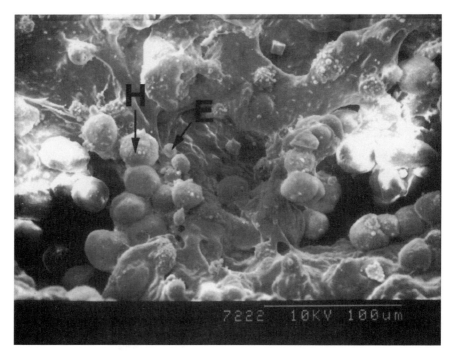

FIGURE 7. Scanning electron micrograph showing a mixture of primary endothelial cells and primary hepatocytes maintained in static culture 12 hours after seeding onto biodegradable polymer scaffolds. Hepatocytes (the larger cells, ~20 microns in diameter, *e.g.,* labeled H) remain mostly rounded, while endothelial cells (the smaller cells, ~12 microns in diameter, *e.g.,* labeled E) show mixed morphology, with many spread over the surface.

the powder bed, it simultaneously begins to dissolve or swell the particles it comes in immediate contact with and also begins to wick out along the surfaces of adjacent particles. A particle at the edge of the advancing solvent front may then become partially embedded in the line created by the chloroform without being completely joined to the particles adjacent to it in the line.

Trace contaminants may be introduced in either the powder preparation or printing steps of the 3DP™ process. Analysis of completed devices with ESCA showed only the expected elements (C, O) in survey scans and revealed trace adventitious aliphatic carbon in high-resolution C1s scans.

Initial experiments with 3DP™ devices were conducted in static culture with primary endothelial cells in order to develop seeding protocols and assure the devices were conducive for cell adhesion and survival. For this purpose, culture was carried out for up to 5 weeks. As observed by light microscopy, cells attached and filled in the channels of the device over the 5 week period (FIG. 5). The uptake of DiI-Ac-LDL (data not shown) demonstrated the presence of viable cells. The cells had a normal cobblestone appearance and covered the surface as observed by SEM (FIG. 6). The polymer devices did not exhibit significant degradation as

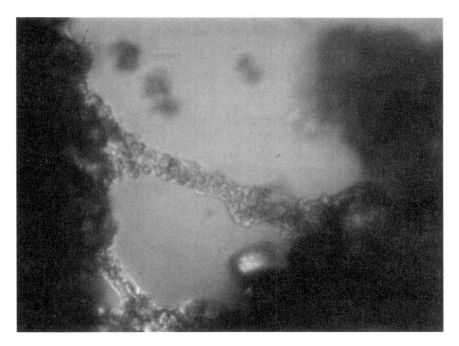

FIGURE 8. Optical micrograph of cell organization in the smallest channels in mixed endothelial cell/hepatocyte cultures after 2 days under static conditions. Cells bridge across the channel forming structures which appear analogous to sinusoids.

assessed by changes in morphology or handling characteristics during the 5-week period. These results suggested that the devices provided a suitable attachment substrate and were conducive to long-term cell survival.

Mixed populations of hepatocytes and endothelial cells seeded onto the devices exhibited substantial reorganization within the first 72 hours. Although a random mixture of cells was attached to the surface of the devices initially (FIG. 7), organization of cells into structures which bridged across the smallest channels was observed by day 3 (FIG. 8) in static culture. FIGURE 9 demonstrates the formation of similar bridging structures in devices adjacent to solid substrata over a one-day period. Endothelial cells sorted to the cell-medium interface, covering the hepatocytes (FIG. 10). This phenomenon has been previously observed on two-dimensional substrata in experiments which showed that mixed cocultures of hepatocytes and non-parenchymal liver cells (NPCs) sort to form spheroidal cellular aggregates consisting of a hepatocyte core surrounded by a continuous layer of NPCs.[18]

The appearance of cells maintained under perfusion conditions (FIG. 11) was similar to that maintained under static conditions (FIG. 7), although perfused scaffolds contained visibly fewer cells at the time of harvest, presumably because the shear forces dislodged clumps of cells while leaving those directly adherent to the surface of the scaffold. We are currently investigating the relationship between flowrate and cell retention.

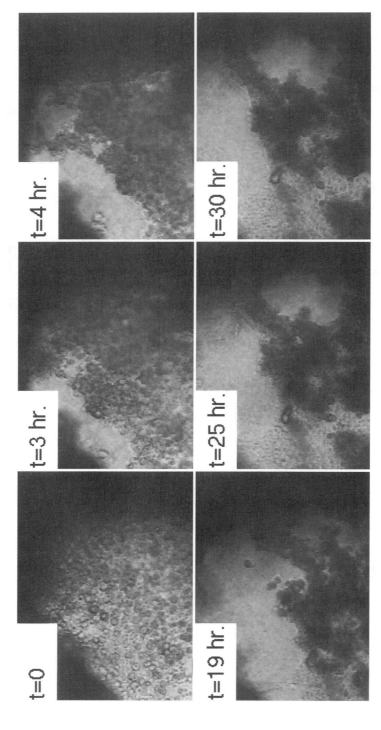

FIGURE 9. Optical micrograph time-line of cell organization in the smallest channels in mixed endothelial cell/hepatocyte cultures beginning immediately after seeding (t = 0). The device (seen on the outer rim of the micrographs) is adjacent to a solid substratum, to which the cells are seen attaching. The formation of a bridging structure is seen on the time scale of 1 day.

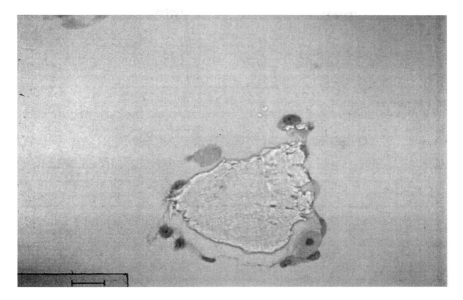

FIGURE 10. Histological appearance of hepatocytes and endothelial cells surrounding a single polymer particle (2 days in static culture). Hepatocytes remain rounded, while endothelial cells are flattened and coat all fluid-contacting surfaces, covering the hepatocytes. Devices were fixed and embedded in JB40 resin, sectioned, and stained with hematoxylin/eosin.

CONCLUSIONS

We have demonstrated the initial feasibility of a new approach to hepatic tissue engineering: *in vitro* organogensis of vascularized tissue. We first constructed scaffolds with a hierarchical structure from biodegradable polyesters using a manufacturing technique amenable to scale-up and commercial production. Our resolution in controlling the structural features in the scaffold is on the order of a few hundred microns. Mixtures of cells (hepatocytes and endothelial cells) showed an intrinsic ability to reform histotypic structures in the channels of the device, suggesting that finer control of resolution may not be necessary to achieve desired tissue structures. We are currently investigating the role of scaffold architecture and culture conditions in achieving hepatic function in long-term perfusion cultures.

SUMMARY

The high metabolic rate of hepatocytes severely limits the mass of cells which can be transplanted without a vascular supply. We are developing an alternative approach in which vascularized tissue is grown *ex vivo* for anastamosis into the portal vein. Here, we discuss the key design issues for *in vitro* organogenesis of vascularized hepatic tissue, describe a fabrication approach for making complex degradable polymer scaffolds to organize cells in three dimensions on the scale of

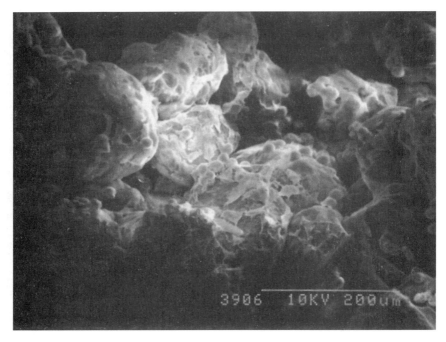

FIGURE 11. Scanning electron micrograph of mixtures of hepatocytes and endothelial cells seeded in biodegradable polymer scaffolds and maintained in a perfusion circuit for 18 hours.

hundreds of microns, and demonstrate the feasbility of using these scaffolds for *in vitro* tissue organization in mixed-cell cultures.

REFERENCES

1. US Transplants Oct. 1, 1985–Dec. 31, 1992: One, two, and three year graft and patient survival rates by organ. United Network for Organ Sharing Scientific Registry, 1994.
2. HOOFNAGLE, J. H., R. L. CARITHERS, C. SHAPIRO & N. ASCHER. 1995. Fulminant hepatic failure: Summary of a workshop. Hepatology **21:** 240–252.
3. ROZGA, J., E. MORSIANI, E. LEPAGE, A. D. MOSCIONI, T. GIORGIO & A. A. DEMETRIOU. 1994. Isolated hepatocytes in a bioartificial liver: A single group view and experience. Biotechnol. Bioeng. 43: 645–653.
4. RHIM, J. A., E. P. SANDGREN, J. L. DEGEN, R. D. PALMITER & R. L. BRINSTER. 1994. Replacement of diseased mouse liver by hepatic cell transplantation. Science **263:** 1149–1152.
5. GROSSMAN, M., S. E. RAPER, K. KOZARSKY, E. A. STEIN, J. F. ENGELHARDT, D. MULLER, P. J. LUPIEN & J. M. WILSON. 1994. Successful ex vivo gene therapy directed to liver in a patient with familial hypercholesterolaemia. Nature Gen. **6:** 335–341.
6. ELIAS, H. & J. C. SHERRICK. 1969. Morphology of the Liver. Academic Press. New York.
7. CIMA, L. G., J. P. VACANTI, C. VACANTI, D. E. INGBER, D. MOONEY & R. LANGER. 1991. Tissue engineering by cell transplantation using biodegradable polymer substrates. J. Biomech. Eng. **113:** 143–151.

8. SMITH, P. F., G. KRACK, R. L. McKEE, D. G. JOHNSON, A. J. GANDOLFI, V. J. HRUBY, C. L. KRUMDEIK & K. BRENDL. 1986. Maintenance of adult rat liver slices in dynamic organ culture. In Vitro Cell. Devel. Biol. **22:** 706–712.

9. SACHS, E., M. CIMA, P. WILLIAMS, D. BRANCAZIO & J. CORNIE. 1992. Three dimensional printing: Rapid tooling and prototypes directly from a CAD model. J. Eng. for Industry **114:** 481–488.

10. WU, B. M., S. W. BORLAND, R. A. GIORDANO, L. G. GRIFFITH-CIMA, E. M. SACHS & M. J. CIMA. 1996. Solid free-form fabrication of drug delivery devices. J. Controlled Rel. **40:** 77–87.

11. STROM, S. C., R. L. JIRTLE, R. S. JONES, D. L. NOVICKI, N. R. ROSENBERG, A. NOVOTNY, G. IRONS, J. R. McCLAIN & G. MICHALOPOULOS. 1982. Isolation, culture, and transplant of human hepatocytes. J. Nat. Canc. Inst. **68:** 771–778.

12. STEINBERG, M. S. 1963. Reconstruction of tissues by dissociated cells. Science **141:** 401–408.

13. POWERS, M. J., R. E. RODRIGUEZ & L. G. GRIFFITH. 1996. Cell-substratum adhesion strength as a determinant of heptocyte aggregate morphology. Biotech. Bioeng. In press.

14. PARK, A. & L. G. GRIFFITH-CIMA. 1996. *In vitro* cell response to differences in poly-L-lactide crystallinity. J. Biomed. Mat. Res. **31:** 117–130.

15. CIMA, L. G., C. R. WILKE & H. W. BLANCH. 1990. A theoretical and experimental evaluation of a novel radial-flow hollow fiber reactor for mammalian cell culture. Bioprocess Eng. **5:** 19–30.

16. SEGLEN, P. O. 1976. Preparation of isolated rat liver cells. Methods Cell Biol. **13:** 29–83.

17. CIMA, L. G., D. E. INGBER, J. P. VACANTI & R. LANGER. 1991. Hepatocyte culture on biodegradable polymeric substrates. Biotech. Bioeng. **38:** 145–158.

18. LANDRY, J., D. BERNIER, C. OULLET, R. GOYETTE & N. MARCEAU. 1985. Spheroidal aggregate culture of rat liver cells: histotypic reorganization, biomatrix deposition, and maintenance of functional activities. J. Cell Biol. **101:** 914–923.

Spheroid Formation of Hepatocytes Using Synthetic Polymer

MASAMICHI KAMIHIRA,[a] KEISUKE YAMADA,
RYUJI HAMAMOTO, AND SHINJI IIJIMA

Department of Biotechnology
Graduate School of Engineering
Nagoya University
Chikusa-ku, Nagoya 464-01, Japan

In recent years, a bioartificial liver support system, in which living hepatocytes are packed in a bioreactor, has attracted a great attention for the treatment of patients with fulminant hepatic failure. Unlike other organs such as heart, lung and kidney, the liver has multiple functions essential to maintain life, including carbohydrate metabolism, synthesis of proteins, amino acid metabolism, urea synthesis, lipid metabolism, drug biotransformation, and waste removal. Owing to their complexity the functions cannot be replaced by fully artificial devices; therefore, living hepatocytes are used for an artificial liver support system. For this purpose, many researchers have investigated maintaining the viability and liver functions of primary hepatocytes.[1-3] From these efforts, the importance of culture conditions including medium components such as growth factors and hormones and cultural substratum has been demonstrated.

Hepatocytes exhibit different morphologies depending on the surface conditions of the cultural substrata. For example, freshly isolated primary hepatocytes are cultured as a monolayer on a collagen-coated dish. On the other hand, the cells form three-dimensional, high cell-density packed, multicellular aggregates called spheroid on proteoglycan-coated or positively charged dishes. The hepatocyte spheroids have been observed to exhibit enhanced liver functions in the long-term compared with monolayer culture.[4-6] Therefore, cell-cell interaction seems to play an important role in the expression of liver function. Many researchers have developed culture methods for forming hepatocyte spheroids.[7-11] In most cases, however, the methods depend on the cultural substratum and require large surface area for initial cell attachment. Therefore, supplement of surface area has been a limiting factor for the preparation of spheroids.

In this regard, we developed a method for the preparation of functional spheroid-like cell aggregates in suspension culture, in which a synthetic polymer was added to the culture medium for inducing liver cell aggregation.

MATERIALS AND METHODS

Hepatocyte Culture

Hepatocytes were isolated from 6–7-week old male Sprague-Dawley rats by the conventional *in situ* collagenase perfusion method[12] and low-speed centrifugation

[a] Author to whom correspondence should be addressed: Tel: +81-52-789-4277; Fax: +81-52-789-3221; E-mail: kamihira@proc.nubio.nagoya-u.ac.jp

procedure. More than 99% of the isolated cells were hepatocytes judging from phase-contrast microscopic observation, and more than 90% were viable based on the trypan blue dye exclusion method. The isolated hepatocytes were cultured in a serum-free hormonally defined medium consisting of Williams' medium E (Gibco Co., New York, NY) supplemented with 0.1 μM CuSO$_4 \cdot$5H$_2$O, 25 nM Na$_2$SeO$_3$, 1.0 μM ZnSO$_4 \cdot$7H$_2$O, 0.1 μM insulin (Sigma Chemical. Co., St. Louis, MO), 1.0 μM dexamethasone (Wako Pure Chemical Co., Osaka, Japan), 20 ng/ml epidermal growth factor (EGF) (Sigma Chemical Co.), 20 μg/ml egg yolk lipoprotein (Wako Pure Chemical Co.), 48 μg/ml gentamicin sulfate (Sigma Chemical Co.), and 100 μg/ml chloramphenicol (Wako Pure Chemical Co.).

A copolymer of methacrylic acid and methylmethacrylate, Eudragit S100 (Röhm Pharma GmbH, Darmstadt, Germany), was added to the medium at various concentrations for promoting cell aggregate formation. Prior to the addition the polymer was solubilized in water adjusting the pH at 7.4 by adding 2M NaOH. The polymer was originally developed as an enteric coating polymer.

For the static petri dish cultures, the cells isolated were seeded at 5.0×10^5 cells per a 35 mm-diameter plastic dish in 2 ml medium. Collagen-coated plastic dishes (catalog no. 4000–010; Iwaki Glass Works Co., Chiba, Japan) were used for monolayer culture of hepatocytes, and positively charged plastic dishes (Falcon Primaria®, catalog no. 3801; Becton Dickinson Co., Bedford, MA), were used for control spheroid culture of hepatocytes. When Eudragit was added to the medium, normal tissue culture plastic dishes (catalog no. 3000–035; Iwaki Glass Works Co.) were used. A half volume of the medium was changed every day.

Spinner Flask Culture

For the spinner flask culture, the freshly isolated hepatocytes were inoculated in a 250 ml spinner flask (Shibata Hario Co., Tokyo, Japan) at 2.5×10^5 cells/ml in 100 ml culture medium. The agitation rate was 50 rpm and the culture temperature was maintained at 37°C by circulating thermo-regulated water into a jacket. A gas containing 95% air and 5% CO$_2$ was provided at a rate of 500 ml/min through the surface of the medium. A small amount of broth was taken from the spinner flask and used for observation of the cells and analyses.

Measurement of Liver Functions

Albumin concentration in the medium was determined by sandwich solid-phase enzyme-linked immunosorbent assay (ELISA), using sheep anti-rat albumin (catalog no. 55729; Organon Teknika Co., Durham, NC) and peroxidase-conjugated anti-rat albumin (catalog no. 55776; Organon Teknika Co.) antibodies for detection and purified rat albumin (Sigma Chemical Co.) as the standard.

Ammonia removal and urea synthesis were measured as follows. First, the medium was carefully removed from the cell-cultured dish, and the fresh medium containing 1.0 mM NH$_4$Cl was added. The dish was cultured for 4 h, then ammonia and urea concentrations in the medium were measured by using diagnostic kits obtained from Wako Pure Chemical Co. (catalog no. 277–14401 and 279–36201, respectively). The rates of ammonia removal and urea synthesis were calculated from the reduction of ammonia concentration and the increase of urea concentration, respectively.

Analyses

The amount of DNA of the cultured cells was determined by DAPI (4',6-diamidino-2-phenylindole dihydrochloride, Wako Pure Chemical Co.)-DNA cytofluorometry method[13] after disruption of the cells by sonication.

The cell activity was measured by MTT (3-(4,5-dimethylthiazol-2-yl) 2,5-diphenyl tetrazolium bromide) (Sigma Chemical Co.) method[14] and expressed as absorbance at 570 nm.

GOT (glutamic oxaloacetic transaminase) activity leaked from hepatocytes to the medium was measured by using a diagnostic kit (catalog no. 275-34101; Wako Pure Chemical Co.).

RESULTS AND DISCUSSION

Effects of Eudragit Concentration on Spheroid Formation and Liver Functions in Petri Dish Culture

In our previous research, we applied Eudragit for specific animal cell separation using an aqueous two-phase system, in which the polymer was used as a ligand-carrier.[15] It was found that the polymer had low cytotoxicity and gave rise to cell aggregation of hepatocytes, whereas other polymers such as chitosan and polyethyleneimine exhibited no such ability or serious cytotoxic effect.

FIGURE 1 shows the photographs of hepatocytes on 1 day and 5 days after inoculation, when the cells were cultured on the various dishes or in suspension containing Eudragit. On a collagen-coated dish, the cells attached, spread out and formed a monolayer within a day. However, the cells gradually detached after 5 days. On a Primaria® dish, the cells initially attached, agglomerated into cell-aggregates on the dish surface, and then formed floating spheroids after 3–4 days, as an earlier researcher described.[7] On the other hand, by the addition of Eudragit, the cells loosely agglomerated from the beginning of the culture, then the cell-cell attachment became tight and formed spheroid-like aggregates after 3 days. The process of spheroid formation was different between the spheroids induced by Primaria® dish and Eudragit addition. However, they were morphologically very similar. In the case of Eudragit addition, normal tissue culture dishes without special surface were used for the culture. Without the polymer, the cells weakly attached on the surface of the dish and did not form spheroids. Hence, the spheroid formation was mediated by the polymer.

FIGURE 2 shows albumin secretion on days 3 and 7. Since the total amount of DNA in the dish did not change much throughout the 7-day culture period (data not shown), the change in albumin secretion was attributable to the change in the ability of cells. The albumin secretion was not different among the cultures on day 3. Although the ability decreased about half for the monolayer culture on day 7, it was almost constant for the spheroid culture using a Primaria® dish. On the other hand, cell morphology and albumin secretion were dependent on Eudragit concentration; the hepatocytes clearly formed floating spheroids with 0.1% Eudragit, but they tended to attach the dish surface above 0.18% Eudragit and the cells formed islets of multicellular aggregates on the dish surface rather than spheroids. The ability of albumin secretion was the highest for 0.1% Eudragit on day 7. From the fact that albumin secretion was not enhanced with monolayer culture using the medium containing Eudragit (data not shown), the expression of the liver function seemed to strongly correlate to the cell morphology.

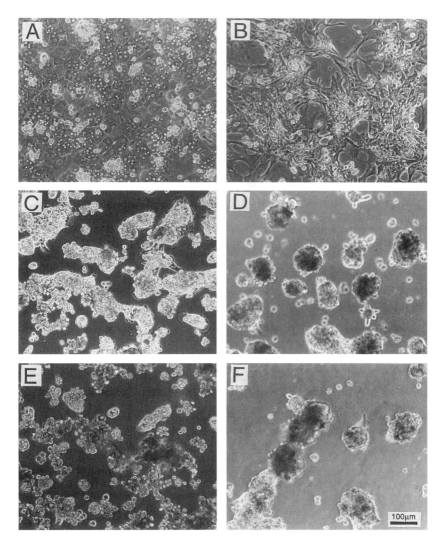

FIGURE 1. Photographs of cultured hepatocytes in static petri dishes on day 1 (**A, C** and **E**) and 5 days (**B, D** and **F**) after inoculation. Hepatocytes were cultured on a collagen-coated dish (**A** and **B**), a Primaria® dish (**C** and **D**), and a normal tissue culture dish in the presence of 0.1% Eudragit (**E** and **F**).

The other liver functions of the spheroids formed by the Eudragit addition, ammonia removal and urea synthesis, were measured on day 4 (FIGs. 3 and 4). Both the functions showed a tendency similar to albumin secretion on day 7. Around 0.1% Eudragit, ammonia removal and urea synthesis were the highest and the values were 4-fold and 1.6-fold those of monolayer culture, respectively. Moreover, the

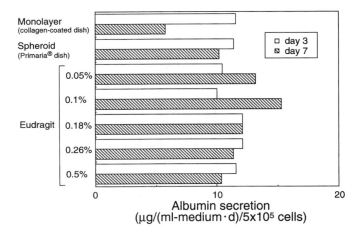

FIGURE 2. Effect of Eudragit concentration on albumin secretion.

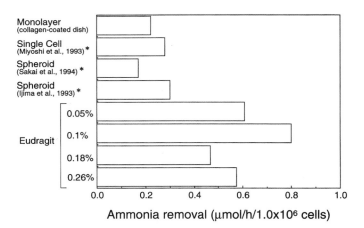

FIGURE 3. Ammonia removal of cultured hepatocytes on day 4. *Culture conditions: (Miyoshi *et al.*[16]) Immobilized in a porous polyvinyl formal resin and cultured in a packed-bed reactor. Ammonium (1 mM) was loaded for 6 h. The rates of ammonia removal and urea synthesis were averaged from the data measured on days 1–7. (Sakai *et al.*[18]) Hepatocyte spheroids were immobilized in follow fiber module. Ammonium (1 mM) was loaded for 2 h. The rate of ammonia removal and urea synhesis were averaged from the data measured on days 2–10. (Ijima *et al.*[17]) Hepatocyte spheroids were immobilized in a polyurethane foam and cultured in pack-bed reactor. Ammonium (3 mM) was loaded for 24 h. The rates of ammonia removal and urea synthesis were averaged from the data on days 6–11.

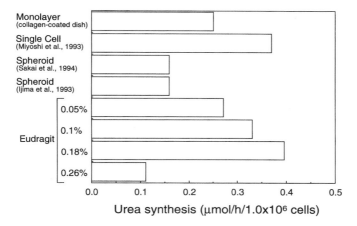

FIGURE 4. Urea synthesis of cultured hepatocytes on day 4. The culture conditions of hepatocytes are the same as in FIGURE 3.

levels of the liver functions with 0.1% Eudragit were higher than those with the spheroids reported previously,[16-18] although the culture conditions were very different. Judging from the above results, 0.1% Eudragit was chosen for spinner flask culture.

The same tendency of enhanced liver functions on Eudragit concentration was observed for the separate isolation of hepatocytes (data not shown).

Spheroid Formation Induced by Eudragit Addition in Spinner Flask Culture

As the next step, the spheroid formation by adding 0.1% Eudragit was performed in a spinner flask. Unlike the static petri dish cultures, the cells were stirred and suspended in the medium in the spinner flask culture. In spite of this difference, hepatocytes formed spheroids effectively 2 days after inoculation (FIG. 5A), when the polymer was added to the medium. Approximately 80% of the cells inoculated agglomerated and became spheroids. The efficiency was higher than that with the static dish cultures described previously.[19] The spheroids formed also exhibited high albumin secretion (data not shown). Therefore, this procedure is promising for the mass preparation of functional hepatocyte spheroids, although the further scale-up study is necessary.

When the polymer was not added in the spinner flask culture, most of hepatocytes seemed to die within a day; the cells were stained with trypan blue dye (FIG. 5D). In order to confirm this, MTT activity and GOT leakage were measured (FIGS. 6 and 7). MTT activity corresponds to cell respiration activity and viability, and GOT concentration in the medium indicates the degree of disintegration of hepatocytes. The MTT activity decreased about half at 12 h for spinner flask culture containing Eudragit compared to those just after isolation from rats (FIG. 6). Since it also decreased to the same level in the static dish cultures, the decrease may be attributable to the culture medium. In the spinner flask culture without the polymer,

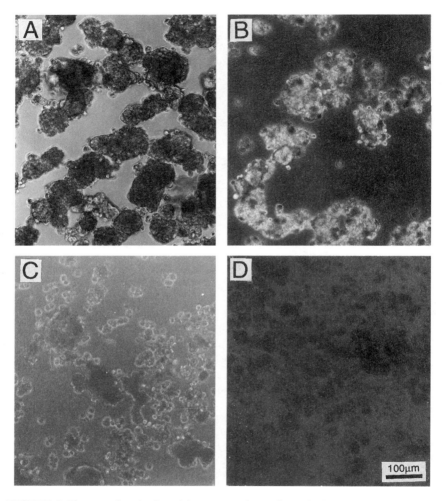

FIGURE 5. Photographs of cultured hepatocytes in a spinner flask on day 2. Hepatocytes were cultured in the presence (**A** and **B**) or absence (**C** and **D**) of 0.1% Eudragit. The cells were stained with trypan blue dye (**B** and **D**).

however, the MTT activity decreased rapidly. The cell viability was about one third of the culture containing Eudragit in this case.

With respect to GOT leakage, it was found that a large amount of GOT leaked from the cells in the spinner flask culture without the polymer. The leaked GOT was 3-fold that of the culture containing the polymer. This change seems to correspond to the decrease in MTT activity. These results suggest that the polymer may have a protective effect for the cells from damage by agitation.

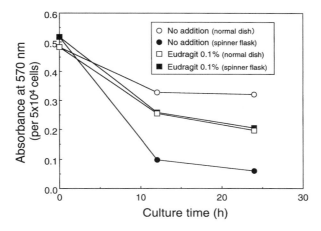

FIGURE 6. MTT activity of cultured hepatocytes.

In conclusion, hepatocytes effectively formed spheroids by the addition of Eudragit in both a static petri dish without special surface modification and a cell-suspended spinner flask with stirring. The spheroids formed exhibited enhanced liver functions such as albumin secretion, ammonia removal and urea synthesis. Thus, the preparation of large amount of functional spheroids is possible by this method and the formed spheroids may be applicable to bioartificial liver support systems.

The modification of the polymer with sugar chains is now under study for obtaining further high efficiency of spheroid formation and enhanced liver specific functions. The results will be described elsewhere.

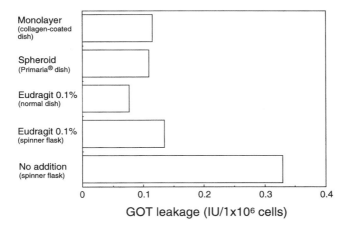

FIGURE 7. GOT leakage in various hepatocyte cultures at 24 h after inoculation.

SUMMARY

It is known that hepatocytes show the different morphology depending on the surface condition of cultural substratum. The cells form a floating cell-aggregate called spheroid on proteoglycan-coated or positively charged dishes. The liver cell functions are generally high and maintained for the long-term in the spheroid culture. Since spheroid morphology is preferable for the construction of a bioartificial liver, it is important to develop an effective method of preparing spheroids. In this regard, we examined a preparation method of functional spheroid-like cell-aggregates, in which a synthetic polymer, Eudragit was added to culture medium for inducing liver cell-aggregation. The cell-cell attachment of the aggregate was loose at the beginning of the culture, but it became tight and spheroids were formed 2–3 days after inoculation. When 0.1% Eudragit was added to the medium, the liver functions such as albumin secretion, ammonia removal and urea synthesis were enhanced compared with monolayer and conventional spheroid cultures. The spheroid formation was also performed with suspension culture in a spinner flask. Approximately 80% of the cells inoculated formed spheroids by the addition of the polymer. Moreover, the polymer showed a protective effect from cell damage by agitation. Since this procedure does not require surface for cell attachment, a large amount of spheroids can be prepared in suspension culture.

REFERENCES

1. ENAT, R., D. M. JEFFERSON, N. RUIZ-OPAZO, Z. GATMAITAN, L. A. LEINWAND & L. M. REID. 1984. Hepatocyte proliferation *in vitro*: Its dependence on the use of serum-free hormonally defined medium and substrata of extracellular matrix. Proc. Natl. Acad. Sci. USA **81**: 1411–1415.
2. DICH, J., C. VIND & N. GRUNNET. 1988. Long-term culture of hepatocytes: Effect of hormones on enzyme activities and metabolic capacity. Hepatology **8**: 39–45.
3. BEN-ZE'EV, A., G. S. ROBINSON, N. L. BUCHER & S. R. FARMER. 1988. Cell-cell and cell-matrix interactions differentially regulate the expression of hepatic and cytoskeltal genes in primary cultures of rat hepatocytes. Proc. Natl. Acad. Sci. USA **85**: 2161–2165.
4. LANDRY, J., D. BERNIER, C. OUELLET, R. GOYETTE & N. MARCEAU. 1985. Spheroidal aggregate culture of rat liver cells: Histotypic reorganization, biomatrix deposition, and maintenance of functional activities. J. Cell Biol. **101**: 914–923.
5. KOIDE, N., T. SHINJI, T. TANABE, K. ASANO, K. KAWAGUCHI, K. SAKAGUCHI, Y. KOIDE, M. MORI & T. TSUJI. 1989. Continued high albumin production by multicellular spheroids of adult rat hepatocytes formed in the presence of liver-derived proteoglycans. Biochem. Biophys. Res. Commun. **161**: 385–391.
6. TONG, J. Z., O. BERNARD & F. ALVAREZ. 1990. Long-term culture of rat liver cell spheroids in hormonally defined media. Exp. Cell Res. **189**: 87–92.
7. KOIDE, N., K. SAKAGUCHI, Y. KOIDE, K. ASANO, M. KAWAGUCHI, H. MATSUSHIMA, T. TAKENAMI, T. SHINJI, M. MORI & T. TSUJI. 1990. Formation of multicellular spheroids composed of adult rat hepatocytes in dishes with positively charged surfaces and under other nonadherent environments. Exp. Cell Res. **186**: 227–235.
8. MATSUSHITA, T., H. IJIMA, N. KOIDE & K. FUNATSU 1991. High albumin production by multicellular spheroids of adult rat hepatocytes formed in pores of polyurethane foam. Appl. Microbiol. Biothechnol. **36**: 324–326
9. SAKAI, Y. & M. SUZUKI. 1991. Formation of spheroids of adult rat hepatocytes on polylysine-coated surfaces and their albumin production. Biotechnol. Tech. **5**: 299–302.
10. TOBE, T., Y. TAKEI, K. KOBAYASHI & T. AKAIKE. 1992. Receptor-mediated formation of multilayer aggregates of primary cultured adult rat hepatocytes on lactose-substituted polystyrene. Biochem. Biophys. Res. Commun. **184**: 225–230.
11. UENO, K., A. MIYASHITA, K. ENDOH, T. TAKEZAWA, M. YAMAZAKI, Y. MORI & T.

SATOH. 1992. Formation of multicellular spheroids composed of rat hepatocytes. Res. Commun. Chem. Pathol. Pharmacol. **77:** 107–120.
12. SEGLEN, P. O. 1976. Preparation of isolated rat liver cells. Methods Cell Biol. **13:** 29–83.
13. HAMADA, S. & S. FUJITA. 1983. DAPI staining improved for quantitative cytofluorometry. Histochemistry **79:** 219–226.
14. MOSMANN, T. 1983. Rapid colorimetric assay for cellular growth and survival: application to proliferation and cytotoxicity assays. J. Immunol. Methods, **65:** 55–63.
15. HAMAMOTO, R., M. KAMIHIRA & S. IIJIMA. 1996. Specific separation of animal cells using aqueous two-phase systems. J. Ferment. Bioeng. **82:** 73–76.
16. MIYOSHI, H., K. YANAGI, K. FURUKAWA & N. OHSHIMA. 1993. Continuous culture of hepatocyte under different medium conditions using a packed-bed reactor with porous resin (in Japanese). Jpn J. Artif. Organs **22:** 147–152.
17. IIJIMA, H., T. MATSUSHITA & K. FUNATSU. 1993. Developement of a hybrid type artificial liver using PUF/spheroid culture system of adult hepatocytes (in Japanese). Jpn J. Artif. Organs **22:** 171–176.
18. SAKAI, Y & M. SUZUKI. 1994. Functional expressions by hepatocyte spheroids entrapped in collagen gel in hollow fiber modules (in Japanese). Jpn J. Artif. Organs **23:** 473–478.
19. PESHWA, M. V., F. J. WU, B. D. FOLLSTAD, F. B. CERRA & W. S. HU. 1994. Kinetics of hepatocyte spheroid formation. Biotechnol. Prog. **10:** 460–466.

Non-Autologous Transplantation with Immuno-isolation in Large Animals— A Review

TRACY L. STOCKLEY[a] AND PATRICIA L. CHANG[a-d]

Departments of [a]Pediatrics, [b]Biology and [c]Biomedical Sciences
McMaster University
Hamilton, Ontario L8N 3Z5 Canada

Transplantation is emerging as a powerful new tool in medicine. Allogeneic transplantation, involving human-to-human transplant of allogeneic non-autologous donor tissue, is currently the only clinically relevant form of human transplantation available to patients. The tissues and organs which are currently amenable to transplantation include kidney, heart, liver, lung, pancreas and bone marrow.[1] However, there is a current shortage of human organs available for transplantations, as the demand continually outstrips the supply of organs suitable for transplantation. The shortage of human organs for transplantation has been the impetus for research into novel methods to achieve replacement of organ functions from xenogeneic donors. This review will discuss one such novel area of research, the use of immuno-isolation devices for non-autologous transplantation.

The major obstacle to successful non-autologous organ transplantation is immune rejection of the newly transplanted organ. This is true for both allogeneic transplantations as well as xenogeneic transplantations, although xenogeneic transplantations are more severely hampered by immune rejection since the greater species disparity between host and donor tissue invokes a more intense immune response known as hyperacute rejection.[2] The immune problem arises as the immune system of the host recognizes tissue antigens of the transplanted tissues as foreign and so mounts an immune response against the transplanted tissues. This immune reaction, if left unchecked, can lead to failure of the transplanted tissues.

Owing to the utility of organ transplantation, techniques designed to overcome the immune barrier to non-autologous transplantation are under intense study. The method that is currently used to prevent immune rejection of allogeneic non-autologous transplants in patients is pharmacological immune suppression. In this situation, drugs that interfere with certain aspects of the immune response are given to patients receiving transplants. These immunosuppressive drugs prevent proper functioning of the immune system in some manner, and so prevent the body from mounting immune responses to the foreign transplanted tissues. For example, cyclosporin A is a commonly used immunosuppressive drug given to transplant recipients. The cyclosporin A inhibits T-cell activation and B-cell mediated humoral response, thus suppressing the immune response of the patient.[3] However, a major drawback with pharmacological immune suppression is that patient must exist in

[d] Author to whom correspondence should be addressed: Department of Pediatrics, Health Sciences Centre Room 3N18, McMaster University, 1200 Main Street West, Hamilton, Ontario L8N 3Z5 Canada; Tel: (905) 521-2100 ext. 3716; Fax: (905) 521-1703; E-mail: changp@fhs. mcmaster.CA

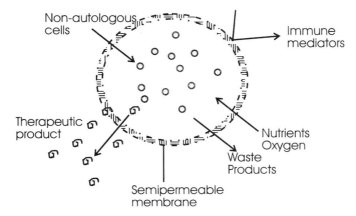

FIGURE 1. Model of immuno-isolation of non-autologous cells using selectively permeable membranes. Non-autologous cells secreting a therapeutic product are placed in immuno-isolation devices fabricated from perm-selective membranes. The capsule membrane allows secretion of the therapeutic product, while preventing access of immune mediators to the cells. The membrane also permits exchange of waste products, nutrients and oxygen between the interior and exterior of the immuno-isolation device.

an immune-compromised state, making the patient more vulnerable to many types of infections.[4]

Owing to the undesirable side effects of pharmacological immune suppression, other ways of blocking immune rejection have been conceived. One method that has gained much interest is the possibility of using genetically engineered donor tissues in xenogeneic transplantations. In this situation, animals that are potentially good donors of organs to humans because of their similar physiology are genetically altered to make their cells more similar to human cells, in the hopes of reducing the immune response to the xenogeneic tissue when transplanted into humans. The majority of this work to date has focused on the production of transgenic swine, which carry an introduced DNA coding sequence containing a gene of interest, resulting in an animal which expresses the modified gene in all tissues. Transgenic swine have been produced that express an inhibitor of human complement so as to protect the porcine tissue from attack by human complement,[5] while other groups are attempting to produce transgenic "knockout" swine which lack the gene coding for an enzyme involved in marking porcine tissues with carbohydrate epitopes that are the major targets of human antibodies involved in rejection.[6] However, this technology is still experimental and has yet to reach human clinical trials.[7]

In comparison, immuno-isolation is a method of overcoming the immune barrier to transplantation which has been proven feasible both in large animals and in recent human clinical trials. Immuno-isolation refers to the process where tissues to be used for transplantation are first enclosed in devices constructed from selectively permeable membranes (for review, see refs. 8–10), and was first conceptualized for production of artificial cells.[11] The permeability of the membrane allows passage of molecules with molecular weights below the threshold cut off, such as the desired therapeutic product secreted by the encapsulated cells (FIG. 1). The membrane also allows for the diffusion of small molecules such as oxygen, nutrients and waste products to maintain the viability of the encapsulated cells. At the same time, the membrane prevents contact between immune mediators with higher molecular weights and the non-autologous cells enclosed in the device, so that the immune response is blocked. Immuno-isolation is currently being studied for its potential with both allogeneic and xenogeneic transplantations of required cell types. As there is no need for general immune suppression while using immuno-isolation devices, this method is an obvious improvement on pharmacological prevention of transplant rejection. As well, immuno-isolation is simpler and more readily achieved than the production of transgenic donor animals with genetically altered tissue antigens. As human clinical trials using immuno-isolation devices for treatment of several human disorders have commenced,[12] immuno-isolation will likely become a clinically relevant procedure.

This review will focus on the use of immuno-isolation for non-autologous transplantation, and in particular will discuss the work that has been accomplished using immuno-isolation in large animals. The application of immuno-isolation to large animals is especially interesting as the data from large animals may be most relevant to human application, and so are indicative of the potential effectiveness of immuno-isolation in treatment of human disorders. The disorders that are potentially treatable with immuno-isolation will be discussed, as well as the types of devices and materials used. The potential application of immuno-isolation technology to disease treatment with gene therapy will also be addressed.

IMMUNO-ISOLATION

Immuno-isolation can be arbitrarily divided into two categories based on the type of cells contained within the immuno-isolation device (TABLE 1). The first category encompasses the use of primary cell types, which are first isolated from an allogeneic or xenogeneic source before encapsulation. This research has focused mainly on potential treatments for endocrine and neurological disorders, which will be discussed in this section. The second category of cells used within the devices are laboratory cell lines. In this case, molecular biology techniques are first used to genetically altered the cells so they produce a desired therapeutic product, and then the genetically engineered cells are placed in immuno-isolation devices. The work on immuno-isolation in gene therapy and its application in large animals will be discussed in the third section.

Endocrine Disorders

The most extensively studied area of endocrine disorder treatment with immuno-isolation has been conducted on diabetes. In this treatment, normal islet cells capable of insulin production are isolated from the pancreas of a normal donor, and then encapsulated in the immuno-isolation device for transplantation. The "artificial pancreas" can then be transplanted into the diabetic individual to achieve control of blood glucose concentrations (for review, see refs 13–17).

Large animal models of diabetes include spontaneously diabetic animals such as canines and monkeys. Diabetes can also be induced in large animals by treatment with drugs such as streptazoin or through surgical removal of the pancreas. Several different types of immuno-isolation devices have been used to demonstrate effective treatment of insulin control in large animal models of diabetes. The first extensive,

TABLE 1. Immuno-isolation Devices Used in Large Animals for Delivery of Therapeutic Products

A. Primary Cell Types

Disorder	Cell Type Used (Product Delivered)	Large Animal Applications	Immuno-isolation Device Used	Allogeneic/Xenogeneic Cells	Ref.
Diabetes	Pancreatic islet cells (insulin)	Canines	Vascular perfusion devices	Allogeneic	18
			Diffusion chambers	Allogeneic	20, 21
			Microcapsules	Allogeneic	29, 30, 31
		Primates	Microcapsules	Xenogeneic	32
		Humans	Microcapsules	Allogeneic	36, 37
Hypoparathyroidism	Parathyroid cells (parathyroid hormone)	*Small animals only*	Microcapsules	Allogeneic	39, 40
Parkinson's disease	PC12 cells (dopamine)	Primates	Microcapsules	Xenogeneic	45
Pain	Chromaffin cells (catecholamines opioid peptides)	Sheep	Tubular devices	Xenogeneic	51
		Humans	Tubular devices	Xenogeneic	52
Liver Failure	Hepatocytes (various)	*Small animals only*	Microcapsules	Allogeneic	53

B. Genetically Modified Cells

Disorder	Cell Type Used/Genetic Modification	Large Animal Applications	Immuno-isolation Device Used	Allogeneic/Xenogeneic Cells	Ref.
Amyotrophic Lateral Sclerosis (ALS)	Baby hamster kidney cells/engineered to secrete ciliary neurotrophic factor	Humans	Tubular device	Xenogeneic	46
Dwarfism	Canine MDCK cells/engineered to secrete human growth hormone	Canines	Microcapsules	Allogeneic	62, 63
Hemophilia B	Mouse myoblasts/engineered to secrete human factor IX	*Small animals only*	Microcapsules	Allogeneic	60
Mucopolysaccharidosis	Mouse fibroblasts/engineered to secrete beta-glucuronidase	*Small animals only*	Microcapsules	Allogenic	61

long-term *in vivo* implantation of immuno-isolation devices containing allogeneic islets into diabetic canines were performed with intravascular perfusion devices. These devices are constructed so that the semipermeable membrane forms an enclosed tube containing the allogeneic canine islets. The tube is then connected to the host's vascular system so that blood flows through the device. The islets release insulin into the blood stream while contact between immune-mediators and the allogeneic cells is prevented. In the first large animal study using these devices, ten pancreatectomized diabetic dogs each received two intravascular perfusion devices containing normal canine islet tissue. Good control of fasting glucose levels was observed in six animals, without the need for exogenous insulin injections. The effect was sustained for up to 5 months, and the devices were tolerated well with little inflammatory response.[18]

In contrast, other devices used to treat diabetes in large animals with immuno-isolation of islet cells do not rely on vascular connections for delivery of insulin. These extravascular devices are implanted either intraperitoneally or intramuscularly, simplifying the implantation procedure. However, the insulin produced by the islet cells within the immuno-isolation device must diffuse from the site of implantation into the vascular system of the animal. These types of non-vascularized immuno-isolation devices which have been used in diabetic large animal models include diffusion chambers and microcapsules.

Several types of diffusion chambers have been evaluated for delivery of insulin. These devices can be either cylindrical or disc-shaped, with the membrane fabricated from various materials, including biocompatible plastics such as polyacrylonitrile-polyvinyl chloride (PAN-PVC), polypropylene and polycarbonate, as well as cellulose nitrate.[19] However, the most common type of diffusion chamber used to date for immuno-isolation in large animal diabetes treatment are short, hollow fiber diffusion chambers in which the islets are placed. A group of hollow fibers containing the islet cells are then implanted intraperitoneally to deliver insulin. In canines, it has been demonstrated that when PAN-PVC hollow fibers containing approximately 300 canine islets were implanted into six totally pancreatectomized dogs, complete insulin independence was obtained in three dogs for up to 4 months. As well, although the other three dogs did not show insulin independence, there was a significant drop in the amount of exogenous insulin that was necessary to control blood glucose levels in these three dogs.[20] A similar decrease in exogenous insulin dependency or total insulin dependence was also seen in an additional six dogs implanted with similar hollow fibers, but receiving an increased number of islets (20,000–40,000 islets/dog).[21]

However, the immuno-isolation device that seems to hold the most promise for eventual clinical application are microcapsules. Microcapsules are small (>1 mm diameter), spherical devices enclosing the allogeneic cells. Although microcapsules are commonly fabricated from alginate,[22,23] a biodegradable and biocompatible polysaccharide extracted from seaweed, microcapsules can also be fabricated from biocompatible plastics.[24,25] Microcapsules have distinct advantages over the vascular devices and hollow fibers. The vascular devices, owing to their larger structural and smaller compartment sizes, cannot contain a large number of islets. Hence, several devices would be needed for each patient, each connected to the vascular system to achieve relevant insulin delivery.[17] The hollow fibers have a better capacity for cells, but are prone to breakage when implanted.[21] In comparison, the microcapsules enjoy many advantageous features. For example, they are more sturdy owing to their smaller size, spherical shape and the fact that the alginate can be further strengthened by lamination of the capsule surface with chemicals such as poly-L-lysine.[26] As well, microcapsules have a greater surface to volume ratio to aid in diffusion. Furthermore, the implantation of microcapsules by injection into the peritoneal cavity is a surgically benign procedure with much reduced morbidity compared to devices requiring vascular shunts.

Several studies in canine models of diabetes have shown the potential usefulness of microcapsules in diabetes treatment. Although initial attempts at application of microencapsulated islets to diabetic canines failed as recently as 1992,[27] it was discovered that some of the initial difficulties in canines were due to an inflammatory response against the alginate caused by the polysaccharide composition of the type of alginate used.[28] When alginate of a less inflammatory type was used, it was shown that glucose independence could be established in spontaneous diabetic dogs, which lasted generally more than 3 months and in some cases up to more than a year. In contrast, canines implanted with non-encapsulated islets rejected the unprotected allogeneic cells within a week.[29,30,31]

Owing to the success seen with microcapsule treatment of diabetes in canines, this technology has moved into primate studies, which are more closely related to humans and so a potentially better indication of human applications. It has recently been demonstrated that implantation of microcapsules containing xenogeneic porcine islets into spontaneously diabetic monkeys allowed for seven of nine monkeys to become insulin independent for a time period ranging from 3 months to more than two years. There was no overgrowth of the capsules upon retrieval at 3 months, the islets remained viable and there was no detrimental effect on the internal organs for up to two years post-implantation. Although this study involved xenotransplantation of porcine islets into primates, there were no anti-porcine islet antibodies produced by the subject animals.[32]

The results of this work with monkeys indicate that this technology may eventually be a useful method with which to treat diabetes. This work also raises the question of whether allo- or xeno-geneic transplants are most potentially promising for humans. Although allogeneic transplants produce a less vigorous immune reaction, Sun's work with microencapsulated xenogeneic cells implanted into monkeys and previous work on discordant xenografts between bovine, canine and rodents using diffusion chambers or microcapsules[33-35] indicate that the immuno-isolation devices may be sufficient in eliminating a severe immune reaction, so that no pharmacological immune suppression is needed. This is important for eventual human application, since the most ideal situation would be one in which non-human sources of islets could be used owing to the shortage of human pancreas donors. As well, the source of islets for humans would not likely be primates, owing to ethical problems and the unsuitability of primate reproduction for obtaining large numbers of animals (long gestation and single births). In contrast, discordant xenografts, such as porcine or bovine islets, would provide a more feasible alternative for implantation into humans.

Microencapsulated islets for treatment of diabetes has also been attempted in two small clinical trials to date. In one case, one type I diabetic patient received microencapsulated human islets. This patient was being treated at the same time with low-dose immunosuppressive agents to maintain a kidney transplant. This patient obtained insulin independence for 9 months post-implantation.[36] In a second study, six patients (3 type I and 3 type II diabetics) received human islets that had been placed within hollow fiber isolation devices implanted subcutaneously. In this case, the study was conducted to see mainly if the fibers would be tolerated and the islets survive, since too few islets were used to achieve insulin independence in a human. The patients were not immunosuppressed and the fibers were in place for only 2 weeks. However, this work demonstrated that encapsulated islets can survive *in vivo* and that the immuno-isolation device protected the allogeneic cells from the host immune system.[37] Further ongoing human clinical trials[38] should indicate the eventual feasibility of microencapsulated islets as a treatment for diabetes.

Immuno-isolation devices have also been investigated for use with other endocrine systems not discussed here. The immuno-isolation of parathyroid cells, which may be useful for treatment of hypoparathyroidism, has been reported.[39,40] As well, encapsulation of adrenal cortical cells has also been reported.[41] These studies have met with various degrees of success, but have not yet reached the stage of large animal trials.

Neurological Disorders

Immuno-isolation also has potential for application to neurological disorders. The situation for neurological disorders is unique, however, as the product delivered from the cells within the immuno-isolation device must be able to reach the neuronal tissues. Since the blood-brain barrier prevents molecules in the systemic circulation from reaching the brain, the immuno-isolation devices cannot be deposited in peripheral sites, but must be placed within the neuronal compartment. This can be achieved by implanting immuno-isolation devices into the space containing the cerebral spinal fluid (CSF) in such a manner that the devices do not cause any neurological or physical problems.[42]

Therapeutic molecules which may be useful in treating symptoms of neurological disorders may be potentially delivered through the use of immuno-isolation. For example, implantation of PC12 cells secreting dopamine may be useful for treatment of Parkinson's disease.[43,44] In one large animal study, it was shown that four out of five hemiparksonian monkeys receiving implantations of immuno-isolated xenogeneic rat PC12 cells showed behavioral improvement for up to 5 months post-implantation.[45] Thus, immuno-isolation may allow the delivery of substances such as dopamine to neuronal tissue in disorders such as Parkinson's disease. Substances which may have survival-promoting effects on neurons can also potentially be delivered by immuno-isolation and may be useful in preventing neuronal death in neurodegenerative diseases, such as the delivery of neuronal growth factors to the CNS of patients with amyotrophic lateral sclerosis (ALS).[46]

As well, substances for treatment of other neurological problems not related to neurodegeneration may be delivered using immuno-isolated cells. One example is the treatment of pain with immuno-isolated cells. Encapsulated adrenal chromaffin cells have been found to significantly reduce the effects of acute and chronic pain in rodent models.[47–49] This effect is thought to be due to the release of pain-reducing substances such as opiod peptides and catecholamines from the transplanted immuno-isolated cells.[50] In a large animal trial which was done as a prelude to human clinical trials, xenogeneic bovine chromaffin cells were encapsulated in 5 cm long hollow tube devices constructed from a perm-selective membrane, and implanted into the lumbar subarachnoid space of sheep. Release of catecholamine was determined after implantation for 4 or 8 weeks, and was shown to be similar to catecholamine release before implantation.[51] Based on these preclinical tests of feasibility in sheep, treatment of chronic pain using xenogeneic immuno-isolated cells has recently moved to human trials. Xenogeneic bovine adrenal chromaffin cells were encapsulated in a hollow fiber and implanted into the CSF of three patients with terminal cancer pain which was not relieved by narcotics. It was found that all three patients showed a reduction in the required level of exogenously supplied pain medication. Autopsy reports showed that there were no adverse effects on the spinal cords of the three patients. The retrieved implants also showed good biocompatibility, with no adherent cells or fibrotic overgrowth observed.[52]

Other Disorders

Another type of cell that has been shown to be successfully encapsulated are hepatocytes. Encapsulated hepatocytes may provide an alternative to liver transplantation in patients with liver failure. Studies have shown promise for the potential usefulness of immuno-isolated hepatocytes, both *in vitro*[53] and *in vivo* in rodents.[54]

Immuno-isolation devices have also been shown to be effective in encapsulation of various cells for other novel applications. For example, encapsulation of hybridoma cell lines producing monoclonal antibodies has been reported, and the hybridoma cells placed within microcapsules showed good viability and continued production of antibodies.[55] Furthermore, immuno-isolation technology may also be adapted to encapsulation of non-mammalian cell types. It has been demonstrated that genetically modified *Escherichia coli* DH5 bacteria contained within microcapsules can lower the plasma urea level in uremic rats with kidney failure.[56] Thus, immuno-isolation of various types of cells may be potentially useful for numerous medical applications.

IMMUNO-ISOLATION IN GENE THERAPY

Immuno-isolation may also play an important role in gene therapy. Gene therapy can be defined as the treatment of a disorder by the introduction of a gene coding for some desired product into an affected individual. The introduced gene allows for the production of the required therapeutic protein in the affected patient, which then allows disease amelioration. The merger of gene therapy and immuno-isolation is based on the fact that before cells are placed within immuno-isolation devices they can first be genetically altered to secrete a recombinant product. Thus, instead of using primary cells such as islet cells within the immuno-isolation devices, recombinant cells secreting a novel product are used. The genetically engineered cells are placed in the immuno-isolation devices and implanted into affected individuals (for review, see ref. 57).

The use of genetically altered cells has several advantages over the use of terminally differentiated tissues. Since well-characterized laboratory cell lines are used, the cellular system can be precisely defined, and cells that tolerate the environment of the immuno-isolation device can be used for maximum cell survival once implanted. As well, since the cultured cells are available in potentially unlimited supply, one cell line can be engineered to secrete a desired product and then grown in sufficient quantities to be used for all patients requiring the same recombinant product. The cultured cells can also be frozen and thawed when required at a later date. These features of cultured laboratory cell lines make them more ideal for immuno-isolation than terminally differentiated tissues, which are difficult to obtain in sufficient quantities and for which the quality control required for good manufacturing practice (GMP) purposes will be more laborious to meet.

This section will discuss the delivery of recombinant products using immuno-isolation in large animals and in human clinical trials. As well, this section will also discuss other large animal models of human disease which may be potential models in which to test immuno-isolation for gene therapy.

Delivery of Recombinant Gene Products

Our laboratory has been investigating the possibility of using immuno-isolation as a means of delivering recombinant therapeutic products for gene therapy. Initial work in our laboratory focused on delivery of products to mice through the use of recombinant cell lines encapsulated in alginate microcapsules. This work demonstrated that this approach to gene therapy was feasible and effective at delivery of recombinant products for the treatment of genetic disorders such as growth hormone deficiency, hemophilia and lysosomal storage disease.[58-61] On the basis of this success, we have begun to develop this technology for application to larger animals such as canines, in order to obtain data which may be more applicable to the ultimate adaptation of this technology to humans.

The initial approach to applying immuno-isolation for gene therapy to canines was to determine the delivery of a marker protein from encapsulated cells in normal canines, before attempting the technique in a canine model of a human disease. We used human growth hormone as a marker protein, a 22 kD protein for which the cDNA has been cloned and which can be distinguished immunologically from canine growth hormone. A canine MDCK cell line engineered to secrete human growth hormone was produced and cells were then encapsulated in alginate microcapsules. The capsules used in previous mouse studies were a hollow core alginate-poly-L-lysine-alginate (**APA**) type, which contains the recombinant cells in a hollow sphere of alginate cross-linked with calcium ions and laminated with poly-L-lysine and alginate to strengthen the outer surface of the capsule[58] (FIG. 2). However, when these capsules were implanted into the peritoneal cavity of normal canines, it was found that the capsules were not durable in the canines, as only ~10% of the implanted volume of capsules could be detected on day 7 and no capsules were detected in the peritoneal cavity at 14 days post-implantation. This mirrored the brief delivery of human growth hormone, which peaked between days 1–5 and then was undetectable by day 10 (FIG. 3).[62] This was a significant difference from our experience with the same type of microcapsules in mice, which last for more than seven months *in vivo*.[60]

Owing to the quick loss of the hollow APA type of capsule in the canines, different capsule formulations were used to determine if a mechanically stronger type of capsule would have a longer life span *in vivo* in canines. The new capsules tested were solid type capsules that did not have a hollow core, and in which the alginate had been cross-linked with barium ions that have a greater affinity for alginate than calcium. These solid core capsule types were then either coated with a layer of poly-L-lysine/alginate (**BPA**) or left uncoated (**BaAlginate**). It was found that when the solid type of capsule containing human growth hormone secreting cells were implanted into canines, there was an increased delivery of human growth hormone to the plasma of the canines (FIG. 3). The human growth hormone could first be detected on day 1, and showed a peak of delivery on day 7 that was ~5 times the peak seen with the APA type of capsule. The human growth hormone was again undetectable at day 10–14. Beginning at day 10 there was also an increase in the antibodies detected in the plasma to human growth hormone, since the human growth hormone is detected as a foreign protein by the immune system of the canine (FIG. 4). The rise in human growth hormone-specific antibodies is the likely cause of the drop in levels of human growth hormone in the plasma, and can be used as an indirect indicator of continued delivery from the encapsulated cells secreting human growth hormone. The antibody level continued to rise until ~day 21, and then in most cases dropped off and were undetectable at day 60 (FIG. 4).[62]

The different formulations of the solid core capsules also had different patterns

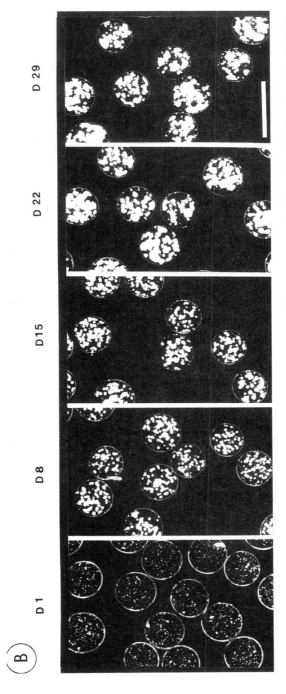

FIGURE 2. Growth of recombinant mouse fibroblasts in alginate-poly-L-lysine alginate microcapsules. Mouse Ltk⁻ fibroblasts transfected with the human growth hormone gene were encapsulated at a concentration of 2×10^6 cells/ml alginate. At various days post-encapsulation, aliquots of the microcapsules were monitored for appearance of the cells within the microcapsules (scale bar = 1000 μ). (From Chang *et al.*[83], reproduced by permission.)

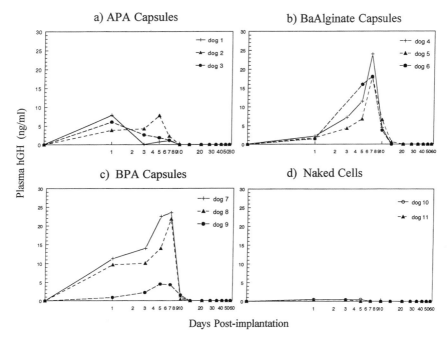

FIGURE 3. Human growth hormone delivered to dog plasma from recombinant canine cells secreting human growth hormone encapsulated in three microcapsule formulations. Human growth hormone-secreting canine MDCK cells were encapsulated in (**a**) APA hollow core microcapsules, (**b**) BaAlginate solid core microcapsules, (**c**) BPA solid core microcapsules and implanted intraperitoneally into 9 dogs. Two control dogs (**d**) were implanted with unencapsulated cells. Human growth hormone in the dog plasma was detected by ELISA.

of delivery of recombinant human growth hormone and showed different duration times *in vivo*. The barium solid core capsules which were coated with poly-L-lysine and alginate (BPA) showed higher levels of delivery of the recombinant product than did the uncoated barium microcapsules (FIG. 3). As well, the coating of poly-L-lysine and alginate gave the capsules a greater mechanical stability. The uncoated capsules lasted less than 14 days *in vivo*, while the coated capsules lasted for greater than two months.[62]

However, all of the capsule types used in the canines showed some biocompatibility problems. All capsules showed an inflammatory response causing mild inflammation of the omentum. Capsules were found embedded in the omentum, although there was no adhesions of capsules to other organs and the retrieved capsules of all types were free of any adherent cells and showed good viability of the encapsulated cells.[62] Although a third capsule formulation using solid capsules cross linked with calcium and coated with poly-L-lysine/alginate was also implanted into canines to determine if this capsule type had improved biocompatibility, these capsules did not show as high a level of delivery of the recombinant product as the barium-poly-L-lysine-alginate capsules.[63] Thus, further investigation into alternate capsule formulations which may be more biocompatible but still allow increased and pro-

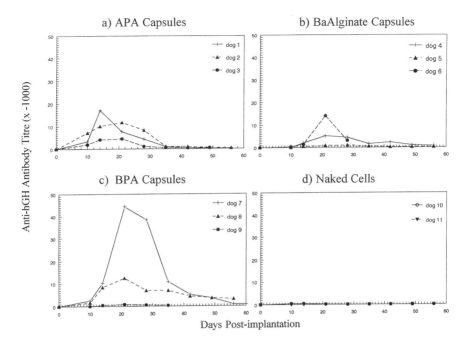

FIGURE 4. Development of anti-human growth hormone antibodies in dogs implanted with microcapsules containing recombinant canine cells. Antibodies against human growth hormone were detected in the dog plasma by anti-human growth hormone specific ELISA. Antibody titer is representative of the dilution of plasma required to give an absorbance reading of 0.65 O.D. at 405 nm. Antibody titers are shown for dogs implanted with (**a**) APA capsules (**b**) BaAlginate capsules, (**c**) BPA capsules, and (**d**) control dogs implanted with naked cells.

longed delivery of recombinant products in larger animals such as canines are required.

Our work with application of gene therapy to larger animals has demonstrated several interesting features. First, the performance of immuno-isolation devices in rodents can not always be applied to a larger animal. This has been shown by our experience with the APA type of capsule, which last for months in mice but are lost within 10 days in canines. Secondly, biocompatibility of the capsules in rodents may not be similar to what is seen in a larger animal. Our experience has indicated that mice implanted with microcapsules do not show the same degree of inflammatory response as seen in canines. Thirdly, regardless of the exact formulation of the microcapsules, they were able to prolong the survival of non-autologous donor cells in canines. In control animals implanted with the same amount of cells but without the protection of microcapsules, no or very little recombinant products or antibodies against them were detected, presumably owing to early demise of the unprotected implanted cells from the host immune rejection (FIGS. 3 and 4). Since a larger animal such as a dog is more comparable to humans in both size and physiology, this work has been most informative in indicating which areas of immuno-isolation for gene therapy need further study for ultimate application to humans.

Gene therapy using immuno-isolation may also be a potential form of treatment for neurological disorders. Similar to the delivery of recombinant products in the systemic circulation, recombinant products can also be delivered to neuronal tissues by implantation of immuno-isolated genetically modified cells into the CSF.

One type of neurological disorder in current clinical trials with immuno-isolation devices is amyotrophic lateral sclerosis (ALS). ALS is a terminal neurodegenerative disease characterized by a progressive loss of motor neurons in the central nervous system. In rodent models, ciliary neurotrophic factor (CNTF) has been shown to reduce the motor neuron cells death similar to the cell death seen in ALS patients.[64] Thus, delivery of CNTF to the neurons of ALS patients may be one method of treatment for this otherwise incurable disorder. However, systemic delivery of CNTF has not been successful owing to its short half-life, the side effects of high systemic doses, and an inability of the CNTF to pass the blood brain barrier to achieve significant levels in the CNS.[65]

Owing to the above problems, the use of immuno-isolation for delivery of CNTF was proposed. Recent trials have begun for treatment of ALS patients with encapsulated cells secreting recombinant CNTF. In this case, xenogeneic baby hamster kidney cells were genetically engineered to secrete human CNTF, and then placed within 5 cm long hollow fibers fabricated from poly-ether-sulfone. One device was then implanted into the CSF of each of 6 ALS patients. It was found that there was detectable hCNTF delivered to the CSF of the patients receiving the implants up to 17 weeks post-implantation. The device was tolerated well and showed no adverse non-biocompatible responses. Although there was no amelioration of the ALS symptoms, the short observation time of 17 weeks may not have been sufficient to see a slowing of the neurodegenerative progress.[46,66]

Genetic Disorders with Large Animal Models Available for Study

The most important test of efficacy for immuno-isolation in gene therapy for human disorders is in animal models which mimic the human disease. As many large animal models of human genetic diseases exist, some with well defined pathology, they provide an essential resource upon which to determine the feasibility of gene therapy in immuno-isolation for humans.

Several large animal disease models currently exist. The large animals that have been observed with diseases that mimic human disorders are primarily dogs, pigs, sheep and primates. Canine disease models comprised the largest group, and include such human disease models as hematological disorders, including hemophilia[67] and von Willebrand's disease,[68] metabolic storage diseases, including mucopolysaccharidosis[69] and Gaucher's disease,[70] neurological disorders, including spinal muscular atropy[71] and ALS[72] and other disorders, such as Wilson's disease[73] and muscular dystrophy.[74] Porcine models include hematological disorders such as von Willebrand's disease,[68] while sheep models include muscular dystrophy[75] and Wilson's disease.[76] Fewer primate models have been found, although certain primate models such as the previously discussed diabetic monkey do exist. As well, several large animal models also exist with various diseases that may have genetic components and may benefit from some types of gene therapy, such as cancers seen in canines, sheep and cattle[77–79] or acquired immune deficiency of primate.[80] Thus, there is a wide range of large animal models on which to test the feasibility of gene therapy with immuno-isolation as appropriate forms of therapy for these diseases.

CONCLUSION

From this review it can be seen that large animals have provided a wealth of feasibility data on the applications of immuno-isolation, both for organ replacement and for gene therapy purposes. Studies of efficacy in large animal models before human trials are important since a large animal is more similar in size and physiology to humans than rodents, and so will provide data that are more relevant to human application. As well, rodent models of human disease do not always mimic the state of the disease in humans. For example, transgenic mice lacking the genes responsible for human disorders such as Tay-Sachs disease[81] and Lesch-Nyhan syndrome[82] do not phenotypically resemble affected humans who are defective in these same genes. Although fewer large animal models exist than do rodent models, the large animal models may mimic more closely the disease state in humans. Thus, there is an importance for large animal model studies of certain treatments as a prelude to human clinical trials.

Furthermore, the trial of a new treatment in large animals can also demonstrate effects that are not readily addressed in small animal models. For example, large animals may be more indicative of the human situation than smaller animals owing to their more complex immune systems and physiology. These features of the larger animals allow us to determine aspects of immunology and biocompatibility that would not be possible in small animals. This has been found in our studies of human growth hormone delivery to canines with immuno-isolation, since the capsule formulation that performed well in mice were not suitable for canines. Further work with large animals should allow insights into what aspects of immuno-isolation need to be improved before human clinical trials can begin.

SUMMARY

Transplantation has become a successful method for the management of functional failure of a variety of tissues or organs. However, the majority of clinical transplantations use non-autologous allogeneic donor tissue implanted from one human to another. In order to prevent rejection of the allogeneic tissue, methods to overcome the immune barrier are necessary. Although prevention of organ rejection is currently achieved with pharmacological immune suppression, the undesirable side effects of this method have incited interest in novel methods to overcome the immune barrier. One such novel method of preventing immune reaction is immuno-isolation, in which the non-autologous tissues are physically isolated from the host tissues by placement in devices with perm-selective membranes. The membranes of these devices allow release of the therapeutic product required from the transplanted tissues, as well as diffusion of nutrients and waste necessary for survival of the non-autologous tissues. The membranes also prevent host immune mediators from contacting the non-autologous cells, thus preventing immune rejection. This technology has been tested for efficacy in large animal models, and is currently in the process of clinical trials in humans. This review will discuss the progress made in using immuno-isolation of non-autologous tissues in large animals.

Immuno-isolation can be subdivided into two major areas of interest based on whether the non-autologous tissue used in the immuno-isolation device is genetically altered (gene therapy) or not. Studies using non-genetically altered non-autologous cells for immune-isolation have been dominated by the use of pancreatic islet cells for the treatment of diabetes. This work has been tested in large animal models of diabetes, including canine and primate model animals, and human clinical trials are underway. As well, there has also been work on treatment of neurological disorders such as Parkinson's disease or chronic pain using non-autologous immuno-isolated adrenal chromaffin cells or dopaminergic PC12 cells in large animals such as sheep and primates. This work will be reviewed in detail as to the types of disorders, immuno-isolation devices used and the type of large animals involved.

Immune-isolation for gene therapy is a more recently developed field of research. In this case, the non-autologous cells used are first genetically altered to secrete a recombinant therapeutic product before placement in the immune-isolation devices. Genetic engineering of the non-autologous cells is beneficial, as it allows the use of a cell type that tolerates well the environment of the immune-isolation device, while still delivering the therapeutic product of interest. This form of gene therapy has been tested in our laboratory for delivery of marker products such as human growth hormone to canines. As several large animal models of human genetic disorders are available, such as canines affected with hemophilia or the lysosomal storage disease mucopolysaccharidosis, testing the efficacy of immuno-isolation for gene therapy in large animal models is an important prelude to human clinical trials.

This review will discuss the topics outlined above, as well as some further considerations of the usefulness of large animal models in studying immune-isolation for non-autologous transplantation. Large animals may be more appropriate model organisms than rodents in which to study immune-isolation, as issues such as biocompatibility and immune response in a larger animal can be addressed. As well, large animal studies of immune isolation may provide data that are more relevant than rodent studies to the eventual application to human clinical trials.

REFERENCES

1. CATTO, G. R. C., Ed. 1987. Clinical Transplantation. Current Practice and Future Prospects. MTP Press. Boston.
2. PLATT, J. L., G. M. VERCELLOTTI, A. P. DALMASSO, A. J. MATAS, R. M. BOLMAN, J. S. NAJARIAN & F. H. BACH. 1990. Transplantation of discordant xenografts: A review of progress. Immunol. Today **11:** 450–456.
3. BOREL, J. F. & H. C. GUNN. 1986. Cyclosporine as a new approach to therapy of autoimmune disease. Ann. N. Y. Acad Sci. **475:** 307–318.
4. GLOVER, S. 1987. Problems of the immunosuppressed patient. *In* Clinical Transplantation. Current Practice and Future Prospects. G. R. C. Catto, Ed. MTP Press. Boston.
5. FODOR, W. L., B. L. WILLIAMS, L. A. MATIS, J. A. MADRI, S. A. ROLLINS, J. W. KNIGHT, W. VELANDER & S. P. SQUINTO. 1994. Expression of a functional human complement inhibitor in a transgenic pig as a model for the prevention of xenogeneic hyperacute organ rejection. Proc. Natl. Acad. Sci. USA **91:** 11153–11157.
6. SANDRIN, M. S. & I. F. C. McKENZIE. 1994. Gal (1,3)Gal, the major xenoantigen(s) recognised in pigs by human natural antibodies. Immunol. Rev. **141:** 170–190.
7. WILLIAMS, N. 1997. Pig-human transplants barred for now. Science **275:** 473.
8. LANZA, R. P., J. L. HAYES & W. L. CHICK. 1996. Encapsulated cell technology. Nat. Biotech. **14:** 1107–1111.
9. LANZA, R. P. & W. L. CHICK. 1997. Immunoisolation: At a turning point. Immunol. Today **18:** 135–139.
10. LYSAGHT, M. J., B. FRYDEL, F. GENTILE, D. EMERICH & S. WINN. 1994. Recent progress in immunoisolated cell therapy. J. Cell. Biochem. **56:** 196–203.
11. CHANG, T. M. S. 1964. Semipermeable microcapsules. Science **146:** 524–525.
12. LANZA, R. P. & W. L. CHICK. 1997. Transplantation of encapsulated cells and tissues. Surgery **121:** 1–9.
13. LANZA, R. P. & W. L. CHICK. 1995a. Encapsulated cell transplantation. Transplant Rev. **9:** 217–230.

14. LANZA, R. P. & W. L. CHICK. 1995b. Encapsulated cell therapy. Sci. Am., July, 16–25.
15. LACY, P. E. 1995. Treating diabetes with transplanted cells. Sci. Am., July, 50–58.
16. LACY, P. E. 1995. Islet cell transplantation for insulin-dependent diabetes. Hospital Practice, June, 41–45.
17. LANZA, R. P. & W. L. CHICK. 1996/1996. Pancreas. In Yearbook of Cell and Tissue Transplantation, R. P. Lanza & W. L. Chick, Eds.: 253–264. Kluwer Academic Publishers. Netherlands.
18. SULLIVAN, S. J., T. MAKI, K. M. BORLAND, M. D. MAHONEY, B. A. SOLOMON, T. E. MULLER, A. P. MONACO & W. L. CHICK. 1991. Biohybrid artificial pancreas: long term implantation studies in diabetic, pancreatectomized dogs. Science 252: 718–721.
19. COLTON, C. K. & E. S. AVGOUSTINIATOS. 1991. Bioengineering in development of the hybrid artificial pancreas. J. Biomech. Eng. 113: 152–170.
20. LANZA, R. P., K. M. BORLAND, P. LODGE, M. CARRETTA, S. J. SULLIVAN, T. E. MULLER, B. A. SOLOMON, T. MAKI, A. P. MONACO & W. L. CHICK. 1992a. Treatment of severely diabetic pancreatectomized dogs using a diffusion-based hybrid pancreas. Diabetes 41: 886–889.
21. LANZA, R. P., P. LODGE, K. M. BORLAND, M. CARRETTA, S. J. SULLIVAN, A. M. BEYER, T. E. MULLER, B. A. SOLOMON, T. MAKI, A. P. MONACO & W. L. CHICK. 1993. Transplantation of islet allografts using a diffusion-based biohybrid artificial pancreas: Long-term studies in diabetic, pancreatectomized dogs. Transplant. Proc. 25: 978–980.
22. LIM, F. & A. M. SUN. 1980. Microencapsulated islets as bioartificial endocrine pancreas. Science 210: 908–910.
23. WINN, S. R. & P. A. TRESCO. 1994. Hydrogel applications for encapsulated cellular transplants. Meth. Neurosci. 21: 387–402.
24. SEFTON, M. V., L. KHARLIP, V. HORVATH & T. ROBERTS. 1992. Controlled release using microencapsulated mammalian cells. J. Controlled Release 19: 289–298.
25. COHEN, S., M. C. BANO, K. B. VISSCHER, M. CHOW, H. R. ALLCOCK & R. LANGER. 1990. Ionically cross-linkable polyphosphazene: a novel polymer for microencapsulation. J. Am. Chem. Soc. 112: 7832–7833.
26. LIM, F. & R. D. MOSS. 1981. Microencapsulation of living cells and tissues. J. Pharm. Sci. 70: 351–354.
27. CALAFIORE, R. 1992. Transplantation of microencapsulated pancreatic human islets for therapy of diabetes mellitus. ASAIO J. 38: 34–37.
28. SOON-SHIONG, P., M. OTTERLIE, O. SKJAK-BRAEK, O. SMIDSROD, R. HEINTA, R. P. LANZA & T. ESPEVIK. 1991. An immunological basis for the fibrotic reaction to implanted microcapsules. Transplant. Proc. 23: 758–759.
29. SOON-SHIONG, P., E. FELDMAN, R. NELSON, R. HEINTZ, N. MERIDETH, P. A. SANDFORD, T. ZHENG & J. KOMTEBEDDE. 1992. Long-term reversal of diabetes in the large animal model by encapsulated islet transplantation. Transplant. Proc. 24: 2946–2947.
30. SOON-SHIONG, P., E. FELDMAN, R. NELSON, J. KOMTEBEDDE, O. SMIDSROD, G. SKJAK-BRAEK, T. EXPEVIK, R. HEINTZ & M. LEE. 1992. Successful reversal of spontaneous diabetes in dogs by intraperitoneal microencapsulated islets. Transplantation 54: 769–774.
31. SOON-SHIONG, P., E. FELDMAN, R. NELSON, R. HEINTZ, Q. YAO, Z. YAO, T. ZHENG, N. MERIDETH, G. SKJAK-BRAEK, T. EXPEVIK, O. SMIDSROD & P. SANDFORD. 1993. Long-term reversal of diabetes by the injection of immunoprotected islets. Proc. Natl. Acad. Sci. USA 90: 5843–5847.
32. SUN, Y., X. MA, D. ZHOU, I. VACEK & A. M. SUN. 1996. Normalization of diabetes in spontaneously diabetic cynomologus monkeys by xenografts of microencapsulated porcine islets without immunosuppression. J. Clin. Invest. 98: 1417–1422.
33. LANZA, R. P., D. H. BUTLER, K. M. BORLAND, J. M. HARVEY, D. L. FAUSTMAN, B. A. SOLOMON, T. E. MULLER, R. G. RUPP, T. MAKI, A. P. MONACO & W. L. CHICK. 1992b. Successful xenotransplantation of a diffusion-based biohybrid artificial pancreas: A study using canine, bovine and porcine islets. Transplant. Proc. 24: 669–671.
34. LANZA, R. P., W. M. KUHTREIBER, D. M. ECKER, J. P. MARSH & W. L. CHICK. 1995a. Transplantation of porcine and bovine islets into mice without immunosuppression using uncoated alginate microspheres. Transplant. Proc. 27: 3321.

35. LANZA, R. P., W. M. KUHTREIBER, D. M. ECKER, J. P. MARSH & W. L. CHICK. 1995b.
     Successful bovine islet xenografts in rodents and dogs using injectable microreactors.
     Transplant. Proc. **27:** 3211.
36. SOON-SHIONG, P., R. E. HEINTZ, N. MERIDETH, Q. X. YAO, Z. YAO, T. ZHENG,
     M. MURPHY, M. K. MOLONEY, M. SCHMEHL, M. HARRIS, R. MENDEZ, R. MENDEZ &
     P. A. SANDFORD. 1994. Insulin independence in a type I diabetic patient after encapsu-
     lated islet transplantation. Lancet **343:** 950–951.
37. SCHARP, D. W., C. J. SWANSON, B. J. OLACK, P. P. LATTA, O. D. HEGRE, E. J. DOHERTY,
     F. T. GENTILE, K. S. FLAVIN, M. F. ANSARA & P. E. LACY. 1994. Protection of
     encapsulated human islets implanted without immunosuppression in patients with
     type I or type II diabetes and in nondiabetic control subjects. Diabetes **43:** 1167–1170.
38. VIRORX. 1997. Beta cell encapsulation. Internet site: http://www.diabetes.com/betacl.
     html
39. DARQUY, S. & A. M. SUN. 1987. Microencapsulation of parathyroid cells as a bioartificial
     parathyroid. Trans. Am. Soc. Artif. Intern. Organs **XXXII:** 356–538.
40. FU, X. W. & A. M. SUN. 1989. Microencapsulated parathyroid cells as a bioartificial
     parathyroid. Transplantation **47:** 432–435.
41. LIM, F. 1984. Microencapsulation of living cells and tissues—theory and practice. *In*
     Biomedical Applications of Microencapsulation. F. Lim, Ed.: 137–154. CRC Press.
     Boca Raton, FL.
42. AEBISCHER, P., S. R. WINN & P. M. GALLETTI. 1991a. Transplantation of neural tissue
     in polymer capsules. Brain Res. **448:** 364–368.
43. WINN, S. R., P. A. TRESCO, B. ZIELINSKI, L. A. GREENE, C. B. JAEGER & P. AEBISCHER.
     1991. Behavioural recovery following intrastriatal implantation of microencapsulated
     PC12 cells. Exp. Neurol. **113:** 322–329.
44. AEBISCHER, P., P. A. TRESCO, J. SAGEN & S. R. WINN. 1991. Transplantation of microen-
     capsulated bovine chromaffin cells reduces lesion-induced rotational asymmetry in
     rats. Brain Res. **560:** 43–49.
45. AEBISCHER, P., M. GODDARD, A. P. SIGNORE & R. L. TIMPSON. 1994. Functional recovery
     in hemiparksonian primates transplanted with polymer-encapsulated PC12 cells. Exp.
     Neurol. **126:** 151–158.
46. AEBISCHER, P., M. SCHLUEP, N. DEGLON, J.-M. JOSEPH, L. HIRT, B. HEYD, M. GODDARD,
     J. P. HAMMANG, A. D. ZURN, A. C. KATO, F. REGLI & E. E. BAETGE. 1996. Intrathecal
     delivery of CNTF using encapsulated genetically modified xenogeneic cells in amyo-
     trophic lateral sclerosis patients. Nat. Med. **2:** 696–699.
47. SAGEN, J. 1992. Chromaffin cell transplants for alleviation of chronic pain. ASAIO
     J. **38:** 24–28.
48. SAGEN, J., H. WANG, P. A. TRESCO & P. AEBISCHER. 1993. Transplants of immunologically
     isolated xenogeneic chromaffin cells provide a long-term source of pain-reducing
     neuroactive substances. J Neurosci. **13:** 2415–2423.
49. AEBISCHER, P., P. A. TRESCO, S. R. WINN, L. A. GREENE & C. B. JAEGER. 1991. Long-
     term cross species brain transplantation of a polymer-encapsulated dopamine-secreting
     cell line. Exp. Neurol. **111:** 269–275.
50. SAGEN, J. & G. D. PAPPAS. 1987. Morphological and functional correlates of chromaffin
     cell transplants in CNS pain modulatory regions. Ann. N. Y. Acad. Sci. **495:** 306–333.
51. JOSEPH, J. M., M. B. GODDARD, J. MILLS, V. PADRUN, A. ZURN, B. ZIELINSKI, J. FAVRE,
     J. P. GARDAZ, F. MOSIMANN, J. SAGEN, L. CHRISTENSON & P. AEBISCHER. 1994.
     Transplantation of encapsulated bovine chromaffin cells in the sheep subarachnoid
     space: a preclinical study for the treatment of cancer pain. Cell Transplant. **3:** 355–364.
52. AEBISCHER, P., E. BUCHSER, J. M. JOSEPH, J. FAVRE, N. DE TRIBOLET, M. LYSAGHT, S.
     RUDNICK & M. GODDARD. 1994b. Transplantation in humans of encapsulated xenoge-
     neic cells without immunosuppression—a preliminary report. Transplantation
     58: 1275–1277.
53. SUN, A. M., A. CAI, A. SHI, F. MA, G. M. O'SHEA & J. GHARAPETIAN. 1986. Microencapsu-
     lated hepatocytes as a bioartificial liver. Trans. Am. Soc. Artif. Organs **XXXII:** 39–41.
54. BALLADUR, P., E. CREMA, J. HONIGER, Y. CALMUS, M. BAUDRIMONT, R. DELELO,

J. CAPEAU & B. NORDLINGER. 1995. Transplantation of allogeneic hepatocytes without immunosuppression: Long-term survival. Surgery **117:** 189–194.

55. BANO, M. C., S. COHEN, K. B. VISSCHER, H. R. ALLCOCK & R. LANGER. 1991. A novel synthetic method for hybridoma cell encapsulation. Biotechnology **9:** 468–471.

56. PRAKASH, S. & T. M. S. CHANG. 1996. Microencapsulated genetically engineered live *E. coli* DH5 cells administered orally to maintain normal plasma urea level in uremic rats. Nat. Med. **2:** 883–887.

57. CHANG, P. L. 1995. Nonautologous somatic gene therapy. *In* Somatic Gene Therapy. P. L. Chang, Ed.: 203–233. CRC Press. Boca Raton, FL.

58. CHANG, P. L., N. SHEN & A. J. WESTCOTT. 1993. Delivery of recombinant gene products with microencapsulated cells in vivo. Hum. Gene Ther. **4:** 433–440.

59. AL-HENDY, A., G. HORTELANO, G. S. TANNENBAUM & P. L. CHANG. 1995. Correction of the growth defect in dwarf mice: A novel approach to somatic gene therapy. Hum. Gene Ther. **6:** 165–175.

60. HORTELANO, G., A. AL-HENDY, F. A. OFOSU & P. L. CHANG. 1996. Delivery of human factor IX in mice by encapsulated recombinant myoblasts: A novel approach towards allogeneic gene therapy of hemophilia B. Blood **87:** 5095–5103.

61. BASTEDO, L., C. J. D. ROSS, M. S. SANDS, G. HORTELANO & P. L. CHANG. Somatic gene therapy on the murine model of mucopolysaccharidosis type VII. In Preparation.

62. PEIRONE, M. A., K. DELANY, J. KWIECIN, A. FLETCH & P. L. CHANG. 1997. Delivery of recombinant gene product to canines with non-autologous microencapsulated cells. Submitted.

63. PEIRONE, M. A., P. FITZGERALD & P. L. CHANG. 1997. Delivery of recombinant gene product to canines using solid core calcium-alginate gel spheres. Submitted.

64. SAGOT, Y., S. A. TAN, E. BAETGE, H. SCHMALBRUCH, A. C. KATO & P. AEBISCHER. 1995. Polymer encapsulated cell lines genetically engineered to release ciliary neurotrophic factor can slow down progressive motor neuronopathy in the mouse. Eur. J. Neurosci. **7:** 1313–1322.

65. BARINAGA, M. 1994. Neurotrophic factors enter the clinic. Science **264:** 772–774.

66. AEBISCHER, P., N. A.-M. POCHON, B. HEYD, N. DEGLON, J.-M. JOSEPH, A. D. ZURN, E. E. BAETGE, J. P. HAMMANG, M. GODDARD, M. LYSAGHT, F. KAPLAN, A. C. KATO, M. SCHLUEP, L. HIRT, F. REGLI, F. PORCHET & N. DE TRIBOLET. 1996b. Gene therapy for amyotrophic lateral sclerosis (ALS) using a polymer encapsulated xenogenic cell line engineered to secrete hCNTF. Hum. Gene Ther. **7:** 851–860.

67. BRINKHOUS, K. M. & T. GAMBILL. 1972. Hemophilia A and B, Model no. 12. *In* Handbook: Animal Models of Human Disease. Fasc. 1. T. C. Jones & D. B. Hackel, Eds. Registry of Comparative Pathology, Armed Forces Institute of Pathology, Washington, D. C.

68. DODDS, W. J. 1977. Von Willebrand's disease, Model no. 110. *In* Handbook: Animal Models of Human Disease, Fasc. 6 T. C. Jones, D. B. Hackel & G. Migaki, Eds. Registry of Comparative Pathology, Armed Forces Institute of Pathology, Washington, D. C.

69. SHULL, R. M., R. J. MUNGER, E. SPELLACY, C. W. HALL, G. CONSTANTOPOULOS & E. F. NEUFELD. 1983. Mucopolysaccharidosis I, Model no. 264. *In* Handbook: Animal Models of Human Disease, Fasc. 12. C. C. Capen, D. B. Hackel, T. C. Jones & G. Migaki, Eds. Registry of Comparative Pathology, Armed Forces Institute of Pathology, Washington, D. C.

70. HARTLEY, W. J. & B. R. H. FARROW. 1982. Gaucher's disease, Model no 241. *In* Handbook: Animal Models of Human Disease, Fasc. 11. C. C. Capen, D. B. Hackel, T. C. Jones & G. Migaki, Eds. Registry of Comparative Pathology, Armed Forces Institute of Pathology, Washington, D. C.

71. SANDEFELDT, E., J. F. CUMMINGS, A. DE LAHUNTA, G. BJORCK & L. P. KROOK. 1977. Infantile spinal muscular atrophy, Werdnig-Hoffman disease, Model no. 99. *In* Handbook: Animal Models of Human Disease, Fasc. 6. T. C. Jones, D. B. Hackel & G. Magaki, Eds. Registry of Comparative Pathology, Armed Forces Institute of Pathology, Washington, D. C.

72. CORK, L. C., J. W. GRIFFIN, R. J. ADAMS & D. L. PRINCE. 1981. Motor neuron disease: spinal muscular atrophy and amyotrophic lateral sclerosis, Model no. 213. *In* Hand-

book: Animal Models of Human Disease. Fasc. 10. C. C. Capen, D. B. Hackel, T. C. Jones & G. Migaki, Eds. Registry of Comparative Pathology, Armed Forces Institute of Pathology, Washington, D. C.

73. OWEN, C. A. JR. & J. LUDWIG. 1982. Wilson's disease, Model no. 249. In Handbook: Animal Models of Human Disease, Fasc. 11. C. C. Capen, D. B. Hackel, T. C. Jones & G. Magaki, Eds. Registry of Comparative Pathology, Armed Forces Institute of Pathology, Washington, D. C.

74. BRAUND, K. G., R. E. MCKERRELL, M. TOIVIO-KINNUCAN, J. R. MEHTA & D. M. VAUGHN. 1989. Muscular dystrophy, Model no. 366. In Handbook: Animal Models of Human Disease. Fasc. 17. C. C. Capen, T. C. Jones & G. Migaki, Eds. Registry of Comparative Pathology, Armed Forces Institute of Pathology, Washington, D. C.

75. MCGAVIN, M. D. 1975. Muscular dystrophy, Model no. 51. In Handbook: Animal Models of Human Disease, Fasc. 4. T. C. Jones & D. B. Hackel, Eds. Registry of Comparative Pathology, Armed Forces Institute of Pathology, Washington, D. C.

76. HOWELL, J. MCC., S. R. GOONERATNE & J. M. GAWTHORNE. 1985. Wilson's disease, Model no. 307. In Handbook: Animal Models of Human Disease, Fasc. 14. C. C. Capen, T. C. Jones & G. Migaki, Eds. Registry of Comparative Pathology, Armed Forces Institute of Pathology, Washington, D. C.

77. MILLER, J. M. 1975. Malignant lymphoma, Model no. 56. In Handbook: Animal Models of Human Disease, Fasc. 4, T. C. Jones & D. B. Hackel, Eds. Registry of Comparative Pathology, Armed Forces Institute of Pathology, Washington, D. C.

78. HUNT, R. D. & L. V. MELENDEZ. 1975. Malignant lymphoma, Model no. 60. In Handbook: Animal Models of Human Disease, Fasc. 5. T. C. Jones & D. B. Hackel, Eds. Registry of Comparative Pathology, Armed Forces Institute of Pathology, Washington, D. C.

79. STRANDBERG, J. D. & D. G. GOODMAN. 1975. Breast cancer, Model no. 54. In Handbook: Animal Models of Human Disease. Fasc. 5. T. C. Jones & D. B. Hackel, Eds. Registry of Comparative Pathology, Armed Forces Institute of Pathology, Washington, D. C.

80. LETVIN, N. L. & N. W. KING. 1984. Acquired immune deficiency syndrome, Model no. 291. In Handbook: Animal Models of Human Disease. Fasc. 13. C. C. Capen, D. B. Hackel, T. C. Jones & G. Migaki, Eds. Registry of Comparative Pathology, Armed Forces Institute of Pathology, Washington, D. C.

81. YAMANAKA, S., M. D. JOHNSON, A. GRINBERG, H. WESTPHAL, J. N. CRAWLEY, M. TANIIKE, K. SUZUKI & R. L. PROIA. 1994. Targeted disruption of the Hexa gene results in mice with biochemical and pathological features of Tay-Sachs disease. Proc. Natl. Acad. Sci. USA 91: 9975–9979.

82. FINGER, S., R. P. HEAVENS, D. J. S. SIRINATHSINGHJI, M. R. KUEHN & S. B. DUNNETT. 1988. Behavioral and neurochemical evaluation of a transgenic mouse model of Lesch-Nyhan syndrome. J. Neurol. Sci. 86: 203–213.

83. CHANG, P. L., G. HORTELANO, M. TSE & D. E. AWREY. 1994. Growth of recombinant fibroblasts in alginate microcapsules. Biotech. Bioeng. 43: 925–933.

Macrophysiologic Roles of a Delivery System for Vulnerary Factors Needed for Bone Regeneration

JEFFREY O. HOLLINGER[a] AND JOHN P. SCHMITZ

[a]Division of Plastic and Reconstructive Surgery
Oregon Health Sciences University
3181 SW Sam Jackson Park Road
Portland, Oregon 97201-3098

[b]Department of Oral and Maxillofacial Surgery
University of Texas
Health Science Center At San Antonio
7703 Floyd Curl Dr
San Antonio, Texas 78284-7823

MACROPHYSIOLOGY

Physiology is a branch of science that "explain(s) the physical and chemical factors . . . responsible for the origin, development, and progression of life.[1]" Progression of life depends upon healthy cells, controlled renewal, and functional harmony. The general physiologic process responsible for sustenance of life is referred to as *homeostasis*. Guyton underscores the significance of *homeostasis* by stating[1]: ". . . the body is a social order of about 100 trillion cells organized into different functional structures. . . . Each functional structure provides its share in the maintenance of homeostatic conditions. . . . As long as normal conditions are maintained in the internal environment, the cells of the body continue to live and function properly. Thus, each cell benefits from homeostasis, and in turn each cell contributes its share toward the maintenance of homeostasis." Therefore, distilled to its simplest form, *homeostasis* equals balance and health among cells.

We define *macrophysiology* as the dynamic, operational framework that addresses functional relationships among cells, tissues, organs, organ systems, and the laboratory-produced clinical product. *Macrophysiology* unites tissue engineering and physiology.

Tissue engineers must focus on the cell as the lynch pin for a laboratory-designed clinical product and the structural and functional significance of cells must be respected and supported to ensure therapeutic efficacy and *homeostasis*. Therefore, a bone regeneration product must fulfill specific *macrophysiological* criteria. For example, the delivery system should deploy and localize bone morphogenetic protein (BMP) in register with cell requirements at the recipient locale and act as a provisional substratum to support cells until they become self-sustaining, express suitable extracellular matrix components, and restore form and function. Furthermore, the delivery system must be conceived with chemical and physical properties

[a] Tel: (503) 494-8426; Fax: (503) 494-8378; E-mail: Hollinge@OHSU.edu
[b] Tel: (210) 567-3462; Fax: (210) 235-3493

to promote entry of the desired phenotype to the wound bed. This chemotactic event heralds a continuum of discrete steps to renew deficient tissue.

A clinical product consisting of poly(α-hydroxy acid) and BMP may fulfill the operational framework fundamental to *macrophysiology* and osseous regeneration.

A KEY GROUP OF BONE REGULATORY MOLECULES

Structurally deficient bone is programmed with the the capacity to regenerate. This cell-driven process operates at tissue (*e.g.*, blood, bone), organ (*e.g.*, liver), and systemic (*e.g.*, skeletal) levels to reconstitute form and therefore function indistinguishable from that derived through embryogenesis. A group of regulatory molecules appear to be key for bone regeneration: the bone morphogenetic proteins (BMPs). To date, twelve BMPs have been reported.[2-5] BMPs (designated BMP-1 through BMP-12) are members of the transforming growth factor beta family.[4] Other molecules in this clan that have close genetic sequence identity to BMPs include dpp (*i.e.*, the Drosophila gene, decapentaplegic), drosophila 60A, vegetal pole-derived gene, growth/differentiation factors (GDFs),[4,6] the inhibins (α, βA, βB), and Mullerian inhibiting substance.[7,8]

BMPs provide essential cues for body patterning during embryogenesis (*e.g.*, limb development) and tissue and organ formation.[4,9-11] Therefore, aside from their localization in skeletal and dental sites, BMPs have been found in hair follicles, heart, kidney, oocytes, and central nervous system.[12,13] Purportedly, a suite of BMPs are operational during embryogenesis and bone regeneration.[6,14-16]

Moreover, different concentrations of BMP evoke multiple phenotypic expression, such as adipocytes, chondrocytes, and osteoblasts from a single mesodermal progenitor cell line such as C3H10T1/2.[17,18] Perhaps it is the differential concentration within various anatomical locales during embryogenesis that causes multiple phenotypes. This concept is consistent with the notion BMPs have broad *morphogenetic* responsibilities.[19]

BMP-2 and BMP-7 are osteoinductive. The principle of osteoinduction, coined over twenty-five years ago,[20,21] is the ability to cause pluripotential cells from a non-osseous environment to differentiate into chondrocytes and osteoblasts, culminating in bone formation.[22] Amazingly little is known about the mechanistic regulation of chondro-osteoblastic lineage expression by BMP; however, functional roles for BMPs are being reported. For example, BMP-2 induces differentiation of committed progenitor cells into either chondroblasts or osteoblasts[23] and is chemotactic for osteoblasts.[24] BMPs 3 and 4 may be involved with chondrogenesis. Messenger RNA for BMP-4 has been detected between 12 to 72 hours after fracture (prior to cartilage and bone formation) and BMP-4 is expressed by osteoprogenitor cells and not by differentiated osteoblasts.[25] BMP-6 appears to regulate chondrocyte calcification during fracture healing and BMP-7 promotes chondrogenic and osteogenic phenotypes from newborn rat calvaria.[26,27] Thus, different BMP combinations probably regulate chondrogenesis, osteogenesis, and fracture repair.

BMP-promoted regeneration of osseous wounds has been explored in a series of preclinical studies that include rat calvaria,[28-30] rabbit ulna[31,32] and radius,[33] sheep long bone,[34] mandibles in dogs,[35] alveolar clefts[36] and long bone in dogs,[37] and long bone in non-human primates.[38] In these preclinical osseous studies, either recombinant human BMP-2 or 7 regenerated ablative wounds that ordinarily would not have healed by new bone formation. (These wounds were critical-sized defects.[39,40])

The reoccurring theme in preclinical BMP studies is the importance of the delivery system. A clinically relevant delivery system for BMP must have specific physical and chemical properties to localize BMP, to ensure interaction with mesenchymal pluripotential cells, and to provide instructional guidance for bone contour renewal.[33,41] Several additional properties will be introduced in the ensuing section.

DELIVERY SYSTEM ENGINEERING

BMP is a nonconstitutive wound healing factor: its expression by osteoblasts is influenced by the environment, *e.g.*, the presence of a wound. Inadequate endogenous BMP can be augmented by exogenous BMP. Therefore, recombinant human BMP (rhBMP) can be administered to patients to regenerate bone. However, it is clinically prudent to introduce the minimal therapeutic quantity of rhBMP for effect. This clinical criterion will be achieved by a delivery system.

The concept of *macrophysiology* relates cell dynamics and bone regeneration with the physical and chemical properties of the delivery system and its vulnerary payload: BMP. Consequently, the last section of our paper cautiously and briefly will integrate osseous wound regeneration with selected *structural and functional* properties of a poly(α-hydroxy acid) delivery system (*i.e.*, the *biomaterial*).

THE WOUND HEALING CONTINUUM: A CHALLENGING LANDSCAPE FOR A DELIVERY SYSTEM

An acceptable venue for scholarly study of osseous wound healing dynamics is the bone fracture model. Identification of events (*e.g.*, spatial and temporal localization of regulatory cell modulators) in a characterized fracture healing model can provide a functional, uncluttered outline to guide wound product development.

The stages and components of fracture repair have been chronicled histologically and with cell and molecular biology techniques.[7,42-45] FIGURE 1 provides a general schematic overview of fracture repair.

During fracture repair, specific cell phenotypes, extracellular matrix components, cytokines, and growth factors appear at discrete, predictable times during the wound healing process, fortifying the notion of a *continuum*. From the onset of wound trauma until regeneration, cell-mediated events throughout the continuum lead to restoration of deficient tissue. Differential BMP expression, different concentration gradients of the BMPs, and temporal variation of their expression throughout the continuum prompt morphodifferentiation of distinct cell phenotypes. Disruption of this synchrony can impair fracture healing. Therefore, a clinically suitable delivery system for BMP-inspired bone regeneration must be engineered to meet the dynamic, challenging landscape of the wound healing continuum. The poly(α-hydroxy acids) may be likely candidates.

POLY(α-HYDROXY ACIDS): DELIVERY SYSTEM CANDIDATES WITH VIRTUES

The poly(α-hydroxy acids) (abbreviated PHAs) have a thirty year history of safety and efficacy as biodegradable, biocompatible sutures and have commanded accolades in the areas of BMP delivery and tissue engineering.[41,46-48]

DEMOLITION PHASE: IMMEDIATE - EARLY INJURY

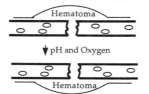

PLATELETS: clotting, growth factors

INFLAMMATION: neutrophils, lymphocytes, monocytes, mast cells, macrophages

RESORPTION: osteoclasts, macrophages

FACTORS: TGF-β, PDGF, FGF, EGF, CYTOKINES, INTERLEUKINS

ADDITIONAL CELLS: pericytes, undifferentiated cells

PROLIFERATION PHASE

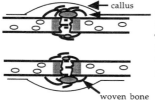

GRANULATION TISSUE: endothelial cells, neovascularization, collagens (I, IV, V, IX, X), fibroblasts

● = CHONDROGENESIS

CELLS: macrophages, endothelial cells, chondrocytes, osteoclasts, osteoblasts

FACTORS: IGF, PDGF, FGF, TGF-β, BMPs

EARLY REMODELING PHASE

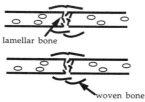

woven bone develops into lamellar bone

FACTORS: PTH, CT, GH, IGF, TGF-β, BMPs

CELLS: osteoclasts, osteoblasts

Type I collagen predominates

LATE REMODELING PHASE

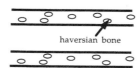

lamellar bone, haversian bone

bone contour restored

FIGURE 1. The set of four panels is a summary schematic of selected components of the healing fracture. KEY: TGF-β: transforming growth factor beta; PDGDF: platelet derived growth factor; FGF: fibroblast growth factor; EGF: epidermal growth factor; IGF: insulin-like growth factors; BMP: bone morphogenetic protein; PTH: parathyroid hormone; CT: calcitonin; GH: growth hormone. (From Hollinger & Wong,[45] published with permission from the editor.)

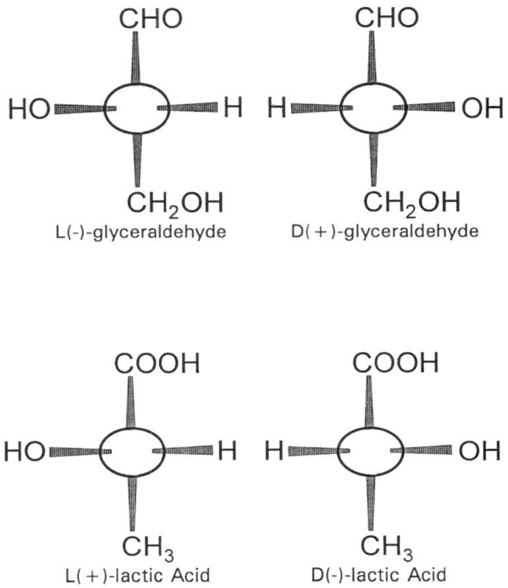

FIGURE 2. The spatial arrangements of atoms and groups of atoms about the chiral carbon (or carbons) are designated as D or L, using glyceraldehyde as a standard. The + and − symbols denote rotation of polarized light to left or right, respectively. Dimerization of these precursors yields the six membered lactide rings. (From Hollinger,[52] published with permission from the publisher.)

Standard ring opening polymerization and step growth polycondensation methodologies are used typically to produce commonly encountered PHA homopolymers such as polylactide and polyglycolide, and their copolymers, poly(lactide-co-glycolide). FIGURES 2–4 depict several variations of synthesis products that are possible. (A limited, noninclusive number of original investigations and reviews on PHAs are provided in the bibliography.[41,49–55])

Synthesis methodologies for PHAs have been described; modifications have been developed; analyses of the post-synthesis products and properties have been assessed; and diverse applications explored.[52]

In keeping with the spirit of this paper, it is timely to discuss some *structural and functional* attributes required for a PHA delivery system destined for the clinic.

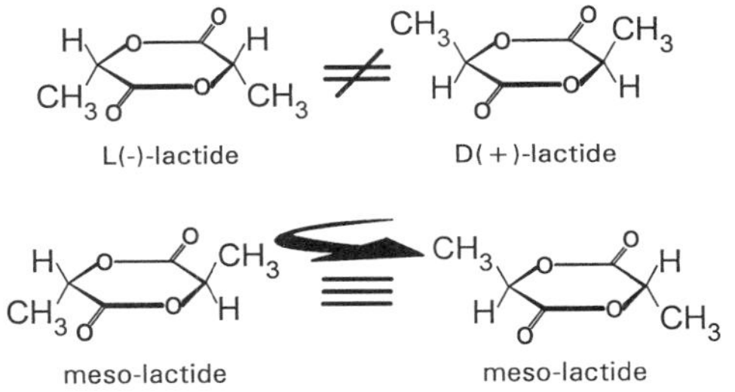

FIGURE 3. There are three forms of lactides: L(−), D(+), and *meso*-lactide. The physical and chemical properties of each lactide are different; therefore, synthesis of polylactides from these combinatorial precursors can yield polylactides with disparate properties. (From Hollinger,[52] published with permission from the publisher.)

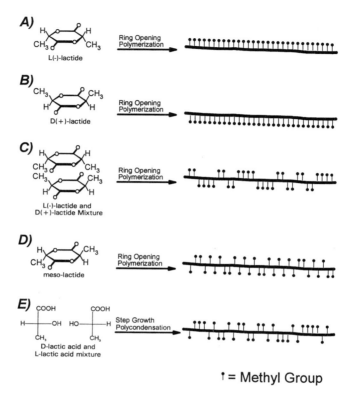

↑ = Methyl Group

FIGURE 4. An illustration of possible multiple combinations of methyl group positions for lactide homopolymers. **A** and **B:** Ring opening polymerization of L(−)-lactide and D(+)-lactide will yield a highly predictable methyl group orientation. Note that for polyL(−)- and D(+)-lactides, the methyl groups are consistently placed on opposite "planes" of the polymer backbone. **C:** Ring opening polymerization of an equimolar mixture of L(−)- and D(+)-lactides will yield a multiplicity of methyl group diads and tetrads. The precise sequence anticipated will be unpredictable. **D:** Ring opening polymerization of *meso*-lactide will produce a polymer with random combinations of methyl group orientations (in "ones" and "twos") on either side of the "plane." **E.** Step growth polycondensation of D- and L-lactic acid mixtures will result in a staggering array of unpredictable permutations of methyl groups. (From Hollinger,[52] published with permission from the publisher.)

General: Biocompatibility and Biodegradability

A fundamental assumption tissue engineers make when they use *biodegradable* PHAs to deliver either cells or vulnerary factors, is the PHA will be *biocompatible*. Definitions for *biocompatibility* and *biodegradability* can arouse heated debate and conjure provocative definitions. A consensus definition for *biocompatibility* is "The ability of a material to perform with an appropriate host response to a specific situation.[56]" We like to include the comment that the implanted material/product, in whole or degrading parts, will do no harm and promote a desired effect.

TABLE 1. Functional Significance of Attributes of a Delivery System and BMP

Attributes	Functions	References
Biocompatibility	". . . to perform with an appropriate host response to a specific situation." The implanted material/product, in whole or its degrading parts, will do no harm and promote a desired effect	56
Biodegradability	The capacity to be removed completely from the recipient by physiologic processes	52
Pharmacokinetics	A release rate for BMP from a delivery system	
Chemoattractant	The attraction of cells to a site in response to a soluble biologic factor, *e.g.,* BMP release from the delivery system	24
Differentiation	Terminal cell expression from a pluripotent progenitor	23
Angiogenesis	Growth of branching capillary networks	57
Surface		
Texture	Requirements for bone cells not known	
Charge	Osteoblast expression inhibited by electronegative charge; electropositive surface probably advantageous.	52
Amorphous Crystalline Hydrophilicity Hydrophobicity	Increase spreading (*i.e.,* decrease surface angle) on a surface, cells tend to loose tissue-specific function; more rounded cells appear able to retain function	54
Internal architecture		
Void size	Optimum void size for bone ingrowth should be greater than 200 μm; cells must enter and attach to establish osteoblast phenotype	51, 61

Whether semantic or physiologic preference drive the choice for the appropriate term that embodies and describes the removal of an implanted biomaterial, within this paper we use the term *biodegradable*. A consensus definition of this attribute is the capacity to be removed from the recipient through physiological processes, *e.g.,* cellularly, hydrolytically, enzymatically.

Specific: Pharmacokinetics, Angiogenesis, Chemotaxis, Cell Attachment, Surface Design, Internal Architecture, Signal Transduction, Phenotypic Expression

We highlight a few specific attributes in TABLE 1 that must be inculcated into the tissue engineer's design of a delivery system for vulnerary factors.

Pharmacokinetics (*i.e.,* release rate of BMP from a delivery system) is an important design property for a bone regeneration product. The pharmacokinetic capacity of the delivery system must coincide with osseous wound healing dynamics. There are additional considerations associated with pharmacokinetics, BMPs, and patients. However, at this time, they only can be presented as questions. Which of the currently identified 12 BMPs should be delivered? Are multiple BMPs required? Is there an optimal temporal sequence for therapeutic effect? At what time following injury should BMP(s) be administered? Immediately? Should there be a delay? What dose(s) is (are) appropriate? Should doses be pulsatile? Sustained? Are anatomical variations a consideration? Is recipient age a consideration? One fact can be stated: No bench mark pharmacokinetic profile is available for a delivery system design to ensure the dose(s) of vulnerary factor is (are) released at the proper time(s) during the wound regenerating continuum.

Cells and their soluble biologic products initiate, modulate intensity, duration, and cessation of wound healing. A key requirement for tissue regeneration is *angiogenesis*: the growth of branching capillary networks.[57] The capillaries are the conduits for passage of nutrients, gases, waste, and cells trafficking to and from the healing wound. Pluripotential cells (*e.g.*, pericytes) transit the neovasculature, are attracted (*i.e.*, by the process of *chemoattraction*) to the wound site by BMP, bind to type IV collagen of the vessels,[58] and under the aegis of BMP, follow a sequential path leading to osteoblast development (*i.e.*, *differentiation*).[59]

Antecedent to angiogenesis is substratum formation: neovessels cannot punch into a vacuum. Immediately post-injury, a hematoma forms; it is followed by granulation tissue, thus providing early foundational support for the neovasculature. The granulation tissue transitions into an organized extracellular matrix (ECM) to direct cell-cell interactions, cell-integrin receptor binding, and cell-cytokine receptor coupling (*e.g.*, serine-threonine kinase receptors for BMP) to promote wound healing.[60] Therefore, a PHA delivery system must function as a provisional ECM until sufficient endogenous components for a substratum are elaborated and consolidated.[61] Through receptor-ligand binding, the mature ECM provides key navigational cues for cell entry to the wound site and modulates cell activity by shape-transduction mechanisms.[57] The cells lured to the treated site (by PHA/BMP) must attach (*i.e.*, *anchor*) to the PHA and cells must penetrate to its internal architecture and alight on internal surfaces. *Anchorage* depends on focal interactions between adhesive substrates such as fibronectin, laminin, vitronectin, osteonectin, tenascin, thrombospondin, and transmembrane receptors, known as integrins.[62] *The ECM exerts local control among adhesive substrates, vulnerary factors, controls cell shape, and therefore, phenotypic expression; it is critical for regulation of cell growth, differentiation, and morphogenesis.*[63-66] *It is imperative a tissue-engineered PHA delivery system fulfills the macrophysiologic roles of an ECM.*

In addition to the array of adhesive regulators and receptor substrates that must synergistically interact with the delivery system, the *chemical and physical* features of that delivery system's *interior* (*e.g.*, *void volume*) *and exterior* will impact on *anchorage and phenotypic expression* of cells. Post-synthesis chemical and physical properties of a manufactured delivery system that affect cells and determine bone regeneration include *surface charge, hydrophilicity, hydrophobicity, surface texture, amorphousness, and crystallinity.*[52,54,67] Integration of these delivery system attributes and functional dynamics of bone regeneration are summarized in TABLE 1.

CONCLUSION

A tissue engineered product for bone regeneration must possess defined structural and functional features. Many, but not all, of the required features have been mentioned. In light of the versatility of the PHAs and the powerful wound healing impact of BMPs, a PHA/BMP combination is a compelling bone regenerating therapy for the clinic. This combination may be a rational therapeutic alternative to traditional treatments such as autograft and allogeneic bank bone, provided it is conceived to oblige a challenging taskmaster: *macrophysiology*.

SUMMARY

Traditional histology identifies three components of bone: cells, an extracellular mineralized organic matrix, and a lymphatic-vascular component. Specialized bone cells known as osteoblasts promote bone regeneration. Clinically, this property has been exploited by surgeons with autografts and bank bone preparations to restore deficient form and function to almost every aspect of the skeleton. Unfortunately, these therapies can be inadequate for patients with panskeletal trauma. Therefore, a suitable alternative may be a laboratory-derived product consisting of a vulnerary factor and delivery system. The integration of a laboratory-engineered product in an osseous wound environment is a formidable challenge demanding a keen appreciation of the product's *macrophysiologic roles* in wound healing biology. Consequently, the purposes for this paper are 1) to define briefly *macrophysiology* relevant to a delivery system for vulnerary molecules and bone regeneration; 2) to review a key family of bone regenerating molecules, the bone morphogenetic proteins (BMPs); and 3) to relate delivery system engineering with bone regeneration.

REFERENCES

1. GUYTON, A. C. 1991. Textbook of Medical Physiology. W. B. Saunders. Philadephia, pp. 2–23.
2. WOZNEY, J. M. 1992. Molecular Reproduct. Develop. **32:** 160–167.
3. CELESTE, A. J., J. J. SONG, K. COX, V. ROSEN & J. M. WOZNEY. 1994. J. Bone Miner. Res. **9:** S137.
4. KINGSLEY, D. M. 1994. Genes Develop. **8:** 133–146.
5. NGUYEN, A. M., M. TRAN, T. OATES, O. ALVARES & D. L. COCHRAN. 1995. J. Dent. Res. **74:** 251.
6. STORM, E. E., T. V. HUYNH, N. G. COPELAND, N. A. JENKINS, D. M. KINGSLEY & S. LEE. 1994. Nature **368:** 639–643.
7. EINHORN, T. A. 1994. Enhancement of fracture healing by molecular or physical means: An overview. *In* Bone Formation and Repair. C. T. Brighton, G. E. Freidlaender & J. M. Lane, Eds.: 223–238. AAOS. Rosemont, IL.
8. ISHIDOU, Y., I. KITAJIMA, H. OBAMA, I. MARUYAMA, F. MURATA, T. IMAMURA, N. YAMADA, P. TEN DIJKE, K. MIYAZONO & T. SAKOU. 1995. J. Bone Miner. Res. **10:** 1651–1659.
9. KINGSLEY, D. 1994. Trends in Genetics. **10:** 16–21.
10. WINNIER, G., M. BLESSING, P. A. LABOSKY & B. L. HOGAN. 1995. Genes Develop. **9:** 2105–2116.
11. KAPLAN, F. S. & E. M. SHORE. 1996. Bone **19**(Suppl): 13–21.
12. ELIMA, K. 1993. Ann. Med. **25:** 395–402.
13. HARRIS, S. E., M. A. HARRIS, P. MAHY, J. WOZNEY, J. Q. FENG & G. R. MUNDY. 1994. Prostate **24:** 204–211.
14. DUBOULE, D. 1994. Science **266:** 575–576.
15. LAUFER, E., C. E. NELSON, R. L. JOHNSON, B. A. MORGAN & C. TABIN. 1994. Cell **79:** 993–1003.
16. TICKLE, C. 1994. Nature **368:** 587–588.
17. AHRENS, M., T. ANKENBAUER, D. SCHRÖDER, A. HOLLNAGEL, H. MAYER & G. GROSS. 1993. DNA Cell Biol. **12:** 871–880.
18. WANG, E. A., D. L. ISREAL & D. P. LUXENBERG. 1993. Growth Factors **9:** 57–71.
19. WOLPERT, L. 1989. Development **107:** 3–12.
20. URIST, M. R., M. F. SILVERMAN, K. BURING, F. L. DUBUC & J. M. ROSENBURG. 1967. Clin. Orthop. **53:** 243.
21. URIST, M. R. & B. S. STRATES. 1971. J. Dent. Res. **50:** 1392–1406.
22. URIST, M. R. 1994. The search for and discovery of bone morphogenetic protein. *In*

Bone Grafts, Derivatives and Substitutes. M. R. Urist, B. T. O'Conner & R. G. Burwell, Eds.: 315–362. Butterworth. London.

23. KOMAKI, M., T. KATAGIRI & T. SUDA. 1996. Cell Tissue Res. **284:** 9–17.
24. LIND, M., E. F. ERIKSEN & C. BÜNGER. 1996. Bone **18:** 53–57.
25. NAKASE, T., S. NOMURA, H. YOSHIKAWA, J. HASHIMOTO, S. HIROTA, Y. KITAMURA, S. OIKKAWA, K. ONO, & K. TAKAOKA. 1994. J. Bone Miner. Res. **9:** 651–659.
26. BOSTROM, M. G., J. LANE, W. S. BERBERIAN, A. A. MISSRI, E. TOMIN, A. WEILAND, S. DOTY, D. GLASER & V. ROSEN. 1995. J. Orthop. Res. **13:** 357–367.
27. CAREY, D. & X. LIU. 1995. J. Bone Mineral Res. **10:** 401–405.
28. KENLEY, R., K. YIM, J. ABRAMS, E. RON, T. TUREK, L. MARDEN & J. HOLLINGER. 1993. Pharm. Res. **10:** 1393–1401.
29. KENLEY, R., L. MARDEN, T. TUREK, L. JIN, E. RON & J. HOLLINGER. 1994. J. Biomed. Mater. Res. **28:** 1139–1147.
30. MARDEN, L. J., J. O. HOLLINGER, A. CHAUDHARI, T. TUREK, R. SCHAUB & E. RON. 1994. J. Biomed. Mater. Res. **28:** 1127–1138.
31. COOK, S. D., G. C. BAFFES, M. W. WOLFE, K. SAMPATH, D. C. RUEGER & T. S. WHITECLOUD. 1994. J. Bone Joint Surg. **76A:** 827–838.
32. BOSTROM, M., J. LANE, E. TOMIN, M. BROWNE, W. BERBERIAN, T. TUREK, J. SMITH, J. WOZNEY & T. SCHILDHAUER. 1996. Clin. Orthop. Rel. Res. **327:** 272–282.
33. ZEGZULA, H. D., D. BUCK, J. BREKKE, J. WOZNEY & J. O. HOLLINGER J. Bone Joint Surg. In press.
34. GERHART, T. N., C. A. KIRKER-HEAD, M. J. KRIZ, M. E. HOLTROP, G. E. HENNIG & E. A. WANG. 1993. Clin. Orthop. Rel. Res. **293:** 317–326.
35. TORIUMI, D. M., H. S. KOTLER, D. P. LUXUNBERG, M. E. HOLTROP & E. A. WANG. 1991. Arch. Otolaryngol. Head and Neck Surg. **117:** 1101–1112.
36. MAYER, M. H., J. O. HOLLINGER, E. RON & J. WOZNEY. 1996. Plastic Reconstr. Surg. **98**(2): 247–259.
37. COOK, S. D., G. C. BAFFES, M. W. WOLFE, T. K. SAMPATH & D. C. RUEGER. 1994. Clin. Orthop. **301:** 302–312.
38. COOK, S. D., M. W. WOLFE, S. L. SALKELD & D. C. RUEGER. 1995. J. Bone Joint Surg. **77-A:** 734–750.
39. SCHMITZ, J. P. & J. O. HOLLINGER. 1986. Clin. Orthop. Rel. Res. **205:** 299–308.
40. HOLLINGER, J. O. & J. KLEINSCHMIDT. 1990. J. Craniofac. Surg. **1:** 60–68.
41. HOLLINGER, J. O. & K. LEONG. 1996. Biomaterials. **17:** 187–194.
42. BOLANDER, M. E. 1992. Proc. Soc. Exp. Biol. Med. **200:** 165–170.
43. STEENFOS, H. H. 1994. Scand. J. Plast. Reconstr. Hand Surg. **28:** 95–105.
44. EINHORN, T. 1995. J. Bone Joint Surg. **77-A:** 940–956.
45. HOLLINGER, J. O. & M. E. K. WONG. 1996. Oral Surg. Oral Med. Oral Pathol. **82**(5): 475–492.
46. VACANTI, C. A., R. LANGER, B. SCHLOO & J. P. VACANTI. 1991. Polymer Preprints **32:** 228–229.
47. MIKOS, A. G., Y. BAO, L. G. CIMA, D. E. INGBER, J. P. VACANTI & R. LANGER. 1993. J. Biomed. Mater. Res. **27:** 183–189.
48. MIKOS, G. A., G. SARAKINOS, S. LEITE, J. VACANTI & R. LANGER. 1993. Biomaterials. **14:** 323–330.
49. HOLLINGER, J. O. & G. C. BATTISTONE. 1986. Clin. Orthop. Rel. Res. **207:** 290–305.
50. RON, E. & R. LANGER. 1992. Erodible systems. *In* Treatise on Controlled Drug Delivery. Fundamentals, Optimization, Applications. A. Kydonieus, Ed.: 199–224. Marcel Dekker, Inc. New York.
51. BREKKE, J. 1995. Architectural principles applied to three-dimensional therapeutic implants composed of bioresorbable polymers. *In* Handbook of Biomaterials and Applications. D. L. Wise, Ed.: 689–731. Marcel-Dekker. New York.
52. HOLLINGER, J. 1995. Biomedical Applications of Synthetic Biodegradable Polymers. CRC Press, Inc. Boca Raton, FL, pp. 1–257.
53. LO, H., S. KADIYALA, S. E. GUGGINO & K. W. LEONG. 1996. J. Biomed. Mater. Res. **30:** 475–484.
54. PARK, A. & L. G. CIMA. 1996. J. Biomed. Mater. Res. **31:** 117–130.

55. SCHUGENS, C., V. MAQUEST, C. GRANDFILS, R. JEROME & P. TEYESSIE. 1996. J. Biomed. Mater. Res. **30:** 449–461.
56. BLACK, J. 1992. Biological Performance of Materials. Fundamentals of Biocompatiblity. Marcel Dekker, Inc. New York, pp. 1–390.
57. INGBER, D. E., P. DEEPA, Z. SUN, H. BETENSKY & N. WANG. 1995. J. Biomech. **28:** 1471–1484.
58. PARALKAR, V. M., A. K. N. NANDEDKAR, R. H. POINTER, H. K. KLEINMAN & A. H. REDDI. 1990. J Biol Chem. **265:** 17281–17284.
59. LYNCH, M. P., J. L. STEIN, G. STEIN & J. B. LIAN. 1995. Exp. Cell Res. **216:** 35–45.
60. RAGHOW, R. 1994. FASEB J. **8:** 823–831.
61. BREKKE, J. 1996. Tissue Eng. **2:** 97–114.
62. HYNES, R. O. 1992. Cell **69**(1): 11–26.
63. SAGE, E. H. & P. BORNSTEIN. 1991. J. Biologic. Chem. **266:** 14831–14834.
64. HARALSON, M. A. 1993. Lab. Invest. **69:** 369–372.
65. SINHA, R. K., F. MORRIS, S. A. SHAH & R. S. TUAN. 1994. Clin. Orthop. Rel. Res. **305:** 258–272.
66. WANG, N. & D. E. INGBER. 1994. Biophys. J. **66:** 2181–2189.
67. DAVIES, J. E. 1996. The Anat. Rec. **245:** 426–445.

Use of an Immunoisolation Device for Cell Transplantation and Tumor Immunotherapy

ROBIN L. GELLER,[a] THOMAS LOUDOVARIS,
STEVEN NEUENFELDT, ROBERT C. JOHNSON, AND
JAMES H. BRAUKER

Gene Therapy Unit
Baxter Healthcare Corporation
Round Lake, Illinois 60073

Immunoisolation, or implantation of tissues in a membrane-enclosed device, is an approach aimed at allowing maintenance of cells in an environment where they are segregated from the host tissues. The transplant device must be well vascularized to support the implanted cells at high densities. Further, encapsulated allogeneic tissues can be protected from immune attack without the need for immunosuppression. Early work on immunoisolation, by Algire and co-workers, showed that allografts could be protected when implanted into mice within diffusion chambers with large pore membranes that prevented entry of host cells.[1-4] We have had similar results.[5] Rejection of allografts occurred only if the pores were sufficiently large to allow entry of host cells.

Over the last decade several groups have investigated immunoisolation using a variety of approaches. Hollow fiber filters have been shown to protect pancreatic islet xenografts in rats[6] and mice.[7] However, these devices utilize low flux membranes that prohibit the implantation of high desities of islets.[8] Another approach is to implant microcapsules of alginate and other hydrogels.[9] This approach has been shown to be effective in many laboratories; however, the capsules are irretrievable after implantation in the peritoneal cavity and are highly fragile.[10] Moreover, rejection responses including severe fibrotic responses were observed whenever microcapsules either empty or containing xenogeneic islets became overgrown or attached to host tissues.[11-14]

We have developed a flat sheet immunoisolation device called the TheraCyte™ system (Fig. 1). The membranes of this device protect allogeneic tissues at high densities[5] but are unable to protect xenogeneic cells from destruction.[5,15] In addition to using the TheraCyte™ system to protect encapsulated tissues from immune destruction, we have taken the unique approach of using the device to deliver antigenic stimuli in order to deliberately induce an immune response outside of the device directed at the destruction of tumor cells. The present manuscript discusses several aspects of the TheraCyte™ system including device vascularization, the immunology of transplantation of allografts and xenografts, and the use of the device for the treatment of cancer.

---

[a] Author to whom correspondence should be addressed: Baxter Healthcare Corp., DF6-2W, One Baxter Parkway, Deerfield, IL 60015; Tel: (847) 948-4434; Fax: (847) 948-4497.

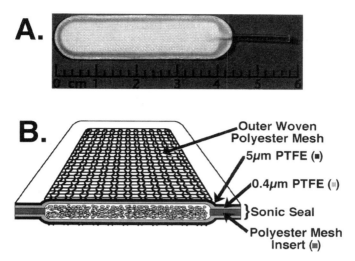

FIGURE 1. TheraCyte™ device **A:** This 1 × 4 centimeter immunoisolation device will hold up to 40 μl of cells or tissues for transplantation. The device contains a polyethylene port to permit access to the device lumen for loading. **B:** A cross-section view features the cells encapsulated in a two-layer polytetraflouroethylene (PTFE) membrane envelope formed using a polyester mesh insert. The 5 μm pore outer vascularizing membrane, the 0.4 μm pore inner immunoisolating membrane, the insert and outer woven polyester mesh are ultrasonically welded to form the device with an internal lumen capacity of either 40 μl, 20 μl or 4.5 μl.

BIOCOMPATIBILITY AND VASCULARIZATION

Efforts at implantation of high density tissues within immunoisolation devices have been carried out for over 60 years. The main hurdles with implanted biomaterials have been the overgrowth of scar tissues, known as the foreign body response.[16,17] It was observed in numerous laboratories that when devices containing pancreatic islets were implanted in animals, diabetes was corrected only transiently. Upon removal of devices and histological examination it was concluded that the device became overgrown by a foreign body response which caused nutritional stress to the islets.[16,17]

We investigated the foreign body response to biomaterials in a rat subcutaneous implant model. Previously, we described a screening study in which various membranes were implanted subcutaneously in rats to observe the host response to the biomaterials.[18] That study revealed a group of membranes that became neovascularized at the membrane-tissue interface and led to the hypothesis that membrane architecture has a pivotal role in driving neovascularization.[18,19] The appearance of this neovascularization response correlated closely with membrane pore size. The effect was seen only when the pores of the membrane were sufficiently large to allow host cells to penetrate into the interstices of the membrane. However, pore size alone was necessary, but not sufficient, to induce neovascularization. Several membranes with pores sufficiently large to allow penetration of host cells did not become vascularized (FIG. 2, TABLE 1). Another important feature of the membranes is the structure of the material that surrounds or defines the pore. Scanning

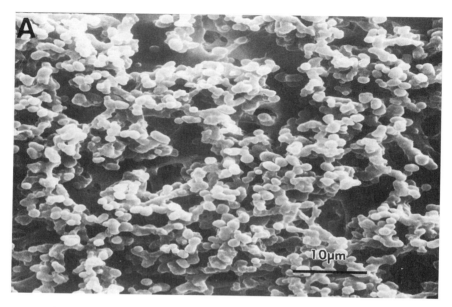

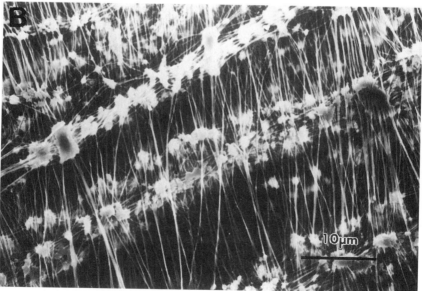

FIGURE 2. Scanning electron micrographs of 5 μm Sartorius cellulose acetate **(A)**, 3 μm Gore teflon **(B)**, 12 μm Nucleopore polycarbonate **(C)**, and 5 μm Milliopore teflon **(D)**. All of these membranes fall within pore size ranges that allow penetration of host inflammatory cells. Note fine structures (<5 mm diameter) that delimit the pores of membranes that do induce close vascular structures **(A** and **B)** in contrast to large surface area structures that delimit the pores of the membranes that do not induce close vascular structures after implantation **(C** and **D)**.

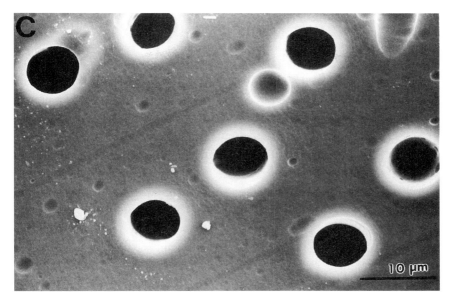

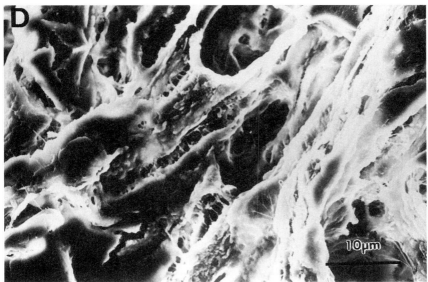

FIGURE 2. (*Continued*)

TABLE 1. Membranes That Were Invaded by Cells after Implantation

Having Close Blood Vessels		Not Having Close Blood Vessels	
Membrane	Pore Size	Membrane	Pore Size
Mixed esters cellulose	1.2	Polyester	3
Mixed esters cellulose	8.0	Polyester	5
Cellulose Acetate	0.8	Polyester	8
Cellulose Acetate	1.2	Nylon	10
Cellulose Acetate	3.0	Nylon	10
Cellulose Acetate	5.0	Nylon	10
Cellulose Acetate	8.0	PTFE	5
PTFE/Polyester[a]	1.0	PTFE	10
PTFE/polypropylene	3.0	Polycarbonate	1
PTFE/polyester	3.0	Polycarbonate	3
Versapore[a,b]	0.8	Polycarbonate	8
Versapore	1.2	Polycarbonate	12
Versapore	3.0		
Versapore	5.0		

Membranes were implanted subcutaneously in rats for three weeks, explanted, processed for histology and stained with hematoxylin and eosin. The number of the close vascular structures were quantitated as described previously.[21] Membranes used include mixed esters of cellulose (Millipore), cellulose acetate (Sartorius), PTFE/polyester (Gore), Versapore® (Gelman), polyester (Tetco), PTFE (Millipore) and Polycarbonate (Nuclepore).

[a] Less than 50% of these membranes had close vascular structures.
[b] Acrylic copolymer on nylon support.

electron microscopy revealed distinguishing characteristics of the geometry of the materials that did or did not induce neovascularization. Membranes that did become vascularized (FIG. 2,A and B) had finer geometric features than membranes that did not become vascularized (FIG. 2,C and D). Among the membranes examined, the material forming the pores (holes large enough for cells to enter) consisted of materials which were no greater than 5 μm in diameter on average. In contrast, membranes that did not become vascularized had materials which defined the pores that were much larger.

Our current hypothesis is that cells are able to flatten on the larger features of the non-vascularizing membranes, and therefore are similar in activity to cells that are flattened on the surface of small pore membranes (FIG. 3B). Thus, this situation is similar to a classical foreign body response. In contrast, the cells that enter vascularizing membranes remain rounded (FIG. 3A). We hypothesize that the differences in cell shape lead to differences in cell biochemistry. Perhaps the rounded cells in the vascularizing membrane release angiogenic factors that cause neovascularization at the membrane tissue interface. A model for this possibility is the release of factors from cultured macrophages.[20] These vascularizing membranes have been incorporated into immunoisolation devices (FIG. 1) for transplantation of living cells at high packing densities.[5,15,21] This device consists of a bilaminar membrane in which the outer "vascularizing" membrane promotes neovascularization at the membrane tissue interface and an inner "immunoisolating" membrane which prevents contact between host tissue and encapsulated tissue. We have used these devices to investigate the immunology of transplantation of allogeneic and xenogeneic tissues as discussed below.

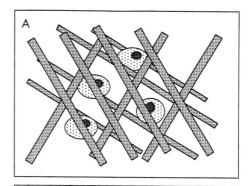

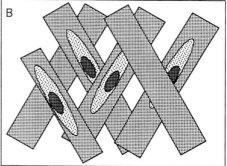

FIGURE 3. Diagrammatic representation of cells penetrating the pores of a memebrane that induces vascularization (vascularizing, **A**) and one that does not (non-vascularizing, **B**). The pore sizes are identical in both membranes, but the structures that delimit the pores are too fine for cells to flatten on the vascularizing membranes **(A)**, whereas the cells can flatten on the larger structures of the non-vascularizing membranes **(B)** as they would on a flat surface. We hypothesize that the rounded cells invading the vascularizing membrane release angiogenic factors that induce neovascularization.

TRANSPLANTATION OF ALLOGRAFTS AND XENOGRAFTS

Immunoisolation, has been shown to protect allografts when the membranes used prevented the entry of host cells into the implanted device (FIG. 4A).[3,5] Rejection of the allografts only occurred if the pores were sufficiently large to allow entry of host cells, *i.e.* when there is direct cell contact with the host's immune system (FIG. 4B). In the case of encapsulated xenografts, even when direct cell contact with the host was prevented, the immunoisolation membranes failed to protect the xenograft (FIG. 4C). The host's immune system is responsible for this rejection since these encapsulated xenografts readily survived in immunologically deficient mice or rats.[5,15] The destruction of xenografts has been observed in CBA and Balb/C mice,[15] rats[5] and dogs (unpublished observations) using the 0.4 μm pore size immunoisolating membrane of our device. Xenografts were shown to survive only when implanted into immunodeficient athymic rats and mice or in one particular mouse strain, C57/BL6,[7] which appears to be a poor responder to xenografts.

Subsequent analysis of the cellular mediators of the destruction of the encapsulated xenografts demonstrated a requirement for CD4[+] T cells, but not CD8[+] T cells, B cells or anti-xenograft antibodies.[15] Reconstitution of SCID mice with CD4[+] T cells alone, (lymph node cells depleted of CD8[+] T cells and B cells) resulted in the destruction of the encapsulated xenografts.[15]

The requirement for CD4[+] T cells and the presence of the cell-impermeable membrane suggests that stimulation of the immune system is through the indirect

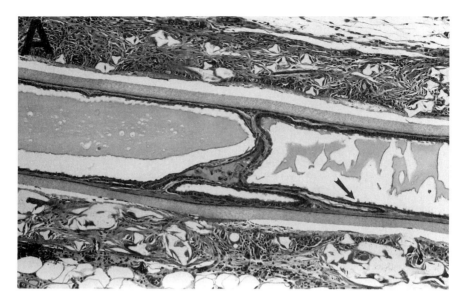

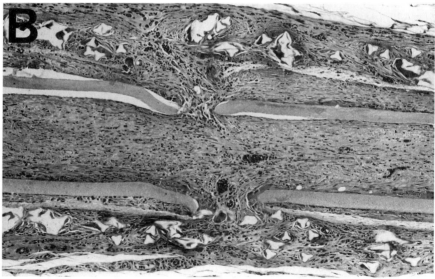

FIGURE 4. Light micrographs of minced embryonic lung tissue from Sprague-Dawley rats implanted into Lewis rats with intact membranes **(A)** or membranes with holes poked in them to allow host cell penetration **(B)** for one month and mouse embryonic lung tissue implanted in intact membranes into Lewis rats for one month **(C)**. Note that ciliated epithelial tissue (*arrow*) was present in the allograft **(A)** in intact membranes but no living epithelial cells were found when holes were poked in the membrane **(B)**. Instead, the devices were filled with host inflammatory cells and vasculature. Implanted xenogeneic tissue **(C)** was necrotic and surrounded by a large halo of inflammatory cells (photographed at lower magnification to show surrounding tissue).

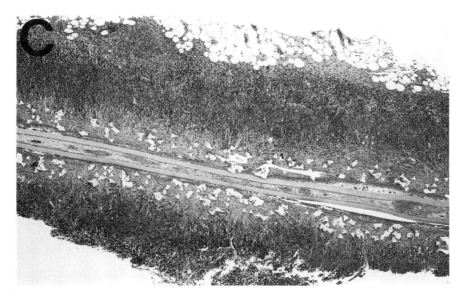

FIGURE 4. (*Continued*)

presentation of xeno-antigens to CD4$^+$ T cells. We hypothesize that the destruction of encapsulated xenografts is due to antigens shed or secreted from the encapsulated xenogeneic cells which can diffuse out through the cell-impermeable membrane. Once outside the device, these xeno-antigens are ingested and processed by antigen presenting cells, such as macrophages or dendritic cells. The processed antigens are then presented to CD4$^+$ T cells which in turn stimulate an inflammatory reaction resulting in the death of the encapsulated cells. It is possible that the destruction of the xenografts is not the result of a specific immune attack. It is clear that non-specific mechanisms are sufficient for the destruction of xenografts within large pore diffusion chambers since even isogeneic tissue is destroyed when mixed with xenogeneic tissue.[5] Starvation due to the local immune response, cellular accumulation and/or the observed decrease in vascular structures around the device could be responsible for the non-specific destruction of the implanted tissue.[5] Specific factors secreted by CD4$^+$ T cells or macrophages such as cytokines, superoxides and/or nitric oxides may be involved in the destruction of the xenogeneic tissue; such factors may prove very difficult to keep out. Whether a specific immune response is also occuring that targets xenografts is, as yet, unknown.

To prevent the destruction of encapsulated xenogeneic tissues the stimulation of the host immune system must be minimized. This could be accomplished either by eliminating immune cell contact with xeno-antigens or via modulation of the host immune response subsequent to the recognition of xeno-antigens. We have found that the use of smaller pore membranes can restrict the release of shed xeno-antigens and thereby protect encapsulated xenografts.[22] However, these more restrictive xenoprotective membranes will nutritionally support lower densities of encapsulated tissues. The practical result is then a therapeutic device too large to be practical. As illustrated in FIG. 5, membranes that allow immune cell access will not support the survival of allografts or xenografts. Once immune cell access is

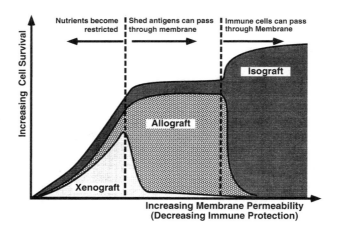

FIGURE 5. Relationship between encapsulated cell survival and increasing membrane permeability. Membranes that allow immune cell access will only support isografts but not allografts or xenografts owing to penetration by immune cells. Once immune cell access is prevented then isografts and allografts are protected but not xenografts. Xenograft protection is achieved only in membranes that restrict the amount of shed antigens being released from the device thereby preventing the inflammatory response surrounding the device. Xenoprotective membranes however, are also restrictive of nutrients required for cell survival, as demonstrated by poor allograft and isograft survival in these membranes.

prevented then allografts but not xenografts are protected. To achieve xenograft protection, membranes must restrict the amount of shed antigens being released from the device. The consequence of this, however, is impaired tissue survival even for allografts and isografts due to nutritional deficit.[8,22]

An alternative to a xenoprotective membrane is the use of current clinical immunosuppressive protocols along with alloprotective membranes for successful implantation of xenografts. Conventional immunosuppressive drugs, such as cyclosporin A can be effective in protecting encapsulated xenografts (unpublished observations). The use of immunosuppression with encapsulated device implants could be used in cases where the treatment of the disease outweigh the adverse side effects of the immunosuppressants. The first use of xenografts with immunosuppression will most likely be in diabetic patients who have been transplanted with a kidney and are already receiving immunosuppression.

TUMOR IMMUNOTHERAPY USING AN IMMUNOISOLATION DEVICE

While the TheraCyte™ system does protect allografts from immune destruction, the protection is not a result of an abrogated immune response. Rather, the device protects allografts in the face of an immune response occuring outside of the device. This led us to test whether the TheraCyte system could be used to induce an anti-tumor response which could effectively eliminate nonencapsulated tumor elsewhere in the body.

Previous studies (see ref. 23 for review) have suggested that irradiated tumor cells modified by introduction of cytokine genes can stimulate an immune response against unmodified tumor at a distal site when such vaccines are administered by injection of the modified cells usually after irradiation of the cells to eliminate the

TABLE 2. Treatment of Pre-existing Tumors

Device Contents	Free Irradiated Cell Injection	Number of Animals Tumor Free at 60 Days
No cells	−	0/3
No cells	+	0/3
Live tumor cells	−	0/4
Live tumor cells	+	1/4
Irradiated tumor cells	−	1/5
Irradiated tumor cells	+	3/5

Tumors were initiated by injection of 1×10^3 MCA-38 cells intramuscularly into C57/B6 mice five days before device implantation. Animals were implanted in the ventral subcutaneous space (21) with two devices each containing either 1×10^6 MCA-38 cells or empty devices. Free injection consisted of 1×10^6 irradiated MCA-38 cells injected at the incision site at the time of surgery.

possibility of tumor formation by the injected cells.[24] Use of an immunoisolation device for the delivery of such cell-based tumor vaccines has several advantages. First, re-introduced tumor cells are sequestered within the device; this may minimize risk to patients with tumors and may also prevent anergy resulting from defective interactions between tumors and components of the immune system.[25–27] Second, by preventing immune-mediated destruction of the encapsulated cells, the immunoisolation device may maximize the period of effective immunization by antigens shed from those cells thereby reducing or eliminating the need for multiple rounds of treatment. Finally, the stimulating cells can be quantitatively removed at the end of the treatment period.

Several groups have previously examined the effects of tumor cells implanted within diffusion chambers and the results have been decidedly mixed. Biggs and Eisen were able to demonstrate induction of immunity to tumor cells implanted within diffusion chambers, but subsequent work revealed that the immune response was generated by the release of viral particles from the encapsulated tumor cells and not by tumor-specific antigens.[28] Stillstom demonstrated anti-tumor immunity in a different tumor model; but the protection observed was transient: the levels of protection dropped dramatically with time.[29] In other cases no systemic immunity was observed[30,31] and in at least one case it was argued that the presence of diffusion chambers containing tumor cells could lead to enhanced tumor growth.[31]

We chose the mouse colon carcinoma cell line, MCA-38 as a model system to test whether the TheraCyte™ system can be effectively used to induce an anti-tumor immune response. The first model we tested was prevention of tumor formation. C57/B6 mice were implanted subcutaneously with two devices containing 10^6 live MCA-38 cells each. After three weeks the animals were challenged with 10^6 MCA-38 cells injected subcutaneously into the left flank. All of the control animals (no implants) developed tumor at the challenge site while 100% of the animals that were implanted with devices remained tumor free after this challenge as well as after a second challenge several weeks later.[32] These results suggested that an immunoisolating device can be used to generate a systemic anti-tumor response in the absence of direct contact between the immunizing cells and the immune system of the host.

Prevention of tumor formation is one measure of an anti-tumor response, a more rigorous model may be to ask whether a pre-existing tumor can be eliminated following implantation of devices containing tumor cells. To test this model we initiated tumors in mice by intramuscular injection of 10^3 MCA-38 cells. Three to five days later the animals were implanted with devices as outlined in TABLE 2. We observed several significant difference when treating pre-existing tumors. First,

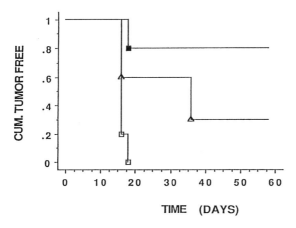

CUM. TUMOR FREE

TIME (DAYS)

FIGURE 6. Tumors were initiated by injection of 1×10^3 MCA-38 cells intramuscularly into C57/B6 mice three days before device implantation. Animals were implanted in the ventral subcutaneous space[21] with devices containing irradiated MCA-38 cells and slow release preparations of IL-2 (■). Animals with implants which did not get cytokine received an injection of irradiated MCA-38 cells outside of the device at the time of implant (△). Control animals received no treatment (□). Animals were monitored for formation of tumors at the challenge site.

devices containing cells alone were not effective against pre-existing tumors unless implantation was accompanied by the deposit of irradiated tumor cells at the device site but outside of the device (free irradiated cell injection). Moreover, live tumor cells within the device were not effective whether or not irradiated cells were present outside of the device. The most effective treatment was the combination of irradiated cells implanted within devices accompanied by the injection of additional irradiated cells outside of the device. In this case, growth of the pre-existing tumor was prevented in up to 60% of the experimental animals. These results are consistent with the work of Dranoff *et al.,*[24] who also demonstrated a need for irradiation of the cells in order to obtain a vigorous anti-tumor response in the face of pre-existing tumor.

These results raise several issues. First, why were irradiated cells more effective than live cells and second why was the free cell injection necessary? A partial answer to both questions may be timing. In the face of a pre-existing, intact tumor the rapid initiation of an immune response is essential. It may be that irradiation of the cells leads to a more rapid immune response due to quantitative and qualitative changes in the molecules released from dead or dying cells. The response may be enhanced by the expression of new molecules as the cells attempt to repair the radiation induced damage or the response may be enhanced by the expression of inflammatory signals from the irradiated cells. It is also possible that the free injection of irradiated cells may further accelerate the immune response via direct contact between the cells of the immune system and the immunizing cells. This direct contact alone is not sufficient for an effective anti-tumor response however; none of the animals implanted with empty devices and inoculated with irradiated tumor cells at the device site were protected from tumor growth.

The results described above suggested that tumor cells alone in an immunoisolation device were not sufficient to mediate an anti-tumor response in the face of a pre-existing tumor and further suggested that direct contact between immunizing tumor cells and the host immune system may be necessary. To probe this further, we asked whether it would be possible to replace the signals provided by the free irradiated cells with a soluble factor. Using a slow release formulation of interleukin-2 (IL-2) we implanted animals having pre-existing tumors with devices containing irradiated MCA-38 and 2000 Units of IL-2. The results of one representative experiment are shown in FIG. 6. The combination of slow release cytokine and cells in

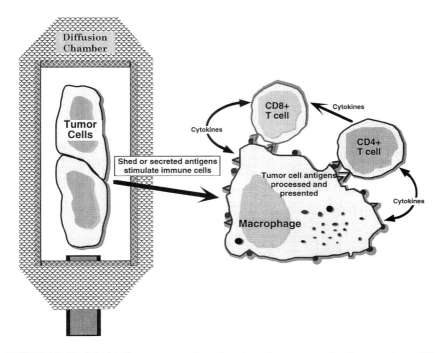

FIGURE 7. Model of indirect presentation of antigens from encapsulated tumor tissue. We hypothesize that antigens are shed from the cells encapsulated within the immunoisolation device. These shed antigens are picked up, processed and presented by antigen presenting cells of the host to both CD4+ and CD8+ cells. This "indirect" presentation of antigen could then lead to the activation of lymphocytes able to mediate anti-tumor activity.

devices was as effective as the combination of devices containing cells and an injection of irradiated cells outside of the device. Thus, direct contact between the cells of the host immune system and the immunizing tumor cells is not essential to generate an anti-tumor response that is effective against pre-existing tumor if activation signals such as IL-2 can be exogenously supplied.

CONCLUSIONS

The data obtained from both the xenograft model and the tumor model suggest that a robust immune response can be engendered without direct contact between the host and the immunizing cells. In the case of xenografts the extent of this immune response is sufficient to lead to the death of the encapsulated cells possibly due to nutritional deficit. In the case of tumor cells, the resulting immune response can eliminate tumor cells elsewhere in the body. These observations are consistent with a number of recent studies on antigen presentation. Matzinger has suggested in the "danger" theory that the immune system is designed to differentiate between harmless and dangerous entities and that the distinction between the two is made by antigen-presenting cells.[33] She has further suggested that while tumors are themselves poor antigen presenting cells it might be possible to actively immunize against tumors by priming antigen-presenting cells (*i.e.*, indirect activation).[33] That such indirect activation is a viable option for initiating anti-tumor responses is further supported by observations from a number of groups suggesting that exogenous antigens can be presented on Class I molecules as well on Class II molecules[34-37] by phagocytes. Experiments have indicated that the presentation occurs when antigen is bound to particles including membrane fragments[34] or is found in association with cellular debris. This process may be particularly applicable to presentation of tumor derived antigens[37] and in fact may serve as the major pathway for generating CTL responses to endogenous tumors.[35] As shown in FIG. 7, such indirect presentation is compatible with release of material from cells encapsulated within an immunoisolation device. These shed antigens would then be picked up and presented by professional antigen-presenting cells leading to the activation of both CD4⁺ and CD8 cells⁺.

REFERENCES

1. WEAVER, J. M., G. H. ALGIRE & R. T. PREHN. 1955. The growth of cells in vivo in difffusion chambers. II. The role of cells in the destruction of homografts in mice. J. Natl. Cancer Inst. **15:** 1737–1767.

2. ALGIRE, G. H., M. L. BORDERS & V. J. EVANS. 1958. Studies of heterografts in diffusion chambers in mice. J. Natl. Cancer Inst. **20:** 1187.

3. ALGIRE, G. H., J. M. WEAVER & R. T. PREHN. 1954. Growth of cells in vivo in diffusion chambers I. Survival of homografts in immunized mice. J. Natl. Cancer Inst. **15:** 493–507.

4. ALGIRE, G. H. 1957. Diffusion-chamber techniques for studies of cellular immunity. Ann. N. Y. Acad. Sci. **69:** 663–667.

5. BRAUKER, J., L. A. MARTINSON, S. K. YOUNG & R. C. JOHNSON. 1996. Local inflammatory response around diffusion chambers containing xenografts. Transplantation **61:** 1671–1677.

6. LANZA, R. P., D. H. BUTLER, K. M. BORLAND, J. E. STARUK, D. L. FAUSTMAN, B. A. SOLOMON, T. E. MULLER, R. G. RUPP, T. MAKI, A. P. MONACO & W. L. CHICK. 1992. Xenotransplantation of canine, bovine, and porcine islets in diabetic rats without immunosuppression. Proc. Natl. Acad. Sci. USA **88:** 11100–11104.

7. LACY, P. E., O. D. HEGRE, A. GERASIMIDI-VAZEOU, F. T. GENTILE & K. E. DIONNE. 1991. Maintenance of normoglycemia in diabetic mice by subcutaneous xenografts of encapsulated islets. Science **254:** 1782–1784.

8. COLTON, C. K. 1995. Implantable biohybrid artificial organs. Cell Transplant. **4:** 415–436.

9. SUN, A. M. 1988. Microencapsulation of pancreatic islet cells: A bioartificial endocrine pancreas. Methods Enzymol. **137:** 575–580.

10. WEBER, C. J., J. AYRES-PRICE, M. COSTANZO, A. BAKER & A. STALL. 1994. NOD mouse peritoneal cellular response to poly-L-lysine-alginate microencapsulated rat islets. Transplant. Proc. **26:** 1116–1119.

11. COLE, D. R., M. WATERFALL, M. McINTYRE & J. D. BAIRD. 1992. Microencapsulated islet grafts in the BB/E rat: A possible role for cytokines in graft failure. Diabetologia **35:** 231–237.

12. CLAYTON, H. A., N. J. LONDON, P. S. COLLOBY, P. R. BELL & R. F. JAMES. 1991. The effect of capsule composition on the biocompatibility of alginate-poly-L-lysine capsules. J. Microencapsul. **8:** 221–233.

13. WIJSMAN, J., P. ATKISON, R. MAZAHERI, B. GARCIA, T. PAUL, J. VOSE, G. O'SHEA & C. STILLER. 1992. Histological and immunopathological analysis of recovered encapsulated allogeneic islets from transplanted diabetic BB/W rats. Transplantation **54:** 588–592.

14. GOTFREDSEN, C. F., M. G. STEWART, G. M. O'SHEA, J. R. VOSE & A. J. MOODY. 1990. The fate of transplanted encapsulated islets in spontaneously diabetic BB/Wor rats. Diabetes Res. **15:** 157–163.

15. LOUDOVARIS, T., T. E. MANDEL & B. CHARLTON. 1996. CD4+ T cell mediated destruction

of xenografts within cell-impermeable membranes in the absence of CD8+ T cells and B cells. Transplantation **61:** 1678–1684.

16. COLTON, C. K. & E. S. AVGOUSTINIATOS. 1991. Bioengineering in development of the hybrid artificial pancreas. J. Biomech. Eng. **113:** 152–170.

17. SCHARP, D. W., N. S. MASON & R. E. SPARKS. 1995. Islet immuno-isolation: The use of hybrid artificial organs to prevent islet tissue rejection. World J. Surg. **8:** 221–229.

18. BRAUKER, J. H., V. CARR-BRENDEL, L. A. MARTINSON, J. CRUDELE, W. D. JOHNSTON & R. C. JOHNSON. 1995. Neovascularization of synthetic membranes directed by membrane architecture. J. Biomed. Mat. Res. **29:** 1517–1524.

19. PADERA, R. F. & C. K. COLTON. 1996. Time course of membrane microarchitecture-driven neovascularization. Biomaterials **17:** 277–284.

20. KNIGHTON, D. R., H. SCHENUENSTUHL, B. J. HALLIDAY, Z. WERB & M. J. BANDA. 1983. Oxygen tension regulates the expression of angiogenesis factor by macrophages. Science **221:** 1283–1285.

21. CARR-BRENDEL, V. E., R. L. GELLER, T. J. THOMAS, D. R. BOGGS, S. K. YOUNG, J. CRUDELE, L. A. MARTINSON, D. A. MARYANOV, R. C. JOHNSON & J. H. BRAUKER. 1997. Transplantation of cells in an immunoisolation device for gene therapy. *In* Methods in Molecular Biology: Expression and Detection of Recombinant Genes. R. Tuan, Ed. Humana. Totowa, NJ. **63:** 373–387.

22. MARTINSON, L., R. PAULEY, J. BRAUKER, D. BOGGS, D. MARYANOV, S. STERNBERG & R. C. JOHNSON. 1995. Protection of xenografts with immunoisolation membranes. Cell Transplant **3:** 249.

23. TEPPER, R. I. & J. J. MULE. 1994. Experimental and clinical studies of cytokine gene-modified tumor cells. Hum. Gene Ther. **5:** 153–164.

24. DRANOFF, G., E. JAFFEE, A. LAZENBY, P. GOLUMBEK, H. LEVITSKY, K. BROSE, V. JACKSON, H. HAMADA, D. PARDOLL & R. C. MULLIGAN. 1993. Vaccination with irradiated tumor cells engineered to secrete murine granulocyte-macrophage colony-stimulating factor stimulates potent, specific and long-lasting anti-tumor immunity. Proc. Natl. Acad. Sci. USA **90:** 3539–3543.

25. TOWNSEND, S. E. & J. P. ALLISON. 1993. Tumor rejection after direct stimulation of CD8+ T cells by B7-transfected melanoma cells. Science **259:** 368–370.

26. GIMMI, C. D., G. J. FREEMAN, J. G. GRIBBEN, G. GRAY & L. M. NADLER. 1993. Human T-cell anergy is induced by antigen presentation in the absence of B7 stimulation. Proc. Natl. Acad. Sci. USA **90:** 6586–6590.

27. CHEN, L., P. S. LINSLEY & K. E. HELSTROM. 1993. Costimulation of T cells for tumor immunity. Immunol. Today **14:** 483–486.

28. BIGGS, M. W. & J. E. EISEN. 1965. Diffusion chamber studies of allogenic tumor immunity in mice. Cancer Res. **25:** 1888–1893.

29. STILLSTROM, J. 1974. Induction of SV-40-tumor immunity by SV-40-transformed cells in diffusion chambers. Acta Pathol. Microbiol. Scand. **82:** 676–686.

30. RUMI, L., C. D. PASQUALINI & S. L. RABASA. 1995. Growth of sarcoma 180 in splenectomized mice bearing diffusion chambers containing spleen or tumor cells. Eur. J. Cancer **7:** 551–555.

31. KLEIN, S., M. A. JASNIS, M. DIAMENT, L. DAVEL, J. AGUIRRE & Y. P. DEBONAPARTE. 1994. Immunomodulation by soluble factors from tumor cells cultured in vivo in diffusion chambers. Tumor Biol. **15:** 160–165.

32. LEVON, S. A., D. A. MARYANOV, S. K. NEUENFELDT, T. J. THOMAS, J. H. BRAUKER & R. L. GELLER. 1995. Cancer immunotherapy utilizing an immunoisolation device. J. Cell. Biochem. **21B:** 9.

33. MATZINGER, P. 1994. Tolerance, danger and the extended family. Ann. Rev. Immunol. **12:** 901–1045.

34. HARDING, C. V. & R. SONG. 1994. Phagocytic processing of exogenous particulate antigens by macrophages for presentation by class I MHC molecules. J. Immunol. **153:** 4925–4933.

35. ROCK, K. L. 1996. A new foreign policy: MHC class I molecules monitor the outside world. Immunol. Today **17:** 131–137.

36. ZAUDERER, M. 1996. Special delivery for peptide-stimulated immunity. Nature Biotechnol. **14:** 703–704.

37. HUANG, A. Y. C., P. GOLUMBEK, M. AHMADZADEH, E. JAFFEE, D. PARDOLL & H. LEVITSKY. 1994. Role of bone marrow derived cells in presenting MHC class I-restricted tumor antigens. Science **264:** 961–965.

Human Fetal Striatal Transplantation in an Excitotoxic Lesioned Model of Huntington's Disease

P. R. SANBERG,[a,c] C. V. BORLONGAN,[a] T. K. KOUTOUZIS,[a]
R. B. NORGREN JR.,[b] D. W. CAHILL,[a] AND
T. B. FREEMAN[a]

[a]Division of Neurological Surgery and the Neuroscience Program
Departments of Surgery, Neurology, Psychiatry and Pharmacology
University of South Florida College of Medicine
Tampa, Florida 33612

[b]Department of Cell Biology and Anatomy
University of Nebraska Medical Center
Omaha, Nebraska 68198

Transplantation of fetal neural tissue into the adult brain was initially investigated to examine the developmental and regenerative capacity of the nervous system.[1,2] Intrastriatal transplantation has been a major focus of neural transplantation research because of the well-characterized anatomy of the normal striatum (or caudate-putamen). With many chemically identified types of striatal neurons and fiber systems, their reaction upon lesioning and transplantation could provide essential information about factors regulating, for instance, neuronal survival and differentiation. Apart from this initial goal of investigating CNS development and plasticity, neural grafting has been demonstrated to ameliorate the functional deficits induced by various brain lesions. Accordingly, it was suggested that neural grafting might be an appropriate treatment for various neurodegenerative disorders.[1,3]

NEURAL TRANSPLANTATION AND EXCITOTOXIC MODELS OF HUNTINGTON'S DISEASE

Neural transplantation has emerged as an alternative therapeutic modality for Parkinson's disease (PD).[4] Concrete evidence detailing functional and neuroanatomical recovery following fetal ventral mesencephalic cell transplantation has been reported in PD patients.[5,6] These promising developments in neural transplantation for PD and the demonstration of survival and efficacy of fetal striatal transplants into animal models of Huntington's disease (HD)[7,8] may validate clinical trials of neural transplantation for HD. Recently, Peschanski and colleagues[9] outlined the rationale for proceeding with clinical trials of fetal neural transplantation as a treatment modality for HD. Since several other research centers worldwide have set-up clinical trials for fetal neural transplantation for HD, the implications of the evidence from animal models should be closely evaluated.

[c] Author to whom correspondence should be addressed: Division of Neurological Surgery, Department of Surgery, University of South Florida College of Medicine, Tampa, FL 33612.

Selective excitotoxic compounds [*e.g.,* kainic acid (KA), ibotenic acid (IA), and quinolinic acid (QA)] have been used extensively to successfully create lesions in the striatum (or caudate-putamen) in humans, which is the primary brain structure damaged in HD[10] and to produce neurobehavioral symptoms similar to HD.[7,8] These excitotoxic animal models have also been used to characterize the potential effects of neural tranplantation. Investigations have shown that rodent fetal striatum transplanted into rodents (allografts)[8,11] or primates (xenografts)[1,2] can produce recovery of function. Further, xenografts of human fetal tissue can grow and integrate in the rodent brain provided immunosuppression is given.[11] However, there has been significant variability in the histological appearance of these grafts, most likely related to differences in the regions of dissection of the donor tissue.[12] Recently, Pakzaban and colleagues[13] demonstrated that selective dissection and transplantation of the rat lateral (but not medial) ganglionic eminence resulted in grafts consisting of primarily striatal-like tissue. The striatal lateral eminence dissected from E15 rat fetuses result in striatal transplants with more resemblance to the adult striatum than a combination of medial eminence and lateral eminences.[13]

Immunohistochemical characterization of the grafted tissue was first described using acetylcholinesterase (AChE) histochemistry.[14] Using specific neuroanatomical markers, AChE-rich (patch or P regions) and -poor (no patch or NP regions) areas have been identified within the grafts.[15] The AChE P regions of the grafts have been demonstrated to correspond to the appearance of neuronal phosphoprotein dopamine- and adenosine-3′,5′-monophosphate-regulated phosphoprotein (DARPP-32).[16] In addition, absence of DARPP-32 immunoreactive patches correspond to AChE NP regions. Together, these two immunohistochemical techniques have become standard ways to identify the grafted striatal tissue. A homogenous striatal-line graft generating a AChE-rich transplant has been demonstrated by selective dissection of striatal lateral eminence.[13]

Transplantation studies on animal models have been carried out using cell suspension or solid tissue transplant paradigms. Investigators who use the cell suspension technique have employed younger donor tissue (E14–15), while many investigators who use solid tissue transplants have utilized older tissue (E17–19).[17] Clinical studies in PD have shown positive results with solid tissue transplants of ventral mesencephalon, and its use may be more efficient in the actual surgical procedure since it requires less handling.[4–6,18] Therefore, it may be advantageous to similarly employ solid tissue transplants of fetal striatal lateral eminence in HD.

While clinical trials of neural transplantation on HD have begun based on preliminary data,[19,20] additional studies need to examine the ability of human fetal striatal tissue to develop in the host brain. The present study provides evidence that transplantation of sub-dissected human fetal striatal tissue derived from the fetal striatal lateral eminence survives and grows within the host brain, and produces gross behavioral recovery of animals with striatal excitotoxic lesions.

MATERIALS AND METHODS

Subjects

Eight week old male Sprague-Dawley rats obtained from Zivic Miller were used as subjects. The animals were housed in Plexiglas cages in a room with controlled temperature and humidity, and maintained on a 12 h light-dark cycle with lights on at 0700 am. Food and water were freely available in the house cage.

Surgery

The surgical procedures were carried out in sterile conditions. Animals were first anesthetized with sodium pentobarbital (60 mg/kg, i.p.) then placed in a Kopf stereotaxic frame. Bilateral (n = 8) or unilateral (n = 8) striatal lesions were made using 240 nmol of quinolinic acid (QA), dissolved in 0.90% saline with a pH of 7.4. Each animal received 1 μl of QA into the dorsolateral aspect of the striatum with coordinates set at AP: 3.0; ML: 1.5; DV: 4.5.[21] Recovery of each animal was constantly monitored following surgery.

Transplantation

Transplantation was performed between 1 and 2 months post-lesion. Tissue was obtained as described elsewhere,[22] and was in accordance with federal, state and local laws and in accordance with NIH guidelines. Selective abortion of fetuses was chosen with target fetal age window set at 7 to 9 weeks post-conception (PC). Dissection and staging for embryonic age was previously described.[12,23] The whole striatal lateral eminence and anterolateral ventricular eminence anterior to the foramen of monroe was dissected and stored in a hibernation medium. The tissue was kept refrigerated with a mean temperature maintained at 8°C.[24] Transplantation was carried out within 24 h to 48 h of the time tissue was obtained. Unilateral solid intraparenchymal transplantation was conducted as follows: a) striatal tissue was minced into 0.75 × 1.25 mm pieces in HBSS medium; b) a Hamilton syringe and 20-gauge spinal needle was used to suction the tissue pieces contained in about 1 μl of HBSS medium; c) the needle was lowered into position (AP: 3.2; ML: 1.5; DV: 4.5)[21] and 1 μl was infused over 1 min. An additional 1 min was allowed for diffusion before the needle was retracted. Eight bilaterally lesioned and 4 unilaterally lesioned animals were randomly selected and each animal received approximately ¼ of the whole striatal lateral eminence. Four other unilaterally lesioned animals received 1 μl of HBSS. Each animal's condition was closely monitored following transplantation and until the animal recovered. For immunosuppression, Cyclosporine-A (10 mg/kg/d, Sandoz Pharmaceutical) dissolved in olive oil was injected intraperitoneally (i.p.) every day starting on the day of surgery until the day the animals were sacrificed for histological purposes.

Behavioral Test

Eight unilaterally lesioned animals were tested for apomorphine-induced rotational behavior 2 weeks and 1 month post-lesion. Each animal was injected with apomorphine (1.0 mg/kg, i.p.) dissolved in normal saline with ascorbic acid. Immediately after injection, each animal was placed in a transparent Plexiglas box (40 × 40 × 35.5 cm) for visual observations of rotational behavior. All eight animals showed at least 8 rotations per min for 30 min at 1 month post-lesion. At 1 month post-transplant and once a month thereafter over a period of 4 months, these animals were again tested for apomorphine-induced rotational behavior.

Histochemistry

The 8 bilaterally lesioned animals that received fetal striatal transplants were sacrificed at 10 weeks post-transplant while the 8 unilaterally lesioned animals that

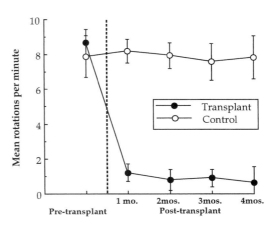

FIGURE   1. Apomorphine-induced rotations. Using Student's *t*-tests, transplanted animals exhibited significantly fewer apomorphine-induced rotations compared to control animals in all post-transplant tests (*t*'s > 26.93, df = 6, *p* < 0.001) or compared to their pre-transplant level (*t*'s > 30.12, df = 6, *p* < 0.001).

received either fetal striatal transplants or HBSS were sacrificed at about 16 weeks post-transplant. Animals were perfused with 300 ml phosphate buffered saline followed by 300 ml 4% paraformaldehyde. Free-floating frozen sections were cut at 10 microns. Sections were stained with cresyl violet or processed for acetylcholinesterase histochemistry.

RESULTS

Behavioral Effects

As early as 1 month post-transplant and continuing during the post-transplantation period, transplanted animals showed significant reductions in apomorphine-induced rotational behavior. Using Student's *t*-tests, transplanted animals exhibited significantly fewer apomorphine-induced rotations compared to control animals in all post-transplant tests (*t*'s > 26.93, df = 6, *p* < 0.001) or compared to their pre-transplant level (*t*'s > 30.12, df = 6, *p* < 0.001) (FIG. 1). For this behavioral measure there appeared to be no correlation with the appearance of AChE patches.

Cellular Changes

As seen in FIGURES 2A and 2B corresponding to brain sections from control animals which were lesioned but received HBSS instead of a transplant, both Nissl and AChE stains were light and revealed ventricular enlargement indicating loss of intrinsic striatal neurons. In lesioned animals which had recovered after receiving fetal striatal tissue, the transplanted tissue grossly resembled normal striatum. In addition, Nissl stains of brain sections from experimental animals revealed that transplanted fetal striatal tissue grows, integrates, and reconstitutes neural tissue that appeared mostly homogenous with densely packed cells and minimal obvious inflammatory/immunological reactions (FIG. 3A). This figure represents one of the largest grafts which grew and survived within the striatal area. In FIGURE 3B however, AChE was much less apparent within the transplanted tissue than in the

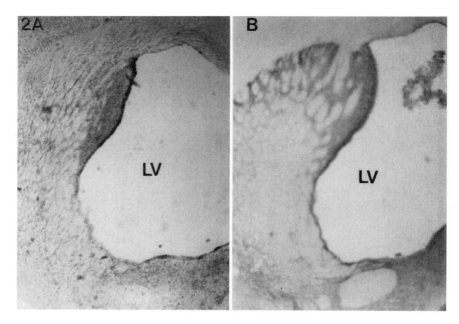

FIGURE 2. Representative brain sections of lesioned animals not receiving transplants. Left panel **(A)** corresponds to Nissl staining while right panel **(B)** corresponds to AChE staining. Both sections show pale stains indicating loss of intrinsic striatal neurons. Enlargement of the lateral ventricle (LV) is also observed.

host brain. Further evidence of graft placement and integration can be seen in FIGURES 3C and 3D. While the sections are more rostral than those indicated in 3A and 3B, the grafts are more compact and demonstrate more positive AChE staining. When AChE was present, there appeared to be an inverse correlation between the density of cells and the amount of AChE labeling in the graft.

DISCUSSION

The observation of behavioral recovery following fetal striatal transplantation in an excitotoxic rat model of HD was similar albeit earlier than that seen by Pundt and colleagues.[7] Of interest, while grafted tissue did not show consistent AChE staining, the observed behavioral recovery of rotational behavior was robust. Other studies have reported AChE-positive neuronal patches in grafted striatal tissue.[7,13,25] The present finding would suggest that, at least for this behavioral task, the functional effects of the graft are not necessarily related to such specific striatal cellular markers, a finding noted previously by Sanberg et al.[26] On the other hand, Dunnett and colleagues[11,27] report that the observation of striatal-like AChE-rich patches in striatal transplants from early rat donors may correlate with recovery of a more complex behavioral task.

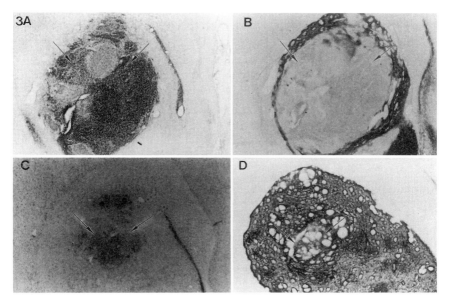

FIGURE 3. Representative brain sections of lesioned animals receiving human striatal transplants. Tissue in left panels (**A,C**) are stained for Nissl substance and right panels (**B,D**) are stained for AChE. The upper panels (**A,B**) correspond to sections through the mid-portion of the graft while the graft in the lower panels (**C,D**) to sections through the anterior pole of the graft. The large grafts are Nissl positive throughout (**A,C**) while AChE staining is more prominent at its anterior pole (**D**).

The absence of AChE stains in many of the present grafts may be due to the following:

1. An early maturation period of 10–16 weeks prior to histological analysis in the present study may have resulted in primarily small densely packed cells, which are likely AChE-negative progenitor cells. A longer post-transplantation period may reveal AChE-positive large neurons as the grafted cells mature and begin "dendritic-arborization." It has been demonstrated by Henderson[28] that in the ferret brain cholinergic pathways form early in the prenatal period but express transmitter function late in postnatal life.
2. The present transplantation technique of solid transplants may have resulted in each animal receiving a different portion of the fetal striatal dissection. It could be assumed that not all tissue areas are as homogeneous in regards to AChE, therefore a suspension technique may provide a better distribution of AChE viable tissue across animals.[18] Finally, assumptions regarding the development of the striatum originating in the lateral ganglionic eminence are based extensively on research from other species.[12]

Recently, Brundin and collegues[25,29] have also shown that a more complex motor and cognitive deficit recovery may be related to increased density of AChE-rich patches in human fetal tissue striatal transplants. They have argued that fetal tissue transplantation should not be performed in HD patients until further studies demonstrate effective behavioral functional recovery with the transplant showing at least 30% AChE-rich like patches. However in their cell suspension transplants of human lateral ganglionic eminence into the rodent model,[29] they have observed no greater than 10% AChE patches similar to the present study.

Nevertheless, early improvement in more generalized motor behavior has been seen in animals given either fetal striatal allografts[26,30,31] or human xenografts (present study) which may not contain AChE-rich patches.

It is possible that such early general motoric behavioral recovery in animals may be related to possible clinically significant improvement in the generalized choreiform movements associated with HD patients. Such movements are exaggerated during arousal and decrease significantly during repose.[16] A decrease in generalized hyperactivity in animals seems to be seen consistently by most fetal striatal transplantation research with or without striatal-like patches. It is possible therefore, that the preliminary reports of early significant recovery described in patients thus far that have received fetal striatal transplantation, if correct, may be related to non-specific effects of the transplants (*e.g.* trophic factors, *etc.*) as compared to specific long-term circuitry changes and concomitant increases in striatal-like patches.[19] While the rationale for commencement of neural transplantation in HD has been outlined,[9] critical evaluation of existing data and further animal experiments are needed to properly direct subsequent clinical trials.[29,32]

REFERENCES

1. BJORKLUND, A. 1991. Neural transplantation–an experimental tool with clinical possibilities. Trends Neurosci. **14:** 319–322.
2. GAGE, F. H. & L. J. FISHER. 1991. Intracerebral grafting: A tool for the neurobiologist. Neuron **6:** 1–12.
3. DUNNETT, S. B. & C. N. SVENDSEN. 1993. Huntington's disease: Animal models and transplantation repair. Curr. Opin. Neurobiol. **3:** 790–796.
4. OLANOW, C. W., J. H. KORDOWER & T. B. FREEMAN. 1996. Fetal nigral transplantation as a therapy for Parkinson's disease. TINS **19:** 102–109.
5. KORDOWER, J. H., T. B. FREEMAN, B. J. SNOW, F. J. G. VINGERHOETS, E. J. MUFSON, P. R. SANBERG, R. A. HAUSER, D. A. SMITH, G. M. NAUERT, D. P. PERL & C. W. OLANOW. 1995. Neuropathological evidence of graft survival and striatal reinnervation after the transplantation of fetal mesencephalic tissue in a patient with Parkinson's disease. New Engl. J. Med. **332:** 1118–1124.
6. FREEMAN, T. B., C. W. OLANOW, R. A. HAUSER, G. M. NAUERT, D. A. SMITH, C. V. BORLONGAN, P. R. SANBERG, D. A. HOLT, J. H. KORDOWER, F. J. C. VINGERHOETS, B. J. SNOW, C. CALNE & L. L. GAUGER. 1995. Bilateral fetal nigral transplantation into the postcommissural putamen in Parkinson's disease. Ann Neurol. **38:** 379–388.
7. PUNDT, L. L., T. KONDOH, J. A. CONRAD & W. C. LOW. 1995. Human fetal striatum exhibits viable tissue and cells for transplantation from donors 7–18 weeks in gestation. Soc. Neurosci. Abstr. **20:** 473.
8. SANBERG, P. R., M. A. HENAULT, S. H. HAGENMEYER-HOUSER, M. GIORDANO & K. H. RUSSELL. 1987. Multiple transplants of fetal striatal tissue in the kainic acid model of Huntinton's disease: Behavioral recovery may not be related to acetylcholinesterase. Ann. N. Y. Acad. Sci. **495:** 781–5.
9. PESCHANSKI, M., P. CESARO & P. HANTRAYE. 1995. Rationale for intrastriatal grafting of striatal neuroblasts in patients with Huntington's disease. Neuroscience **68:** 273–285.
10. NEILL, D. B., J. F. ROSS & S. P. GROSSMAN. 1974. Effects of lesions in the dorsal and ventral striatum on locomotor activity and on locomotor effects of amphetamine. Pharmacol. Biochem. Behav. **2:** 697–702.
11. BJORKLUND, A., K. CAMPBELL, D. J. S. SIRINATHSINGHJI, R. A. FRICKER & S. B. DUNNETT.

1994. Functional capacity of striatal transplants in the rat Huntington model. In Functional Neural Transplantation. A. Bjorklund & S. B. Dunnett, Eds. Raven Press. New York, pp. 157–195.

12. FREEMAN, T. B., P. R. SANBERG & O. ISACSON. 1995. Development of the human striatum for fetal striatal transplantation in the treatment of Huntington's disease. Cell Transplant. **4:** 539–545.

13. PAKZABAN, P., T. W. DEACON, L. H. BURNS & O. ISACSON. 1993. Increased proportion of acetylcholinesterase-rich zones and improved morphological integration in host striatum of fetal grafts derived from the lateral but not the medial ganglionic eminence. Exp. Brain Res. **97:** 13–22.

14. ISACSON, O., D. DAWBARN, P. BRUNDIN, F. H. GAGE & A. BJORKLUND. 1987. Neural grafting in a rat model of Huntington's disease: Striosomal-like organization of striatal grafts as revealed by immunocytochemistry and receptor autoradiography. Neuroscience **22:** 481–497.

15. GRAYBIEL, A. M., F. C. LIU & S. B. DUNNETT. 1989. Intrastriatal grafts derived from fetal striatal primordia. I. Phenotypy and modular organization. J. Neurosci. **9:** 3250–3271.

16. WICTORIN, K. & A. BJORKLUND. 1989. Connectivity of striatal grafts implanted into the ibotenic acid lesioned striatum. II. Cortical afferents. Neuroscience **30:** 297–311.

17. WICTORIN, K. 1992. Anatomy and connectivity of intrastriatal striatal transplants. Prog. Neurobiol. **38:** 611–639.

18. FREEMAN, T. B., P. R. SANBERG, G. M. NAUERT, B. D. BOSS, D. SPECTOR, C. W. OLANOW & J. H. KORDOWER. 1995. The influence of donor age on the survival of solid and suspension intraparenchymal human embryonic nigral grafts. Cell Transplant. **4:** 141–154.

19. KURTH, M. C., O. KOPYOV & D. B. JAQUES. 1996. Six month follow-up of motor function after fetal transplantation in a patient with Huntington's disease. Amer. Soc. Neur. Transplant. Abstr. **3:** 15.

20. MADRAZO, I., R. E. FRANCO-BOURLAND, H. CASTREJON, C. CUEVAS & F. OSTROSKY-SOLIS. 1995. Fetal striatal homotransplantation for Huntington's disease: First two case reports. Neurol. Res. **17:** 312–315.

21. PAXINOS, G. & C. WATSON. 1984. The Rat Brain In Stereotaxic Coordinates. Sydney. Academic Press.

22. NAUERT, M. & T. B. FREEMAN. 1994. Low pressure aspiration abortion for obtaining embryonic and early gestational fetal tissue for research purposes. Cell Transplant. **3:** 147–151.

23. FREEMAN, T. B., M. S. SPENCE, B. D. BOSS, D. H. SPECTOR, R. E. STRECKER, C. W. OLANOW & J. H. KORDOWER. 1991. Development of dopaminergic neurons in the human substantia nigra. Exp. Neurol. **113:** 344–353.

24. FREEMAN, T. B. & J. H. KORDOWER. 1991. Human cadaver embryonic substantia nigra grafts: Effects of ontogeny, pre-operative graft preparation and tissue storage. *In* Intracerebral Transplants in Movement Disorders. O. Lindvalle & A. Bjorklund, Eds.: 163–170. Elsevier Science Publishers, B.V. Amsterdam.

25. NAKAO, N., E. M. GRABSON-FRODI, H. WIDNER & P. BRUNDIN. 1996. DARP-32 rich zones in grafts of lateral ganglionic eminence govern the extent of the functional recovery in skilled-paw-reaching in an animal model of Huntington's disease. Am. Soc. Neural Transplant. Abstr. **3:** 39.

26. SANBERG, P. R., M. A. HENAULT & W. A. DECKEL. 1986. Locomotor hyperactivity: Effects of multiple striatal transplants in an animal model of Huntington's disease. Pharmacol. Biochem. Behav. **25:** 297–300.

27. FRICKER, R. A., E. M. TORRES, S. P. HUME & S. B. DUNNETT. 1994. Functional striatal grafts: Correlations between positron emission tomography in vivo, graft survival, and recovery of reaching behavior. Soc. Neurosci. Abst. **20:** 473.

28. HENDERSON, Z. 1991. Early development of the nucleus basalis-cortical projection but late expression of its cholinergic function. Neuroscience **44:** 311–324.

29. BRUNDIN, P., R. A. FRICKER & N. NAKAO. 1996. Paucity of P-zones in striatal grafts prohibits commencement of clinical trials in Huntington's disease. Neuroscience **71:** 895–897.

30. SANBERG, P. R. & J. T. COYLE. 1984. Scientific approaches to Huntington's disease. CRC Rev. Clinic. Neurobiol. **1:** 1–44.
31. SANBERG, P. R., K. WICTORIN & O. ISACSON. 1994. O. Cell transplantation for Huntington's disease. Medical Intelligence Unit, R. G. Landes, Co., CRC Press. Boca Raton, FL.
32. BORLONGAN, C. V., S. POLGAR, T. B. FREEMAN, D. W. CAHILL, R. A. HAUSER & P. R. SANBERG. 1996. Will fetal striatal transplantation correct the akinetic stage of Huntington's disease? Neurodegeneration. **5:** 189–195.

Microcapsules as Bio-organs for Somatic Gene Therapy[a]

PATRICIA L. CHANG[b]

Departments of Pediatrics, Biology and Biomedical Sciences
McMaster University
Hamilton, Ontario L8N 3Z5 Canada

Treatment of human diseases with gene therapy is a technological breakthrough that has been touted to be the ultimate medicine. As of September, 1990 when the first human clinical trial was initiated, the number of human gene therapy trials has been increasing at an exponential rate. Currently, over 150 clinical protocols involving gene transfer have been approved by the NIH Recombinant DNA Advisory Committee, and over 1000 patients worldwide have been recruited for these studies. The NIH spends about \$200 million a year to fund gene therapy-related work while the biotechnology private industry spends about an equal amount for similar purposes.[1] As the human genome project is scheduled to be completed ahead of the projected date of 2005, the potential for therapeutic application within the next decade is likely to be substantial.

In spite of the tremendous potential of this new medical technology, gene therapy either through the *ex vivo* (genetic alteration of the patient's explanted tissue followed by re-implantation), or through the *in vivo* (direct injection of DNA encoding desired therapeutic gene) route has not demonstrated definitive clinical efficacy.[2] Many technological problems (lack of efficient and effective vectors, insufficient levels of expression, unpredictable outcomes) have yet to be overcome.[3] Furthermore, the potentially high cost for patient-specific genetic modification required for the above procedures has not even been assessed. To address some of these concerns, we have proposed an alternative strategy of non-autologous somatic gene therapeutics.[4] Instead of engineering patient-specific recombinant cells each time a patient is treated, we envisioned creating a universal recombinant cell line expressing a desirable gene product for implantation in all patients suffering from the same product deficiency. Such a universal cell line can be thoroughly evaluated for safety, stored in liquid nitrogen, and restored to grow in culture whenever a patient is to be treated. The elimination of patient-specific genetic modification may thus lower the cost of such gene therapy treatment. The use of the same recombinant cell line will also ensure a more predictable outcome in different patients.

To protect the recombinant cells from immune rejection after implantation, we have adopted the technique of immuno-isolation used in tissue transplantation.[5] Microcapsules fabricated from biocompatible material are used as micro bio-organs to enclose the recombinant cells for re-implantation. The permeability threshold

[a] The author is grateful to the NSERC for a strategic grant, the Ontario Mental Health Foundation, the Canadian Hemophilia Society and the Miles/Canadian Red Cross Society for support.
[b] Address for correspondence: Department of Pediatrics, Room 3N18, McMaster University Medical Centre, 1200 Main Street West, Hamilton, Ontario L8N 3Z5 Canada; Tel: (905) 521-2100 Ext. 3716; Fax: (905) 521-1703; E-mail: changp@fhs.mcmaster.ca

461

TABLE 1. Construction of Cell Lines Secreting Proteins of Different Molecular Weights

Secreted Protein	Molecular Weight	Plasmid Vector	Parental Cell Line	Recombinant Cell Line
Human growth hormone (hGH)	27,100	pNMG3	Mouse Ltk⁻	LhGH1 (1C5)
Rat serum albumin (rSA)	68,000	Rldn 10b-cALB	Mouse Ltk⁻	LRSA-1 (3D5)
Human arylsulfatase A (hASA)	120,000	Rldn 10b-cARA	Mouse Rec⁻	RASA-1 (1B1)
Mouse β-hexosaminidase (β-HEX)	120,000	(constitutive)	Mouse Rec⁻	2A50
Human immunoglobulin (IgG)	154,000	EBV	Human B Cells	JU-EBV
Mouse β-glucuronidase (β-GLU)	300,000	pMSXND-MβG	Mouse Rec⁻	2A50

Plasmid vector DNA that encoded the cDNA for the different recombinant gene products was transfected into their parental cell lines by calcium phosphate precipitation. The IgG-producing cell line was transformed with Epstein-Barr Virus (EBV) only. After selection with G418, the resistant transfected clones were isolated and screened for expression of the various recombinant gene products. (Data from Awrey et al.,[12] with permission.)

of these microcapsules is thought to limit the diffusion of molecules >150 kD such as the immunoglobulins and the host's lymphocytes, which are responsible for tissue rejections. Hence, recombinant products smaller than this molecular weight cut-off are thought to be appropriate targets for delivery while those with larger molecular weights are excluded on theoretical grounds. We have now succeeded in demonstrating the principle of this approach both *in vitro* and *in vivo*, and gained further insights into the role of permeability in such immuno-isolation devices.

IN VITRO STUDIES

Microcapsules fabricated from the sea-weed extract alginate composed of repeating blocks of L-guluronic and D-mannuronic acids[6] have been used successfully in many *in vitro* and *in vivo* studies.[7–10] They are biocompatible and capable of maintaining the appropriate permeability characteristics of a desirable immuno-isolation device. To verify the permeability of these capsules to recombinant gene products, we constructed a series of cell lines expressing recombinant gene products of molecular weights ranging from ~27 to 300,000 (TABLE 1). Cells secreting these gene products were encapsulated in microcapsules fabricated from alginate, cross-linked with calcium ions and laminated on the surface with poly-L-lysine and alginate.[11] As expected, molecules of lower than 150 kD such as human growth hormone and albumin were readily recovered from the cultured media of these encapsulated cells (FIG. 1,A and B). However, molecules of sizes including the desired limit of 150 kD were also readily recovered in the culture media (IgG, FIG. 1D). When the alginate microcapsules were reinforced with an additional coat of poly-L-lysine and alginate membrane on the surface, the permeability threshold was sufficient to prevent the exit of large recombinant molecules such as β-glucuronidase (300 kD).

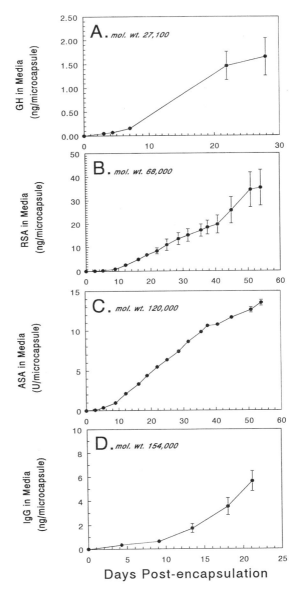

FIGURE 1. Accumulation of recombinant gene products of different sizes from microencapsulated recombinant cells. The total amounts of marker proteins secreted by the recombinant cells and accumulated in the cell culture media were ascertained by assaying aliquots in triplicate at the indicated time points, (Av. ± S.D.). (Data from Awrey et al.,[12] with permission.)

    A: hGH—human growth hormone;
    B: RSA—rat albumin;
    C: ASA—human arylsulfatase A;
    D: hIgG—human IgG.

However, this improvement was transient. After two weeks in culture, the double-coated microcapsules were no longer able to prevent the leakage of such high-molecular weight molecules into the media (FIG. 2). Hence, when the traditional type of alginate microcapsules was used as an immuno-isolation device for recombinant cells, the expected permeability threshold of <150 kD was not maintained.[12]

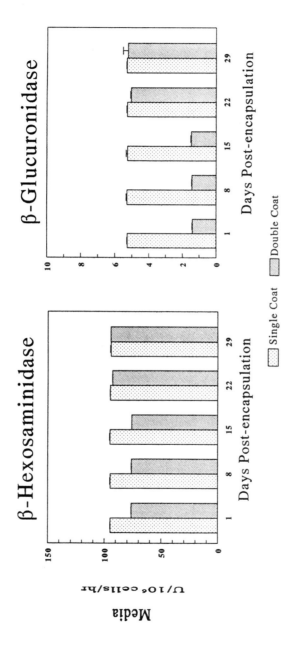

FIGURE 2. Effect of the number of membrane coats on permeability of microcapsules to secreted gene products. The recombinant cell line 2A50 secreting β-hexosaminidase (MW 120,000) and β-glucuronidase (MW 300,000) was encapsulated according to the routine procedure except before the liquefaction step with sodium citrate, half of the microcapsules were subjected to an additional round of polylysine and alginate wash. This created an additional coat of membrane and the microcapsules were considered as double-coated. The microcapsules processed regularly with a single round of polylysine and alginate wash were considered as single-coated. On various days post-encapsulation, aliquots of the microcapsules were removed for determination of the rate of the enzyme secretion into the media. (Data from Awrey et al.,[12] with permission.)

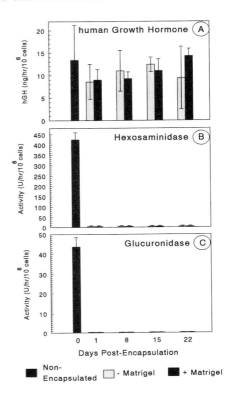

FIGURE 3. Secretion of marker proteins from HEMA-MMA microcapsules. Mouse fibroblasts engineered to secrete human growth hormone **(A)** or mouse lysosomal enzymes **(B, C)** were encapsulated in HEMA-MMA microcapsules, in the presence(+) or absence(−) of the matrix material Matrigel. Secretion rates of gene products from encapsulated cells were determined in triplicate (average ± S.D.) and compared to the non-encapsulated cells on day 0. On the day of the assay, the capsules were washed and incubated with pre-equilibrated fresh medium. Aliquots were removed at timed intervals for the determination of the secretion rates of the gene products. (From Tse *et al.*,[13] reprinted with permission.)

However, when an alternate biomaterial, a synthetic thermoplastic fabricated from hydroxyethyl methacrylate-methyl methacrylate (HEMA-MMA) was used to encapsulate these recombinant cells,[13] molecules of high molecular weights such as β-hexosaminidase (120 kD) or β-glucuronidase (300 kD) were totally impeded from passage through the membranes. The small molecular weight species such as human growth hormone (27 kD) were readily secreted to the external medium (FIG. 3). The loss of a clear molecular weight cutoff in the alginate microcapsules[12] may be related to the process of encapsulation. When the alginate capsules were first extruded together with the cells as a suspension, some of the cells may have lodged in the periphery of the gelled spheres. These sites of cellular protrusion will interrupt the subsequent laminating steps, thus creating pores in the membrane.[14] In comparison, the method of encapsulating cells within HEMA-MMA microcapsules by interfacial precipitation does not require mixing cells with the membrane-forming constituents.[15] Therefore, the membrane integrity is not perturbed and the permeability is thus maintained (FIG. 4).

DELIVERY OF RECOMBINANT GENE PRODUCTS TO RODENTS

Since recombinant gene products can be produced from encapsulated cells, the feasibility of delivery *in vivo* was tested by intraperitoneal implantation of the

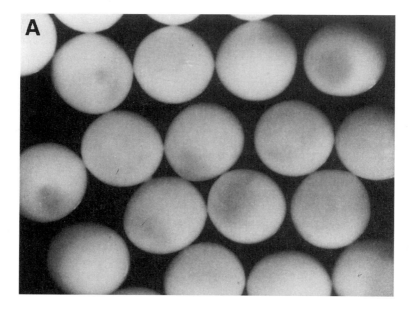

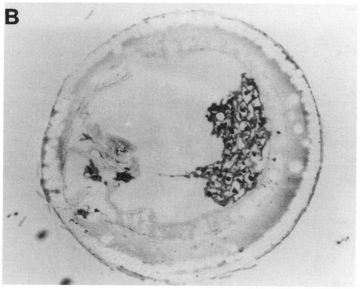

FIGURE 4. Morphology and histology of the HEMA-MMA microcapsules. The thermoplastic microcapsules fabricated from thermoplastic HEMA-MMA were photographed under light microscopy to show the smooth and spherical opaque surface of the capsules **(A)**. The microcapsules containing 2A50 cells in Matrigel were sectioned, stained with toluidine blue, and examined with light microscopy at day 22 post-encapsulation, magnification : 100 × **(B)**. The continuity of the outer membrane and the confinement of the inner stained cell mass were evident. (From Tse et al.,[13] reprinted with permission.)

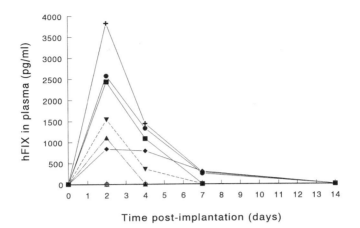

FIGURE 5. Human FIX delivered to mouse plasma. Four normal C57BL/6 mice (+, ●, ◆, ■) were implanted intraperitoneally with 5×10^6 and two mice (▲, ▼) with 8×10^5 microencapsulated recombinant myoblasts (MLhFIX-5D5). Four control mice (+, ○, △, ◇) were injected with 5×10^6 unencapsulated MLhFIX-5D5 myoblasts. Human FIX secretion into mouse plasma was detected by ELISA with a sensitivity of ≥ 200 pg/ml of human factor IX. (Data reproduced from Hortelano *et al.*[17] with permission.)

alginate-poly-L-lysine-alginate microcapsules into mice. It was demonstrated that mouse fibroblasts (Ltk⁻) engineered to secrete human growth hormone can deliver physiological level of the human growth hormone to the mice.[16] This method of delivery was further refined to deliver human clotting factor IX, the coagulation factor whose deficiency is responsible for hemophilia B.[17] The important modifications included the use of an alternate form of alginate to improve the stability of the microcapsules and change of cell type from fibroblasts to mouse myoblasts (C2C12). The advantage of using myoblasts is that they can potentially be differentiated terminally into myotubes under appropriate growth conditions from the proliferative myoblasts.[18] The proliferative capability of fibroblasts and myoblasts is necessary for gene transfer and genetic modification. However, their indefinite growth in the limited space of the microcapsules would have caused eventual cell death and necrosis when space and nutrient exchange became limiting. With this strategy of implanting encapsulated myoblast-myotube, human factor IX was detected in the plasma of the mouse. However, as was observed before in the delivery of a xenogenic protein, human growth hormone, to mice,[16] the factor IX also subsided to undetectable levels after 14 days (FIG. 5). However, this disappearance was not due to the loss of microcapsule function or gene expression from the encapsulated cells. Microcapsules recovered from the implanted animals even up to day 213 post-implantation still remained intact and continued to secrete human factor IX *in vitro*.[17] It appeared that the human factor IX provoked an antigenic response from the murine recipients, thus causing it to become cleared from the circulation at accelerated rates (FIG. 6). Therefore, the lack of detectable human factor IX in the circulation after two weeks was not due to the lack of factor IX delivery but rather due to the development of anti-factor IX antibodies. This was further supported by the detection of high titer of mouse anti-human factor IX antibodies in the

FIGURE 6. Increased clearance of hFIX from plasma of mice implanted with encapsulated hFIX-secreting myoblasts. Intraperitoneal injections of 6 μg of purified hFIX were administered to each of **(A)** three mice (mouse **B, C,** and **D** from FIG. 5) implanted seven months earlier with encapsulated hFIX-secreting myoblasts (MLhFIX-5D5), **(B)** three mice implanted with the same volume of encapsulated cells not secreting hFIX, and **(C)** three naive mice as controls. Blood samples were drawn at 3, 6 and 24 h post-injection. ELISA was performed on samples to determine hFIX in plasma. (Data are averages ± SEM, reproduced from Hortelano et al.,[17] with permission.)

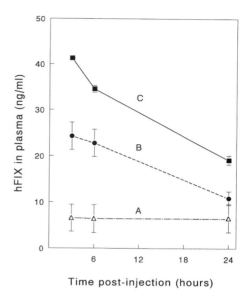

animals implanted with the encapsulated recombinant cells even up to day 213 (FIG. 7). Thus, it was clear that micro-encapsulated recombinant cells are capable of long-term delivery of a recombinant gene product in vivo.

TREATMENT OF ANIMAL MODELS OF HUMAN GENETIC DISEASES

Since growth hormone is species specific, its growth-enhancing biological activity could not be demonstrated when human growth hormone was delivered to the mice from the encapsulated cells.[16] However, when the Snell dwarf mice deficient in growth hormone production[19] were implanted with encapsulated mouse myoblasts engineered to secrete *mouse* growth hormone, the growth enhancing effects were clearly demonstrated (FIG. 8). Both the body weight and body length of the treated animals increased significantly over those of the controls implanted with either unencapsulated recombinant cells or encapsulated but non-transfected myoblasts.[20]

Although the clinical efficacy of this non-autologous gene therapy is demonstrated in this model of growth-hormone deficiency, this model is unlikely to be useful in clinical practice. Recombinant purified human growth hormone is readily available for patient treatments and the intricate circadian rhythm of growth hormone secretion is difficult to reproduce. However, the potential use of this approach is highly appropriate for diseases that do not require tight metabolic regulation, that are devastating, and that can be improved with low constitutive delivery of a recombinant product. The lysosomal storage diseases appear to be ideal models for this treatment protocol. They are catastrophic illnesses caused by deficient lysosomal enzymes; they have few treatment strategies that are clinically effective; and even individuals with less than 10% of normal enzyme activity can be clinically quite normal. In addition, these enzymes are present in almost all tissues in the

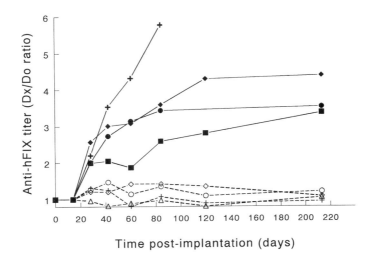

Time post-implantation (days)

FIGURE 7. Development of anti-hFIX antibodies in the implanted mice. Four C57BL/6 mice (+, ◆, ●, ■) were implanted with 5×10^6 microencapsulated MLhFIX-5D5 and four control mice (+, ○, △, ◇) were injected with 5×10^6 unencapsulated recombinant myoblasts. One mouse (+) died on Day 78 from accidental anesthetic overdose. Antibodies against hFIX in plasma were detected by ELISA. The ratio of absorbance for a particular day and mouse (Dx) over that of the same mouse at day 0 (D0) was used to indicate antibody titer. Plasma from mice immunized with purified hFIX (Dx/Do = 9.17 ± 0.39) was included in all assays as a positive control. (Data reproduced from Hortelano et al.,[17] with permission.)

body and their production does not appear to be tightly regulated. Since the gus^{mps}/gus^{mps} mouse is an authentic model of the human lysosomal storage disease mucopolysaccharidosis type VII or Sly disease,[21,22] it was an ideal model to test the clinical efficacy of the above strategy. When microcapsules enclosing mouse cells engineered to secrete the missing lysosomal enzyme β-glucuronidase were implanted intraperitoneally into these mutant mice, within 2–4 weeks significant levels of the enzymes were recovered from plasma, liver, spleen and kidney (TABLE 2). The typical lysosomal inclusions observed in the untreated mutants were also greatly reduced to almost normal appearance on histological examination.[23] Hence, the implantation of micro-encapsulated recombinant cells secreting lysosomal enzymes was effective in delivering the enzyme to the circulation as well as to various peripheral organs. The enzyme appeared to be adequately endocytosed into the relevant target organelles so that the accumulated substrates in the lysosomes could be cleared. These results appear promising for further clinical evaluation of non-autologous implantation as a strategy for the treatment of lysosomal storage diseases.

In conclusion, using microcapsules as bio-organs for gene therapy is a novel approach that has now been demonstrated to be clinically effective. However, the success with treating rodent models of human genetic diseases still has to be translated to larger animal models closer to the human species. For this endeavor, much work remains to study the structural and the biocompatible properties of the implant material, the efficacy and safety of the cell lines, the performance of the transfecting vectors, and finally the host's immune response to such implants. However, clinical

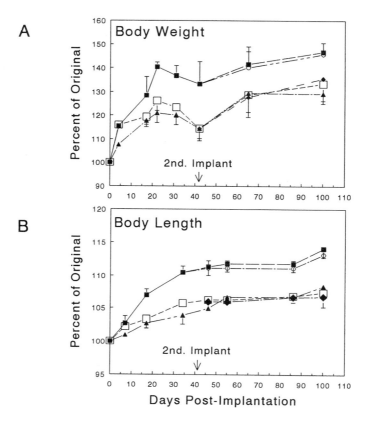

FIGURE 8. Encapsulated mouse growth hormone-secreting myoblasts enhanced the growth of Snell dwarf mice. On day 0, three groups of 6–7 week-old Snell dwarf mice (male) were implanted intraperitoneally with either 3 ml of microcapsules containing 7.2×10^5 mGH-secreting **Myo-45** myoblasts (Group A: ■, N = 5) or 2 ml of microcapsules containing 2.4×10^5 of non-transfected C_2C_{12} myoblasts (Group B: □, N = 6 , or $\sim7 \times 10^5$ mGH-secreting Myo-45 myoblasts without encapsulation (Group C: ▲, N = 3). On day 42, one Group A and two Group B mice were sacrificed for autopsy studies and retrieval of microcapsules. The remaining four mice in each of groups A and B were subdivided into two groups and re-implanted with 3 ml of microcapsules containing either 4×10^5 mGH-secreting Myo-45 myoblasts (■ or ◆, N = 2) or 5.6×10^5 non-transfected C_2C_{12} myoblasts (□ or ○, N = 2). **(A)** The body weights are represented as means ± SD (N ≥ 3) or range (N = 2). The slight weight loss between days 22–42 coincided with an accidental rise in ambient temperature in our animal facilities. **(B)** The body lengths were measured under anesthesia as the distance between the tip of the nose and the end of the tail (Mean ± SD or range if N < 3). Significant differences in weight ($p < 0.025$) and length ($p < 0.0005$) between Group A and Group B or C were found at day 17 post-implantation and thereafter (Student's t-test). (Data reproduced from Al-Hendy *et al.*,[20] with permission.)

TABLE 2. The Levels of β-Glucuronidase Restored in the Various Organ Systems of the Gus^{MPS}/Gus^{MPS} Mouse by 4 Weeks Post-implantation

% of Normal	Liver	Spleen	Kidney	Brain
Mutant Control (N = 3)	0.01	0.01	0.01	0.23
Treated Mutant				
week 2 (N = 3)	11.3	18.0	60.0	3.0
week 4 (N = 3)	43.5	65.8	20.2	11.5

Five ml of alginate microcapsules enclosing an MPR⁻ mouse fibroblast cell line transfected with the mouse β-glucuronidase cDNA and secreting 510 U/10^6 cells/h were implanted intraperitoneally into each of 9 MPSVII mice. At week-2 and -4 post-implantation, the treated mice were sacrificed for biochemical, histological and histochemical studies. (Data from Bastedo et al.,[23] with permission)

trials using either terminally differentiated cells or recombinant cells in either alginate or thermoplastic capsules have already been initiated.[24,25] With the high level of interest from the biotechnology sectors, the potential benefit to the patients, and possible reduction in such health care costs, this strategy of bio-organ implantation for gene therapy is likely to become a useful addition to modern medicine.

SUMMARY

Current human gene therapy relies on genetic modification of the patient's own cells. An alternate non-autologous approach is to use universal cell lines engineered to secrete therapeutic products. Protection with immuno-isolation devices would allow the same recombinant cell line to be used for different patients, thus potentially lowering the cost of treatment. The feasibility of this idea has now been demonstrated *in vitro* and *in vivo*. Recombinant gene products with potential therapeutic applications (human growth hormone, factor IX, lysosomal enzymes, adenosine deaminase) have been expressed from genetically modified cells after encapsulation with alginate-poly-L-lysine-alginate or hydroxyethyl methacrylate-methyl methacrylate. We have also demonstrated the feasibility of this idea *in vivo*. After intraperitoneal implantation, genetically modified mouse Ltk⁻ fibroblasts or C2C12 myoblasts encapsulated in alginate-poly-L-lysine-alginate could deliver recombinant gene products (human growth hormone, human factor IX) to the systemic circulation of mice. The clinical efficacy of this novel approach to gene therapy has now been shown in murine models of human diseases. In the Snell dwarf mice deficient in growth hormone production, implantation of encapsulated mouse myoblasts engineered to secrete mouse growth hormone resulted in increases in body weight, length and organ sizes, some to >25% above those of the controls. In the Gus/Gus mice suffering from the lysosomal storage disease mucopolysaccharidosis type VII due to deficient β-glucuronidase, implantation of encapsulated mouse fibroblasts engineered to secrete mouse β-glucuronidase resulted in delivery of normal levels of the enzyme in the plasma and significant correction of the organ histopathology. Hence, delivery of recombinant gene products through bioartificial devices appears to be a promising strategy for the treatment of genetic diseases.

ACKNOWLEDGMENTS

The author would like to thank the many students, associates and colleagues who have helped in developing this program, in particular Ms. L. Bastedo, Ms. M. Tse, Drs. D. Awrey, A. Al-Hendy, G. Hortelano, M. V. Sefton and M. Sands, and Dr. Tracy Stockley for reading the manuscript.

REFERENCES

1. WADMAN, M. 1995. Hyping results 'cold damage' gene therapy. Science **378:** 655.
2. NIH Report. 1995. Report and Recommendations of the Panel to Assess the NIH Investment in Research on Gene Therapy.
3. CRYSTAL, R. G. 1995. Transfer of genes to humans: Early lessons and obstacles to success. Science **270:** 404–410.
4. CHANG, P. L. 1995. Nonautologous somatic gene therapy. In Somatic Gene Therapy. P. L. Chang, Ed.: 203–223. CRC Press Inc. Boca Raton FL.
5. CHANG, T. M. S. 1964. Semipermeable microcapsules. Science **146:** 524–525.
6. SMIDSRØD, O. 1974. Molecular basis for some physical properties of alginates in the gel state. Faraday Disc. Chem. Soc. **57:** 263.
7. GOOSEN, M. F. A., G. M. O'SHEA, H. GHARAPETIAN, S. CHOU & A. M. SUN. 1985. Optimization of microcapsulation parameters: Semipermeable microcapsules as a bioartificial pancreas. Biotechnol. Bioeng. **27:** 146.
8. KING, G. A., A. J. DAUGULIS, P. FAULKNER & M. F. A. GOOSEN. 1987. Alginate-polylysine microcapsules of controlled membrane molecular weight cutoff for mammalian cell culture engineering. Biotechnol. Prog. **3:** 231.
9. LIM, F. & A. M. SUN. 1980. Microencapsulated islets as bioartificial endocrine pancreas. Science **210:** 908–910.
10. CHANG, T. M. S. 1995. Artificial cells with emphasis on bioencapsulation in biotechnology. Biotechnol. Ann. Rev. **1:** 267–295.
11. LIU, H.-W., F. A. OFOSU & P. L. CHANG. 1993. Expression of human factor IX by microencapsulated recombinant fibroblasts. Hum. Gene Ther. **4:** 291–301.
12. AWREY, D. E., M. TSE, G. HORTELANO & P. L. CHANG. 1996. Permeability of alginate microcapsules to secretory recombinant gene products. Biotechnol. Bioeng. In press.
13. TSE, M., H. ULUDAG, M. V. SEFTON & P. L. CHANG. 1996. Secretion of recombinant proteins from hydroxyethyl methacrylate-methyl methacrylate capsules. Biotechnol. Bioeng. **51:** 271–280.
14. WONG, H. & T. M. CHANG. 1991. The microencapsulation of cells within alginate poly-L-lysine microcapsules prepared with the standard single step drop technique: Histologically identified membrane imperfections and the associated graft rejection. Biomater. Art. Cells Immobil. Biotechnol. **19:** 675–86.
15. ULUDAG, H. & M. V. SEFTON. 1993. Microencapsulated human hepatoma cells: In vitro growth and protein release. J. Biomed. Mater. Res. **27:** 1213–1224.
16. CHANG, P. L., N. SHEN & A. J. WESTCOTT. 1993. Delivery of recombinant gene products with microencapsulated cells in vivo. Hum. Gene Ther. **4:** 433–440.
17. HORTELANO, G., A. AL-HENDY, F. A. OFOSU & P. L. CHANG. 1996. Delivery of human factor IX in mice by encapsulated recombinant myoblasts: a novel approach towards allogeneic gene therapy of hemophilia B. Blood **87:** 5095–5103.
18. BLAU, H. M., J. DHAWAN & G. K. PAVLATH. 1993. Myoblasts in pattern formation and gene therapy. Trends Genet **9:** 269–27.
19. LIN, C., S. C. LIN, C. P. CHANG & M. G. ROSENFELD. 1992. Pit-1-dependent expression of the receptor for growth hormone releasing factor mediates pituitary cell growth. Nature **360:** 767–768, 1992.
20. AL-HENDY, A., G. HORTELANO, G. S. TANNENBAUM & P. L. CHANG. 1995. Correction of the growth defect in dwarf mice with nonautologous microencapsulated myoblasts—an alternate approach to somatic gene therapy. Hum. Gene Ther. **6:** 165–175.

21. BIRKENMEIER, E. H., M. T. DAVISSON, W. G. BEAMER, R. E. GANSHOW, C. A. VOGLER *et al.* 1989. Murine mucopolysaccharidosis type VII—Characterization of a mouse with β-glucuronidase deficiency. J. Clin. Invest. **83:** 1258–1266.
22. SLY, W. S., B. A. QUINTON, W. H. MCALISTER & D. L. RIMOIN. 1973. β-Glucuronidase deficiency: Report of clinical, radiologic and biochemical features of a new mucopolysaccharidosis. J. Pediatr. **82:** 249–257.
23. BASTEDO, L., M. S. SANDS, G. HORTELANO, A. AL-HENDY & P. L. CHANG. 1994. Partial correction of murine mucopolysaccharidosis VII with micro-encapsulated non-autologous recombinant fibroblasts. Am. J. Hum. Genet. **55:** A211.
24. SOON-SHIONG, P., R. E. HEINTZ, N. MERIDETH, Q. X. YAO, Q. YAO, T. ZHENG, M. MURPHY, M. K. MOLONEY, M. V. SCHMEHL, M. HARRIS, R. MENDEZ & P. A. SANDFORD. 1944. Insulin independence in a type 1 diabetic patient after encapsulated islet transplantation. Lancet **343:** 950.
25. AEBISCHER, P., M. SCHLUEP, N. DÉGLON, J. JOSEPH, L. HIRT, B. HEYD, M. GODDARD, J. P. HAMMANG, A. D. ZURN, A. C. KATO, F. REGLI & E. E. BAETGE. 1996. Intrathecal delivery of CNTF using encapsulated genetically modified xenogeneic cells in amyotrophic lateral sclerosis patients. Nat. Med. **2:** 696–699.

Index of Contributors

Date Due →

Books returned after due date are subject to a fine.

Fairleigh Dickinson University Library
Teaneck, New Jersey

T001-15M
11-8-02